MECHANISMS OF DISEASE
A Textbook of Comparative General Pathology

SECOND EDITION

David O. Slauson, D.V.M., Ph.D.
Diplomate, American College of Veterinary Pathologists,
Distinguished Professor of Comparative Medicine,
Chairman, Department of Pathobiology,
College of Veterinary Medicine,
University of Tennessee,
Knoxville, Tennessee

Barry J. Cooper, B.V.Sc., Ph.D.
Diplomate, American College of Veterinary Pathologists,
Associate Professor of Pathology,
Department of Pathology,
College of Veterinary Medicine,
Cornell University,
Ithaca, New York,

With a Contribution by
Maja M. Suter, Dr.med.Vet., Ph.D.
Diplomate, American College of Veterinary Pathologists,
Assistant Professor of Pathology,
Department of Pathology,
College of Veterinary Medicine,
Cornell University,
Ithaca, New York

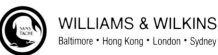

WILLIAMS & WILKINS
Baltimore • Hong Kong • London • Sydney

Editor: Jonathan W. Pine, Jr.
Associate Editor: Linda Napora
Copy Editor: Anne K. Schwartz
Designer: JoAnne Janowiak
Illustration Planning: Lorraine Wrzosek
Production Coordinator: Adèle Boyd

Copyright © 1990
Williams & Wilkins
428 East Preston Street
Baltimore, Maryland 21202, USA

Accurate indications, adverse reactions, and dosage schedules for drugs are provided in this book, but it is possible that they may change. The reader is urged to review the package information data of the manufacturers of the medications mentioned.

Printed in the United States of America

First Edition 1982

Library of Congress Cataloging in Publication Data

Slauson, David O.
    Mechanisms of disease : a textbook of comparative general
pathology / David O. Slauson, Barry J. Cooper with a contribution
from Maja M. Suter.—2nd ed.
        p.   cm.
    Includes bibliographies and index.
    ISBN 0-683-07743-0
    1. Pathology, Comparative.   I. Cooper, Barry J.   II. Suter, Maja
M.   III. Title.
    [DNLM: 1. Pathology.   2. Pathology, Veterinary.   QZ 33 S631m]
RB114.S58   1990
636.089′607—dc20
DNLM/DLC
for Library of Congress   89-16539
                                                    CIP

                                                                        93
                                                            6 7 8 9 10

Preface

Our aim for this book remains to introduce students to disease concepts inherent in clinical medicine through the study of pathogenetic mechanisms. Although written for beginning students of pathology who will ultimately become clinicians, we hope the book will also be a sourcebook of basic material for residents and graduate students, as well as a compact review of disease mechanisms for persons preparing for national board examinations. We have been gratified by the reception given to the first edition and have made a genuine effort to keep the character of the book intact in this revision.

Pathology is a changing science. Disease is still often caused by various microbes and toxins, but our continuing fascination with **how** disease occurs has produced markedly increased levels of resolution and an enriched understanding of the complex mechanisms by which mammals become sick. Accompanying this increased comprehension has been an explosion of detailed information that confounds even purposeful efforts to master it. A partial list of newer, relevant, explanatory items in contemporary pathology might include fibronectin, plasminogen activators, interleukins, leukotrienes, protein C, acumentin, phospholipase A_2, defensins, integrins, gelsolin, f-actin, tumor necrosis factor, perforins, prions, protein kinase C, interferon, NADPH-oxidase, antithrombin III, PAF, lipomodulin, the MAC, profilin, thrombomodulin, calcisomes, HMW kininogen, NK cells, superoxide anion, G proteins, the Mo1/LFA-1/Leu M5 complex, RGD sequences, leucine zippers, and the TATA box. Is this pathology? Whatever happened to pneumonia and mastitis?

The questions beg answers, and the answers beg explanations. Pneumonia and mastitis are still with us; our contemporary molecular brilliance has yet to be translated into truly effective therapy for many clinical situations, but this is changing rapidly. It is changing because advances in the biological understanding of disease have allowed therapy to be more specific and less empirical. We always knew that pneumonia and mastitis could be caused by bacteria; Koch's postulates told us so. The real story, however, was not the bacteria themselves but their molecular products and the influence of those products on host tissues and defense mechanisms. Now we are beginning to understand disease in some detail, and we must rethink many of the old explanations regarding pathogenesis; they were not incorrect, but simply inadequate.

Disciplinary lines have blurred. Contemporary pathology is a blend of the disease-oriented aspects of what used to be the intellectual provinces of such diverse disciplines as immunology, cell biology, biochemistry, medicine, and physiology. Does this mean that pathology has lost its identity as a discipline? Not at all. Pathologists have both contributed to and profited from the advances in all of these various areas of science. This blending of disciplines has produced much progress and a few problems for the authors of textbooks. One relates to organization.

Should we discuss the activation of the complement system under inflammation, in which complement activation is clearly of importance, or should it be discussed as part of the immunopathogenesis of the hypersensitivities? We have had to do some blending and to make some arbitrary decisions in such matters.

A second problem relates to deciding how much detail is appropriate for contemporary students. We continue to believe that modern students require sophisticated explanations of disease mechanisms in order to best equip them for the future, but simultaneously we recognize the curricular limitations of time and the obstacles to learning created by information overload. Teachers must act as guides and provide appropriate road maps. Students have neither the time nor the inclination for resplendent exercises in scientific trivial pursuit. Nor do we.

The role of the teacher of pathology has also changed. It is clearly insufficient to merely relate the traditional stories of disease at a simplistic level, but good judgment must prevail in selecting the borders that define an appropriate level of detail. We must be prepared to filter and summarize the bounteous available knowledge in order to present a contemporary picture of disease that avoids the hazard of accidental information drowning. We must simultaneously recognize that much of what we now teach may be obsolete within the professional lifetimes of our students. We therefore stress the importance of "lifelong learning" and hope to convey a sense of the excitement of discovery and the pleasure of independent thinking. We must make students aware that "the pathobiology of disease" is inspiring largely because "the biology of health" is so exciting. The conflict for contemporary pathology lies not in whether the study of lesions is still appropriate, but in how best to present lesions in the modern light of how those lesions came to be. We must make the lesions come to life.

> "Bitzer," said Thomas Gradgrind, "your definition of a horse." "Quadruped. Gramnivorous. Forty teeth, namely twenty-four grinders, four eye-teeth, and twelve incisive. Sheds coat in the spring; in marsh countries sheds hoofs too. Hoofs hard, but requiring to be shod with iron. Age known by marks in mouth." Thus (and much more) Bitzer. "Now . . . ," said Mr. Gradgrind, "you know what a horse is."
>
> Charles Dickens, *Hard Times*

If we approach the teaching of pathology the way Mr. Gradgrind approached the defining of *Equus caballus,* our students will respond similarly, and all of the fascinating biology of the diseased state will be reduced to a list of lesions which might be used to merely define, say, infectious bovine rhinotracheitis. But Thomas Gradgrind was wrong, and Bitzer's definition of a horse came from a dictionary. It classified a horse, but it did not capture the inherent excitement of the beast. No racing fan ever bet on a "gramnivorous quadruped," no jockey ever rode one, and no artist ever painted one. One of our challenges is to capture for students the excitement of disease mechanisms.

An additional challenge can be illustrated by even a quick trip to the library. The constant and unending flow of published observations germane to the study of disease mechanisms has become almost unmanageable, and all of us have had to become innovative in facing the dilemma of "keeping up." We are pleased to recognize in this regard that "three minds are better than two"; Dr. Maja Suter of Cornell University has joined us on this edition with an extensively rewritten chapter on immunopathology.

A major goal for the Second Edition was to reflect current knowledge about disease mechanisms without a major expansion in volume. This required a substantial rewriting of much of the text material.

We have occasionally had to be ruthless about what was included and what was left behind. What we have chosen to present reflects our best collective wisdom regarding the needs of contemporary students; we assume full responsibility for our decisions.

Lastly, we have made a substantial effort to present a contemporary synopsis of disease pathogenesis in a palatable and readable way. We continue to believe that no more exciting blend of science can be found than that which is aimed at an understanding of disease.

David O. Slauson
Barry J. Cooper

Acknowledgments

It is a pleasure to be able to record a measure of thanks to the many individuals who have directly or indirectly contributed to the completion of this book. Our families have been generous in their support and understanding of the substantial "night work" associated with the completion of this task, and they have grown accustomed to seeing us hovered over the word processor. We are grateful to our colleagues who have patiently read and reread certain portions of the text in an effort to make things as current as possible. We have also been fortunate to have had the skilled and critical input of current and former pathology residents and graduate students such as Drs. Phil Bochsler, Bruce Car, Charlie Clifford, Beth Valentine, and Erby Wilkinson. With these and others coming behind us, the future of pathology is secure indeed.

Several of our colleagues have again been kind enough to share important micrographs with us, and their individual contributions are noted in the text. The many line drawings came from the skilled hands of Jane Jorgensen who showed once again that she could make outstanding drawings from rough sketches made on various pieces of paper. Mitsu Suyemoto provided considerable skilled photographic assistance.

Williams & Wilkins has been tenacious for excellence from the beginning, and our editors, Jonathan Pine and Linda Napora, have been unfailingly patient with our penchant for altering deadlines.

Finally, it would be wrong to fail to mention the numerous unseen contributions made by our students of pathology over the years. In a very real way, it has been their probing questions, effusive spirit, indefatigable good humor, and consistent enthusiasm for pathology that caused this book to be written. Students always think that we are their teachers, but it is we who learn from them.

David O. Slauson
Barry J. Cooper

Contents

Preface to the Second Edition .... *vii*

Acknowledgments .... *xi*

Chapter 1

Pathology—The Study of Disease 1

Chapter 2

Disease at the Cellular Level 19

Chapter 3

Disturbances of Blood Flow and Circulation 89

Chapter 4

Inflammation and Repair 167

Chapter 5

Immunopathology 302
Maja M. Suter, Dr.med.Vet., Ph.D.

Chapter 6

Disorders of Cell Growth 377

Chapter 7

**Nature and Causes of Disease: Interactions of Host,
Parasite, and Environment** 472

Index *521*

1
Pathology—The Study of Disease

What Is Pathology?
What Do Pathologists Do?
Tools of Pathology
Language of Pathology
Approach to the Study of Pathology
  Injury versus Reaction to Injury

Biology versus Pathobiology
Causes and Pathogenesis of Disease
Continuity, Interactions, and Lesions
Role of Cell Biology in Contemporary Pathology
Reference Material

The study of pathology is an important and exciting milestone for students of biomedical science. For them it is an introduction to the study of disease and the mechanisms which underlie it. From the study of pathology should emerge the concepts upon which a satisfying career in medicine can be built. We are firmly committed to the idea that the best medical practice, both diagnostic and therapeutic, is based on a thorough understanding of the mechanisms of disease. Pathology is concerned with these mechanisms.

Students must rationalize and comprehend many apparent conflicts on their route to an understanding of disease. The vital host defenses linked together in the inflammatory response also constitute the major pathways of tissue injury. The same coagulation factors that produce the beautiful and life-saving hemostatic plug are responsible for the ugly and life-threatening thrombus. The injured endothelial cell produces both tissue thromboplastin to start the clot and plasminogen activators to initiate clot removal. Macrophages and neutrophils perform phagocytic heroics on our behalf while simultaneously releasing enzymes that degrade our tissues. To gain an understanding of these things is to acquire an appreciation of **how** and **why** diseases are complicated affairs.

Disease is a manifestation of physiology gone wrong, and it ultimately reflects some structural or functional alteration in the cells of which all living things are made. To understand disease, we must turn our attention toward understanding the changes that occur in living tissues in response to various kinds of stimuli. Students often first encounter pathology with some apprehension, feeling that they are poorly prepared to study disease when in fact they are usually well equipped. They are well versed in the normal structure and function of tissues. The typical student, however, generally feels that **finally** all of that basic material has been surmounted so that something applicable to medicine can now be learned. Students usually consider pathology a worthwhile pursuit, but all too often they do not seem to appreciate that understanding normal structure and function is the ultimate basis for understanding disease, and that it is in no sense irrelevant to medicine.

Students seem surprised to discover that, in the disease state, there are, with rare exceptions, no new cellular functions or new metabolic pathways at work. Rather, existing pathways are accentuated, di-

Table 1.1
Statements of the Obvious[a]

The proportions and organization of both cellular and extracellular constituents of a tissue determine the structural and functional characteristics of the tissue.

The structural and functional characteristics determine the adaptability of each tissue. Tissue adaptability decreases with aging and in many disease states.

Any agent or condition that exceeds a tissue's capacity to adapt results in an injury or disease process.

Understanding the mechanism and site of action of a disease-producing agent or condition should allow one to predict the effects of this perturbance on the host.

Knowing the structural and functional changes occurring in the tissues allows one to predict the clinical presentation.

The clinical presentation, conversely, allows us to draw conclusions about the structural and functional changes that have occurred in the tissue. These conclusions can then be used to decide on a differential list of causes for each disease process.

---

[a] Courtesy of Dr. R. R. Minor.

minished, or lost. The same is largely true for structural changes. Only rarely are truly new structures involved in disease states; rather there are increases, decreases, or alterations in structures already present in the normal animal. Even the grossest lesion is produced by the same rigorous, lawful, molecular and cellular interactions that govern normalcy. Disease is difficult to understand, but our success or failure in doing so more often lies in the realm of logic than in the realm of application. The Statements of the Obvious in Table 1.1 may help to place this in perspective.

WHAT IS PATHOLOGY?

Broadly speaking, pathology is the study of disease. According to the dictionary, it is the "study of the essential nature of disease, especially the structural and functional consequences thereof." Pathology, however, is different things to different people. To the student it is an introduction to disease, an introduction to the abnormal processes that manifest themselves as signs and symptoms in sick animals. The clinician sees pathology as one of the means by which a diagnosis can be made. To the pathologist it is the study of lesions associated with disease and the

mechanisms that underlie them. These various views of pathology are not incompatible. They simply reflect the varied interests of individuals. Pathology is the study of disease. It is the study of morphologic lesions (i.e., structural abnormalities) that characterize particular diseases. Most importantly in the context of this book, it is the study of how and why these lesions develop and their functional consequences.

As a subject for study, pathology bridges the gap between the basic sciences and clinical medicine. it has one foot in the sciences of tissue structure and function, anatomy and histology, physiology and biochemistry. The other foot is in the clinics.

At the simplest level, pathology identifies lesions and often can provide a diagnosis for clinicians. The science of pathology, however, did not grow simply from a need to recognize and name lesions and diseases. It arose from the attempts of practicing clinicians to **understand** disease. The first pathologists were clinicians who studied the structural abnormalities of the tissues in an attempt to explain the illnesses of their patients. Gradually pathology evolved into a specialty, but today it still retains its roots in morphology and in understanding the nature of disease. General pathology, the subject of this book, involves the study of the mechanisms by which tissues are injured. It provides the basic principles that allow us to understand specific diseases, whether they involve the lung, the liver, the kidneys, or any other organ system.

The study of disease can be approached in many different ways. We can emphasize the expressions of various disease processes as they lead to the recognizable alterations in tissues which we call **lesions.** We can emphasize the study and classification of these lesions into recognizable patterns and forms useful in understanding disease and in making definitive diagnoses. We can emphasize the causative agents, the bacteria, viruses, fungi, toxins, and so on, responsible for causing disease. We can emphasize the functional consequences of various kinds of organic diseases, and thus emphasize **pathophysiology.** All of these are important, but these approaches are by their very nature too often aimed at asking "what is it?" rather than "why is it?" or "how is it?"

Students beginning to learn about disease must emphasize the **how** and the **why** over the **what** if they are to become flexible clinicians able to think their way through disease problems encountered in clinical patients. A fascinating world of disordered structure and function lies before us in any diseased creature if we can only have the eyes to see it. To enumerate a list of clinical signs and then a list of lesions is not enough, for it is the relation of one to the other that counts. Sometimes this is easy, sometimes difficult, and sometimes impossible to determine. Sometimes our ignorance, however we might try to mask it in attractive scientific phraseology, still sounds like ignorance. But if we try to understand disease as to its **hows** and **whys,** we undertake a persistent endeavor that is the ultimate challenge of medicine.

Pathology can never be purely a science; it is made up of too many variables and immeasurables. The dog with verrucose mitral endocardiosis and the cow with viral rhinotracheitis are not internal combustion engines. We can interpret them but we cannot memorize their circuitry and replace their spark plugs. Our best effort is to try to understand **why** their systems failed by knowing **how** such systems fail. In other words, knowing **what** disease they have is ultimately less useful than understanding the mechanisms by which that disease came to be. The former approach gives a name to the disease to help us communicate among ourselves, but the latter forces a reconstruction of the moving series of events involved in the disease process itself.

WHAT DO PATHOLOGISTS DO?

Clearly, not all of the many people who study disease would call themselves pathologists. Traditionally, pathologists have been regarded as those who study the morphologic manifestations of disease. To some extent this is still true. Most pathologists today are trained to study the morphologic manifestations of disease, but they are also vitally interested in the functional changes with which such lesions are associated. Most are interested in **why** such lesions develop. Pathologists are medical specialists who have spent a number of years in specific training, often leading to **specialty board certification.** In North America, veterinary pathologists are certified by the **American College of Veterinary Pathologists,** the oldest and largest specialty group recognized by the American Veterinary Medical Association.

Many pathologists have particular interests, and a number of subspecialties have developed within the field of pathology. **Medical pathology** deals with the diseases of man, and **veterinary pathology** with the diseases of animals other than man. Many veterinary pathologists would regard themselves as **comparative pathologists** as their interests encompass the diseases of all species, including man. The study of the pathogenesis of animal diseases often allows considerable insight into similar disease processes in man, and information gained from the study of human diseases is usually pertinent to veterinary medicine as well. **Diagnostic pathologists** study tissue abnormalities, using either **gross** pathology or **histopathology** (microscopic pathology) or both, in order to identify the nature of the disease. They may study the whole animal, in the case of the postmortem examination (necropsy), or they may study samples of tissue taken from the living patient as a diagnostic procedure (biopsy). **Surgical pathologists** specialize in the study of biopsy material. **Specialty pathologists** might have a specific interest in particular organ systems and would, for example, be recognized as neuropathologists, pulmonary pathologists, or renal pathologists. Other specialty pathologists might be experts in **environmental pathology, toxicologic pathology,** or **zoo and wildlife pathology.**

Such specialization is a natural outcome of the virtual explosion of information available about disease and disease mechanisms. It is a tough chore even for specialists to keep up with their fields in today's world, and pathologists who believe they know all of the answers probably do not understand all of the questions. One beneficial outgrowth of specialization is **consultation.** The renal pathologist asks the neuropathologist to examine the brain lesions in a case awaiting a final diagnosis, and the neuropathologist seeks the opinion of the renal pathologist on a difficult kidney case. Both individuals profit from the knowledge of the other. Most pathologists try to keep up with the entire field of pathology in a broad sense, and most have recognized the necessity for specialization.

Immunopathologists are particularly interested in tissue injury that is associated with or caused by the immune system. **Clinical pathologists** are especially important in the laboratory analysis of disease as it occurs in living patients. They provide a wide variety of investigative tests and help to interpret them to support or deny diagnoses. They utilize hematology, cytology, serum chemistry, clinical endocrinology, and similar procedures to help make specific diagnoses. **Experimental pathologists** manipulate, analyze, and sometimes recreate abnormalities of structure and function so that we may better understand the mechanisms that underlie disease. Of course, there is some overlap in these interests. Diagnostic pathologists may utilize the techniques of immunopathology, for instance, and experimental pathologists also may be diagnostic pathologists.

General pathology is a traditional academic subdivision of pathology that remains in use to distinguish it from **special pathology,** or the pathology of specific diseases as they affect specific organs and organ systems. As such, general pathology deals with common denominators of disease and the mechanisms of disease production. The topics of general pathology include cellular degeneration and death, circulatory disorders common to many tissues, inflammation and repair, immunopathology, growth disturbances and neoplasia, and the nature and causes of disease, including genetic influences on disease. These are the subjects of general pathology because they have common mechanistic features useful to a general understanding of specific disease states. All tumors have some features in common. Inflammation, whether it affects the heart or the lungs or the kidneys, has a large number of common features. Hence, what is learned in general pathology is applicable to disease problems involving any organ system. As such, it is a mechanism-oriented discipline.

TOOLS OF PATHOLOGY

The wide range of interests covered by pathology necessitates the use of a wide variety of tools, or techniques, to study lesions. While highly sophisticated and expensive equipment is necessary for some special procedures, the best pathologic examination usually begins with rather simple tools indeed; the **eyes** and the **hands** of the pathologist. A great deal can be learned from a specimen by the fundamental processes of careful examination and inspection, and most good pathologists are quite astute observers. Skillful palpation and visual scrutiny are often learned talents, and experience can be an invaluable teacher. Individuals preparing for careers in pathology spend years in training before they are "eligible" to take the American College of Veterinary Pathologists' examination for Board Certification in Veterinary Pathology.

The **light microscope,** familiar to all, remains the basic tool of the pathologist. It provides magnification of tissue changes up to a maximum of about 1000 times normal, and it is most commonly used to study sections of tissues taken from animals. The sections used in histopathology are simply very thin slices of tissue prepared from larger pieces of tissue preserved in formaldehyde or other fixative and embedded in a medium such as paraffin wax. The sections are stained with dyes that allow the various components of the tissue to be visualized. The usual stain for routine sections is **hematoxylin** and **eosin** (H&E) (Fig. 1.1), but a wide variety of special stains may be used to illustrate special components of the tissue. For example, the periodic acid-Schiff (PAS) reaction is used to demonstrate carbohydrate substances such as glycogen. Toluidine blue stain can be used to illustrate mast cell granules and so distinguish these cells from others. A number of different stains can illustrate organisms in tissues. There are many special

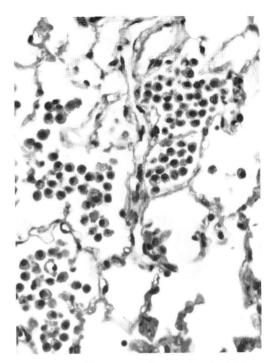

Figure 1.1. Tissue section stained with hematoxylin and eosin (H&E). In this routine preparation, nuclei stain dark with the hematoxylin while cytoplasmic and extracellular elements stain light with the eosin. This section of lung from a dog contains many alveolar macrophages.

stains, each of which has special usefulness to the pathologist (Table 1.2).

Histochemical stains are those that react with specific chemical groups or substances in the tissue. For instance, stains are available that can identify iron in tissues and distinguish it from other substances. Enzyme histochemical stains identify specific enzymes in the tissue. These are widely used, for example, in the study of muscle lesions to distinguish different types of muscle fibers (Fig. 1.2). For some of these techniques, sections cut from fresh, frozen (rather than fixed) tissue are required.

Other special techniques utilizing the light microscope are **darkfield, phase contrast,** and **fluorescence** microscopy. The latter technique is especially useful

Table 1.2
Commonly Used Stains in Pathology

Stain	Use
Hematoxylin and eosin (H&E)	Routine staining
Phosphotungstic acid-hematoxylin (PTAH)	Cross-striations in muscle, fibrin
Masson trichrome	Connective tissues, collagen
van Gieson stain	Elastin fibers, connective tissues
Oil red O (frozen sections)	Lipid
Periodic acid–Schiff reaction (PAS)	Carbohydrate
Best carmine	Glycogen
Congo red	Amyloid
Crystal violet	Amyloid
Acid-fast	Bacteria, mycobacteria
Brown-Brennan (B&B; Gram stain)	Bacteria
Levaditi method	Spirochetes
Von Kossa	Calcium salts
Luxol fast blue (LFB)	Myelin
Gomori silver	Fungi
Toluidine blue	Mast cell granules

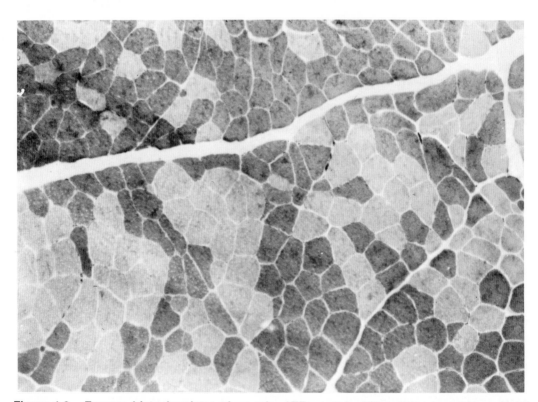

Figure 1.2.   Enzyme histochemistry of muscle. ATPase stain differentiates type I fibers (light) from type II fibers (dark). In this case there is abnormal grouping of fiber types typical of denervation followed by reinnervation. The lesion in this dog could not be appreciated without enzyme histochemistry.

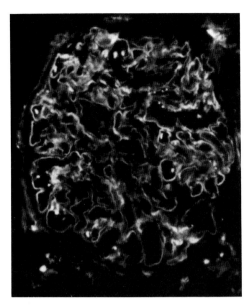

Figure 1.3. Fluorescence microscopy. This section of kidney has been stained with fluorescein-labeled antibody against equine IgG. It demonstrates linear deposition of host IgG in the glomerulus. (Micrograph courtesy of Dr. R. M. Lewis).

in immunopathology where deposits of immunoglobulin, complement proteins, or other substances can be detected. If, for example, we wanted to illustrate deposits of IgG in the glomeruli of a horse with glomerulonephritis, we would apply a specific antiserum against equine IgG which binds to the IgG in the renal tissue (Fig. 1.3). The antiserum is conjugated to a dye such as fluorescein, which is fluorescent under ultraviolent (UV) light. The suspect tissue is examined in a microscope fitted with UV illumination, and the IgG deposits, if present, are revealed by fluorescence against a dark background. This technique has been modified by labeling antisera with the enzyme horseradish peroxidase so that instead of fluorescence, a colored reaction product of a substrate oxidized by the enzyme is detected, and can be seen in the ordinary light microscope. Any substance against which an antiserum can be raised can be detected by these techniques, and they are now widely used in pathology.

Electron microscopy is also an important method for examining the morphologic changes in diseased tissues. Its major advantage is high resolution, which greatly exceeds that of light microscopy, and magnification of well over 100,000 is possible. Structures far too small to be seen in the light microscope can thus be resolved by the electron microscope (Fig. 1.4). For **transmission** electron microscopy, small pieces of fixed tissue are embedded in special plastics and extremely thin sections are cut. Stains are used which are electron dense, and the image formed by the beam of electrons is recorded on photographic film. **Scanning** electron microscopy is used to study the three-dimensional structure of tissue (Fig. 1.5). It is particularly useful in demonstrating surface microanatomic changes that cannot easily be appreciated with the transmission electron microscope.

Finally, special methods of preparation can be used for electron microscopy. Deposition of substances such as immunoglobulins can be demonstrated by **immuno-electron microscopy** using antisera linked to electron-dense substances or to enzymes using methods that produce an electron-dense product. These techniques are similar to those used in light microscopy, but they provide much higher resolution.

Tissues embedded in plastic also can be used for high-resolution light microscopy. Because sections can be cut from plastic which are much thinner than the 4–5 μm usually provided by paraffin-embedding techniques, a much better level of resolution is provided (Fig. 1.6).

Pathologists, especially experimental pathologists, use many other techniques to measure the functional consequences of lesions. These include essentially all the techniques of contemporary investigative biology. As the answers to research questions become more and more compli-

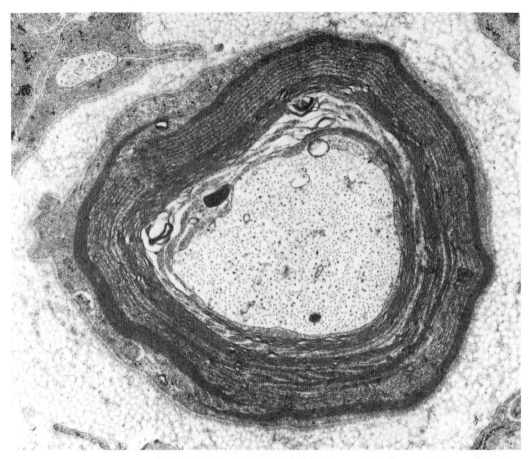

Figure 1.4. Transmission electron micrograph. In this peripheral nerve from a dog with inherited neuropathy there is abnormal compaction of myelin lamellae. The increased resolution provided by electron microscopy allows such lesions to be visualized.

cated, experiments in modern pathology increasingly involve studies at the cellular and molecular levels of resolution. The data generated by such research are very important, for they provide the basis on which we eventually are able to first understand and then predict the clinical consequences of particular morphologic lesions.

LANGUAGE OF PATHOLOGY

The study of pathology will introduce the student to an extensive new vocabulary. Many of these terms will become evident throughout this book. Here we will limit ourselves to a few particular terms that are of general importance. A **lesion** is an abnormality in a tissue. Generally when we use this term we are referring to a structural abnormality, but sometimes the word refers to a functional abnormality. We might, for instance, use the term "biochemical lesion" to describe a functional abnormality. Such a lesion may or may not have a morphologic counterpart. **Pathogenesis** is the term used to describe the way in which a disease or lesion develops. That is, it is the sequence of events and mechanisms that underlie a disease process. The lesion itself is an observation, its pathogenesis is the explanation of how and why it developed.

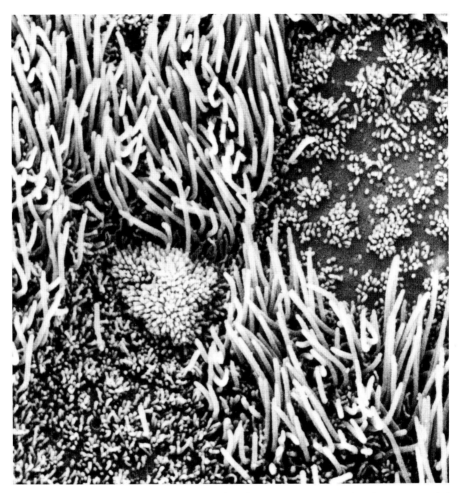

Figure 1.5. Scanning electron micrograph (SEM). The three-dimensional structure of these ciliated bronchial epithelial cells is revealed here, as are the microvilli on adjacent goblet cells. SEM is a useful high-resolution means of studying cell surfaces. (Micrograph courtesy of Dr. W. L. Castleman.)

Disease itself is hard to define. What does it mean to be sick? It is the culmination of those various defects, abnormalities, excesses, deficiencies, and injuries occurring at the cell and tissue level which ultimately result in clinically apparent dysfunction. Disease may sometimes go undetected at the clinical level even though the lesions underlying the disease have been present in the tissues for a long time. Most of us can recall from our experience some situation where a person "suddenly" became ill, but the underlying lesions had in fact been present for months. Cancer often presents in this way.

Diseases, and indeed lesions, are often difficult to categorize, and the terminology can be confusing. Let us take the specific example of leptospirosis in a dog. Leptospirosis names the disease and as such it is the **definitive diagnosis.** The dog probably has subacute nonsuppurative interstitial nephritis, which names the lesion and gives us a **morphologic diagnosis.** As the **etiology,** or cause, in

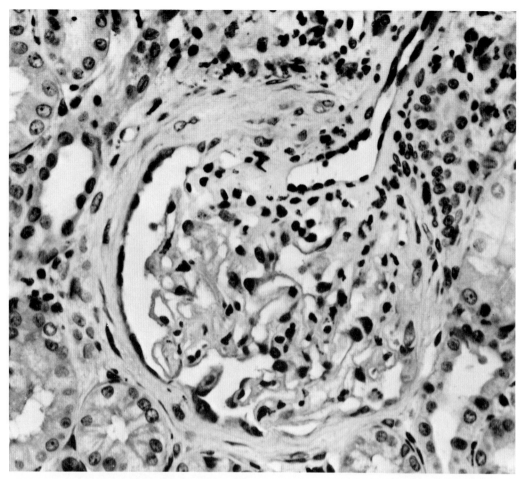

Figure 1.6. Plastic embedded tissue. In this 2μm thick section of a glomerulonephritic dog kidney, the thickened capillary walls in the glomerulus and the adhesions to Bowman's capsule are clearly evident. These changes are often hard to evaluate in routine material.

our example is *Leptospira canicola,* the **etiologic diagnosis** for the renal lesions would be leptospiral nephritis.

Other examples can be given. *Escherichia coli* (the etiology) results in colibacillosis (the disease), which is basically an acute to subacute catarrhal enteritis (the morphologic diagnosis). *Mycobacterium paratuberculosis* (the etiology) produces a chronic granulomatous enterocolitis (the morphologic diagnosis) in cattle which have Johne's disease (the name of the disease and the definitive diagnosis). One of the important jobs of diagnostic pathologists is to find, interpret, and name such changes in order to reach a diagnosis. In some situations, particularly with surgical biopsies, this information will allow the pathologist to offer a **prognosis,** or estimate of the future behavior of any lesion or change in tissue with respect to its influence on the whole organism.

APPROACH TO THE STUDY OF PATHOLOGY

Pathology, and in fact medicine as a whole, can be approached in two ways. We can learn to **recognize** disease entities and to treat them by certain set maneuvers. Unfortunately, disease varies in its manifestations and such an approach is bound to fail frequently. Alternatively, we can try to **understand** the disease process and to make logical diagnoses and formulate treatments based on the functional abnormalities that we have shown to be present. In practice we utilize both methods, but it is essential that we understand, as well as we can, the biologic processes which underlie disease.

If we can understand basic pathobiological mechanisms, we can dissect our way through new or unfamiliar disease syndromes. If we understand, we can generate rational rather than empirical methods to treat disease. We need only to look at the recent history of medicine to see that our attempts to understand disease have led to much more effective means to control it.

We can appreciate disease at any one of a variety of levels, ranging from the whole animal, or organismal level, to the molecular level. Between these extremes we might understand any particular disease process at the level of the organs, the tissues, the cells, or the subcellular organelles involved. Consider, for example, a dog that is presented with the disease diabetes mellitus (Fig. 1.7). At the crudest level of understanding we have a sick or possibly even a dead dog. If we

look at the organ level we find that the animal has a large, yellow liver, which we recognize as fatty change, or the accumulation of lipid in the liver cells. If we look in more detail we find that the islets of Langerhans in the pancreas are vacuolated. These are observations. They allow us to make a probable diagnosis of diabetes mellitus. However, it is only the appreciation of molecular, or functional changes in this case, which allows us to really understand the basis of this disease. Diabetes mellitus was recognized for many years as a disease syndrome before its basis was understood. It was not until the discovery of insulin and its role in controlling blood glucose levels that we really began to understand diabetes mellitus. With this understanding came the opportunity to treat the disease with exogenous insulin. As a result many people and animals enjoy a relatively normal life despite having this disease.

It is a basic tenet of pathology that all disease is essentially a manifestation of cellular injury. Such injury leads to changes in the structure and function of tissues and organs. The changes in function are what we recognize as symptoms and clinical signs. The changes in structure are what we recognize as morphologic lesions. To understand disease we must understand the changes in structure

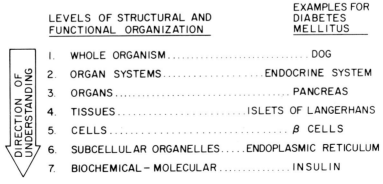

Figure 1.7. **Levels of tissue organization.** Our ability to understand disease mechanisms depends on the level of resolution where reliable information is available. For diabetes Mellitus, the molecular basis in known. This is not true for many diseases.

and function which occur in response to a variety of stimuli. In reading this book the student may sometimes wonder about the relevance of such detailed discussions of disease mechanisms. We would suggest that, at such times, the example of diabetes mellitus be reconsidered. It is on the basis of detailed understanding that future advances in medicine, including therapy, will be made.

Injury *versus* Reaction to Injury

We also should make a distinction between injury and the reaction to injury. Very often it is the reaction to injury, rather than the injury itself, that produces the clinical manifestations of disease. Take for example a simple, focal, bacterial infection in the skin. We perceive such an infection as local swelling, heat, redness, and pain. These changes are for the most part not brought about by the bacteria themselves, but by the host reaction that we call inflammation. The bacteria may or may not be capable of injuring host tissues, but they are recognized by host defense systems and, through a variety of complex mechanisms, the local blood flow is increased, fluid and plasma proteins leak out of vessels, and phagocytic cells migrate into the lesion. It is the latter changes that we appreciate, not the presence of the bacteria or their direct effects.

Biology *versus* Pathobiology

In beginning the study of pathology the student is not entering a strange new world. Pathology is a subdiscipline of biology. With rare exceptions there are no new metabolic or biochemical pathways involved in disease, nor are new structures usually involved. Rather structures and functional pathways that **already exist** are altered, either accentuated, diminished, or lost altogether. It is the departure from the normal day-to-day balance or steady state that produces disease. From this observation the concept of pathophysiology emerges. **Pathophysiology** is the alteration of normal functions that constitutes the disease process.

Consider, for example, the rather common clinical problem of uremia (renal failure). If a dog presented in uremia dies, and a necropsy is performed, the pathologist might find a number of lesions. These might include chronic inflammation of the kidneys, mineralization of a variety of tissues, softening of the bones, and enlargement of the parathyroid glands. However, it was not this list of lesions which led to the dog entering the hospital. It was the pathophysiology of the disease which did that. What the owner of the dog observed was abnormal function, that is **clinical signs.** The complaint of the owner might well have been that the dog had bad breath, difficulty in eating, increased water consumption, and polyuria manifested by nightly urination on the living room carpet.

It is the job of the clinician to understand how the pathophysiology of renal disease can lead to these signs. In this case, the pathophysiology of the disease relates to the function of the kidneys in electrolyte and water homeostasis. Loss of functional kidney tissue leads to loss of body water and to calcium and phosphorus imbalances. The animal becomes dehydrated and drinks more (polydipsia), which is often accompanied by frequent urination (polyuria), often at night (nocturia). The calcium-phosphorus imbalance leads to stimulation and hyperplasia of the parathyroid glands. The parathyroid hormone secreted leads to removal of calcium from bones in an attempt to maintain blood calcium homeostasis. As a result, the bones become soft. Loss of renal function also leads to accumulation of nitrogenous wastes. These contribute to the offensive ammoniacal breath odor common to animals in renal failure. The measurement of nitrogenous wastes in the blood, particularly urea nitrogen, is a common aid to the diagnosis of renal failure. This whole pathophysiologic syndrome is called uremia.

As students of disease, therefore, we should direct our attention toward understanding the phenomena that lead to the disease state (that is, towards its pathogenesis), its morphologic expressions, and its functional consequences (or pathophysiology). There is no more exciting detective work than starting with a sick animal and working backward through clinical signs and clinicopathologic tests of organ function to arrive at an understanding of the disease and its lesions which permits an accurate diagnosis. A thorough understanding of disease mechanisms gained from the study of pathology will be of great value in supporting this satisfying approach to clinical medicine.

It is our sincere hope that this book will help students to be excited by the prospect of understanding disease. The attitudes formed by students now will influence their whole future. Those who appreciate trying to understand disease will enjoy their professional life; those who are willing to settle for dogma will miss much of the challenge and pleasure of a medical career. It is a matter of learning how to think and how to interpret. There are fewer absolutes and more uncertainties. The "art" and the "science" of medicine become united. To see how enjoyable this kind of medical thinking can be, Lewis Thomas's superb little book *Lives of a Cell* is highly recommended.

Causes and Pathogenesis of Disease

Disease can be caused by a great variety of agents. These include infectious agents (viruses, bacteria, fungi, and parasites), chemical agents, and physical agents such as heat, cold, radiation, and direct trauma. There are literally thousands of individual etiologic agents that can be the cause of disease. It is important to realize, however, that this long list is not reflected by an equally long list of host reactions, and regardless of how long the list of individual etiologic agents becomes, mammalian organisms have really only six basic forms of expression of injury (Table 1.3). In other words, the pathogenetic mechanisms and morphologic and functional expressions of disease are limited, regardless of the cause.

Many agents cause disease through common pathways. For example, the virus that causes feline infectious enteritis, a parvovirus, attacks mitotically active cells in the intestinal glands. These same cells are particularly susceptible to radiation injury. The result of each of these injuries, therefore, is the same. There is necrosis of intestinal gland cells, and the lesions are essentially the same in each case despite having quite different causes. This is not to say that there are not still a bewildering variety of mechanisms that may be involved in disease processes. The variety, however, reflects the complexity of **normal** biologic processes, not the number of potential causes of diseases.

The complexity of biological interactions that occur in the whole animal makes the study of disease very difficult. Often we can identify a cause and observe the effect, namely the disease. The pathobiological processes connecting the two, however, may present a puzzle that is impossible to understand when working with the whole animal. For this reason most detailed research these days is done on isolated tissues or cells *in vitro*. Much of our understanding of immunologic phenomena, for example, is derived from studying lymphocytes and macrophages *in vitro*. In this way we can assemble small parts of the puzzle without the confusion of interactions that occur in the whole animal. Nevertheless, the objective is essentially to understand these processes in the intact animal. The puzzle is not yet complete and, essentially, it never will be. There always will be new questions about normal and abnormal biological processes. Presumably the answers

Table 1.3
Classes and Causes of Tissue Lesions[a]

Classes	Causes
Disruptive defects	**Genetic abnormalities**
Incision (a cut) not a laceration	Autosomal
Abrasion (friction lesion)	Sex-linked
Excoriation (friction lesion)	Dominant
Laceration (stretch lesion)	Recessive
Contusion (stretch lesion deep in tissues)	Polygenic, etc.
Fracture (stretch lesion of bone)	**Physical injury**
Constriction or dilation	Trauma
Rupture	Obstruction
Degenerative defects	Pressure
Degeneration	Ionizing radiation
Hydropic	Ultrasonic vibration
Fatty	UV light, etc.
Hyaline	**Thermal injury**
Fibrinoid	Heat ($> +5°C$)
Necrosis	Superficial
Coagulation	Deep
Liquefaction	Electric current
Caseous	Microwaves
Fat	Cold ($< -15°$ C), etc.
Mineralization	**Chemical injury**
Metastatic	Exogenous
Dystrophic	Toxins
Vascular defects	Poisons
Hyperemia	Drugs
Congestion	Food substances
Edema	Endogenous
Thrombosis	Metabolites
Ischemia	Cytolytic or inhibitory substances (AgAb
Hemorrhage	+ complement)
Inflammation	Free radicals
Acute	Oxidants, etc.
Subacute	**Infections or infestations**
Chronic	Bacterial
Suppurative	Fungal
Nonsuppurative	Viral
Granulomatous	Protozoal
Focal	Parasitic
Multifocal	Mycoplasmal, etc.
Diffuse	**Metabolic abnormalities**
Defects of growth and differentiation	Hormone imbalance
Atrophy	Enzyme defects
Hypertrophy	Membrane defects
Aplasia	Structural protein defects, etc.
Hypoplasia	**Nutritional injury**
Hyperplasia	Undernutrition
Metaplasia	Overnutrition
Neoplasia	Nutritional imbalance
Developmental (congenital defects)	Nutritional deficiencies, etc.
All of above	

[a] Courtesy of Dr. R. R. Minor.

will provide the same sort of advances in our ability to modify or treat disease that we have experienced in the past.

Continuity, Interactions, and Lesions

Emerging from our discussions of the complexity of the disease process is an important concept. It is that **when we look at lesions we are seeing a static representation of a dynamic process.** In other words, the disease process is composed of continually evolving, interacting mechanisms. Lesions may be progressing and becoming more severe, they may be resolving, or their severity may be relatively constant. However, they are rarely static. They rarely remain exactly the same over long periods of time. This con-

cept is analogous to a motion picture film (Fig. 1.8). If we look at a single frame we see a still picture. But we know that this is only a representation of a moment in a continuum. In the same way, when we look at a histologic slide we are seeing one moment in the continuum of the development of the lesion.

How do we interpret this "still"? Can we tell in what direction it was evolving? The answer often is yes, we can. Consider again the motion picture frame. Let us assume it showed a person running. We can tell easily from a single frame whether the person was running forward or backward. Why? Because our **experience** has taught us to recognize these things. We have seen many people running and we

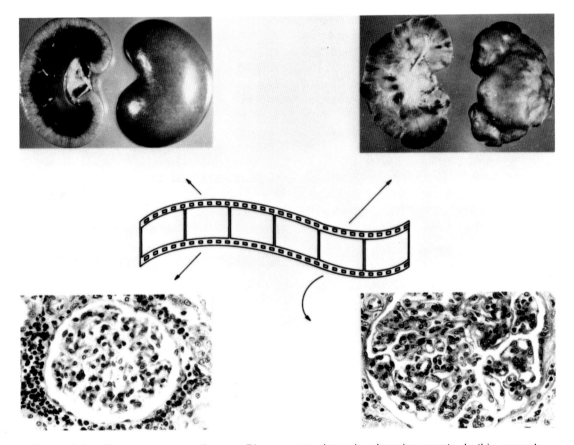

Figure 1.8. Disease as a continuum. Diseases are dynamic, changing events. In this example, glomerulonephritis progresses from the acute stages to the chronic stages, and the disease looks different at different stages in its pathogenesis.

know from experience **how** and **why** a person running forward would look different from one running backward. If we had never seen a person running we would **not** be able to make these assumptions. The interpretation of lesions is the same. We learn from experience to interpret the "still" picture we see as a lesion, as part of a dynamic disease process. The role of experimental pathology is, partly, to teach us these things. By looking at multiple samples taken at different points in time, for example, we can learn how lesions evolve. These lessons allow us to interpret the likely progress of naturally occurring lesions and to predict the likely outcome of a disease process. In other words, we can suggest a prognosis.

Returning to our opening question, what is pathology? It is pathobiology, the study of biologic functions that, for some reason, are not proceeding normally. It is **not** just morbid anatomy, **not** just the recognition of lesions or the recognition of what the disease is. It is the **understanding** of disease processes, their morphologic expression, and, most importantly, their functional expression and significance. To be good pathologists we must first become good biologists. To be students of pathology, we must be good students of biology. We must never forget that, whatever the disease, we are basically looking at normal processes functioning in an abnormal way.

ROLE OF CELL BIOLOGY IN CONTEMPORARY BIOLOGY

The concept of a cell evokes varied images in various minds: a subunit of Hooke's sections of cork, blue-green algae floating in a saline sea, polygonal structures scraped from the belly of a frog, neurons as long as your arm, leukocytes packed with granules. All of these are highly specialized responders to external stimuli, which carry from cell generation to cell generation a unique biological history. Tossed into a hostile environment

by the pressures of evolution, the cell still struggles against disease. How do its secrets relate to present day pathology? To disease?

Things used to be less complicated. In the not too distant past, cells enjoyed our relative ignorance and lived out their lives with little investigative intervention. We viewed their contents hazily, and speculated about their workings. As pathologists, we were often more concerned with lesions at the tissue level and we spoke a language largely unfettered by molecular dialects. We tried to accumulate a common knowledge, and we probed disease mechanisms with rather uniform tools and beautifully simple techniques. Our purpose seemed to be the reproducible recognition of the altered state and the creation of explanatory dogma.

Disease no longer seems willing to settle for such historical innocence. We all have witnessed the emergence of a medical science of bewildering complexity. Disciplinary lines have blurred. Contemporary pathology now includes the disease-oriented aspects of what used to be the intellectual provinces of such diverse disciplines as immunology, cell biology, biochemistry, medicine, and physiology. Some of the old truths about disease pathogenesis seem so poorly applicable in the new world that they have become more a hindrance than an aid, not because the old truths have become false, but because it is now clear that we do not fully understand them. They have become facts without a purpose; observable phenomena without a palatable explanation.

Through it all, the cell has remained central. We have investigated cells and they have repeatedly provided several new questions for each of our singular answers. We have been persistent. We have x-rayed their surfaces and we have cleaved their proteins; we have probed their cytoplasmic depths, and we simultaneously have probed our minds. Small wonder we are still sometimes confused. But we refuse, quite simply, to abandon the idea that an understanding of disease is within our reach. The **goal of pathology** here is explicit. It is simply **to understand life in the abnormal state** and thus to form a central bridge in the entire arch of medicine. Pathology is not "morbid anatomy," the science of lesions found in the dead. It exists largely because of its applicability to life. There is no limit to its scope, but its hallmark ultimately must continue to be the cell and its domains, its functions, and perhaps most importantly, the controls over its behavior in the abnormal state.

It may be that the best way to mentally visualize the importance of the cell and its intracellular control mechanisms is to imagine what things would be like if no controls existed. The long list of successive chemical transformations that make up the metabolic pathways would proceed in an undirected and useless fashion, using too much here and leaving behind too little there. The machinery of biosynthesis and degradation would do its tricks oblivious to the real needs of the cell. The failure of these cooperative systems would lead to a markedly reduced ability to respond to adverse changes in the surrounding extracellular environment. In the end, these alterations in normal cellular control phenomena would lead to biochemical anarchy followed, in many cases, by the overthrow of the central governing systems. Cell death would be followed by tissue death. Lesions would occur.

Many of us are familiar with the analogy between the cell and a city. Surrounding it is a freeway (the cell membrane) with rather specific exit and entrance sites to and from the interior. City hall (the nucleus) houses the many administrative officials and is connected to the outlying freeway by a complicated maze of streets and roads (the cytoskeleton) which are difficult to map. Scattered along the streets are various buildings essential to the overall well-being of the metropolitan region: gas and electric company power plants (the mitochondria), various industrial factories for the manufacture of useful products (synthetic regions like the endoplasmic reticulum), sanitation engineering districts (detoxifying mechanisms), warehouses and storage sites (glycogen, lipids), and a post office for packaging and mailing (Golgi apparatus). In the city, food must be brought in, used, and then the resulting garbage and sewage removed. Products fabricated in specific parts of town must be transported throughout the city, and some things may even be packaged for exportation. A complicated communication system is needed to keep all of this running smoothly. When communications break down, traffic jams are likely and robbery, smuggling, suicide, murder, and other illegal activities increase. Catastrophes can occur if the public transportation and sanitation workers go on strike, and life in the city becomes uncomfortable if not unbearable. The point is simple: the organism is dependent on tissue integrity, tissue integrity is linked ultimately to cellular integrity, and the cell is the functional sum of its parts, all of which must be perfectly integrated if homeostasis is to be maintained. We see diseases at the level of the whole organism, but we should not lose sight of the fact that **virtually all diseases are ultimately reflections of cellular biology gone wrong.**

If we wish, therefore, to learn how life begins and ends, we must study it at its greatest level of functional resolution. We must begin with the unit of life structure itself, the cell, and understand the environment in which it lives, its structure and function, its control mechanisms, and how its disturbances are expressed as disease. In its ultimate form, disease is merely a mirror that reflects to the outside changes in internal cellular function. We will therefore begin our study of disease by examining fundamental changes as they occur at the cellular level.

Reference Material

Alberts, B., Bray, D., Lewis, J., Raff, J., Roberts, K., and Watson, J. D.: *Molecular Biology of the Cell,* ed. 2. Garland Publishing, New York, 1989.

Cheville, N. F.: *Cell Pathology,* ed. 2. Iowa State University Press, Ames, Iowa, 1983.

Cheville, N. F.: *Introduction to Veterinary Pathology.* Iowa State University Press, Ames, Iowa, 1988.

Cotran, R., Kumar, V., and Robbins, S. L.: *Pathologic Basis of Disease,* ed. 4. W. B. Saunders, Philadelphia, 1989.

Frost, J. K.: *The Cell in Health and Disease: An Evaluation of Cellular Morphologic Expression of Biologic Behavior,* ed. 2. Karger, Basel, 1986.

Jones, T. C., and Hunt, R. D.: *Veterinary Pathol-ogy,* ed. 5. Lea and Febiger, Philadelphia, 1983.

Sodeman, W. A., Jr., and Sodeman, T. M.: *Pathologic Physiology: Mechanisms of Disease,* ed. 7. W. B. Saunders, Philadelphia, 1984.

Smith, L. H., and Thier, S. O.: *Pathophysiology: The Biological Basis of Disease,* ed. 2. W. B. Saunders, Philadelphia, 1985.

Thomas, L.: *Lives of a Cell; Notes of a Biology Watcher.* Bantam Books, New York, 1975.

Thomas, L.: *The Medusa and the Snail: More Notes of a Biology Watcher.* Viking Press, New York, 1979.

Thompson, R. G.: *General Veterinary Pathology,* ed. 2. W. B. Saunders, Philadelphia, 1984.

Weiss, L.: *Histology: Cell and Tissue Biology,* ed. 5. Elsevier Biomedical, New York, 1983.

2
Disease at the Cellular Level

Normal Cells and Cellular Adaptation
  Plasma Membrane
  Nucleus
  Cytoplasmic Organelles
    Mitochondria
    Endoplasmic Reticulum and Golgi Apparatus
    Lysosomes
    Cytoskeleton—Microtubules and Cytoplasmic Filaments
    Peroxisomes
  Cytocavitary Network and Movement of Cell Membranes
  Cellular Adaptation
    Cellular Atrophy
    Hypertrophy
Cell Injury
  Morphology of Cell Injury
    Reversible Cell Injury
    Ultrastructural Changes in Injured Cells
    Lethal Cell Injury and Necrosis
    Classification of Necrotic Lesions
    Apoptosis
  Consequences of Cell Injury
  Pathogenesis of Cell Injury
    Causes of Cell Injury
    Hypoxic Cell Injury
      Sequence of Changes in the Injured Cell

    Mitochondria in Cell Injury
    Cell Membrane in Cell Injury
    Endoplasmic Reticulum in Cell Injury
    Lysosomes in Cell Injury
    Other Organelles in Cell Injury
  Cell Injury Due to Membrane Damage
    Causes of Membrane Damage
    Mechanisms of Membrane Injury
    Free Radicals, Lipid Peroxidation, and Membrane Injury
    Functional and Morphologic Consequences of Cell Membrane Injury
  Reversibility and Irreversibility
    Role of Calcium in Cell Injury
    Relationship of Membrane Damage to Calcium and Cell Death
    Cell Injury, Calcium, and Membrane Damage: A Recapitulation
  Hepatic Fatty Change as a Model of Nonlethal Cell Injury
Pigments and Other Tissue Deposits
  Intracellular Lipid Accumulation
  Intracellular Protein Accumulation
  Pigments
  Calcification
  Amyloid and Amyloidosis
Cellular Pathology in Perspective
Reference Material

In order to understand disease in the whole animal, the level at which we usually study it as clinicians, it is important to realize that animals become diseased because some of their cells are not functioning normally. This might be stated in another way by saying that sick cells result in sick animals. Thus, the present day study of disease attempts to understand how cells react to injury, and how this is manifested in the whole animal. We cannot claim, however, that this concept of the cellular basis of disease is a modern one. In fact, **cellular pathology** dates from the mid-19th century and originated largely from the ideas of Rudolf Virchow. Relatively recently, however, we have acquired many sophisticated techniques that allow us to probe ever more deeply into the workings of the cell. As a result many diseases are now understood at the subcellular and, in some cases, at the molecular level. In this chapter we will discuss the ways in which cells react to injury, providing a basis for subsequent chapters and, hopefully, for future clinical experience.

NORMAL CELLS AND CELLULAR ADAPTATION

Before describing how cells react to injury, we should briefly review the structure and function of the normal cell. Of course, differentiated cells differ from one

19

another, depending on their specialized function, but all cells have in common the basic organelles necessary for synthesis of lipids, proteins, and carbohydrates; for energy production; and for transport of ions and other substances (Fig. 2.1). Here we will concentrate on these shared features.

Plasma Membrane

It is difficult to argue that any one cell component is more important to the well-being of the cell than any other, but, from the point of view of cellular pathology, the plasma membrane occupies a special niche. It is critical to the well-being of the cell, and, as we shall see in this and in following chapters, interactions at the cell surface are of tremendous importance

in disease processes. Physically, the plasma membrane forms a barrier between the cell and its environment and all of the interactions of the cell with other cells, bacteria, viruses, hormones, and other substances involve the plasma membrane.

Ultrastructurally the plasma membrane has a trilaminar appearance, with two electron-dense layers separated by an electron-lucent layer. Chemically it is known to be composed predominantly of lipid and protein with some carbohydrate. The tendency when viewing electron micrographs is to think of the plasma membrane as a rather static structure but current evidence indicates that it is dynamic and that it can be modulated in response to a variety of stimuli. The modern concept of the structure of the plasma

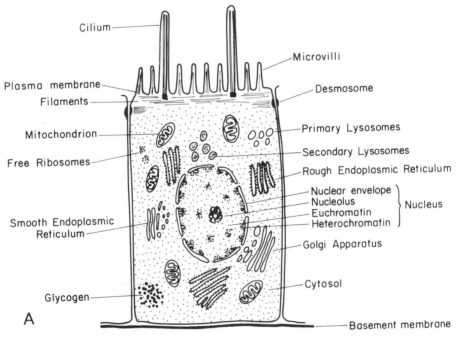

Figure 2.1. Typical mammalian cell. *A*, the features found in mammalian cells are shown schematically. Not all cells rest on a basement membrane and desmosomes, cilia, and microvilli are surface specializations found on only some cells. *B*, a normal heptocyte of a mouse is shown. Most of the organelles found in mammalian cells can be identified. Desmosomes *(arrows)* are present on either side of the canaliculus *(C)* into which microvilli protrude. *M*, mitochondria; *RER*, rough endoplasmic reticulum; *SER*, smooth endoplasmic reticulum; *L*, lysosomes; *Gl*, glycogen; *N*, nucleus; *Nu*, nucleolus; *G*, Golgi apparatus.

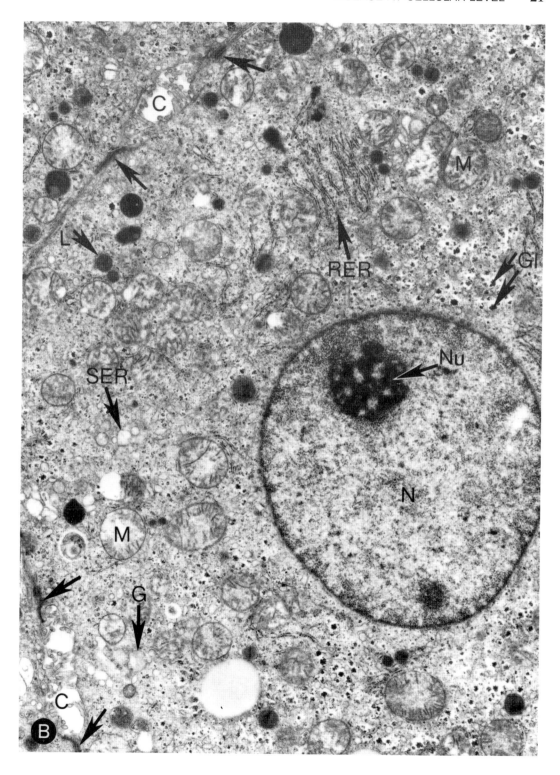

membrane, resulting from this knowledge, is known as the **fluid mosaic model.** In this model the membrane is considered to consist of a lipid bilayer in which are embedded various protein molecules and protein-carbohydrate complexes. The lipid molecules, predominantly phospholipids, are **amphipathic.** In other words, they have a polar and a nonpolar end. The polar ends of the molecules are hydrophilic, and the nonpolar ends are hydrophobic. As shown in Figure 2.2, they are arranged in the membrane with their hydrophilic ends in contact with the aqueous phase of the cytoplasm or of the extracellular fluid.

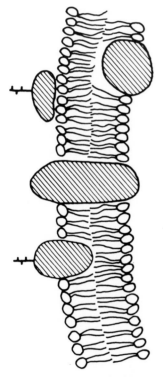

Figure 2.2. Structure of the plasma membrane. Shown schematically is the lipid bilayer made up of lipid molecules with their hydrophilic ends in contact with the cytosol or the extracellular fluid. Embedded in the bilayer are peripheral and integral proteins. Some bear carbohydrate side chains that project from the cell surface and contribute to the glycocalyx.

Associated with the lipid bilayer are a variety of protein molecules (Fig. 2.2). These are mostly globular and are of two types. **Peripheral** membrane proteins are present on the external surface of the membrane and are fairly easily removed. **Integral** membrane proteins are embedded in the membrane but project from either the external or cytoplasmic surfaces. These can be removed only with difficulty. Currently no protein molecules are thought to be buried completely in the lipid bilayer. The protein molecules associated with the plasma membrane are thought to correspond to the tiny bumps that can be visualized when the membrane is examined *en face* in the electron microscope using the freeze fracture technique.

The lipid bilayer is thought to be fluid in the sense that both the lipid and the protein molecules embedded within it can move laterally, but not throughout the depth of the membrane. In particular, proteins may move about on the surface of the cell so that their distribution may alter from diffuse to clustered or *vice versa.* However, this movement is regulated by the cell, and protein molecules can be immobilized or directed. A good example of this phenomenon is provided by the "capping" that is observed in lymphocytes allowed to contact specific antigen or treated with antibody against immunoglobulin. The immunoglobulin molecules on the surface of cells thus treated move to one pole of the cell to form a "patch" or cap. The plasma membrane, therefore, is a dynamic structure able to respond to a variety of stimuli and insults.

The plasma membrane has a variety of specialized functions too complex to more than summarize here. As already mentioned, it separates the interior of the cell from its environment. As such, it acts as a semipermeable membrane, critical to cell homeostasis, which allows passive diffusion of some molecules, energy-dependent active transport of others, and completely prevents the entry of still others. Active transport processes are particularly important in maintaining differences in concentration of sodium, potassium, and other ions between the intracellular and extracellular fluids. As a consequence of this function, the cellular water content also is controlled. The fact that the cell membrane is central to the regulation of ionic homeostasis, a phenomenon dependent on cellular energy, is important in the pathogenesis of cell injury, as will be described below.

The proteins in and on the plasma membrane are important as cellular antigens, as receptors for hormones and other substances, and for cell-to-cell and cell-to-substrate interactions. Intercellular recognition and interaction is important in a variety of ways. For example, platelets and polymorphonuclear leukocytes interact with endothelial cells, B lymphocytes interact with T lymphocytes, and macrophages interact with lymphoid cells. In addition some cells, such as macrophages and sensitized lymphocytes, can recognize and interact with cells such as bacteria, parasites, or virus-infected cells. All of these phenomena are believed to involve functions of the cell surface. Changes in the plasma membrane therefore may be of great importance when we consider disease at the cellular level. As described in Chapter 6, alterations in the plasma membrane may be important in the pathogenesis of neoplasia where intercellular interactions and the control of growth are very abnormal.

Many cells are surrounded by a cell coat or **glycocalyx,** a carbohydrate-rich layer believed to be at least partly composed of the glycoprotein terminals of membrane proteins. Many of the antigens and receptors already mentioned are in this layer. One particular surface protein, **fibronectin,** is thought to be important in the interaction of cells with one another and with connective tissue matrix components. Fibronectin binds to colla-

gen, fibrinogen, actin, and glycosaminoglycans and is thought to be very important in the attachment of cells to the connective tissue substrate. It is also thought to be involved in wound healing (Chapter 4) and possibly plays a role in opsonizing material for phagocytosis (Chapter 4). There is some evidence, described in Chapter 6, that fibronectin binding is abnormal in cells that have undergone neoplastic transformation, which may be important in determining their ability to invade.

Finally, the plasma membrane may show a variety of morphologic specializations. These include microvilli, interdigitations, caveolae, and myelin, all specializations related to specific functions of the cell bearing them. Many cells also show specialized intercellular attachments. These include tight junctions, gap junctions, and desmosomes.

Nucleus

The nucleus might be thought of as the "brain" of the cell. It contains the genetic information that ultimately directs all of the cell's activities. DNA is located and replicated in the nucleus and RNA is synthesized there for transport to the cytoplasm. It is beyond the scope of this chapter to deal in detail with the functions of the nucleus. Instead, we will concentrate on a discussion of its structure and the changes that it can undergo in response to alterations in cellular function.

The **nuclear envelope** surrounds the nucleus and separates the nuclear contents from the cytoplasm (Fig. 2.3). It is made up of a double membrane enclosing a space, 10–15 nm wide, called the **perinuclear cisterna.** In many cells a **fibrous lamina** is present immediately adjacent to the inner aspect of the nuclear envelope. This layer is made up of filamentous proteins and is thought to provide structural support for the nuclear membranes. The outer membrane of the nuclear envelope bears ribosomes on its

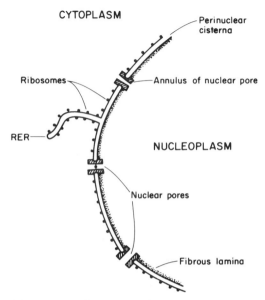

Figure 2.3. Structure of the nuclear envelope. The arrangement of the nuclear envelope and its relationship to the endoplasmic reticulum are shown.

outer surface and sometimes can be seen to be contiguous with the endoplasmic reticulum. For these reasons many people believe that the nuclear membranes and the perinuclear cisterna are a specialization of the endoplasmic reticulum. At regular intervals, the nuclear membranes are penetrated by **nuclear pores** 50–70 nm in diameter. Associated with the pore, a transmembrane cylindrical structure called an **annulus** also has been described, and across the pore a diaphragm sometimes can be visualized. Both the annulus and the diaphragm are thought to play a role in regulating the passage of substances across the nuclear envelope. The nuclear pores are possibly the site of transport of RNA molecules from the nucleus into the cytoplasm.

The characteristic blotchy appearance of the nucleus in stained histologic or cytologic preparations is due to its content of **chromatin,** which contains DNA and associated proteins. Two types of chromatin are recognized. **Heterochro-**

matin is condensed and intensely basophilic in light microscopic preparations. **Euchromatin** is dispersed, and, as a result, stains relatively lightly. It is, however, the metabolically active chromatin and therefore is prominent in cells actively synthesizing protein and RNA. This point is important in recognizing rapidly dividing cells, such as in neoplasia or hyperplasia.

The **nucleolus** forms a roughly spherical substructure of the nucleus. It contains 5–10% RNA and a little DNA, the balance being mostly protein. The nucleolus is the site of synthesis of most of the components of ribosomal RNA, and cells that are actively synthesizing protein usually have one or more prominent nucleoli. Again this is of significance in interpreting the histopathologic appearance of neoplasms.

Cytoplasmic Organelles

The cytoplasm of the cell is made up of a number of different organelles suspended in an aqueous gel called the **cytosol** (Fig. 2.1). The latter is the fluid matrix of the cell and is itself a dynamic component. It contains many different soluble enzymes, transfer RNA, and other substances important in cell metabolism. The staining characteristics of the cytoplasm depend on the relative concentrations of protein and nucleic acids dissolved or suspended in the cytosol. The higher the concentration of nucleic acids, mainly present in ribosomes, the more basophilic the cytoplasm appears with conventional H&E stains.

Mitochondria

The mitochondria are the site of production of most of the ATP, which forms the cell's major energy source. As such, they are critical to the normal function of the cell, and, as discussed later in this chapter, they play a central role in cell injury. Drastic damage to the mitochondria usually heralds the death of the cell.

Mitochondria vary greatly in shape and size depending on the type of cell and, to some degree, on their functional status. As shown in Figure 2.4 they are bounded by two membranes, the inner one of which is thrown into many folds called **cristae.** Two compartments are thus formed, the outer one lying between the outer and inner membranes and the inner one (the mitochondrial matrix) inside the inner

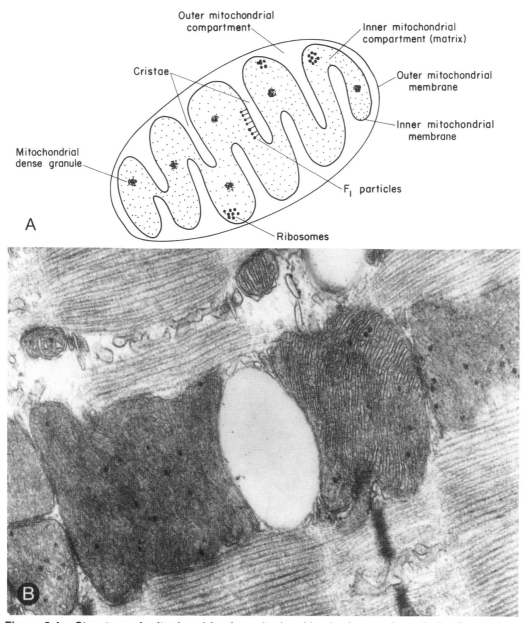

Figure 2.4.   Structure of mitochondria. *A,* a mitochondrion is shown schematically. *B,* mitochondria from a skeletal muscle fiber of a mouse are shown. The outer membrane, the cristae arising as infoldings of the inner membrane, and mitochondrial dense granules are clearly evident. A lipid droplet lies between two large mitochondria.

membrane. Electron-dense granules, which contain divalent cations and are called, appropriately enough, **mitochondrial-dense granules,** also are located in the mitochondrial matrix.

There is a highly ordered structure-function relationship in mitochondria, specific enzymes being localized in one or the other of the compartments or closely associated with one of the membranes (Table 2.1). Those which concern us most are those involved in energy production. The enzymes of the tricarboxylic acid cycle, with the exception of succinate dehydrogenase, are located in the matrix, while those of the respiratory chain and succinate dehydrogenase are located on the inner membrane. Other enzymes also are present in the mitochondria. For a detailed review the reader should consult a textbook of cell biology.

Mitochondria are dynamic structures, not only in terms of their metabolic activity but in their size, shape, and numbers. They are able to replicate and are apparently continually destroyed and replaced in the cell. They may increase or decrease in number according to demands made on the cell. Mitochondria also contain their own DNA, which can be replicated locally, and they can synthesize RNA and protein. Defects in mitochondrial genes can result in diseases showing a maternal pattern of inheritance. This is because the ovum contributes all of the mitochondria to the zygote. Mitochondria are not independent of nuclear genetic information, however, and many of their proteins are coded for by nuclear DNA. Mitochondrial adaptation to injury will be considered further later in this chapter.

Endoplasmic Reticulum and Golgi Apparatus

The **endoplasmic reticulum** (ER) (Figs. 2.1 and 2.5) is an important membranous organelle system that is involved in various synthetic and metabolic processes. Two types of ER are recognized: rough or granular endoplasmic reticulum (RER) and smooth endoplasmic reticulum (SER).

In most cells the rough endoplasmic reticulum consists of a series of flattened, membranous sacs, known as cisternae, in

Table 2.1
Distribution of Enzymes in Mitochondria

Outer membrane	Monoamine oxidase
	Fatty acyl-CoA ligase
	Kinurenine hydroxylase
	Rotenone-insensitive NADH–cytochrome C reductase
Outer compartment	Adenylate kinase
	Nucleoside diphosphokinase
Inner membrane	ATP synthetase
	Succinate dehydrogenase
	Respiratory chain enzymes
	β-hydroxybutyrate dehydrogenase
	Carnitine fatty acid acyl transferase
Matrix	Malate and isocitrate dehydrogenases
	Citrate synthetase
	Fumarase
	Aconitase
	α-keto acid dehydrogenases
	β-oxidation enzymes

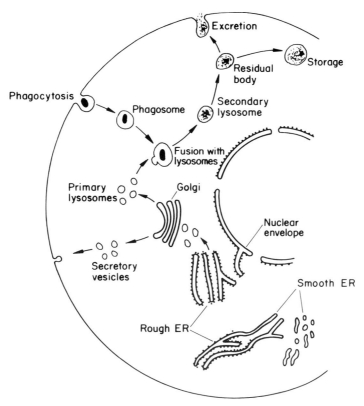

Figure 2.5. Cytocavitary network. The relationships of the subcellular components of the cyto-cavitary network are illustrated (*see* text).

which protein-rich material sometimes can be visualized. In some cells the ER takes the form of tubules or small vesicles. Attached to the cytoplasmic surface of the RER, producing the granular ultrastructural appearance that gives it its name, are large numbers of **ribosomes.** As the RER and ribosomes both are involved in the synthesis and secretion of protein, we will consider them together here.

Ribosomes are small (approximately 20 nm) dense granules that occur either free in the cytoplasm or, as already indicated, attached to the RER. They usually are present as aggregates called **polysomes** and on the RER often are arranged in a spiral pattern. When examined by suitable ultrastructural techniques they can be seen to be arranged along a "thread" thought to be mRNA. Ribosomes, of course, are rich in RNA and

therefore impart basophilic staining properties. Cells that are actively synthesizing a lot of protein, then, tend to have intensely basophilic cytoplasm. As a general rule free cytoplasmic ribosomes produce protein for use in the cell, whereas ribosomes attached to the RER are involved in the synthesis of protein for export from the cell.

A series of experiments in the last few decades have clarified the role of the RER in the synthesis and packaging of secretory proteins. Polypeptide molecules are synthesized on the bound ribosomes, and, somehow, are passed directly to the lumen of the RER, where they often can be visualized in electron micrographs as finely granular material. The nascent peptide chains apparently pass through the membrane of the ER and serve a role in holding the polysome to the ER. Although in a few cases the secretory product is concentrated in the RER, it usually is transferred to the Golgi apparatus where final processing takes place.

The **Golgi apparatus** (Fig. 2.5) is made up of a series of closely associated cisternae arranged something like a stack of coins. Associated with one face, the so-called forming face, is a series of small vacuoles or vesicles. Adjacent to the opposite face, the mature face, are somewhat larger vacuoles, often called condensing vacuoles. The membranes of the Golgi apparatus are smooth, having no attached ribosomes, but are frequently fenestrated near their edges and have many protrusions or irregularities that are thought to represent vacuoles in the process of fusion with the cisternal membrane.

The function of the Golgi apparatus is to modify, concentrate, package, and sort proteins for secretion from the cells. Many of these are glycoproteins, and although the initial carbohydrate moieties may be added in the RER, most carbohydrates are added in the Golgi apparatus. The general process of secretion is thought to involve the budding of vesicles from the RER, transport to the Golgi apparatus, and fusion with its cisternae. The product moves through the cisternae, where it is processed and eventually budded off as condensing vacuoles. In secretory cells these form secretory granules, the contents of which are released from the cell in response to the appropriate stimulus. Lysosomes, the structure and function of which are described below, are formed in a similar way.

The **smooth, or agranular, endoplasmic reticulum** is distinct from the RER in lacking attached ribosomes. Most commonly, it consists of a series of tubular or vesicular membranous structures. It varies greatly in amount depending on the type of cell. It is most abundant in hepatocytes and cells that secrete steroid hormones, such as those of the adrenal cortex and the Leydig cells of the testis. The SER sometimes can be seen to be connected to the RER, and it is believed that it is derived from the latter.

The SER has a variety of functions. In essence it acts as a membranous carrier on which are displayed enzymes that carry out biosynthetic or metabolic processes. In hepatocytes it is associated with enzymes that metabolize a variety of toxins and drugs. In steroid-secreting cells, many of the enzymes that synthesize the hormones are located on the membranes of the SER. Finally, the amount of SER and its associated enzymes can vary depending upon the demands made upon the cell. This has certain implications in the pathogenesis of some types of cell injury and is discussed in greater detail later in this chapter.

Lysosomes

Lysosomes (Figs. 2.5 and 2.6) are membrane-bound organelles that are important in the digestion of biological material in the cell. They contain a wide variety of enzymes capable of breaking down all types of cellular components including lipids, proteins, and nucleic acids. Lysosomal enzymes generally have their optimal activity at an acid pH and therefore are known as acid hydrolases. Lysosomes are referred to by different terms depending on their functional state. **Primary lysosomes** are those which have not yet become involved in any digestive process, while **secondary lysosomes** are those which contain material undergoing active digestion. **Residual bodies** (Fig. 2.7) are the end point of the lysosomal digestive process. They contain the remaining indigestible debris and little, if any, enzyme activity. Much of this material is lipid, and it gives rise to the pigment **lipofuscin** sometimes found in aging or injured cells.

Generally, lysosomal enzymes are thought to be synthesized on the RER and finally packaged in the Golgi apparatus.

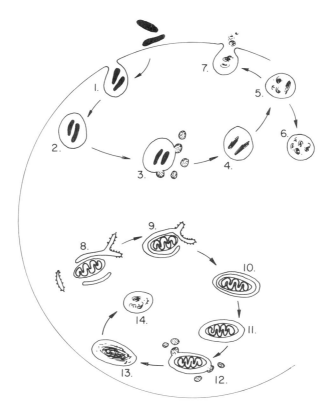

Figure 2.6.   Heterophagy and autophagy. In heterophagy, or phagocytosis, extracellular material is taken up by an infolding of the plasma membrane *(1)* to form a phagocytic vacuole *(2)*. The latter fuses with lysosomes *(3)* to produce a phagolysosome, or secondary lysosome, in which the contents are digested *(4, 5)*. The end products of digestion may be stored as residual bodies *(6)* or sometimes excreted from the cell *(7)*. In autophagy, effete or injured organelles are initially surrounded by a double membrane thought to be derived from endoplasmic reticulum (ER) *(8, 9, 10)*. The inner of the two membranes is lost *(11)* and the vacuole fuses with lysosomes to form a secondary lysosome *(12)*. The remainder of the digestive process is identical to heterophagy *(13, 14)*.

Morphologically, lysosomes vary in appearance depending on the cell in which they are found and on their functional state. Primary lysosomes contain no ingested material and therefore often are difficult to distinguish from other membrane-bound vesicles. They can be demonstrated using histochemical stains that reveal their hydrolytic enzymes, the usual one used being acid phosphatase. Of course, once secondary lysosomes are formed, they can be recognized by their content of ingested material. Residual bodies sometimes contain whorled membrane-like material frequently referred to as "my-

elin bodies." In some cells, lysosomes are given special names. The best example is the azurophil granules of the neutrophil, which are in fact primary lysosomes (Chapter 4).

The material digested by lysosomes can originate from within the cell or from ingested material. **Autophagy** refers to the process by which part of the cell's own cytoplasm and its organelles can be sequestered and digested. In this process the material to be digested is first surrounded by a membrane (Fig. 2.6), which is thought to be derived from the endoplasmic reticulum. This vacuole then fuses

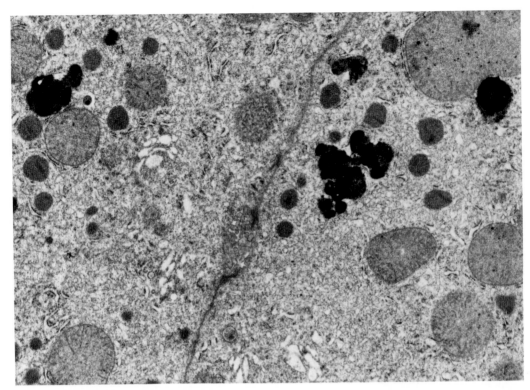

Figure 2.7.   Residual bodies. The dense material represents residual bodies in two adjacent hepatocytes. (Micrograph courtesy of Dr. W.L. Castleman.)

with a primary or a secondary lysosome, the contents are exposed to the acid hydrolases, and digestion begins. Other studies have shown autophagic vacuoles to be formed directly from lysosomes in an energy-dependent process that apparently involves microfilaments. Autophagy is seen in degenerating cells, in cells treated with certain drugs, and in cells undergoing atrophy as well as in apparently healthy, active cells. It is presumed that autophagy is a mechanism by which injured or otherwise effete organelles can be removed and by which normal turnover of organelles can occur.

Heterophagy is a process by which material taken up from outside the cell is digested. Such material is ingested by the process known in more general terms as **endocytosis.** It is first entrapped in an infolding of the plasma membrane, which

is then pinched off to form a vacuole. Again the cytoskeleton is intimately involved in this process. Localized aggregation of microfilaments has been shown to occur shortly after the attachment of a particle to be ingested. This energy-dependent process is presumably necessary for the local membrane movements required to form the pseudopodia that engulf the particle. When the material ingested is relatively large and particulate the process is referred to as **phagocytosis,** and the vacuole formed is a **phagosome.** Fluid material, often containing solids in suspension, is taken up by **pinocytosis.** Despite the distinction made in naming these processes, they are mechanistically the same, differing only in the size of the vacuoles or vesicles formed. Pinocytotic vesicles are relatively small. The subsequent steps of fusion with primary or secondary lysosomes are essentially identical to those already described for autophagy.

A third mechanism for internalization of material from the exterior is called **receptor-mediated endocytosis.** This is a more specific mechanism in which the substance in question, such as a peptide hormone, interacts with receptors on the cell surface which are associated with coated pits. Coated pits are depressions in the cell membrane lined by electron-dense material containing a unique protein, **clathrin.** Coated pits, with their bound material, are internalized as vesicles. Material internalized in this way appears to be able to follow a different route than that internalized by phagocytosis or pinocytosis. Instead of fusing with lysosomes, the material apparently may pass directly to elements of the Golgi apparatus or ER or to an intermediate compartment where the contents may be transferred for further transport. The contents of the vesicles and the membrane components can be separated, and the membrane, together with receptors, can be returned to the surface of the cell.

Phagocytosis is an important part of the defense armamentarium of the animal. Both neutrophils and macrophages are capable of recognizing foreign material, including invading organisms, and ingesting it. These cells add a special adaptation to the process by secreting additional enzymes, which are capable of killing organisms, into the phagosome. In the case of neutrophils, the enzymes are contained in the **specific granules** that fuse with the phagosome along with lysosomes. The role of lysosomes in host defenses and in disease in general is further discussed later in this chapter and in Chapters 4 and 7.

Cytoskeleton—Microtubules and Cytoplasmic Filaments

It is now evident that the complex, dynamic spatial organization of essentially all cells involves the interaction of three classes of filaments which collectively are referred to as the **cytoskeleton.** These are **microfilaments, microtubules,** and **intermediate filaments.** The cytoskeleton is considered to be important in the maintenance of cell shape and in cell movement.

Microfilaments are about 6 nm in diameter, are based on **actin,** and are most familiar as the classic thin filaments in muscle cells. However, nonmuscle cells also contain actin as well as a number of actin-associated proteins involved either in contraction and cell movement or in the regulation of microfilament formation. Microfilaments are involved in several distinct fiber systems. **Stress fibers** contain bundles of microfilaments and are thought to be involved in anchoring the cytoplasmic matrix to the substrate, although they are also contractile. They are most commonly found in cultured cells, and only rarely *in vivo,* although they have been found in certain pathological conditions, including in endothelial cells of rats with experimental hypertension. Stress fiber–like filaments have also been described in the Schwann cells of dogs with an inherited demyelinating neuropathy. Microfilaments also form thinner bundles and mesh-like arrangements, which seem to be involved in maintaining the gel-like state of the cytoplasm. The microfilament system is complex from the molecular point of view. At least six molecular forms of actin are known, and actin exists in the cell either in its filamentous form, as F-actin, or as the monomeric, or globular, G-actin. There are at least 12 different regulatory proteins involved in the control of actin polymerization and the form that the resulting filaments adopt in the cell.

Microtubules are narrow cylinders, about 25 nm in diameter, formed by polymerization of the protein tubulin. They can be rapidly assembled and disassembled, making them a dynamic component of the cytoskeleton. They are of variable length but may be quite long, perhaps 50 μm or more. Microtubules are also associated with other proteins, the so-called **microtubule-associated proteins,** which are thought in many cases to cross-link them to other cytoskeletal components. Microtubules are prominent components of flagella, cilia, and the mitotic spindle, as well as of neurotubules in axons. However, they are present in all cells. They generally are considered to be important in the maintenance of cell shape, in the beating movement of flagella and cilia, and in the movement of chromosomes in cell division. They are important in the internal organization of the cell and the movement of cytoplasmic organelles and granules. For this reason they are intimately involved in the process of cellular secretion. Microtubules also are thought to play a role in cell movement by interacting with microfilaments. In particular, they seem to be important in coordinating directional movement. For example, if microtubules are destroyed (using the drug colchicine), the treated cells retain the ability to move but lose the ability to respond to directional stimuli. Microtubules are obviously important in the function of phagocytes such as neutrophils, and are therefore important to the defense of the host. Their importance is illustrated in the **Chediak-Higashi syndrome,** in which there is a possible defect in microtubular function. Patients with this disease are unusually susceptible to infection (Chapter 7). Defects in microtubules, or their associated proteins, are also known to cause abnormalities in the function of cilia in man and in dogs. Because of the role of cilia in pulmonary clearance and defense (*see* Chapter 7), these defects commonly result in chronic respiratory infections.

Intermediate filaments form the third group of cytoskeletal filaments. They have a diameter of 7–11 nm and are thought to play an important role in the mainte-nance of the cell's three-dimensional shape. There are five types of intermediate filaments made up of biochemically and antigenically related, yet distinct, proteins. The different intermediate filaments are tissue specific. **Cytokeratins,** which include the keratin of keratinizing stratified epithelia, are found in epithelial cells of all types, and are the constitutional protein of the tonofilaments. Epithelia may even be subclassified based on the types of cytokeratins they contain. **Vimentin** is found in mesenchymal cells such as fibroblasts and certain other nonepithelial cells. **Desmin** is found in skeletal and cardiac muscle cells, as well as in visceral smooth muscle cells. Some vascular smooth muscle cells contain vimentin. **Glial fibrillary acidic protein** (GFAP) is found in astrocytes, intestinal glial cells, and apparently in some Schwann cells. Astrocytes may coexpress GFAP and vimentin. Finally, the triplet of **neurofilament proteins** is found in neuronal neurofilaments in the central and peripheral nervous systems. Using appropriate specific antibodies and immunocytochemistry it is possible to classify cells according to their content of intermediate filaments. This is particularly important in the classification of neoplasms (*see* Chapter 6). For example, carcinomas arising from epithelial cells contain cytokeratins, astrogliomas contain GFAP, and rhabdomyosarcomas, arising from skeletal muscle cells, contain desmin. Because tissue-specific intermediate filament type seems to be preserved even in poorly differentiated neoplasms, intermediate filament proteins can act as **markers** allowing classification of neoplasms that might be otherwise difficult to recognize.

The various components of the cytoskeleton are also linked to the plasma membrane and its proteins. They are thought to be important in the regulation of the movement of surface molecules and in such plasma membrane functions as phagocytosis. In addition the various components of the cytoskeleton are linked by "linker proteins" that are as yet poorly defined.

Peroxisomes

Peroxisomes are small roughly spherical organelles up to 1.5 μm in diameter. They are bounded by a single membrane and have a fairly homogeneous, moderately electron-dense internal structure. Morphologically, peroxisomes, which apparently are derived from ER, resemble lysosomes but can be distinguished from the latter by their enzyme content. Also, they often contain a structure called a **nucleoid,** which is not found in lysosomes. Peroxisomes contain several enzymes related to the metabolism of hydrogen peroxide. Urate oxidase, D-amino acid oxidase, and α-hydroxy acid oxidase produce hydrogen peroxide, and catalase destroys it.

The role of peroxisomes in disease is not clear, but their enzyme content suggests that they may be involved in the destruction of hydrogen peroxide, a substance that may injure cells.

This review of the structure of the normal cell and the essential functions of its organelles is intended to be only a brief summary. The student who feels unfamiliar with this material should read a text in medical cell biology. It is a truism, but worth stating anyway, that we cannot appreciate the abnormal before we adequately understand the normal.

Cytocavitary Network and Movement of Cell Membranes

Many of the membrane-bound cytoplasmic organelles that we have just discussed are considered to belong to a functionally contiguous system referred to as the **cytocavitary network.** This includes lysosomes, phagosomes, residual bodies, secretory granules, the Golgi apparatus, the endoplasmic reticulum (both SER and RER), peroxisomes, and the nuclear envelope (Fig. 2.5).

These organelles are interconnected functionally by a series of membrane fusions and buddings, which provide a directed traffic of membranes and contents of vesicles within the cell. For example, many proteins synthesized in the RER are transported to the Golgi for modification. This is accomplished by vesicles that bud from the ER and move to the Golgi, where they fuse. Similarly, phagosomes transport phagocytosed material to the lysosomes, and secretory vesicles transport material to the cell surface. There is now much evidence that the membrane involved in this traffic is recycled. For example, membrane that fuses with the plasma membrane in a secretory event is internalized and transported back to the Golgi for reuse. In this way the cell avoids a great deal of wastage. Both the Golgi and coated vesicles appear to play major roles in directing the movement of intracellular membrane traffic.

Presumably the cytoskeleton is important in providing direction to this membrane traffic. Integral proteins are limited in their lateral movement in the plasma membrane, and this seems to be due to connections with the cytoskeleton. It is thought that cytoskeletal elements can control the movement of membrane proteins, such as receptors, which would be important in such phenomena as capping and patching.

Dr. B. F. Trump and his colleagues have introduced the terms **esotropy** and **exotropy** to describe the processes involved in fusion and budding of membranes. As shown in Figure 2.8, esotropy involves the turning in of the membrane into the cell sap, followed by membrane fusion and the formation of a new membrane-bound vesicle. The inside of the vesicle is therefore topologically equivalent to the extracellular space. Exotropy involves the turning out of the membrane toward the extracellular space or the cytocavitary space followed by fusion to form a budded-off particle containing cell sap. Each of

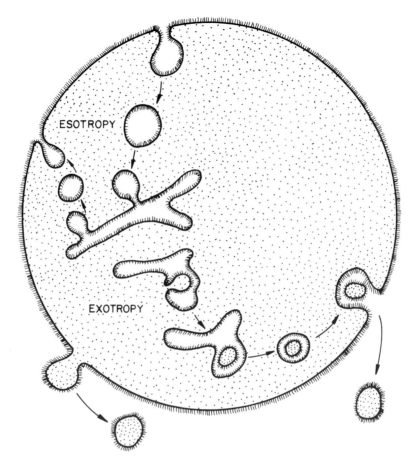

Figure 2.8.   Esotropy and exotropy. The process of esotropy involves the formation of membrane-bound structures in which the orientation of the membrane is reversed. The inside of such structures is equivalent to the extracellular surface of the plasma membrane. The process of exotropy maintains the orientation of the membrane and results in a structure containing cell sap. (Adapted from B.F. Trump, E.M. McDowell and A.U. Arstila. Cellular reaction to injury. In *Principles of Pathobiology*, edited by R.B. Hill and M.F. LaVia. Oxford University Press, New York, 1980.)

these processes can occur in either the forward or the reverse direction.

Forward esotropy includes such processes as pinocytosis and phagocytosis, the formation of vesicles from the ER for transport to the Golgi, and the formation of secretory granules from the Golgi. Reverse esotropy includes the fusion of secretory vesicles with the plasma membrane and the fusion of the phagosome with the lysosome. Examples of forward exotropy are autophagy, cell division, some forms of secretion (such as the secretion of lipid from mammary epithelial cells),

and the budding of many enveloped viruses into the extracellular space or the cytocavitary space. Reverse exotropy is encountered in cell fusion such as occurs in the formation of multinucleate giant cells from macrophages or in the formation of multinucleate skeletal muscle cells from myoblasts during embryogenesis or repair of skeletal muscle.

Cellular Adaptation

Cells normally exist and carry out their functions within a fairly narrow range of physicochemical conditions. The pH of the cell sap, the concentration of electrolytes, and a host of other factors are closely controlled by the cell. The maintenance of these conditions, that is those compatible with cell survival and function, is called **homeostasis,** and serious departure from the norm in some of them results in damage to the cell. In response to unusual stimuli or altered demands, however, the cell can undergo adaptation. Thus, to accommodate these changed conditions, the cell establishes new levels of metabolic or other functional activity without impairing its ability to survive. Usually these functional changes can be correlated with morphologic alterations in the cell. Adaptive changes very often are seen as a response to altered work load. A frequently cited example is the increase in muscle mass which accompan-

ies physical work such as weight lifting. This is a very obvious example, but much more subtle alterations may occur. The hepatocyte, for instance, if subjected to increased need to detoxify drugs or toxins, as explained below, can increase its capacity to do so. The ability of the entire animal to respond to changes in its environment is, therefore, largely accounted for by the adaptive capacity of its constituent cells. Cells may respond by either increasing or decreasing their content of specific organelles.

Cellular Atrophy

When a tissue or organ undergoes a reduction in mass the process is known as **atrophy.** Such a loss of substance can be due to loss of cells (Fig. 2.9) or, of more concern here, to reduction in the size of

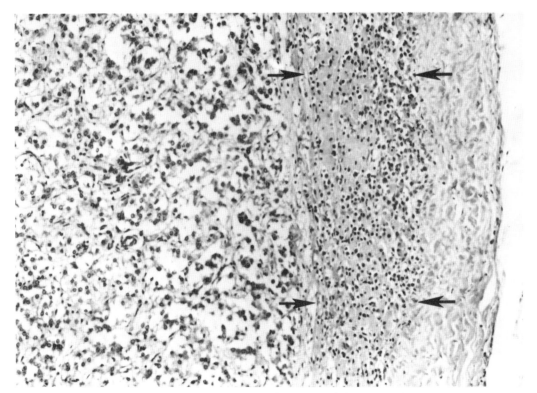

Figure 2.9. Atrophy due to necrosis. In this adrenal gland the cortex *(arrows)* is markedly reduced in thickness due to necrosis of adrenal cortical cells. The cells remaining are macrophages and a few infiltrating lymphocytes.

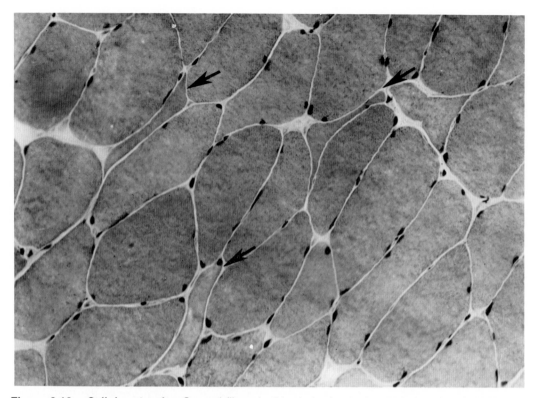

Figure 2.10.   Cellular atrophy. Several fibers in this skeletal muscle are reduced in diameter and angular in shape *(arrows)*. Atrophy of muscle fibers in this case was due to denervation. The atrophic cells are still viable.

individual cells (Fig. 2.10). In the latter case, atrophy is an adaptive response to altered demands on the cell, often a reduction in work load. In addition, loss of innervation or of hormonal stimulation, reduced blood supply, or inadequate nutrition all can lead to atrophy of cells. Thus muscles that are denervated or, for some reason, used less than usual will undergo atrophy accounted for by shrinkage of their constituent cells (Fig. 2.10). The adrenal gland deprived of stimulation by ACTH will undergo adrenocortical atrophy, and the animal deprived of an adequate food supply will be thin, partly due to atrophy of muscle cells. It is of great significance that **atrophic cells are not dead** or really even severely injured. They have reduced functional capacity but retain the ability to control their internal environment and to produce sufficient en-

ergy to suit their new level of activity. Because they are still alive they can adapt again if subjected to more normal functional demands. Therefore, the muscles that have undergone atrophy due to immobilization, for instance, will, given time, regain their normal bulk and strength when returned to use. This phrase "given time" is of considerable potential importance to the clinical consequences of some lesions involving atrophy. A common cause of adrenal cortical atrophy, for instance, is excessive, prolonged treatment with corticosteroids. Because these drugs inhibit the release of ACTH from the adenohypophysis, the adrenal cortical cells are not normally stimulated and undergo atrophy. It is very important to realize that the sudden withdrawal of the exogenous corticosteroids will produce a situation in which atrophic adrenal cortical cells suddenly are called upon to secrete sufficient cortisone to meet the needs of the animal, a demand which they simply may not be able to meet. The result may be acute adrenal cortical insufficiency, a highly dangerous clinical syndrome known as "Addisonian crisis." In contrast, gradual withdrawal of the drug will allow the adrenal glands to respond and adapt to progressively increasing functional demands and avoid a potentially lethal situation.

The mechanisms by which cells undergo atrophy, in particular the signals that trigger the process, are poorly understood. There is, however, actual loss of substance from the cell. In the case of muscle cells undergoing atrophy, for example, there is loss of myofilaments, mitochondria, and endoplasmic reticulum as well as reduced metabolic activity. In other words catabolic processes exceed anabolic processes. One morphologic manifestation of this process is the formation of increased numbers of autophagic vacuoles, formed as the cell breaks down the redundant organelles.

Finally, atrophy may involve the death of some of the affected cells. In many cases, especially in physiological circumstances, this involves the process of **apoptosis** (*see* below). In other cases loss of cells is a late-stage event. For example, in denervated muscle, the long-term loss of the trophic influences of innervation eventually leads to actual loss of myocytes even though their blood supply is adequate. Once that has happened, of course, it may be impossible to fully reverse the process. In other cases, atrophy may be reversed by the process of physiological hyperplasia.

Hypertrophy

When cells are subjected to increased functional demands, or increased work, they may enlarge, and, as a result, the whole organ or tissue mass also enlarges. Hypertrophy, then, is an adaptive response by which organs are increased in size due to an increase in cell size without cellular proliferation. The most striking example again occurs in skeletal muscle that is subjected to an unusual work load. We are all familiar with the increased muscle mass that results from weight lifting. A similar process occurs in the heart, so that highly trained athletes may have hearts that are enlarged due to the increased physiologic demands placed on them. Myocardial hypertrophy also, of course, can be due to pathologic conditions that impose an abnormal workload on the heart. Most commonly this is seen with stenotic valvular disease in which the blood must be ejected through an abnormally narrow valvular opening. This requires more work from the myocardium, and hypertrophy results (Fig. 2.11).

Cellular hypertrophy is not simply a case of cell swelling or enlargement. Although the nature of the signal to the cell is again poorly understood, the net result is an increase in total cellular proteins, including myofibrils in muscle cells as well as organelles such as mitochondria and ER. There is increased synthesis of cellular constituents, and anabolic processes exceed catabolic ones.

Hypertrophy, as an adaptive change, may not always be to the advantage of the animal. In the case of the heart, in particular, there seems to be some limit beyond which hypertrophy cannot compensate for an underlying lesion or disease process. Hypertrophy may, in addition, produce conformational changes in the heart which lead to inefficient pumping. There is some evidence that, despite the increased numbers of mitochondria, the energy metabolism of the hypertrophied myocytes is unable to meet the demands of the increased work load placed on the heart. All of these factors can contribute to eventual heart failure despite the attempt of the individual cells to adapt to the altered circumstances.

In some cases there are more subtle

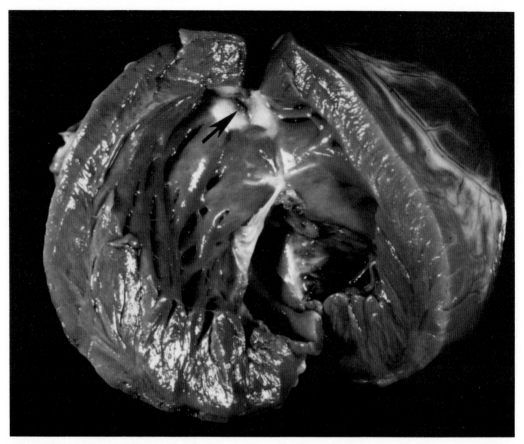

Figure 2.11. Myocardial hypertrophy. Heart from a dog with pulmonic stenosis. The wall of the right ventricle, the cut surface of which is shown, is greatly thickened due to the increased work required to force blood through the stenotic pulmonary valve *(arrow).*

changes in which cellular adaptation leads to hypertrophy of a specific organelle system. This is most dramatically illustrated in the liver by the induction, or hypertrophy, of smooth endoplasmic reticulum in animals treated with certain drugs or toxins. It was pointed out earlier in this chapter that the SER is associated with certain enzyme systems. These include a complex of enzymes known as the **mixed function oxidase** system, which is responsible for the metabolism of a variety of drugs and toxins. Continued exposure to a drug such as phenobarbital induces increased levels of these enzymes, a phenomenon manifested morphologically by a dramatic proliferation of the SER (Fig. 2.12). The inducing drug is more rapidly destroyed and, as a result, often has a more transient effect on the treated animal.

When proliferation of the SER occurs in response to a particular drug there is also an enhanced capacity to detoxify other substances metabolized by the same system. Often this is advantageous to the animal but, when the intermediate products of metabolism are themselves highly toxic, it can be extremely harmful. A classic example is the enhanced toxicity of carbon tetrachloride in animals pretreated with drugs such as phenobarbital. The toxicity of carbon tetrachloride is due to free radicals produced as intermediate

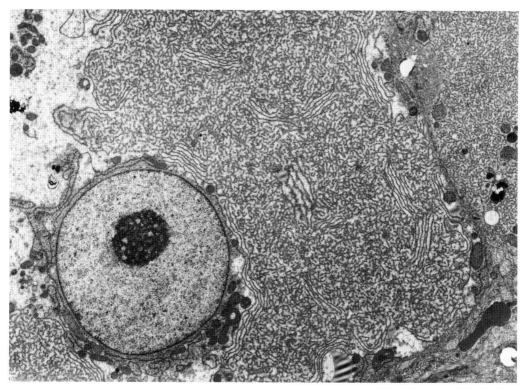

Figure 2.12. Hypertrophy of smooth endoplasmic reticulum. In this liver cell most of the cytoplasm is occupied by smooth endoplasmic reticulum. This increase was induced by prolonged treatment of a dog with the drug primidone. (Micrograph courtesy of Dr. W.L. Castleman.)

metabolites *(see below)*, and the more rapid production of these in the animal with hypertrophy of the SER results in much more extensive hepatocellular damage. Some carcinogens must be metabolized before they are able to induce neoplasia (*see* Chapter 6). Presumably, this activity also is enhanced by hypertrophy of the SER.

Hyperplasia and metaplasia also may be adaptive responses. As such they may involve changes in synthetic activity in the altered cells. Because they involve alterations in patterns of proliferation and differentiation, we have chosen to discuss them, together with other disorders of growth, in Chapter 6.

CELL INJURY

So far, we have reviewed the structure and function of the normal cell and have seen how it can adapt, within limits, to changes in the demands made on it. When these demands reach the point at which there is impairment of the cell's overall functional capacity, the cell is said to be injured. **Cell injury** can be defined simply as any change that results in a loss of the ability to maintain the normal or adapted homeostatic state. Injured cells therefore are unable to keep in balance all of the processes that normally regulate their internal environment. As a result, a variety of morphologic changes occur which we recognize as indications of cell injury.

The extent of injury to the cell can vary and depends on its severity, the cause, the type of cell involved, and its metabolic state at the time of the insult. In the case of sublethal injury, the changes in the cell may be relatively mild and compatible with its continued survival. Such injury often is reversible, and with removal of the stimulus the cell may revert to normal structure and function. The distinction between marked adaptation and mild injury, therefore, is difficult to draw.

Reversible cell injury is sometimes referred to as **degeneration,** and, traditionally, various forms of degeneration have been given specific names such as cloudy swelling, hydropic degeneration and fatty degeneration, according to the microscopic appearance of the affected cells. These designations will be clarified when we consider the morphologic changes that occur in injured cells. For now, suffice it to say that current understanding of pathogenetic mechanisms indicates that they do not represent distinct processes, and it is preferable to abandon these terms and use the simpler "cell injury" or "degeneration."

If the insult is more severe, or if it continues for long enough, the injury may progress to the point where **irreversible cell injury** occurs and the cell dies. **Cell death,** unfortunately, is no more easily defined than is somatic death or the death of the individual animal. Conceptually, cell death means that the changes in the cell can no longer be reversed, but in practice it is impossible to recognize the precise point at which this occurs.

The rate at which the changes in injured cells occur can vary widely. Acute injury produces rapid changes that may be lethal if not quickly reversed, whereas chronic injury may persist for months or even years without killing the cell.

Necrosis is the term used to describe the overall process that occurs when cells that are part of a living organism die. The morphologic changes that we recognize microscopically as necrosis, however, are the result of **degradation** of the contents of the dead cell. Most pathologists therefore use the word necrosis to include cell death *and* the degradative changes that follow it. The initial degradative changes in the dead cell occur as a result of the action of endogenous enzymes derived largely from the lysosomes. This process is referred to as **autolysis** (self-digestion). This term also is used often to describe the changes that occur in all of the cells after an animal has died. There is no real mechanistic difference between these processes, and the latter should be referred to as **postmortem autolysis** to distinguish it from the former.

Morphology of Cell Injury

The traditional tool that the pathologist uses to evaluate changes in cells is the light microscope. For this reason we will first consider the changes that occur in injured cells as they appear at the light microscopic level, followed by those seen with the electron microscope. However, before discussing these changes we should remind ourselves that we are looking at images of cells frozen at one point in time during a dynamic process. We cannot always tell how rapidly the changes were progressing or even whether they were, in fact, progressing or regressing. When we see a cell that shows histologic evidence of injury we cannot be certain how far the change would have progressed if not interrupted by fixation. We cannot tell whether the cell would have gone on to die, would have recovered, or would remain static. The morphologic changes that occur in injured cells always lag behind the functional changes. In particular, the changes associated with necrosis always occur after the cell is biologically dead. Clearly, when we see necrotic cells, we see those in which cell death has occurred some time ago. Equally clearly, some cells that are apparently injured may, in fact, be dead. Without the changes associated with necrosis, however, it is impossible to distinguish recently dead cells from injured, but viable, cells.

Reversible Cell Injury

There are two basic changes that occur in sublethally injured cells. **Cell swelling** is an early and almost universal manifestation of injury. In the light microscope, affected cells are enlarged. This is particularly evident when the swelling compresses adjacent structures. In the liver, for example, hepatocellular swelling may compress sinusoids sufficiently to obliterate their lumina (Figs. 2.13, 2.14). In mildly swollen cells the staining characteristics are altered, producing a somewhat cloudy appearance. This lesion used to be called "cloudy swelling." As the process progresses, many vacuoles of variable size appear in the cytoplasm giving rise to the appearance sometimes called "hydropic degeneration" or "vacuolar degeneration."

Some caution should be exercised in making assumptions about the nature of vacuoles in injured cells. Commonly they represent distended organelles, most often distended ER, but in other cases they may be small lipid droplets or non-membrane-bound areas devoid of cytoplasmic organelles. Special techniques may be required to demonstrate the real nature of vacuoles. Special stains can identify lipids in vacuoles, and electron microscopy can identify distended organelles.

Cell swelling results from loss of the cell's normally precise control of movement of ions and water across the cell membrane. This results in a net uptake of water by the injured cell. The mechanisms involved are discussed later in this chapter. Cell swelling *per se* is not incompatible with survival of the cell. In fact, it often reflects relatively mild, reversible injury.

Cells that are severely injured also

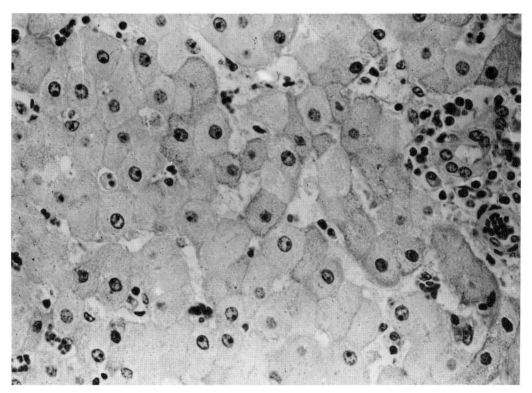

Figure 2.13. Mild cell swelling. The hepatocytes shown here are swollen, and sinusoids are compressed. The cytoplasm of the cells is finely vacuolated. Such vacuoles usually represent dilated cisternae of the endoplasmic reticulum, but very small lipid droplets also might be present.

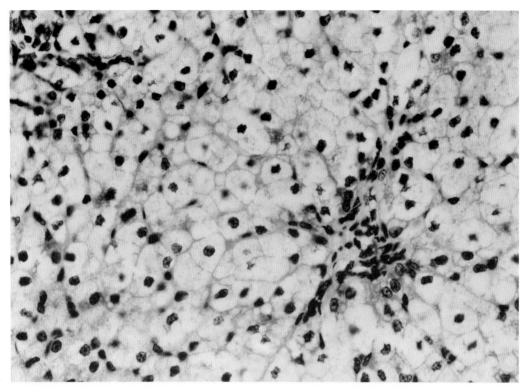

Figure 2.14. **Severe cell swelling.** These hepatocytes are severely swollen and vacuolated. As a result, the sinusoids are obliterated. The vacuoles mostly reflect markedly distended cisternae of the endoplasmic reticulum, but an increase in lipid vacuoles contributes to this appearance.

undergo swelling, and some of them may die. Again, no certain distinction can be made, at the light microscopic level, between a cell swollen because of reversible injury and one fortuitously fixed during its progression to cell death, or even one fixed just after cell death has occurred. From the diagnostic viewpoint, however, the assessment of lesions in the light microscope is not quite as imprecise as this discussion might make it seem. In injured tissues, cells are present in various stages of injury. If, for instance, the majority of cells are swollen and many are actually necrotic we would assume the injury to be more serious than one in which most cells are swollen without evidence of necrosis. The presence of necrotic cells, in other words, would suggest that many of the accompanying swollen, injured cells

were dying or already dead (*see* Fig. 2.35).

In addition to cell swelling, injured cells may exhibit changes in staining characteristics. Cytoplasmic constituents, such as glycogen, may be depleted in injured cells, such changes being associated with altered affinity for certain stains.

Fatty change, the accumulation of excessive intracellular lipid, is also a common manifestation of reversible injury. It is seen most often in cells that normally metabolize a lot of fat. Fatty change often affects renal tubular epithelial cells, myocardial cells, and, in particular, hepatocytes. Morphologically it is characterized by the presence of lipid-filled vacuoles in the cytoplasm of affected cells (Fig. 2.15). Fatty change is most easily recognized when the cytoplasm contains single, large, clearly demarcated vacuoles, but, in some

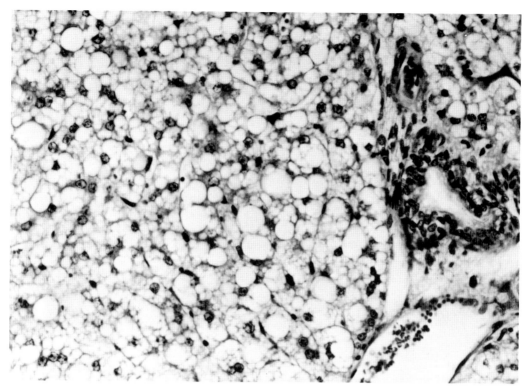

Figure 2.15. Fatty change. These hepatocytes contain increased intracellular lipid producing the sharply demarcated vacuoles seen here. Fatty change may produce single large cytoplasmic vacuoles (macrovesicular) or multiple small vacuoles (microvesicular). Both types of vacuolation are present in this micrograph.

cases, the vacuoles may be small and multiple. The presence of fat in vacuoles may be confirmed by staining frozen sections of the tissue with an oil-soluble dye such as "oil red O." Frozen sections are necessary to avoid extraction of the fat by solvents used in conventional histologic preparations. The pathogenetic mechanisms responsible for the accumulation of fat in injured cells are considered in more detail later in this chapter.

Finally, injured cells may show alterations in nuclear morphology. In sublethal injury these changes are relatively subtle and consist of some clumping in the distribution of chromatin. Dramatic changes in nuclear morphology are usually indicative of necrosis.

Ultrastructural Changes in Injured Cells

The morphologic changes that occur in injured cells can be appreciated at an earlier stage and can be better understood when their ultrastructure is studied. With the electron microscope changes can be detected in individual organelles, and it can be appreciated that some are affected before others. For the moment we will consider only the nature of the changes that occur in each organelle system. Later we will consider the sequence in which such changes occur and how they are thought to be related to the pathogenesis of cell injury.

In the plasma membrane, the major

change seen is the loss of surface specializations. Microvilli or cilia may be lost (Fig. 2.16), and intercellular attachments may break down. In addition, changes in cell outline such as the formation of cytoplasmic blebs may be seen.

Mitochondria commonly are altered in injured cells. Early in the process they may be condensed, with contraction of the inner mitochondrial compartment. This phase is transient, however, and they soon undergo swelling (Fig. 2.17) and even may rupture. Injured mitochondria lose their normal dense granules, but abnormal dense amorphous deposits may appear. In addition, deposits of calcium salts may be formed in damaged mitochondria.

Another common change seen in injured cells, and one that often accounts for the vacuolated appearance seen by light microscopy, is dilatation of the endoplasmic reticulum (Fig. 2.18). Like cell swelling, it is presumably due to changes in the movement of ions and water across membranes, in this case those of the ER. In addition, ribosomes disaggregate and detach from the surface of the RER. Not surprisingly, this change is associated with impaired protein synthesis.

As injury progresses, the membranes of organelles may be disrupted and may lose phospholipids. Because of their amphipathic nature these molecules tend to reaggregate in the cytosol and spontaneously form membrane-like whorls often called **myelin figures** (Fig. 2.19).

Fairly late in cell injury, lysosomes also may be altered. They may swell and, eventually, rupture. Lysosomes tend to retain their functional capacity until late

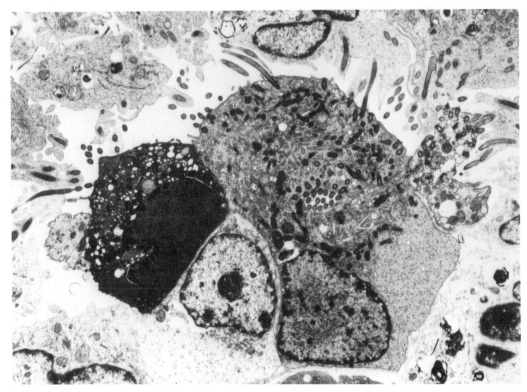

Figure 2.16. Loss of surface specializations. In this injured, ciliated, bronchiolar epithelial cell, cilia have been lost by internalization. Cilia can be seen free in the cytoplasm. The very dark cell on the *left* is necrotic. (Micrograph courtesy of Dr. W.L. Castleman.)

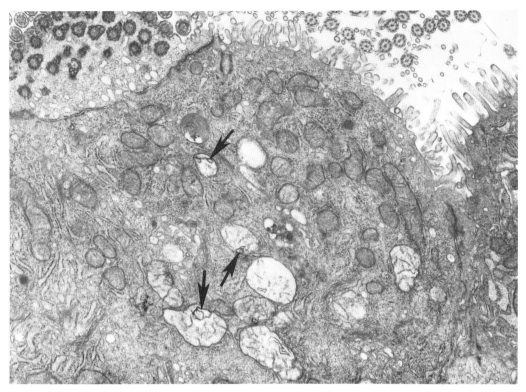

Figure 2.17. High-amplitude swelling of mitochondria. Several of the mitochondria in this cell have undergone high-amplitude swelling. The presence of membranous arrays in some of them *(arrows)* suggests damage to the inner mitochondrial membrane. (Micrograph courtesy of Dr. W.L. Castleman.)

in the process of cell injury. As a result, they fuse with vacuoles containing the remains of injured cell organelles, and many autophagosomes may be found in injured cells. The enzymes released from damaged lysosomes are partly responsible for the breakdown of cell constituents that characterizes necrosis. However, it is generally believed that, in most forms of cell injury, by the time lysosomal enzymes escape into the cytoplasm, the cell is already dead. In certain cases, lysosomal enzymes may contribute actively to the injury to the cell.

Lethal Cell Injury and Necrosis

Irreversibly injured cells can exhibit all of the changes already described. Once cell death has occurred, however, degradation of cell components begins. The morphologic patterns that we recognize as necrosis, therefore, are the result of denaturation and dissolution of proteins and other cellular constituents.

At the light microscopic level, necrosis is characterized by increased eosinophilia of the cytoplasm associated with enhanced binding of the stain eosin to altered proteins, and with loss of ribosomes. The cytoplasm also may be hyalinized (having a homogeneous glassy appearance), or it may be vacuolated. Swollen mitochondria may be evident as eosinophilic cytoplasmic granules. As its contents are broken down, the cytoplasm becomes more vacuolated and "moth-eaten" in appearance. Under the right conditions, discussed below, the necrotic cells also may undergo calcification.

The nucleus also undergoes character-

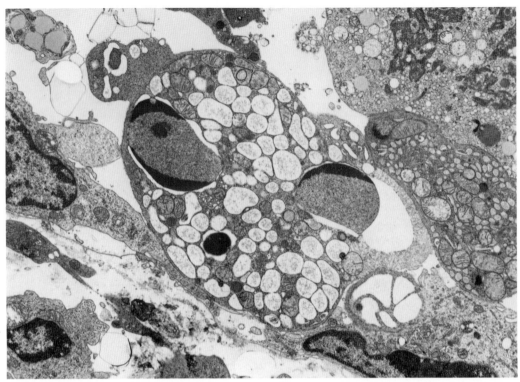

Figure 2.18.   Dilatation of the endoplasmic reticulum. In this injured bronchiolar cell the cisternae of the rough endoplasmic reticulum are dilated. (Micrograph courtesy of Dr. W.L. Castleman.)

istic changes in the necrotic cell. Initially, in injured cells, the chromatin in the nucleus becomes clumped. In cells that have died, the nuclei initially shrink and become densely basophilic, a process called **pyknosis** (Fig. 2.20). They may then break up into fragments, that is undergo **karyorrhexis** (Fig. 2.21), or they may be dissolved **(karyolysis)** (Fig. 2.20). Whatever route it follows, eventually the nucleus disappears. Pyknosis, karyorrhexis, and karyolysis are sure signs of necrosis and, therefore, of preceding cell death.

Necrosis is appreciated most readily microscopically, but before leaving our discussion of the appearance of necrotic cells we should mention that necrosis is discernable grossly as well. In other words, tissue necrosis is often visible to the naked eye. When relatively large numbers of cells undergo necrosis in focal areas,

they may be visible as tissue that is lighter in color than the surrounding normal tissue. This is due to coagulation of their cytoplasmic proteins and, frequently, to reduced blood flow in the necrotic area. In this way infarcts (in the kidney, for example) are often readily visible (Fig. 2.22). Another example is hepatocellular necrosis in the disease **necrobacillosis** (*see* Fig. 7.15). In this particular example the lesions are unusually distinct, but they are very typical of this disease. Necrotic tissue also may be swollen, due to swelling of the individual cells, or it may be reduced in volume, producing a depression on the surface of the organ. It may be softer to the touch than the normal tissue, a change referred to as **malacia.** In addition a local reaction to the necrotic tissue may be apparent as a reddened zone of vascular congestion adjacent to

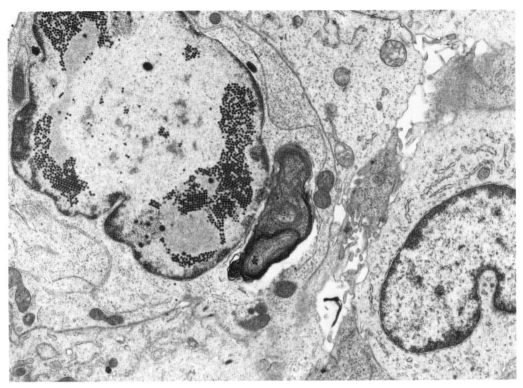

Figure 2.19.   Myelin figure. In this injured bronchiolar epithelial cell from a dog, a large myelin figure, with concentric swirls of membranous material, is present in the cytoplasm. Adenovirus particles can be seen in the nucleus. (Micrograph courtesy of Dr. W.L. Castleman.)

the lesion (Fig. 2.22). Once one is able to recognize these changes it often is possible to detect necrosis during the gross postmortem examination or during surgery.

Classification of Necrotic Lesions

The gross and histologic appearance of necrotic cells may vary somewhat depending on local conditions, in particular on how much fluid or blood flow is present in the lesion.

In the case of **coagulation necrosis** the dead cells take on the appearance of an eosinophilic "shadow" of the original cells (Figs. 2.23 and 2.24). In other words, the original cellular shape and tissue organization is still apparent histologically, but cellular detail is lost, and the nucleus is either gone or apparent only as small basophilic fragments. This appearance often is seen when the blood supply is suddenly and completely cut off or when the cytoplasmic proteins are denatured and resistant to digestion. Necrotic skeletal muscle fibers often show this coagulated appearance, probably because the living cells contain relatively few lysosomes (Fig. 2.24). Eventually these cells are phagocytosed by cells derived from the circulation which are involved in the local reaction. The latter, mostly macrophages, release enzymes into the tissue which can liquify the necrotic cells. Once phagocytosed the remnants are digested in phagolysosomes.

In **liquefaction necrosis,** as the name implies, the affected tissue is liquified. As a result, it is very soft and even may be quite fluid. It is seen characteristically in inflammatory lesions containing a lot of neutrophils, a good example being an ab-

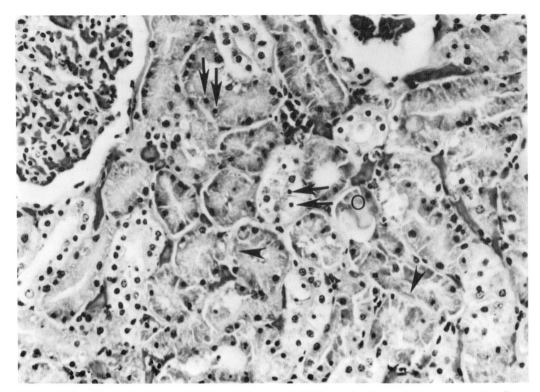

Figure 2.20.   Necrosis. Many of the renal tubular epithelial cells shown here are necrotic. Some contain small, dense nuclei (nuclear pyknosis, *arrows*). In others the nuclei have completely disappeared (karyolysis, *arrowheads*). This was a case of acute ethylene glycol poisoning in a cat. An oxalate crystal *(O)* is present.

scess. When an abscess is cut open the contents often ooze out. The lysosomal enzymes, derived from neutrophils as well as from autolytic digestion, contribute to the process of liquefaction. Some tissues are more likely to show liquefaction necrosis than others. For instance, the parenchyma of the central nervous system typically liquifies when necrotic. Such lesions are referred to as **encephalomalacia** in the brain and **myelomalacia** in the spinal cord. The word malacia means softening and describes the gross appearance and consistency of the affected tissue.

Caseous necrosis is the term applied to describe necrotic tissue that, due to local conditions, is soft and pasty. In the past it was likened by some pathologists to cheese, hence the name. This type of

reaction is likely to be associated with certain bacterial infections. In some species, including man, it is seen in lesions due to *Mycobacterium tuberculosis,* and in the sheep *Corynebacterium ovis* produces similar lesions. In the latter case the disease is even called **caseous lymphadenitis,** because the infection commonly causes caseous necrosis in lymph nodes.

Gangrene is a somewhat archaic term applied to ischemic necrosis of extremities such as limbs, digits, or the tips of the ears (Fig. 2.25). From it the term **gangrenous necrosis** is derived. In reality, there is no distinction between this and either coagulation or liquefaction necrosis, depending again on local conditions. In **dry gangrene** the histologic appearance is one of coagulation whereas in

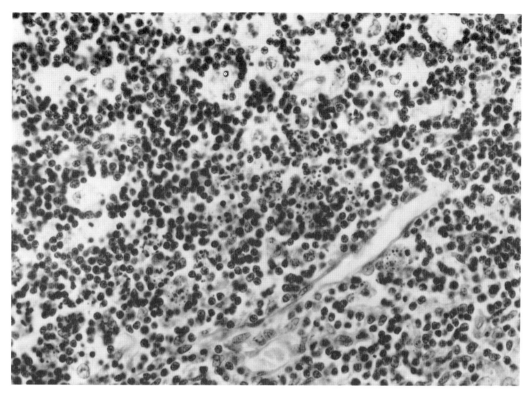

Figure 2.21. Necrosis. In this thymus, the nuclei of a number of necrotic cells have undergone karyorrhexis, producing many small dense fragments of nuclear debris.

wet gangrene, where the actions of bacterial enzymes may be important, it is one of liquefaction.

Especially when focal masses of tissue undergo necrosis, there is often a local response in the surrounding normal tissues. This may include vascular engorgement and congestion and, where there is vascular damage, hemmorrhage. This vascular reaction gives rise to the red zone that often surrounds a necrotic lesion such as an infarct. In addition, the necrotic tissue can evoke an inflammatory response with an associated infiltration of neutrophils and macrophages, in particular, and lesser numbers of lymphoid cells. As already explained, these cells contribute hydrolytic enzymes, derived from lysosomes, which help to break down the dead tissue. They act as phagocytes, ingesting the necrotic debris, removing it from the tissue, and completing its digestion. This process paves the way for healing to occur. The defect left after the removal of dead tissue is repaired in one of a variety of ways depending on the tissue involved. In some the parenchyma can be replaced. In others a scar is formed. Mechanisms involved in the repair of injured tissues are discussed in detail in Chapter 4.

Apoptosis

A distinctive form of cellular destruction, termed **apoptosis,** has also been described. Morphologically, this process is characterized by rapid condensation of nuclear chromatin and cytoplasm, convolution of the cell, and subsequent separation of fragments of the cell into **apoptotic bodies** (Fig. 2.26). These usually consist of nuclear fragments contained

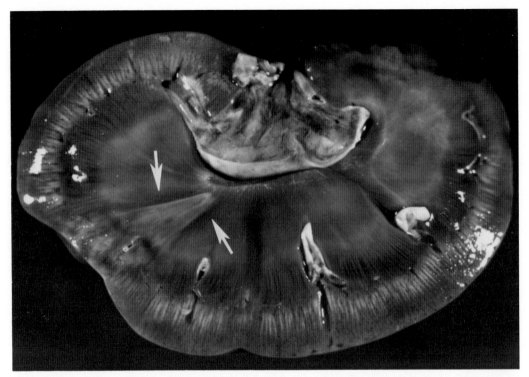

Figure 2.22. Renal infarct. A wedge-shaped segment of pale necrotic tissue can be seen in this kidney from a dog. Its surface is depressed due to collapse of the tissue. The dark borders represent a vascular response to the necrotic tissue *(arrows)*.

within a cytoplasmic mass in which organelle integrity is initially maintained and enclosed within plasma membrane which is initially functionally and morphologically intact. The condensation of chromatin results in peculiar dense masses that abut the nuclear membrane. Apoptotic bodies are phagocytosed by adjacent cells, both macrophages and tissue cells such as epithelial or neoplastic cells, and degraded within phagolysosomes. Although the process of apoptosis may be frequently difficult to distinguish from "conventional" cell injury and necrosis in the usual histopathological preparations, some authors have suggested that apoptosis and necrosis should be separately defined. According to this view necrosis should be applied to the degenerative phenomena that follow irreversible injury, while apoptosis should refer to sit-

uations that suggest cellular self-destruction.

Typically, apoptosis is encountered in processes that involve physiological destruction of cells. It is seen in cells undergoing programmed cell death during development, in cells undergoing normal turnover in postnatal tissues, in normal involution, in some forms of pathological tissue atrophy, and in regression of hyperplasia. It is also commonly seen in malignant neoplasms and in situations in which cell destruction is induced by cell-mediated immune reactions. For example, apoptosis has been observed in a number of diseases in which cell-mediated immunity is believed to be of pathogenetic importance in the destruction of tissues (*see* Chapter 5). Certain toxins, drugs, mild hyperthermia, and irradiation can also induce apoptosis.

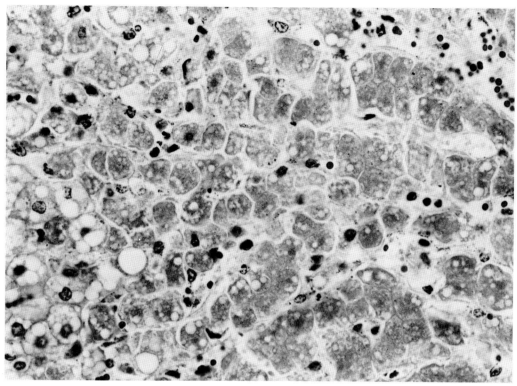

Figure 2.23. Caogulation necrosis. Many of the cells shown in this micrograph lack nuclei and are obviously necrotic. They have retained their shape and are easily recognizable as liver cells. Even lipid vacuoles in their cytoplasm still can be recognized.

Apoptosis appears to be an active, physiological process. In particular, active protein synthesis is necessary for its occurrence, but the nature of the particular proteins involved is unknown. It also seems to involve specific nucleolytic events in which there is double-stranded cleavage of DNA at internucleosomal linker regions. This may relate to the peculiar pattern of change in nuclear chromatin that is characteristic of apoptosis. Perhaps the most compelling reason for distinguishing necrosis from apoptosis is that recognition of the former should point to severe cellular injury, while the latter should suggest selective elimination of cells, whether that be physiological or pathological. In the context of this chapter we are concerned with tissue injury, but in chapter 5 apoptosis is discussed in relation to certain kinds of immune-mediated injury.

Consequences of Cell Injury

This chapter began with the observation that illness of the whole animal can be attributed to functional abnormalities at the cellular level. Here we briefly consider some of the functional consequences of cell injury.

When injured cells are examined while alive, they show a number of abnormal functions. These are initially abnormal, violent cell movements, blebbing of the plasma membrane, and, of course, cell swelling. These changes reflect loss of control of certain mechanisms by the cell. Abnormal cell shape and movement presumably involve altered function of the cytoskeleton, the intracytoplasmic micro-

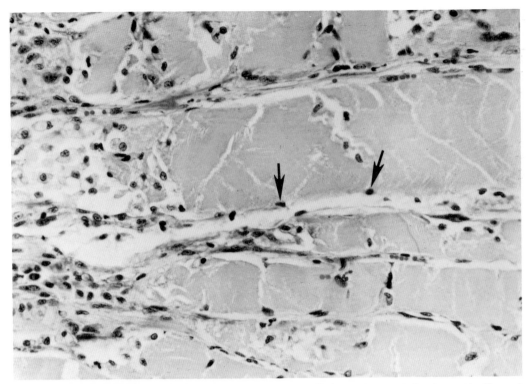

Figure 2.24. Coagulation necrosis. The cytoplasm of these necrotic skeletal muscle fibers is hyalinized and fragmented. The cells lack muscle nuclei or have pyknotic nuclei *(arrows). On the left* macrophages have invaded the tissue to phagocytose the necrotic cellular material. This is the typical appearance of necrotic muscle cells.

tubules, and filaments. Some of these changes are due to loss of energy production in the cell and influx of calcium ions, but there are alterations in protein synthesis and other functions as well. Altered protein synthesis can lead to secondary changes in the cell such as the accumulation of lipids. These aspects are considered in more detail below. The importance of the injury to the whole animal depends in part on the tissue involved, as well as the extent and the severity of the injury. If the myocardium is involved, for example, the consequences can be quite grave. On the other hand if skeletal muscle is involved, a similar degree of tissue injury probably would be of little overall functional consequence. The **prognosis** (that is, the likely outcome of the disease process) is dependent on such factors, and

the clinician needs to assess what tissues are involved and to what extent during his evaluation of the patient.

One result of cell injury that is useful in establishing a diagnosis and prognosis is the measurement of cellular enzymes in body fluids. When cells are injured severely or die, the plasma membrane becomes leaky, and, among other things, enzymes can escape into the circulation (Fig. 2.27). These can be measured by the clinician, and the study of serum enzymes forms a very important diagnostic aid. As an example, consider a horse that is clinically suspected of having necrosis of skeletal muscle. Measurement of the activity in the serum of an enzyme that usually is found only in skeletal muscle can confirm (or deny) this possibility. Such an enzyme is **creatine kinase** (CK) found in

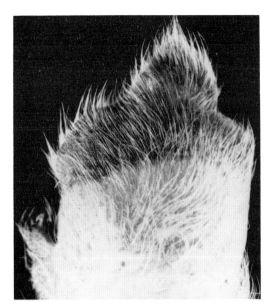

Figure 2.25. Dry gangrene. The necrotic tip of this ear from a pig is dry and sharply demarcated from the viable tissue.

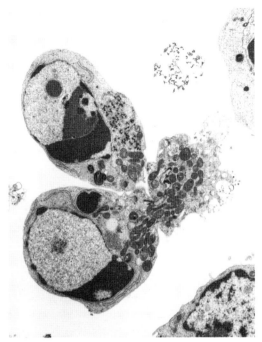

Figure 2.26. Apoptosis. The process of apoptosis is shown in the NS-1 mouse myeloma cell line. Note the constriction of the cell to form lobes containing organelles and nuclear fragments with characteristic dense chromatin masses. These lobes will bud off to form apoptotic bodies. (Micrograph courtesy of N.I. Walker *et al., see: Meth. Achiev. Exp. Pathol. 13:*18–54, 1988).

quantity only in skeletal muscle, myocardium, and brain. Therefore, if the levels of CK in the serum are very high, and if myocardial or brain injury can be excluded clinically, the diagnosis is confirmed. An understanding of the relative amounts of certain enzymes in different tissues and the relative half-lives of the enzymes in the circulation therefore allows us to evaluate injury to a variety of tissues.

Pathogenesis of Cell Injury

Having discussed the appearances of injured cells and the consequences of such injury, we might now ask ourselves what mechanisms are involved in their generation. Why, for example, do injured cells swell? Why do some cells survive injury and others die? What are the critical changes that result in cell death? It soon will become clear that definite answers are available for only some of these questions. Analysis of the molecular events that occur in cell injury is difficult because they cannot be studied in isolation.

The various biochemical changes interact, so that changes in one must be associated with changes in others. As a result it is extremely difficult to single out any one change and say "this is the critical event in cell injury and cell death."

It is clear, however, that despite the variety of tissues which may be involved, and despite the plethora of potential causes, **cell injury is mediated *via* two main mechanisms.** The first is interference with the energy supply of the cell, and the second is direct damage to cell membranes. Even this observation is an oversimplification because it is becoming apparent that membrane damage is a common factor in most, if not all, kinds of cellular injury, including anoxia. These

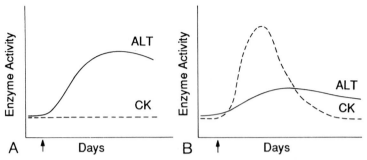

Figure 2.27. Changes in serum enzymes after cell injury. Following severe injury or necrosis to a tissue (indicated here by *arrows*) cellular enzymes may be released and appear in the serum. *A,* when liver cells, which are rich in alanine aminotransferase (ALT) and poor in creatine kinase (CK), are injured much ALT, but little CK, appears in the serum. *B,* when muscle cells, which are rich in CK but have little ALT, are injured much CK, but little ALT, appears in the serum. A knowledge of the tissue specificity of these and other enzymes makes serum enzymology a valuable diagnostic technique.

matters are considered in some detail below. In addition, we briefly discuss injury to specific subcellular organelles.

Causes of Cell Injury

Cells can be damaged by a wide variety of agents too numerous to list here. However, we can consider certain groups into which most of these causes fall. They include hypoxia, chemical agents, physical agents including trauma, genetic abnormalities, biologic agents, immune mechanisms, and nutritional abnormalities.

Hypoxia is one of the most common causes of cell injury. It usually is associated with **ischemia,** or interruption of the supply of blood to the tissue, when it results in infarction. It also may be associated with reduced oxygen-carrying capacity of the blood or with interference with the respiratory chain. **Infarction,** or death of tissue due to interruption of its blood supply, can result from a variety of causes which are discussed in Chapter 3. Reduced oxygen-carrying capacity of the blood may occur whenever the effective levels of hemoglobin are reduced significantly. This may happen in severe anemia, in methemoglobinemia due to nitrite poisoning, or in carboxyhemoglobinemia due to carbon monoxide poisoning.

The best known example of interference with the respiratory chain is cyanide poisoning. Cyanide inactivates cytochrome oxidase thus blocking the transfer of electrons on the respiratory chain. All of these phenomena have the effect of interfering with the energy supply of the cell, and this probably occurs in many forms of cell injury.

Physical agents that can injure cells are diverse. They include direct trauma, such as lacerations or crush injuries, heat, cold, and radiation. The extent of such injuries may be increased by tissue hypoxia associated with local vascular damage. Radiation injury may be caused by x-rays, radioactive isotope emissions, and, most commonly, ultraviolet (UV) light. Many of us have suffered cell injury due to UV radiation, in the form of sunburn. Animals also may be sunburnt, and those with unpigmented, poorly haired skin are particularly susceptible. In both animals and man, long-term exposure to UV and other forms of radiation may cause cancer, a phenomenon discussed in Chapter 6.

Chemical agents are present in our environment in a bewildering variety and many of them are more or less toxic. Even those which are essential for the health of our cells can, paradoxically, be injurious when present in excess. Examples include sodium chloride, selenium, copper, and iron salts to name only a few. Other chemicals are very potent toxins, minute quantities of which can injure cells and cause illness or death of the animal. Chemical toxins act in a wide variety of ways, but most either injure membranes directly (we include those that interact with receptors) or interfere with the energy metabolism of the cell.

Genetic abnormalities can produce a wide variety of disease entities. They are discussed with injuries to DNA in Chapter 8.

Biologic agents also may injure cells in a number of ways. The agents involved include viruses, bacteria, protozoa, fungi, and even algae. Viruses, for instance, can alter the metabolism of host cells, bacteria can elaborate toxins (*see* Chapter 7), and a number of these agents can cause cell injury mediated by the actions of the host's own immune response. The ways in which the immune response can cause cell injury are discussed in Chapters 5 and 7, but we can point out here that the mechanism usually involves damage to the cell membrane or hypoxia associated with vascular injury. The binding and activation of complement, for instance, punches tiny "holes" in the plasma membrane of the target cell. The target cells may be bacteria, other organisms, or infected or otherwise abnormal host cells.

Malnutrition is a major cause of cell injury in many species. Deficiencies of protein, carbohydrate, or vitamins result in abnormal metabolic and synthetic processes. Overnutrition also can result in injury.

Because, as we have emphasized, membrane damage or interference with energy metabolism represent the major pathways of cell injury, they have been studied in some detail. Interference with energy metabolism has been most commonly studied using anoxic cell injury

produced by ischemia. In the case of membrane injury, models using chemical toxins have been used, one of the best characterized of which is injury to the liver by carbon tetrachloride. In the following section, the information obtained from these studies is discussed, with emphasis on the correlation of structural and functional changes.

Hypoxic Cell Injury

Injury due to hypoxia, in particular that associated with ischemia, is possibly the single most common cause of cell injury. Tissue cells vary in their susceptibility to hypoxia. Some can withstand relatively long periods of hypoxia without permanent injury, but others are lethally injured by brief periods of oxygen deprivation. In part, this is dependent on the capability of cells to utilize anaerobic glycolysis as a source of energy. Glycolysis, however, is a relatively inefficient mechanism of energy production compared to oxidative phosphorylation, and it generates lactic acid, which, as we will see, can contribute to cell injury. Interference with the major energy supply of the cell has, of course, many functional consequences, and many biologic processes fail. These vary in importance in terms of their contribution to cell injury. Here we will pay most attention to those which are significant in this regard.

SEQUENCE OF CHANGES IN THE INJURED CELL. During the progression of cell injury, alterations occur in many of the organelles. While changes are occurring in the mitochondria, for instance, alterations also are occurring in the endoplasmic reticulum, the nucleus, the cytosol, and the plasma membrane. Some changes, however, are characteristic of early cell injury and others of the later stages.

In the cell deprived of oxygen there is rapid, severe impairment of oxidative phosphorylation. As a result, intracellular levels of ATP quickly fall and the

ADP:ATP ratio increases. As ATP is utilized and depleted there is a concomitant rise in inorganic phosphate. This activates anaerobic glycolysis as an alternative source of energy. Therefore, an early morphologic manifestation of cell injury is depletion of glycogen. Associated with this, there is a fall in intracellular pH, which in turn leads to clumping of nuclear chromatin. These changes occur within 15 min of the initiation of hypoxia.

By about 15 min, early changes appear in the mitochondria. There is loss of mitochondrial matrix granules, and the mitochondria begin to undergo conformational changes known as **low-amplitude swelling.** Such mitochondria have a condensed or contracted inner compartment and a relatively expanded outer compartment.

Between 15 and 30 min there is distortion of the outline of the plasma membrane with loss of specialized structures such as microvilli. The mitochondria continue to show low-amplitude swelling at this stage. At the same time, dilatation of the endoplasmic reticulum becomes apparent.

Between 30 min and 1 h there is disaggregation and detachment of polyribosomes from the surface of the RER, the cytosol becomes pallid, and the cell swells. At the same time the mitochondria begin to swell. This change, called **high-amplitude swelling,** is characterized by distension of the inner mitochondrial compartment. Dense amorphous deposits may begin to appear in the mitochondria.

From 2 to 4 h after the onset of anoxia, the mitochondria continue to swell and may be dramatically increased in volume. There are increased numbers of flocculent densities in the matrix, and breaks in the outer mitochondrial membrane may occur. Swelling of the endoplasmic reticulum continues, and it becomes fragmented. Breaks in the plasma membrane can occur. By this stage, the nuclear chromatin is more severely clumped, and early karyolysis becomes evident.

From this time on the changes continue to become more severe. Organelle membranes fragment, chromatin undergoes lysis (karyolysis), and myelin figures derived from membrane components appear in the altered cytoplasm. During the later stages of cell injury lysosomes swell, release enzymes into the cytosol, and the process of autolysis begins. Soon the cell is recognizable in the light microscope as being necrotic.

The changes described above are those seen in cells subjected experimentally to sudden, complete anoxia. In real life, of course, the severity of the insult may vary and the changes in the cell may be modified by local environmental conditions. The rate of progression of changes seen in individual cases therefore also varies. The general progression of acute lethal cell injury is, however, as we have described and is summarized in Figure 2.28.

MITOCHONDRIA IN CELL INJURY. Changes in mitochondrial structure and function are early indicators of hypoxic cell injury. Many of these changes are a direct consequence of altered mitochondrial function. The mitochondria themselves require ATP to continue to work. However, it is known that isolated mitochondria can withstand anoxia without permanent injury for longer periods than can those subjected to anoxia *in vivo*. The accelerated changes that occur in mitochondria *in vivo* are probably partly the result of altered intracellular environmental conditions such as decreased pH and changes in ion concentrations, particularly calcium ions.

Initially mitochondria undergo low-amplitude volume changes (Fig. 2.29). This reaction is reversible and is essentially a physiologic adaptation to altered levels of ADP and ATP in the cell. When the ADP:ATP ratio is increased, the mitochondria adopt this conformation. How-

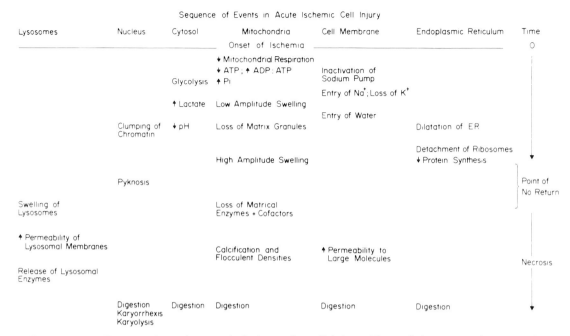

Sequence of Events in Acute Ischemic Cell Injury

Lysosomes	Nucleus	Cytosol	Mitochondria	Cell Membrane	Endoplasmic Reticulum	Time
			Onset of Ischemia			0
			↓ Mitochondrial Respiration			
			↓ ATP ; ↑ ADP : ATP	Inactivation of Sodium Pump		
		Glycolysis	↑ Pi			
				Entry of Na⁺; Loss of K⁺		
		↑ Lactate	Low Amplitude Swelling			
				Entry of Water		
	Clumping of Chromatin	↓ pH	Loss of Matrix Granules		Dilatation of ER	
					Detachment of Ribosomes	
			High Amplitude Swelling		↓ Protein Synthesis	↓
	Pyknosis					Point of No Return
Swelling of Lysosomes			Loss of Matrical Enzymes + Cofactors			
↑ Permeability of Lysosomal Membranes						
			Calcification and Flocculent Densities	↑ Permeability to Large Molecules		Necrosis
Release of Lysosomal Enzymes						
	Digestion Karyorrhexis Karyolysis	Digestion	Digestion	Digestion	Digestion	↓

Figure 2.28. Progression of acute lethal anoxic cell injury. The cellular events that occur in injured cells are arranged here so that their temporal sequences and relationships to one another can be appreciated.

ever, mitochondrial contraction depends on some ATP being present. When ATP is no longer available, the mitochondria begin to undergo high-amplitude swelling (Figs. 2.17 and 2.29). This appears to be associated with damage to the inner mitochondrial membrane. Some ATP apparently is required to maintain the integrity of this membrane. Changes that occur include the loss of the F_1 particles, thought to be the morphological correlate of magnesium-activated ATPase. These changes are associated with a loss of potassium and magnesium ions by the mitochondria and an increase in sodium and calcium ions. Increased membrane permeability and uptake of water account for the swelling that occurs.

Up to this point cell injury is usually still reversible. That is, cells containing significant numbers of mitochondria with early high-amplitude swelling still can recover if a source of oxygen is restored.

In the mitochondria themselves, however, some functions may be lost while others are intact. In other words, the various functional systems in the mitochondria show a variable susceptibility to injury. Pyruvate kinase and α-ketoglutarate dehydrogenase, for example, are matrix enzymes, which are drastically reduced in activity as an early event in mitochondrial injury. Oxidative phosphorylation also is greatly reduced early in the process. In contrast, succinate dehydrogenase, a tightly membrane bound enzyme system, and the electron transport system are much more stable and persist even after the cell is irreversibly injured.

The susceptibility of matrix enzymes to early injury probably is due to their loss, together with cofactors such as NADH, by diffusion from the mitochondria. Thus, as the capacity for oxidative phosphorylation is lost, the inner mitochondrial membrane is altered, ion and water shifts

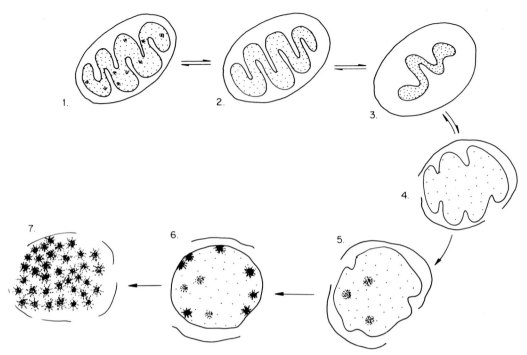

Figure 2.29. Progression of mitochondrial injury. When cells are subjected to sudden anoxic injury, the mitochondria undergo a change from normal conformation *(1)* to the contracted conformation *(3)*. This change is called low-amplitude swelling. More or less at the same time, the mitochondrial dense granules disappear *(2)*. With progression the mitochondria undergo high-amplitude swelling *(4)* and defects in the outer membrane may appear. Up to this point, and even when high-amplitude swelling has begun, the changes are reversible. As the injury progresses, the mitochondria continue to swell, and develop matrical flocculent deposits *(5)* and changes in the inner mitochondrial membrane. Such changes are associated with loss of reversibility. Under some conditions the injured mitochondria may become calcified *(6, 7)*.

occur, and enzymes and their substrates and cofactors are lost as the mitochondria swell. *In vitro* studies have confirmed that mitochondria that undergo swelling do lose components from the matrix. Presumably, when these changes become severe enough, mitochondrial function cannot be restored even if a supply of oxygen is reestablished, but there are more important factors involved in the failure of mitochondria to recover from injury, as discussed below.

As high-amplitude swelling progresses the matrix granules disappear, the matrix takes on a clarified appearance, and dense amorphous deposits of denatured proteins and lipoproteins form, corre-

sponding to the flocculent densities described above. As already mentioned, calcium ions enter the injured mitochondria, and under some conditions enough enter for the deposition of insoluble calcium salts to occur. This is most striking when the flow of blood to the injured tissue is at least partly preserved or when it is restored after a period of ischemia.

CELL MEMBRANE IN CELL INJURY. Alterations of the plasma membrane are amongst the earliest changes to occur in the hypoxic cell. These are manifested morphologically as blebbing and loss of specialized structures. Such distortions may reflect abnormal cytoskeletal function as much as alterations in the plasma membrane, as cytoskeletal components are dynamic and sensitive to changes in ion concentrations, especially calcium.

One of the fundamental properties of the cell membrane is the maintenance of ion and water homeostasis in the cell, and through these processes the maintenance of cell volume. The sodium pump is an energy-dependent system located in the plasma membrane, which is responsible for the active transport of sodium ions out of, and potassium ions into, the cell.

An early manifestation of hypoxia in the cell is the failure of this ion pump to operate. When this happens the ions in the cytoplasm and in the extracellular fluid attempt to reach Gibbs-Donnan equilibrium. In other words, ions attempt to reach an equilibrium where the product of the ionic strengths inside and outside the cell (*i.e.*, on either side of a semipermeable membrane) are equal. The net result is that sodium ions enter the cell, potassium ions leak out, each moving along a concentration gradient, and the cell swells. The cell also tends to lose magnesium and accumulate calcium ions. Similar ion fluxes occur between compartments in the cell, such as between the endoplasmic reticulum or the mitochondria and the cytoplasm.

At first it may not be clear why such free diffusion of ions into and out of the cell should cause the cell to swell. To understand this we must temporarily divert our attention to the way in which the sodium pump regulates cell volume. The basic problem is this: how can sodium chloride contribute to the osmotic effect that is responsible for maintaining cell volume if the cell membrane is freely permeable to it? The answer is that the colloid osmotic pressure of the protein molecules inside the cell is the critical element in this equilibrium. Protein is in higher concentration inside the cell than outside, and therefore there is a net positive colloid osmotic pressure inside the

cell. To balance this, some osmotically active particles must be maintained in relative excess outside the cell. In a passive situation freely permeable ions could not accomplish this, but the sodium pump is able to maintain a high concentration of sodium ions outside the cell and a low concentration inside. In other words, as long as the sodium pump is working, sodium ions function as a nondiffusible external cation that balances the effect of the truly nondiffusible protein molecules inside the cell. When the pump stops, sodium ions enter the cell (accompanied by chloride), moving along their electrochemical gradient. This increases the internal osmotic pressure relative to the outside and draws water into the cell.

The rate of loss of potassium ions may initially exceed that of sodium loss, and the cell may transiently shrink. However, entry of sodium ions into the cell soon exceeds the loss of potassium, and the cell swells. This again is exacerbated by the relatively high intracellular colloid osmotic pressure. As water is drawn into the cell, intracellular potassium is diluted, moving it closer to equilibrium with the outside. Intracellular sodium also is diluted, but this moves it away from equilibrium with the outside and favors further entry of sodium ions. Therefore, the driving force for cell swelling is, in fact, the gradient of colloid osmotic pressure which exists across the cell membrane. At least initially, the water that enters the cell is not distributed uniformly throughout the cytoplasm. Most of it seems to enter the cisternae of the endoplasmic reticulum producing the vacuolated appearance typical of cell injury at the light microscopic level.

The rate and degree of cellular swelling depend on a number of factors, including the relative permeability of the plasma membrane to the major ions, sodium and potassium, the availability of extracellular water, the degree of hypoxia, and constraining viscoelastic forces provided by the supporting connective tissues. In complete ischemia there may be relatively little extracellular water available to be taken up by the cell, thus limiting swelling. The most explosive swelling usually is seen in ischemic tissue in which the blood flow is restored.

As the cell swells and injury progresses, physical damage to the cell membrane occurs, resulting in a true increase in its permeability. This serves only to exacerbate the process. Furthermore, the accumulation of cellular metabolites may also contribute to the osmotic pressure inside the cell, and thus to swelling. If such products accumulate during complete ischemia, they may contribute to the dramatic swelling that follows restoration of blood flow.

Eventually, the membrane becomes permeable to even large molecules, and enzymes and other proteins can leak out of (or into) the cell. This change forms the basis for dye exclusion tests as a means of determining cell viability. When severely injured cells are incubated in solutions of dyes such as trypan blue, their damaged cell membranes are permeable to the dye, and the cell is stained. Viable cells do not take up the dye and therefore are not stained. In this way, severely injured or dead cells can be distinguished from live cells.

Although cell swelling undoubtedly is a dependable marker for cell injury, its role in contributing to the death of the cell is less certain. Cell death can occur in the absence of appreciable cell swelling, depending on the factors already mentioned, and dramatic swelling can occur in reversibly injured cells. However, it is quite clear that prevention of cellular swelling can contribute to the survival of injured cells. This has been demonstrated both *in vivo* and *in vitro,* usually using mannitol as a nonpermeable solute in the extracellular fluid. Even in cultured cells subjected to injury the prevention of cell swelling reduces the incidence of cell death.

This may be attributable to a reduction in the distortion of the plasma membrane associated with swelling. On the other hand, mannitol is a known scavenger of the hydroxyl radical, and its action in alleviating cell swelling and cell death may be due instead to prevention of lipid peroxidation in ischemic cells, as discussed below. Whatever the mode of action, this principle is sometimes applied clinically in the intravenous administration of impermeant solutes such as mannitol to protect against cellular and tissue swelling.

The changes in ion permeability just described have profound effects on the function of excitable cells such as nerves, skeletal muscle cells, and myocardial cells. In the case of anoxic myocardial cell injury (a common enough event, especially in man), the injury can be detected by use of the electrocardiogram (Fig. 2.30). The changes that occur are a reflection of the altered electrophysiological functions associated with ionic shifts in these cells. In addition, products of abnormal lipid metabolism have been shown to be important in alterations of the electrophysiological function of the ischemic heart.

ENDOPLASMIC RETICULUM IN CELL INJURY. The endoplasmic reticulum undergoes dilatation (Fig. 2.18) and fragmentation early in the progression of acute lethal injury due to anoxia. In fact the ER seems to act as a reservoir for much of the water initially taken up by the injured cell. Dilatation of the ER is associated with the movement of both water and sodium ions across the membrane into the cisternal lumen. Associated with dilatation of the ER, there is disaggregation and detachment of ribosomes from the surface of the RER. Early in the course of anoxic cell injury, ribosomes are lost but apparently retain their membrane-binding capacity, as the defect can be repaired by the addition of certain artificial polymers. Later this is not possible, suggesting that, besides initial damage to

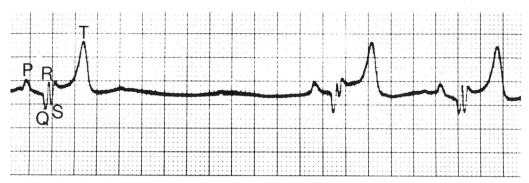

Figure 2.30. Electrocardiographic changes in hypoxic myocardial injury. This lead II EKG is from a dog with aortic stenosis. There is elevation of the *ST* segment and an abnormally large T wave. The configuration of the *QRS* complex is abnormal suggesting a conductive disturbance. (Paper speed = 50 mm/sec, 1 cm = 1 mV; EKG Courtesy of the late Dr. Gary Bolton.)

the membranes of the ER, later changes in ribosomal proteins and nucleic acids take place. At any rate, as a consequence of ribosomal loss, protein synthesis is impaired. This can have important effects on the cell, typified by the development of fatty change, the pathogenesis of which is discussed later in this chapter.

LYSOSOMES IN CELL INJURY. Lysosomes contain a variety of potent hydrolytic enzymes that are capable of digesting essentially all components in the cytoplasm of the cell. It has long been argued, therefore, that the release of enzymes from damaged lysosomes in injured cells could be important in the pathogenesis of cell injury and might in fact be responsible for cell death. This concept of self-digestion is known as the "suicide bag" hypothesis. Its validity has been vigorously debated over the years, but there is surprisingly little direct evidence that the intracellular release of lysosomal enzymes plays a direct role in causing or exacerbating cell injury.

Without doubt lysosomes, like other cell organelles, undergo swelling in injured cells. This is presumed to be due to abnormal fluxes of ions and water and usually occurs before cell injury becomes irreversible. In addition, there is evidence that substrates normally excluded from the lysosome can enter it early in the process of cell injury. The problem remains, however, to demonstrate **leakage of enzymes** from the lysosome into the cytosol before cell injury becomes irreversible. One approach to this has been to sediment lysosomes from homogenates of injured cells in order to determine if lysosomal enzymes are present in the supernatant. If they were, one might assume that they had been released from lysosomes in the injured cells. In fact, such super-natants often do contain lysosomal enzymes, but currently it is believed that these reflect increased fragility of the isolated lysosomes rather than release of enzymes *in vivo*. This is in contrast to the situation with phagocytic cells such as the neutrophil and the macrophage in which lysosomal enzymes can be released to the exterior from living cells as a secretory event (*see* Chapter 4).

Against the suicide bag hypothesis are the following observations: (1) In injured cells ultrastructural changes occur earlier in organelles such as mitochondria and the endoplasmic reticulum than in lysosomes. (2) If release of lysosomal enzymes were important, we might expect that changes in the cytoplasm and its organelles would be more severe near lysosomes. This cannot be demonstrated. (3) If lysosomes are labeled with a phagocytosed marker, such as ferritin, and the cell then is injured, release of the marker occurs late in the progression of injury.

On the other hand there is some evidence that lysosomes can be injured as a primary event, and that this does result in cell injury and cell death. If cells are allowed to phagocytose silica or sodium urate crystals, for example, the crystals enter lysosomes and directly damage them. Crystals can be seen free in the cytoplasm during the early stages of cell injury, and the treated cells die soon after. If phagocytosis is prevented the exposed cell is not injured, suggesting that the injury is due to lysosomal damage rather than a direct effect on the plasma membrane.

In conclusion, therefore, we cannot altogether rule out a role for release of lysosomal enzymes into the cytosol. It may be important in some forms of cell injury, and there is evidence that this may be so in some viral infections and in diseases involving abnormal copper metabolism, as discussed later. However, the overall evidence indicates that in most forms of cell injury, including hypoxia, the release of lysosomal enzymes is a relatively late event and apparently plays no part in causing cell injury. Lysosomal enzymes are eventually released, however, and, after cell death has occurred, they play an important role in producing the changes that characterize necrosis.

OTHER ORGANELLES IN CELL INJURY. As we have already mentioned, injured cells initially may show abnormal cell motility, formation of surface blebs and distortion of microvilli and other surface specializations. The basis of these changes is not well defined, but they may reflect altered function of the cytoskeleton associated with impaired energy metabolism, changes in concentration of calcium and other ions, and changes in pH.

In the cytosol, glycogen is depleted and myelin figures may appear. The latter are thought to be derived from components of damaged cell membranes. In particular, phospholipids "leached" from membranes may spontaneously reaggregate, forming the laminar arrays that characterize myelin figures.

From our discussions so far, it is becoming clear that cell injury due to ischemia or anoxia revolves around damage to cellular membranes. There is mounting evidence that, paradoxically, a good deal of this damage is caused by reactive metabolites derived from oxygen itself. These products are free radicals and are discussed in more detail below. For now, suffice it to say that they can cause extensive damage to many cellular systems, amongst which membranes are prominent. This leads us to a discussion of membrane injury, free radicals, and lipid peroxidation. Finally, we will discuss an overall concept of cell injury involving hypoxia, free radicals, membrane injury, and calcium ions.

Cell Injury Due to Membrane Damage

Direct damage to cell membranes, both the plasma membrane and those of organelles, is the second major pathway through which cell injury can occur. In fact we will argue later that, in the final analysis, anoxic injury is itself mediated through alteration of cell membranes. The concept has emerged that there is a final common pathway through which cell injury occurs, regardless of its cause. Thus, it is not surprising to find that, regardless of cause, injured cells express very similar morphologic and functional alterations. Despite the similarities, however, there are some differences in the morphologic expression of cell injury due to membrane damage and that due to hypoxia. Here we will consider the changes seen in cells injured by damage to their membranes, stressing those lesions that are characteristic of this type of injury.

CAUSES OF MEMBRANE INJURY. A great variety of agents cause injury to cells by damaging their membranes. They include irradiation, many chemical toxins and drugs, bacterial toxins such as the phospholipases produced by some species of *Clostridia* (*see* Chapter 7), and complement (an important immune and inflammatory effector mechanism; *see* Chapters 4 and 5). In addition, some nutritional deficiencies, in particular deficiency of vitamin E or selenium, cause call damage by increasing cellular susceptibility to membrane damage. Hepatocellular necrosis due to intoxication by the solvent carbon tetrachloride (CCl_4) is one example of this type of injury, which has been studied widely. We will use this model as a basis for our discussion of injury to cell membranes, not because it is commonly encountered, but because it is well characterized.

MECHANISMS OF MEMBRANE INJURY.   Toxic agents injure membranes in various ways, commonly by direct interaction with them or by the formation of free radicals that cause peroxidation of membrane lipids. Mercuric chloride, for instance, is able to combine directly with sulfhydryl groups in the cell membranes, whereas CCl_4 acts through membrane peroxidation. Regardless of the exact mechanism involved, the end result is increased membrane permeability and loss of specialized membrane functions.

Carbon tetrachloride toxicity is a classic example of the way in which the metabolic activity of the host can produce intermediates that are the ultimate toxic agents. Carbon tetrachloride is metabolized by the mixed-function oxidase enzyme system in the liver. During this process the free radicals $CCl_3\cdot$ and $Cl\cdot$ are produced. As pointed out earlier in this chapter, this enzyme complex is found in the SER. It can undergo dramatic hypertrophy as an adaptive response to repeated exposure to drugs metabolized by this system. Thus, an animal that has been treated with primidone, for instance, would have hypertrophied SER and would be expected to metabolize CCl_4 more rapidly than usual. It would therefore produce greater concentrations of toxic metabolites of CCl_4 and so enhance its toxicity. Because so many substances are metabolized by the mixed-function oxidase system, there is considerable potential for this sort of enhancement of toxicity. Another example worth mentioning, and one of more specific interest in clinical medicine, is intoxication by acetaminophen. This commonly used antipyretic and analegsic drug is also metabolized by the mixed-function oxidase system. It, too, generates toxic intermediates that, if present in high enough concentrations, can cause lethal hepatocellular injury. Obviously, patients who have been taking drugs that can induce hypertrophy of the SER will be unusually susceptible to these toxic effects. The drugs whose toxic effects can be enhanced in this way are too numerous to list here, but these observations should leave the prospective clinician with a healthy respect for the potential effects of drug interactions. Because the liver is a major site of chemical modification of drugs and toxins, it is peculiarly susceptible to drug- and toxin-induced injury. This should not be surprising if the concept of metabolic activation of toxins is considered.

FREE RADICALS, LIPID PEROXIDATION, AND MEMBRANE INJURY.   The generation of free radicals is a fairly common mechanism of cell damage, and many toxic chemicals and drugs act this way. The toxicity of high concentrations of oxygen to alveolar pneumocytes probably is due to free radical formation, and some forms of ionizing radiation may cause injury through the formation of the radicals $H\cdot$ and $OH\cdot$ from the water in tissues and cells.

There are many sources of free radicals in the cellular environment. The most biologically important free radicals, however, arise as a consequence of cellular metabolism. They are derived from cellular oxidation-reduction reactions involving enzymes such as xanthine oxidase, aldehyde oxidase, flavine dehydrogenases, and peroxidases, or nonenzymatic reactions such as autooxidation reactions and "leakage" from the mitochondrial electron transport system. Cellular sources of free radicals are summarized in Figure 2.31.

Important reactants in this context include superoxide anion (O_2^-), hydroxyl radical ($\cdot OH$), and hydrogen peroxide (H_2O_2). Hydrogen peroxide itself is not a free radical, but it can generate hydroxyl radicals through reaction with ferrous or cupric ions, or by reaction with superoxide anion. The latter reaction is catalyzed by trace amounts of iron.

Free radicals, particularly the hydroxyl radical, are substances that have unpaired electrons and are therefore generally highly reactive. Because of this, most exist only briefly and in low concentrations, and do not travel far from the site at which they are formed. Thus the initial reaction of a free radical in a biologic system will be close to its site of formation. However, free radical chain reactions, such as lipid peroxidation, and the action of products of free radical reactions can produce cellular damage at some distance to the initial event. Free radicals are able to combine with unsaturated lipids in cell membranes, resulting in the formation of organic free radicals (lipid radicals). These in turn rearrange and combine with oxygen to form lipid hydroperoxyl radicals, which then undergo further reaction to form another lipid radical and lipid peroxides, the whole process being called **lipid peroxidation.** The peroxides formed in this reaction are un-

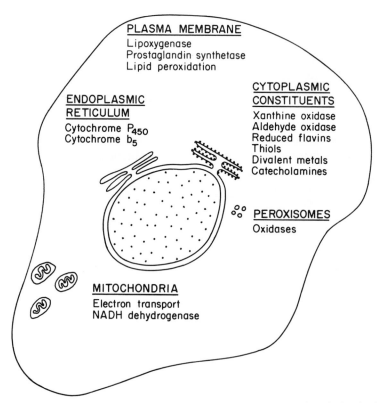

Figure 2.31. Cellular sources of free radicals. Free radicals can be derived *via* a number of cellular metabolic functions.

stable and break down to produce aldehydes (including malondialdehyde) and other compounds as well as generating additional organic free radicals. This reaction, once started, is self-propagating, and limited interaction with the initiating free radicals can led to rapid widespread membrane damage.

Associated with free radical reactions and lipid peroxidation there may be damage to DNA, enzymes, and structural proteins. Chemical changes can occur in amino acids, polypeptide chains can be cleaved, and, in particular, polymerization of protein molecules can occur. The product of lipid peroxidation responsible for the cross-linking that produces protein polymerization is thought to be malondialdehyde. Proteins containing sulfhydryl groups are more susceptible to damage by lipid peroxidation than others. Clearly the damage produced by lipid peroxidation can result in loss of function of enzymes and other proteins in cell membranes and can be devastating for the cell.

The major site of damage caused by lipid peroxidation is in membranes, especially those of subcellular organelles. The membranes of organelles, in particular those of mitochondria and endoplasmic reticulum, contain relatively high levels of unsaturated fatty acids, making them very susceptible to lipid peroxidation. In addition, certain metals such as copper and iron, including iron-containing proteins, can act as catalysts for peroxidation reactions. In the mitochondria, therefore, the presence of cytochromes further enhances their susceptibility to damage by lipid peroxidation.

The membranes of lysosomes, in contrast, are relatively resistant to peroxidation, a consequence of their relatively low content of unsaturated fatty acids. As in hypoxia, lysosomal damage probably is a relatively late event in cell injury due to membrane damage associated with lipid peroxidation. In one special case, however, lysosomal damage may be an important factor in causing cell injury. In Wilson's disease in man and in a similar disease in certain breeds of dogs, there is abnormal copper metabolism and storage of large amounts of copper in hepatocellular lysosomes. In these cases it is thought that the ability of copper to catalyze lipid peroxidation may cause primary lysosomal damage with release of enzymes and injury to the cell. This may be important in the pathogenesis of the extensive hepatocellular necrosis that occurs in these diseases. Massive liver necrosis also is common in chronic copper poisoning, another condition in which there is storage of copper in hepatocytes.

The consequence of all this membrane damage is, of course, abnormal membrane function. Most importantly, protein synthesis is disturbed due to damage to the RER, membrane permeability is disrupted, both in the plasma membrane and in organelles, and abnormal ion fluxes similar to those described in anoxic cell injury occur. Mitochondrial respiration is impaired due to membrane damage and an influx of calcium ions. Mitochondria provide an interesting example of a structure-linked enzyme activity, namely oxidative phosphorylation. This is a closely membrane-associated system, and it has been shown that lipid peroxidation inhibits the coupling of phosphorylation to oxidation. The morphologic and functional manifestations are enlarged upon below.

It would not be fair to leave our discussion of membrane damage induced by free radicals without mentioning the mechanisms the cell has available to protect itself. In fact, the very presence of these defense mechanisms is evidence of the prevalence of free radical–generating reactions in biological systems. Important amongst these defenses are superoxide dismutases, which catalyze the conversion of superoxide anion to hydrogen peroxide, catalases, which break down hydrogen peroxide, and "endogenous antioxidants" such as vitamin E, glutathione, and ascorbate. Vitamin E, a lipid-soluble antioxidant that partitions into cellular membranes, and ascorbate, an aqueous-phase antioxidant, appear to be able to inactivate free radicals and prevent lipid peroxidation of membranes. Glutathione, in its reduced form (GSH), reacts with hydrogen peroxide to form oxidized glutathione (GSSG). This reaction is catalyzed by the selenium-containing enzyme glutathione peroxidase. This enzyme also catalyzes the reduction of lipid peroxides by glutathione, thus preventing the propagation of lipid peroxidation reactions. Vitamin E and selenium can reduce the toxicity of some substances that act through free radical formation. Deficiency of either vitamin E or selenium or both is an important nutritional cause of disease in pigs, cattle, sheep, chickens, and other animals. In all of these species, cell necrosis is a prominent feature of the disease. Presumably deficiency of vitamin E and selenium makes cell membranes unusually susceptible to free radical injury and lipid peroxidation, which in turn results in cell injury.

It should also be added that the consequences of free radical generation are not all bad. In particular, their damaging effects have been very effectively exploited by phagocytic leukocytes as mechanisms for killing microorganisms. This phenomenon is thought to be mediated by superoxide and other radicals, and is discussed in more detail in Chapters 4 and 7.

ROLE OF FREE RADICALS IN ANOXIC CELL INJURY. Although it might seem rather paradoxical, a large body of evidence now suggests that a significant amount of the damage occurring during ischemia or anoxia is mediated by oxygen-derived free radicals. Most of this evidence comes from experimental models in which myocardial or intestinal ischemia is induced, often followed by reperfusion or reoxygenation. It is clear from a number of studies that the reestablishment of perfusion in ischemic tissue is followed by an exacerbation of cell injury. In the myocardium this is accompanied by the development of cell swelling and contraction bands. The concept has developed that a transient period of ischemia causes the death of some cells. Others are "at risk" due to metabolic changes, but not yet dead and are, in fact, potentially able to be rescued. Reperfusion can rapidly induce cell death in a proportion of these cells. This phenomenon has been termed **reperfusion injury,** and the generation of oxygen-derived free radicals seems to be important in this setting.

The evidence for the involvement of oxygen-derived free radicals is both direct and indirect. A number of studies in various species have shown that scavengers of these radicals, such as superoxide dismutase and catalase, can reduce infarct size. It has also been shown that a sudden increase in free radical production and the formation of by-products of lipid peroxidation accompany ischemia and reperfusion. A number of potential sources of these radicals has been proposed, including the metabolism of catecholamines by monoamine oxidase, the "leakage" of oxygen free radicals from mitochondria, arachidonic acid metabolism, the action of the enzyme **xanthine oxidase** on hypoxanthine, and generation by leukocytes (primarily neutrophils and macrophages) that infiltrate the ischemic lesion.

Xanthine oxidase is a potentially important source of oxygen-derived free radicals. The enzyme does not exist as such in normal tissues, but is derived by sulfhydryl oxidation or limited proteolysis of xanthine dehydrogenase. It is hypothesized that activation of proteases by increased cytosolic calcium levels in ischemic cells leads to the conversion to the oxidase form of the enzyme. Evidence for this is that the reaction is irreversible, it occurs in the calcium paradox, and it can be inhibited by soybean trypsin inhibitor. This conversion can occur after only brief periods of ischemia. At the same time its substrate, hypoxanthine, is generated by the degradation of ATP. In the presence of molecular oxygen, xanthine oxidase acts on hypoxanthine to produce urate and superoxide anion (O_2^-). These interactions are summarized schematically in Figure 2.32. It has been shown in a number of experimental models of myocardial or intestinal ischemia that infarction can be limited by treatment with allopurinol, an inhibitor of xanthine oxidase. Additionally, the level of the xanthine oxidase form of the enzyme in ischemic myocardium has been shown to be about three times that of the normal tissue.

There is, therefore, clear evidence for a role of xanthine oxidase in generating free radicals in ischemic tissue. However, this appears to be limited to certain species. For example, the enzyme, in either form, has been demonstrated in tissues of dogs, cats, rats, and bovines, but it is absent from those of humans and rabbits. In experimental myocardial ischemia in the rabbit, free radical inhibitors such as SDO and catalase reduce infarct size, while allopurinol does not. Furthermore, allo-purinol plus SDO is more effective than allopurinol alone in those species that do have the enzyme, suggesting that additional sources of oxygen free radicals are important.

Infiltrating leukocytes are a second potentially important source of oxygen-derived free radicals in ischemic and reperfused tissue. As discussed in chapter 4, macrophages and neutrophils, in particular the latter, generate abundant amounts of superoxide anion during phagocytosis. It has been shown that factors chemotactic for neutrophils, including cleavage products of complement, are generated in ischemic myocardial tissue, and there is a correlation between infarct size and the degree of neutrophil infiltration. Furthermore, depletion of neutrophils by antiserum to cobra venom can reduce infarct size. Finally, drugs that inhibit the generation of superoxide by neutrophils have a similar effect.

FUNCTIONAL AND MORPHOLOGIC CONSEQUENCES OF CELL MEMBRANE INJURY. Not surprisingly, because both mechanisms of cell injury eventually pro-

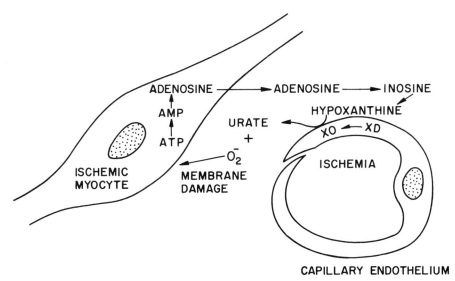

Figure 2.32. Generation of superoxide radical by xanthine oxidase. Xanthine oxidase derived from xanthine dehydrogenase in endothelial cells acts on hypoxanthine to generate oxygen-derived free radicals.

duce membrane alterations, the morphologic and functional changes that accompany cell injury due to membrane damage do not differ substantially from those due to anoxic cell injury. There are some differences, which reflect differences in the most susceptible organelles in each case. The differences will be stressed here rather than repeating the general features of cell injury already discussed.

The earliest changes detectable in hepatocytes injured with CCl_4 are found in the RER. They consist of disaggregation and detachment of polysomes, presumably due to lipid peroxidation of the membranes of the ER. There is evidence, however, that CCl_4 can also interfere directly with the interaction between ribosomes and mRNA.

Soon after this, there is disturbance of ion and water homeostasis, which is expressed first as dilatation of the cisternae of the RER and eventually as cell swelling. Again there is an influx of sodium ions and a loss of potassium. There also is an influx of calcium ions at about this time, which occurs rapidly in this form of injury due to the free access of calcium ions from the blood. As is the case in anoxic cell injury, calcium ions, being potent uncouplers of mitochondrial respiration, damage mitochondria and exacerbate the effects on the cell. The alterations in sodium ion transport which occur are correlated closely with reduced intracellular levels of ATP. This occurs *before* any ultrastructural evidence of damage to mitochondria appears and while oxidative phosphorylation is still intact. Thus, it may represent increased utilization or destruction of ATP rather than reduced production. *In vitro,* CCl_4 can enhance the activity of mitochondrial magnesium-activated ATPase, which might support this contention.

Because disaggregation of polysomes and their detachment from the RER occurs early in CCl_4 poisoning, reduction of protein synthesis can be detected within a few hours of onset of the injury. One consequence of this in the liver is a reduction in the availability of lipid carrier protein, normally synthesized in hepatocytes. This protein is necessary for the export of triglycerides from the liver. Thus, lipids accumulate in hepatocytes injured in this way, and fatty change is a characteristic of CCl_4 toxicity, although it certainly is not specific for it.

All of the changes described above for CCl_4 intoxication are probably primarily the result of lipid peroxidation with subsequent membrane dysfunction. The features that distinguish this form of injury from anoxic cell injury are the early involvement of the RER and the relatively late involvement of the mitochondria. Once these initial changes have occurred, however, cell injury progresses in a manner analogous to that occurring in anoxia. Once again, the critical event determining loss of reversibility is not clear. Certainly neither the reduction in protein synthesis nor the increase in triglycerides kills the cell. Presumably, irreparable membrane damage caused by the agent, coupled with the resultant interference with energy production, is responsible.

Reversibility and Irreversibility

As cell injury progresses to its later stages the changes in the various organelles remain qualitatively similar but become more severe. Eventually organelles break down, cytoplasmic proteins are denatured, and the organelles of the necrotic cell may be barely recognizable at the ultrastructural level. Without doubt such cells are dead, but what is the critical change in the cell which determines that injury is irreversible? To answer that question honestly we must say: nobody really knows. However, we can at least rule out some of the phenomena that we have discussed, and suggest that others might be important.

Changes in the structure and function of the nucleus are probably not of primary importance. Certainly we know that erythrocytes live for over 100 days without a nucleus. Similarly, loss of the ability to synthesize protein due to injury to the nucleus and RER is not critical. Agents that specifically block protein synthesis, for instance, do not cause immediate cell death. Similarly, inhibition of anaerobic glycolysis does not prevent cell death. Reduced intracellular pH, therefore, is apparently not the critical change that we are looking for.

In anoxic cells, despite the importance of adequate supplies of ATP to the cell, reduction of cellular ATP is, in itself, unlikely to be the sole event that results in irreversibility of cell injury. If restored in time, transient reduction in ATP levels does not kill the cell, although prolonged reduction does. In addition, metabolic poisons that interfere with mitochondrial synthesis of ATP can produce low levels of ATP in the cell, similar to those found in anoxia, but they do not produce a comparable degree of necrosis. The important change, therefore, is likely to be some immediate consequence of sufficiently prolonged reduction in intracellular energy levels. Some change occurs which apparently cannot be repaired. One event very likely to be of prime importance in precipitating cell death is irreversible damage to mitochondria such that they cannot regenerate ATP. Such damage is associated with all of the changes described above, and we know that after a certain period of anoxia, and in the usual cellular milieu, the mitochondria are unable to resume the production of energy even when oxygen again becomes available. As a result none of the energy-dependent functions of the cell can be reestablished. Thus, it has been argued that anoxic cells die because a point is reached when the mitochondria are irreversibly damaged. It is presumably for this reason that severe ultrastructural changes in mitochondria correlate best with the onset of irreversible injury.

ROLE OF CALCIUM IN CELL INJURY. In recent years evidence has accumulated which suggests that this view of cell death is too simple an interpretation, and attention has been focused on the role of calcium ions in injured cells. As we have already pointed out, an increase in intracellular calcium ions is a consistent feature of necrosis, and necrotic cells may even contain deposits of calcium salts. This is due to redistribution from intracellular compartments such as the ER to the cytoplasm, and to the influx of calcium ions which results from membrane dysfunction. Of course, the presence of increased quantities of calcium in necrotic cells is not in itself proof that they are of importance in the pathogenesis of the injury. However, there are several lines of evidence which do suggest that this is so. To begin with, there is a good temporal relationship, most easily observed in experimental systems, between the accumulation of calcium in injured cells and cell death.

This question has been extensively studied experimentally, both *in vivo* and *in vitro*. The most common systems that have been used are ischemic heart or liver. Such studies have confirmed that, after a period of anoxia, the intracellular levels of energy stores, in particular ATP, fall dramatically; and that, when the tissue is reperfused or reoxygenated, the mitochondria fail to regenerate ATP. In other words the injury is irreversible, and many of the cells die. This is correlated with a large increase in mitochondrial calcium content. The relationship of the latter to the irreversibility of the injury has been tested in several ways. For example, when the overloading of the mitochondria with calcium is prevented, by initially reperfusing with a low calcium solution or by prior treatment with calcium-antagonist drugs such as chlorpromazine or verapamil, the mitochondria are able to regain their functional capacity to generate ATP, and most of the cells recover. It is very interesting to note that such treatments do not prevent the occurrence of the ultrastructural changes that we have described as typical of irreversible cell injury, including high-amplitude swelling of mitochondria. Thus, even this hallmark of irreversible injury is **not** irreversible, and such changes regress as the cell recovers.

If the influx of calcium into injured cells and their mitochondria is in fact of primary importance in determining irreversibility, it should be possible to test the hypothesis by causing increased entry of calcium as a primary event. This has been done using the so-called **calcium paradox.** If heart tissue, for example, is perfused first with a solution very low in calcium, then with one with normal levels of calcium, there is a massive influx of calcium ions into the cells. This leads to extensive mitochondrial uptake of calcium, loss of ATP generating capacity, and depletion of cellular ATP. In this case, therefore, the disruption of mitochondrial function is the **result** of calcium influx, rather than the reverse.

Similar observations have been made *in vitro,* where the effects of both anoxia and toxic cell injury, in which there is direct attack on the cell membrane, have been tested. Such studies have shown that, for many different drugs, cell death is dependent on the concentration of calcium ions in the external medium. In addition, treatment of cultured cells with calcium ionophores, which allow the influx of calcium ions into the cells, causes cell death. Calcium ionophores can also enhance the toxic effect of other drugs on cultured cells, presumably by amplifying the uptake of calcium ions. Thus, cell death associated with either anoxia or direct membrane damage involves the influx of calcium ions and their deleterious effect on mitochondrial function.

RELATIONSHIP OF MEMBRANE DAMAGE TO CALCIUM AND CELL DEATH.   We have already discussed the fact that damage to cellular membranes in injured cells results in an increased permeability to ions, an influx of sodium and calcium ions, and a loss of potassium and magnesium ions. In addition, redistribution of ions within the cell, importantly, leads to release of calcium ions from the sarcoplasmic reticulum and other cellular compartments into the cytoplasm. Calcium ions are known to be an important intracellular messenger, capable of modulating and activating many different cellular functions. In terms of the present discussion, important amongst these are the calcium-activated ATPases, proteases, and endogenous phospholipases. Activation of ATPases by increased levels of calcium ions further depletes cellular energy stores. Activation of phospholipases further damages the already leaky cellular membranes, including the plasma membrane. There is clear evidence of loss of membrane phospholipids in ischemic liver and myocardium, reflecting membrane damage that affects both plasma membranes and those of the endoplasmic reticulum. Such phospholipid loss can be prevented by prior treatment with chlorpromazine, suggesting that calcium ions are involved in the membrane damage. Other factors are also apparently involved in producing membrane damage in anoxic cells. One of these is the accumulation of potentially harmful metabolites in anoxic cells. We have already discussed the role of free radicals in ischemic cell injury and the fact that these can be generated by calcium-activated phospholipases and proteases. Long-chain acyl-CoA esters and long-chain acyl carnitine also accumulate in ischemic cells, and have been proposed to have a detergent effect that can damage cellular membranes. In addition, there is evidence that lack of oxygen itself is important in contributing to the membrane damage in ischemic or anoxic cells. When cells are treated with metabolic poisons that block the synthesis of ATP, there is little effect on cell viability during the time when actual anoxia produces extensive cell death. Thus the effects of anoxia involve more than just the depletion of cellular energy supplies. Oxygen is also utilized by a number of oxygenases, in particular the fatty acid desaturases, enzymes involved in the synthesis of polyunsaturated fatty acids required for the maintenance of cell membranes. These enzymes are blocked by cyanide, a metabolic poison that also blocks electron transport in the mitochondria, and which does mimic the lethal effects of anoxia on cells. Inhibition of these enzymes therefore is another route by which membrane damage could result from anoxia.

As a consequence of all this it has been argued that the truly critical factor in producing irreversible cell injury is membrane damage. It is apparent that membrane damage is central to such injury, whether it is due to anoxia or to direct attack on cell membranes. However, this picture can be made even more complicated. Certain drugs, such as galactosamine, can induce membrane damage that, in the presence of calcium ions, causes extensive cell death. The effects of galactosamine can be reversed by treatment with uridine. If cells are treated with galactosamine in the absence of calcium, in which case they are not killed, then washed and treated with uridine, and then placed in medium containing calcium, they are not killed. In contrast cells not treated with uridine are killed when exposed to calcium ions. Thus, the membrane damage that led to calcium-mediated cell death was also reversible. As membrane components are continually turned over, it is reasonable to assume that a degree of damage to the cell membranes can be repaired as long as the necessary metabolic energy is supplied. The final outcome of the insult presumably depends on the relative contributions and interactions of these various factors. If we can learn to manipulate these, we may be more successful in treating infarction and other causes of cell death.

CELL INJURY, CALCIUM, AND MEMBRANE DAMAGE: A RECAPITULATION. The arguments that we have presented are summarized in Figure 2.33. Dysfunction of cellular membranes is an early feature of cellular injury, regardless of the cause. As a result there is a redistribution of cellular ions and an influx of sodium and calcium ions from the extracellular fluid. Calcium ions are avidly taken up by the mitochondria, where they are potent inhibitors of oxidative phosphorylation. They also activate ATPases, further reducing cellular ATP supplies, and they activate endogenous lipases and proteases, adding, via several mechanisms, to membrane injury. Cells which by the usual morphologic criteria (which we have already described) would be regarded as irreversibly injured, can recover if this influx of calcium ions is prevented. Thus, the changes in the mitochondria at this stage and those in the cellular membranes, in particular the plasma membrane, are potentially reversible. The influx of calcium ions can be regarded as a critical event in determining that cellular injury is irreversible.

There are, therefore, two central events that contribute importantly to cell death due to a variety of causes. One is damage to cell membranes. In the normal environment of the cells this leads to the second central event, the abnormal uptake of calcium ions by the cell as a whole and by the mitochondria in particular. This is turn prevents the cell from regenerating its ATP supplies, even if the cause of the injury is removed. In the usual situation existing *in vivo*, the uptake of calcium ions can be regarded as a critical event in irreversible injury, without ignoring the importance of membrane injury. It

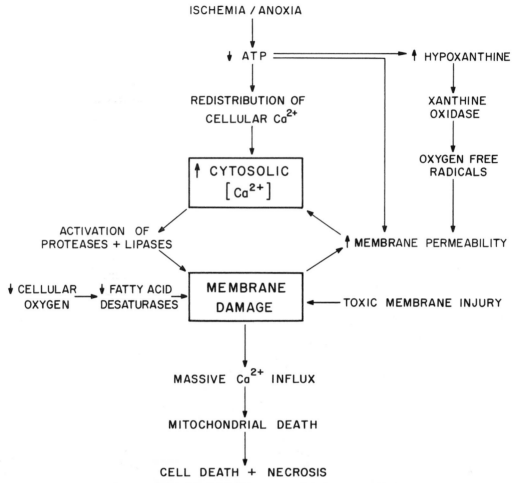

Figure 2.33.   Interactions of hypoxia, membrane damage, and calcium in cell injury. Damage to cell membranes and abnormalities of cellular calcium homeostasis are central to most forms of cell injury.

might be said that the influx of calcium ions provides the *coup de grace* for the injured cells, but this discussion makes it apparent that essentially all forms of cell injury also involve membrane damage. Finally, it cannot be denied that cells deprived of oxygen or exposed to toxic chemicals will eventually die, even if protected from an influx of calcium ions. Prolonged anoxia or intoxication will lead to progressive degeneration of cell membranes and organelles, which will become irreversible even without the participation of calcium ions. In real life situations, however, the interplay of membrane damage, loss of cell energy supplies, and calcium influx are of central importance.

Hepatic Fatty Change as a Model of Nonlethal Cell Injury

Cell injury, no matter what its cause, is not always lethal. Often, cells are injured and cannot adequately carry out their normal functions, but are able to maintain homeostasis and stay alive. **Fatty change,** the name given to abnormal accumulation of lipids in the cell, is a good example with which to illustrate this point. Fatty change can occur in a variety of cells, but is most often seen in the liver, renal tubular epithelium, and the myocardium. In the liver, which we will consider in some detail here, it represents a common nonspecific response that may be seen in a number of diseases.

Morphologically, fatty change may impart a yellow color to the liver. If most cells are affected, the liver will be diffusely yellow. If cells are affected in a zonal pattern, a reticular pattern will be seen grossly (Fig. 2.34). Histologically the lipid in the cells will be evident as vacuoles. Often these are large, sharply demarcated single vacuoles, but at other times vacuoles are smaller and multiple (Fig. 2.15). Although the large single vacuoles are fairly distinctive and characteristic of fatty change, vacuoles in the cell

cytoplasm do not necessarily contain fat. Vacuoles also may represent dilated cisternae of the ER, areas of the cytoplasm depleted of organelles, or stored material in lysosomes. Special stains or electron microscopy may be required to identify their contents.

Fatty change was, in the past, referred to as fatty degeneration or fatty infiltration. These terms are best not used, as the presence of intracellular lipid does not necessarily indicate any degenerative change in the cell, and the fat is not an infiltrate. Abnormal fat vacuoles do indicate an **absolute increase in intracellular lipid** which may be due to abnormalities of synthesis, utilization, or mobilization (export) of fat. Fatty change is sometimes an expression of cell injury, and, when it is, it may be preceded or accompanied by cell swelling. In addition,

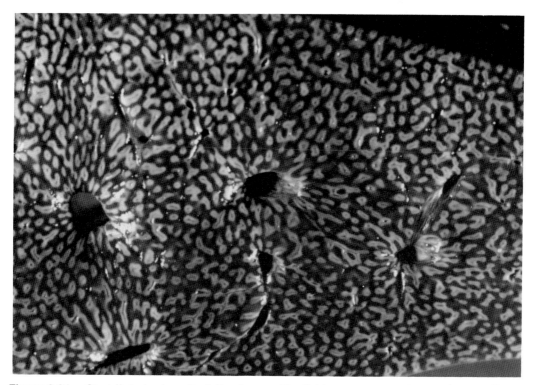

Figure 2.34. Centrilobular hepatic fatty change. The light areas represent parenchyma, adjacent to central veins, which has undergone fatty change due to hypoxia. They contrast with the darker normal tissue.

fatty change can occur as an expression of injury in cells that are destined to die. In the example of CCl$_4$ poisoning, for instance, cells undergoing fatty change may be observed adjacent to cells that are obviously necrotic. Presumably many of the cells containing lipid are severely injured and destined to die. A lesion of this type is shown in Figure 2.35.

In the liver cell, which is particularly susceptible to fatty change, a number of mechanisms may be involved in the accumulation of lipids. In order to understand them, we must review briefly the normal metabolism of fats in the hepatocyte. This is summarized in Figure 2.36. Briefly, lipids enter the liver cells as free fatty acids (FFA), which are mostly esterified to form triglycerides (TG). Some, however, are utilized in the synthesis of cholesterol esters or phospholipids, and some are degraded to produce ketone bodies. The hepatocyte also is capable of synthesizing some fatty acids from acetate. In order to be exported from the hepatocyte, TG must be complexed with a protein called lipid-acceptor protein to form lipoproteins. In theory at least, accumulation of intracellular lipid can occur due to abnormalities in any of these steps. Abnormal amounts of FFA may be delivered to the liver when body fats are rapidly mobilized as occurs, for example, in starvation. As well, experimental models

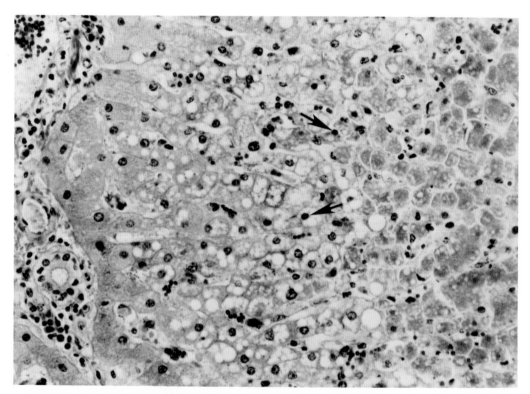

Figure 2.35. Progression of cell injury. In this liver, the progression of cell injury can readily be appreciated. Near the portal area at *left* the hepatocytes show only mild cell swelling. Progressing toward the central vein (which is out of the picture to right), the cells show fatty change, then more severe swelling with nuclear changes such as pyknosis *(arrows)* and eventually coagulation necrosis. This lesion was caused by hypoxia associated with methemoglobinemia. The hepatocytes near the central vein are more susceptible to such insults and, thus, are injured first, resulting in the sequence shown here.

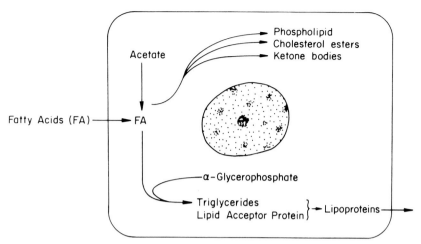

Figure 2.36. Metabolism of fats in the hepatocyte. Fatty acids may be synthesized in the hepatocyte or be taken up from the blood. Some are converted to triglycerides. Lipid carrier protein is essential for their export from the cell.

have shown that interference with the incorporation of FFA into phospholipids, impaired complexing of TG with acceptor protein, or impaired export of the complex from the liver all can result in the accumulation of lipid in the liver cell. In man, chronic alcoholism commonly is associated with fatty liver and is thought to be due to increased availability of α-glycerophosphate, thus enhancing TG synthesis. This accounts for almost all the potential pathways for fatty change in the liver, but, in the context of our discussion of cell injury, the last and most important is the accumulation of TG due to an inability to synthesize the lipid-acceptor protein. The formation of lipoprotein is mandatory for the export of TG from the liver, and the protein moiety (the acceptor protein) is synthesized in the hepatocyte itself. Therefore, any cell injury resulting in a reduction of protein synthesis will impair export of TG and result in fatty change. As pointed out earlier, reduced protein synthesis is an early consequence of injury due to membrane damage, and fatty change is a characteristic finding in the liver injured by toxins such as CCl_4 and phosphorus, and a number of other insults.

The reduction in protein synthesis and the accumulation of lipid are in themselves not lethal to the cell, and cells with fatty change sometimes can survive for a long time. Obviously, as they survive, they can maintain at least minimal homeostatic mechanisms, but functions other than lipid-acceptor protein synthesis also may be impaired. As a result, the animal may show signs of clinical illness.

PIGMENTS AND OTHER TISSUE DEPOSITS

Many pathologic processes are accompanied by the accumulation, either inside cells or in the interstitium, of a variety of abnormal substances. These are known as **deposits,** and many of them, being colored, are **pigments.**

Intracellular Lipid Accumulation

One of the most common of such substances, namely triglycerides, we already have discussed. Triglyceride lipids may accumulate in injured cells and are visible microscopically as clear vacuoles. Other lipids can accumulate producing a similar appearance. These include substances stored in the inherited storage diseases, the **lipidoses,** and phagocytosed lipids. When adipose tissue or the lipid-rich tissues of the central nervous system undergo necrosis, the lipid and other debris is phagocytosed by macrophages, imparting a vacuolated appearance to their cytoplasm. This appearance can be so dramatic that the cells are called foam cells or foamy macrophages.

Cholesterol is another lipid substance that can accumulate in tissues. It deserves special mention because of its involvement in vascular disease and myocardial infarction in man. Atherosclerosis is a lesion of arteries and arterioles in which cholesterol accumulates in smooth muscle cells in the walls of the vessels. The affected cells are vacuolated, appear foamy, and may contain crystallized cholesterol which produces a characteristic needle-like cleft in the tissue (Fig. 2.37A). A comprehensive discussion of atherosclerosis is not appropriate here, but suffice it to say that it is a common lesion in man that predisposes to other problems such as myocardial infarction. In dogs, atherosclerosis is sometimes seen as a complication of hypothyroidism. This condition is associated with hypercholesterolemia, or increased blood cholesterol levels, and affected animals often have widespread atherosclerotic lesions (Fig. 2.37B). Atherosclerosis is, in general, much less important in animals than it is in man.

Occasionally adipose tissue infiltrates the interstitium of skeletal muscle, the myocardium, and other tissues. This process should be distinguished from intracellular lipid accumulation and is of considerably less importance. It is characterized by the presence of histologically normal fat tissue in the interstitial connective tissue and is usually not associated with a functional disturbance.

Intracellular Protein Accumulation

Cells, of course, normally contain a great variety of proteins, but, in a few circumstances, unusual amounts of protein occur which may be apparent histologically as eosinophilic droplets or bodies. In the kidney, protein lost into the ultrafiltrate due to glomerular disease is taken up to some extent by epithelial cells of the proximal tubules. This produces droplets in the cytoplasm of these cells which represent protein in secondary lysosomes. The immunoglobulins produced by plasma cells can accumulate in cisternae of the RER, again producing eosinophilic masses, usually called in this case, "Russell bodies." These changes are of little consequence in terms of cell injury.

The terms **hyalin** and **fibrinoid** are commonly used and should be mentioned here. These descriptive terms coined by histopathologists are really of limited use, because they describe only the appearance of certain deposits rather than their true nature. Hyalin is the name given to any substance, intracellular or extracellular, which has a homogeneous, glassy, eosinophilic appearance. It is not a specific substance but often is protein in nature. For example, plasma proteins that leak through damaged endothelium may give the vessel wall a hyalinized appearance, thickened basement membranes may be hyalinized, and amyloid (discussed more fully below) also has this histologic appearance. Fibrinoid is also a nonspecific term that indicates a fibrin-like appearance. Like hyaline, fibrinoid material is variable in composition, but is often protein in nature and may in fact contain fibrin or degradation products of fibrin.

Pigments

Pigments are substances that are inherently colored. A variety of pigments may accumulate in tissues, either inside or outside cells. They are often subdivided into two groups, endogenous and exogenous pigments. **Endogenous pigments** originate in the affected animal, while **exogenous pigments** come from the external environment.

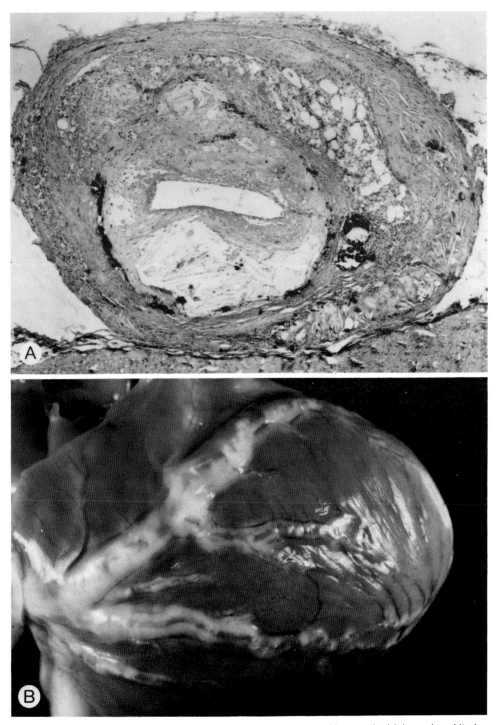

Figure 2.37.   Atherosclerosis. *A,* the wall of this coronary vessel is greatly thickened and its lumen reduced due to atherosclerosis. The light-colored vacuoles represent areas of lipid deposition and the angular clefts, cholesterol deposition. The dark material is calcified tissue. *B,* In this heart the coronary vessels are prominent and light in color due to atherosclerosis. These lesions are from a dog with hypothyroidism.

Exogenous pigments include carbon or soot and other dusts. In special circumstances they may be predominantly silica dust, asbestos dust, or other relatively homogeneous substances. These are often special contaminints of the environment of people or animals. Silicosis, the deposition of silica dust in the lungs, is a special problem for miners, while anthracosis, the deposition of carbon particles, is a special problem of city dwellers. Such inhaled dust particles are found in macrophages in the lungs and in draining lymph nodes. In the case of anthracosis, the pigment gives these tissues a black discoloration. The pigment itself is usu-

ally relatively harmless, but, if present in large quantities, it may cause chronic injury leading to pulmonary fibrosis. Of course the dust we inhale in large industrialized cities usually is accompanied by other substances that can be harmful. In particular, many are potential carcinogens (*see* Chapter 6) and may cause cancer.

Endogenous pigments include a number of substances that may be normal cell products or result from the breakdown of normal substances. **Lipofuscin** already has been mentioned in our discussion of cell injury. In tissue sections it appears as a golden brown, finely granular, intra-

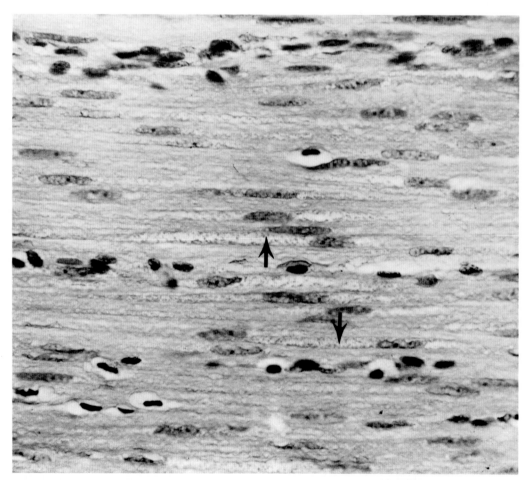

Figure 2.38.   Lipofuscinosis. In these smooth muscle cells, from the intestinal wall of a dog with vitamin E deficiency, there are accumulations of fine granular lipofuscin pigment *(arrows)*.

cellular pigment (Fig. 2.38). It is derived chiefly from the breakdown products of lipids, usually those derived from cell membranes. Therefore it is found most commonly in aged cells, in particular myocardial cells and neurons of old people or animals, or in chronically injured cells. It is, in fact, commonly referred to as "aging pigment" or "wear-and-tear" pigment. Because it is the end result of breakdown of lipid-containing membranes in the lysosome, it essentially is the light microscopic equivalent of residual bodies.

Lipofuscin is increased in certain cells where there is increased turnover of organelles or increased membrane injury. In some species it is increased as a consequence of vitamin E or selenium deficiency. In the dog, for instance, such deficiencies lead to **lipofuscinosis** of the smooth muscle of the intestine, which imparts a distinct yellow-brown discoloration of the organ. Lipofuscin also can be increased by a diet rich in unsaturated fatty acids.

Lipofuscin apparently consists of a complex of lipids, phospholipids, and some protein. It is somewhat variable in composition, presumably reflecting not only its variable origins but the degree to which lysosomal substrates have been broken down. For this reason its staining characteristics are also variable. **Ceroid** is a variant of lipofuscin which is acid-fast and autofluorescent.

Melanin is a normal pigment that usually is found in melanocytes, in epidermal cells, and in the pigmented epithelial cells of the eye. Less commonly, other tissues such as the intestine, the kidney, or the leptomeninges contain melanin. Histologically it has a brown, finely granular, appearance. Melanin is produced by melanocytes, cells of neural crest origin. In the skin it is transferred from these cells to basal cells of the epidermis, where it provides some protection from ultraviolet light. In some pathologic conditions melanin also is found in macrophages. In these cells it is the result of phagocytosis of pigment derived from injured melanocytes or epithelial cells. **Psuedomelanosis** is a term used to describe an artifactual discoloration of tissues which produces an appearance similar to melanin pigmentation. It occurs as a postmorten event when hydrogen sulfide produced by bacteria reacts with iron in the tissues to produce iron sulfide.

Hemosiderin is an iron-containing yellow-brown granular pigment very frequently found in tissue sections. In cells, iron usually is stored, bound to the protein apoferritin, as **ferritin.** When large amounts of ferritin are present aggregates form, producing the granules that we recognize histologically as hemosiderin. Hemosiderin commonly is seen in areas of congestion or hemorrhage, or anywhere where there is excessive breakdown of red blood cells. In almost any section of spleen, for example, it is possible to find at least some hemosiderin (Fig. 2.39). This pigment, therefore, represents stored iron (in the ferric form), which is salvaged from the hemoglobin derived from erythrocytes that have been destroyed.

In sections, hemosiderin is a yellow-gold, granular, intracellular pigment. It increases when there is enhanced absorption of iron or, as we already have mentioned, when there is enhanced breakdown of erythrocytes. Because this occurs mostly in phagocytes in the spleen, this is the most common tissue in which we see hemosiderin. It also can be found in macrophages in other tissues, however. In animals with congestive heart failure it is commonly found in alveolar macrophages in the congested lung (*see* Fig. 3.3) and may impart a grossly apparent light brown color to the tissue. In most cases hemosiderin causes no damage to the cell. There is some evidence that iron can catalyze lipid peroxidation of membranes, but it is not clear whether iron in hemosiderin can contribute to this process.

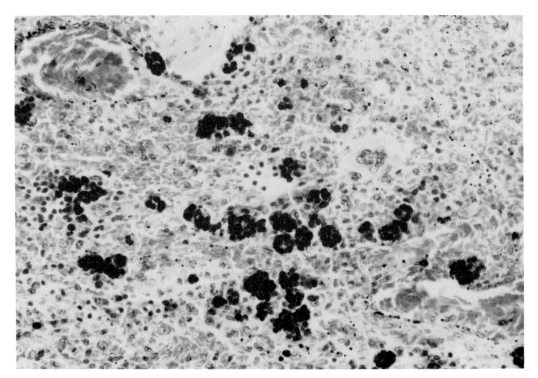

Figure 2.39. Hemosiderosis. In this spleen the dark granular material represents hemosiderin. This is a common finding in the spleen.

Less commonly, copper may be stored in tissues, particularly in hepatocytes. This is seen in animals with chronic copper poisoning, most commonly in sheep, and in some breeds of dogs which have an inherited defect in copper metabolism. Storage of large amounts of copper is toxic to the hepatocyte, and affected animals often have relatively sudden onset of acute hepatocellular necrosis. What precipitates this event is not clearly understood. Copper, however, also is capable of catalyzing lipid peroxidation, and damage to lysosomal membranes may be involved in this form of hepatocellular injury.

Bile pigments, including **bilirubin,** are normal products of the breakdown of the heme portion of hemoglobin. Because red blood cells are continually being destroyed and replaced, there is continual production of bilirubin. It is conjugated in the hepatocyte to its glucuronide, which makes it soluble in water, and then ex-creted into the bile. Bilirubin may accumulate in the blood or in tissues when there is increased breakdown of erythrocytes, such as in hemolytic diseases, or when there is hepatic disease. In the latter case it may accumulate due to failure of either conjugation or excretion. Accumulation of bilirubin in the blood produces a generalized yellow discoloration of the tissue, known clinically as jaundice or icterus. In sections, bilirubin is a green-brown to yellow-brown granular pigment. It is found most commonly in hepatocytes and renal tubular epithelium. In the latter it is thought to be toxic, producing the so-called bile nephrosis or renal tubular necrosis seen in jaundiced animals. Occasionally, at sites of previous hemorrhage, a yellow-brown pigment called hematoidin accumulates. It is thought to be locally precipitated bilirubin, and, unlike hemosiderin, it is negative in special stains for iron.

It is clear from this discussion that a number of pigments, namely hemosiderin, bile pigments, copper, melanin, and lipofuscin, all have a similar appearance in tissues. In practice it often is necessary to use special staining procedures to identify them. In addition, pigment-like material may be deposited as an artefact of preparation. Most troublesome among these is **acid-hematin,** a derivative of hemoglobin produced in tissues fixed in improperly buffered formalin. Superficially it resembles hemosiderin, but it usually can be seen to overlie cells instead of being **in** them.

Calcification

As we have already discussed, calcification is a common manifestation of lethal cell injury, but it is sometimes also seen when there is no apparent preceding cell death. When calcification occurs in injured tissues it is said to be **dystrophic,** and when it occurs in apparently normal tissues it is said to be **metastatic.**

Dystrophic calcification is not associated with hypercalcemia or other disturbances of calcium homeostasis. It occurs in cells injured in a variety of ways including vascular, toxic, metabolic, or inflammatory causes, but, as already mentioned, it is most prominent when a good blood supply is present in the injured tissue. In sections stained with hematoxylin and eosin, the calcium deposits have a finely granular appearance and are basophilic (Fig. 2.40). In necrotic fat cells, calcium often is deposited in the form of insoluble calcium soaps derived from the interaction of calcium ions and fatty acids produced in the necrotic cells.

The pathogenesis of dystrophic calcifi-

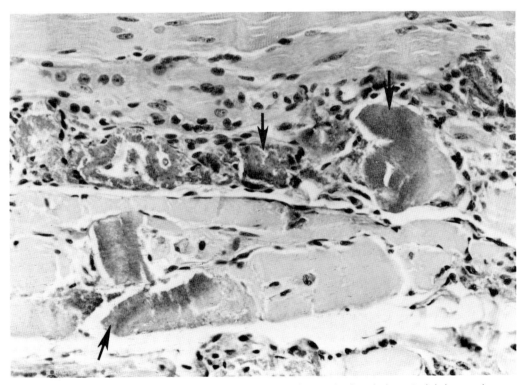

Figure 2.40.   Dystrophic calcification. In this skeletal muscle the dark material *(arrows)* represents calcification of necrotic fibers. The striated appearance seen in some areas is due to the orientation of the mitochondria, the primary site of calcium deposition, with the sarcomeres.

cation is poorly understood. However, like its physiological counterpart, the process may involve the deposition of calcium on or in so-called **matrix vesicles.** These are membranous vesicles probably derived, in physiological situations, by budding of the plasma membrane, and, in pathological processes, as products of cellular disintegration. Acidic phospholipids in these membranous vesicles, in particular phosphatidylserine, may serve as binding sites for calcium. As we have already discussed in this chapter, mitochondria also serve as foci for calcium deposition in injured cells.

Metastatic calcification commonly is associated with hypercalcemia or disturbances of calcium metabolism. For instance it may be seen in primary hyperparathyroidism, hypervitaminosis D, renal failure, and certain neoplastic diseases. The calcium salts may be deposited in a number of sites, but are most commonly seen in the gastric and intestinal mucosae, the interstitium of blood vessel walls, the lung, and the kidney. Very often they are deposited along basement membranes (Fig. 2.41). Why these sites are more susceptible than others to metastatic calcification is poorly understood.

The distinction between dystrophic and metastatic calcification, although useful for classification, may be somewhat artificial. Calcium ions, when present in excess, are potent uncouplers of oxidative phosphorylation and are toxic to cells. Metastatic calcification therefore can cause cell injury, and it is sometimes difficult to distinguish dystrophic from metastatic calcification.

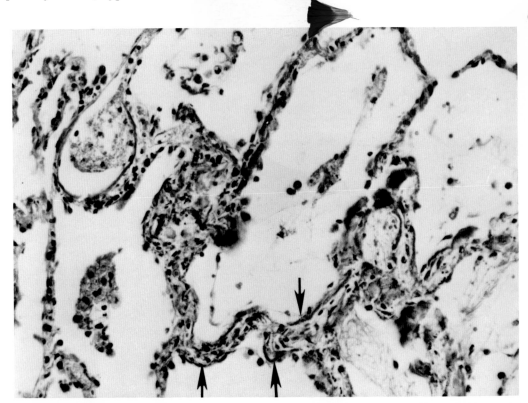

Figure 2.41.   Metastatic calcification. The dark material deposited in this lung represents calcification in a case of chronic renal failure in a cat. This type of calcification often shows a predilection for basement membranes. This can be appreciated here in a blood vessel *(upper left)* and in some alveolar septa *(arrows).*

Amyloid and Amyloidosis

Probably the most important of all tissue deposits is amyloid, so named by Virchow because he believed it to be of polysaccharide, or starch-like, composition. Actually it is now known to be protein in nature.

Amyloid may be deposited locally or systemically, and the disease resulting from deposition of this material is known as **amyloidosis.** Histologically amyloid is a lightly eosinophilic, amorphous, hyaline material that is deposited extracellularly. Frequently it is present in or around the walls of vessels. At other times it may be more diffuse in its distribution. When extensive, amyloid deposits may compress or distort adjacent tissues and cause dysfunction. A common example is amyloidosis of the renal glomeruli. In this case the amyloid is deposited within the walls of glomerular capillaries (Fig. 2.42A and 2.43), leading to leakage of proteins from the plasma into the urine.

Amyloid is distinguished from other deposits of similar appearance by the use of special stains. The most commonly used is **Congo red,** which stains amyloid orange-red and renders it birefringent under polarized light (Fig. 2.42B). Ultrastructurally, amyloid is made up of masses of linear, nonbranching fibrils 7.5–10 nm in diameter (Fig. 2.43).

The deposition of amyloid is a rather ubiquitous response to a variety of pathologic conditions. Frequently it is associated with chronic inflammatory disease, and it also may be found associated with neoplasms, especially those of endocrine origin. At other times amyloid is deposited in the absence of an identifiable predisposing cause. Traditionally, the latter is referred to as **primary amyloidosis** (most commonly seen in man), while the form associated with other diseases is known as **secondary amyloidosis.**

Amyloid now is known not to be a specific chemical substance. Rather, the characteristic appearance and staining reactions of amyloid are due to a particular conformation of the constituent polypeptides known as the **β-pleated sheet.** Therefore, any polypeptide molecules that can adopt this confirmation can produce fibrils that, although chemically variable, are, in fact, amyloid. Because of this, Dr. G. G. Glenner has called the complex of syndromes involving amyloid deposition the **β-fibrilloses.** This peculiar conformation apparently confers the tinctorial properties of amyloid, and makes it rather resistant to enzymatic degradation. Although amyloid seems to persist in tissues for a long time, its stability has never been rigorously proven.

Chemically, amyloid has been shown to occur in two major forms. One form is composed of immunoglobulin light chains and is referred to as **prot___ ___.** The other form contains a protein ___ **protein AA.** The primary form ___ amyloidosis is associated with deposition of amyloid of the AL type. This protein also is deposited in amyloidosis associated with multiple myeloma (plasma cell neoplasia), and it appears that most patients with primary amyloidosis have plasma cell dyscrasias. Amyloid protein of the AL type apparently is composed of homogeneous light chains, of the λ or κ type, or their N-terminal fragments, or both. In addition, circulating proteins that are immunologically cross-reactive with the amyloid deposits often can be demonstrated.

It also has been shown that *in vitro* treatment of λ–Bence Jones proteins (circulating light chains often found in patients with multiple myeloma) with proteolytic enzymes can yield fibrils which are indistinguishable from amyloid. They are composed of a small fragment of the N-terminal variable region of the light chain. However, not all Bence Jones proteins yield amyloid fibrils when so treated.

Primary amyloidosis, at least in man, therefore appears to be associated with

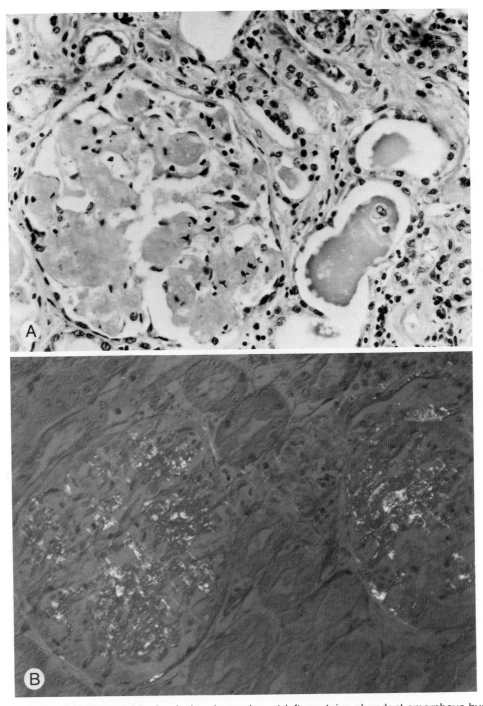

Figure 2.42.   Renal amyloidosis. *A,* the glomerulus, at *left,* contains abundant amorphous hyaline material typical of amyloid. Two tubules to the *right* contain proteinaceous material reflecting the loss of protein through the affected glomeruli. *B,* under polarized light, affected glomeruli stained with Congo red are birefringent and appear light in this photomicrograph.

Campbell, A.K.: Intracellular calcium: friend or foe?. *Clin. Sci. 72:*1–10, 1987.

Cheung, J.Y., Bonventre, J.V., Malis, C.D., and Leaf, A.: Calcium and ischemic injury. *N. Engl. J. Med. 314:*1670–1676, 1986.

Cheville, N.F.: *Cell Pathology,* ed. 3. Iowa State University Press, Ames, 1983.

Clark, I.A.: Tissue damage caused by free oxygen radicals. *Pathology 18:*181–186, 1986.

Cohen, A.S., and Connors, L.H.: The pathogenesis and biochemistry of amyloidosis. *J. Pathol. 151:*1–10, 1987.

Comporti, M.: Lipid peroxidation and cellular damage in toxic liver injury. *Lab. Invest. 53:*599–623, 1985.

De Groot, H., and Littauer, A.: Hypoxia, reactive oxygen, and cell injury. *Free Rad. Biol. Med. 6:*541–551, 1989.

Downey, J.M., Hearse, D.J., and Yellon, D.M.: The role of xanthine oxidase during myocardial ischemia in several species including man. *J. Mol. Cell. Cardiol. 20 (Suppl. 3):*55–63, 1988.

Ericsson, J.L.E., and Brunk U.T.: Alterations in lysosomal membranes as related to disease processes. In *Pathobiology of Cell Membranes, Vol. 1,* edited by B. F. Trump and A.U. Arstila. Academic Press, New York.

Farber, J.L.: Membrane injury and calcium homeostasis in the pathogenesis of coagulative necrosis. *Lab Invest. 47:*114–123, 1982.

Farber, J.L., Chien, K.R., and Mittnacht, S.: The pathogenesis of irreversible cell injury in ischemia. *Am. J. Pathol. 102:*271–281, 1981.

Farber, J.L., and Gerson, R.J.: Mechanisms of cell injury with hepatotoxic chemicals. *Pharmacol. Rev. 36:*71–75, 1984.

Ferrari, R., Ceconi, C., Curello, S., Cargnoni, A., and Medici, D.: Oxygen free radicals and reperfusion injury; the effect of ischemia and reperfusion on the cellular ability to neutralise oxygen toxicity. *J. Mol. Cell. Cardiol. 18:*4–67, 1986.

Flaherty, J.T., and Weisfeldt, M.L.: Reperfusion injury. *Free Rad. Biol. Med. 5:*409–419, 1988.

Freeman, B.A., and Crapo, J.D.: Free radicals and tissue injury. *Lab. Invest. 47:*412–426, 1982.

Glenner, G.G.: Amyloid deposits and amyloidosis. The β-fibrilloses. *N. Engl. J. Med. 302:*1283–1292, 1980.

Gorevic, P.D., and Buhles, W.C.: Amyloidosis. *Ann. Rev. Med. 32:*261–271, 1981.

Gutteridge, J.M.C.: Lipid Peroxidation: Some problems and concepts. In *Oxygen Radicals and Tissue Injury,* B. Halliwell. Fed. Am. Soc. Exp. Biol., Bethesda, 1988.

Halliwell, B.: Oxidants and human disease: some new concepts. *FASEB J. 1:*358–364, 1987.

Hawkins, H.K.: Reactions of lysosomes to cell injury. In *Pathobiology of Cell Membranes, Vol. 2,* edited by B.F. Trump and A.U. Arstila. Academic Press, New York, 1980.

Hess, M.L., and Manson, N.H.: Molecular oxygen: friend and foe. The role of the oxygen free radical system in the calcium paradox, the oxygen paradox and ischemia/reperfusion injury. *J. Mol. Cell. Cardiol. 16:*969–985, 1984.

Jennings, R.B., Ganote, C.E., and Reimer, K.A.: Ischemic tissue injury. *Am. J. Pathol. 81:*179–198, 1975.

Jennings, R.B., and Reimer, K.A.: Lethal myocardial ischemic injury. *Am J. Pathol. 102:*241–255, 1981.

Kim, K.M.: Pathological calcification. In *Pathobiology of Cell Membranes, Vol. 3,* edited by B.F. Trump and A.U. Arstila. Academic Press, New York, 1983.

Kisilevsky, R.: Amyloidosis: A familiar problem in the light of current pathogenetic developments. *Lab. Invest. 49:*381–390, 1983.

Macknight, A.D.C.: Cellular response to injury. In *Edema,* edited by N.C. Staub and A.E. Taylor. Raven Press, New York, 1984.

Marzella, L., Ahlberg, J., and Glaumann, H.: Autophagy, heterophagy, microautophagy and crinophagy as the means for intracellular degradation. *Virchows Arch. [Cell Pathol.] 36:*219–234, 1981.

McCord, J.M.: Oxygen-derived free radicals in postischemic tissue injury. *N. Engl. J. Med. 312:*159–163, 1985.

McCord, J.M.: Superoxide radical: a likely link between reperfusion injury and inflammation. *Adv. Free Rad. Biol. Med. 2:*325–345, 1986.

McCord, J.M.: Free radicals and myocardial ischemia: overview and outlook. *Free Rad. Biol. Med. 4:*9–14, 1988.

McNutt, N.S., and Hoffstein, S.: Membranes and cytoskeleton: role in pathologic processes. *Fed. Proc. 40:*206–213, 1981.

Minotti, G.: Metals and membrane lipid damage by oxy-radicals. *Ann. NY Acad. Sci. 551:*34–46, 1988.

Moll, R., and Franke, W.W.: Intermediate filaments and their interaction with membranes. *Pathol. Res. Pract. 175:*146–161, 1982.

Nayler, W.G., Panagiotopoulos, S., Elz, J.S., and Daly, M.J.: Calcium-mediated damage during postischaemic reperfusion. *J. Mol. Cell. Cardiol. 20(Suppl. 3):*41–54, 1988.

Naylor, W.G.: The role of calcium in the ischemic myocardium. *Am. J. Pathol. 102:*262–270, 1981.

Naylor, W.G.: Calcium and cell death. *Eur. Heart J. 4:*33–41, 1983.

Naylor, W.G., Poole-Wilson, P.A., and Williams, A.: Hypoxia and calcium. *J. Mol. Cell. Cardiol. 11:*683–706, 1979.

Robbins, S.L., and Cotran, R.S.: *Pathologic Basis of Disease,* ed. 3. W.B. Saunders, Philadelphia, 1984.

Robinson, J.R.: Colloid osmotic pressure as a cause

of pathological swelling of cells. In *Pathobiology of Cell Membranes, Vol. 1,* edited by B.F. Trump and A.U. Arstila. Academic Press, New York, 1975.

Rungger-Brandle, E., and Gabbiani, G.: The role of cytoskeletal and cytocontractile elements in pathologic processes. *Am J. Pathol. 100:*361–392, 1983.

Scarpelli, D.G., and Trump, B.F.: *Cell Injury.* Upjohn Co., Kalamazoo, Mich., 1971.

Shine, K.I.: Ionic events in ischemia and anoxia. *Am. J. Pathol. 102:*256–261, 1981.

Simpson, P.J.: Myocardial ischemia and reperfusion injury: Oxygen radicals and the role of the neutrophil. In *Oxygen Radicals and Tissue Injury,* edited by B. Halliwell. Fed. Am. Soc. Exp. Biol., Bethesda, Md., 1988.

Simpson, P.J., and Lucchesi, B.R.: Free radicals and myocardial ischemia and reperfusion injury. *J. Lab. Clin. Med. 110:*13–30, 1987.

Smuckler, E.A., and James, J.L.: Irreversible cell injury. *Pharmacol. Rev. 36:*77–91, 1984.

Southorn, P.A., and Powis, G.: Free radicals in medicine. I. Chemical nature and biologic reactions. *Mayo Clin. Proc. 63:*381–389, 1988.

Southorn, P.A., and Powis, G.: Free radicals in med-icine. II. Involvement in human disease. *Mayo Clin. Proc. 63:*390–408, 1988.

Tappel, A.L.: Lipid peroxidation and fluorescent molecular damage to membranes. In *Pathobiology of Cell Membranes,* edited by B.F. Trump and A.U. Arstila. Academic Press, New York, 1975.

Trump, B.F., and Arstila, A.U.: Cell membranes and disease processes. In *Pathobiology of Cell Membranes, Vol. 1,* edited by B.F. Trump and A.U. Arstila. Academic Press, New York, 1975.

Trump, B.F., McDowell, E.M., and Arstila, A.U.: Cellular reaction to injury. In *Principles of Pathobiology,* ed. 3, edited by R.B. Hill and M.F. LaVia. Oxford University Press, New York, 1980.

Walker, N.I., Harmon, B.V., Gobé, G.C., and Kerr J.F.R.: Patterns of cell death. *Methods Achiev. Exp. Pathol. 13:*18–54, 1988.

Ward, P.A.: Role of toxic oxygen products from phagocytic cells in tissue injury. *Adv. Shock Res. 10:*27–34, 1983.

Weiss, S.J.: Tissue destruction by neutrophils. *N. Engl. J. Med. 320:*365–376, 1989.

Werns, S.W., and Lucchesi, B.R.: Leukocytes, oxygen radicals, and myocardial injury due to ischemia and reperfusion. *Free Rad. Biol. Med. 4:*31–38, 1988.

3
Disturbances of Blood Flow and Circulation

Hyperemia and Congestion
  Types of Hyperemia
    Physiologic Hyperemia
    Pathologic Hyperemia
      Acute Local Active Hyperemia
      Acute Local Passive Hyperemia
      Chronic Local Passive Hyperemia
      Chronic Generalized Passive Hyperemia
    Appearance of Hyperemia
Hemorrhage
  Causes of Hemorrhage
  Clinical Significance and Outcome of Hemorrhage
  Resolution of Hemorrhage
Thrombosis
  General Background
  Overview of Blood Coagulation
  Mechanisms of Blood Coagulation
    Activation Process and Early Steps in Coagulation
    Formation of Activated Stuart-Prower Factor (Xa)
    Formation of Thrombin
    Formation of Fibrin
      Proteolysis of Fibrinogen
      Polymerization of Fibrin Monomers
      Stabilization and Cross-Linking of Fibrin
    Regulatory Mechanisms in Hemostasis and Thrombosis
    Perspectives on Coagulation
  Pathogenesis of Thrombosis
    Vascular Mechanisms in Thrombosis
    Role of the Endothelial Cell
    Rheological and Hemodynamic Mechanisms of Thrombosis
    Basic Mechanisms in the Blood Related to Thrombosis

Role and Properties of Platelets in Hemostasis and Thrombosis
    Platelet Adhesion
    Platelet Aggregation
    Platelet Secretory Events: the Platelet Release Reaction
  Morphology and Morphogenesis of Thrombi
    Arterial Thrombosis
    Venous Thrombosis
    Fate of Thrombi
    Propagation of Thrombi
    Embolism
    Fibrinolysis and Thrombolysis
      Fibrinolysis: Activation of Plasminogen
        Hageman Factor-Dependent Activity
        Extrinsic Plasminogen Activators
        Degradation of Fibrinogen/Fibrin Clots
    Organization of Thrombi
Infarction
  Determinants of Infarction
    Ischemic Susceptibility
    Anatomy of the Vasculature
    Overall Cardiovascular Function
    Clinical Significance of Infarction
Edema
  Interstitium and Extracellular Matrix
  Microvascular Physiology
  Pathophysiology of Edema
    Decreased Plasma Colloidal-Osmotic Pressure
    Increased Blood Hydrostatic Pressure
    Lymphatic Obstruction
    Increased Vascular Permeability
  Appearance of Edema
  Clinical Significance of Edema
Reference Material

All of the cells and tissues of the body are quite explicit about their requirements for a normal blood supply and an adequate fluid milieu in which to bathe. A wide variety of disease settings, unfortunately, disturb these critical support systems. Imbalances of the fluid microenvironment or of the microvasculature itself can cause shifts in the location of normally intravascular water, electrolytes, and plasma proteins. Such abnormalities are commonplace and result in the accumulation of fluids in the extracellular space and other extravascular sites. This is known as **edema.** The blood is an essential and important tissue critical to normal homeostasis but it can cause severe clinical problems when it forms unnecessary blood clots or fails to remain within the conduit profiles of the vascular system. In a large number of clinical settings, blood escapes from the vascular system and enters the tissues or the outside world as **hemorrhage.**

Even while still within the vascular system, blood responds to various physiological and pathological cardiovascular alterations, with the result that too much blood is actively or passively forced into different tissue sites as **hyperemia.** The delicately balanced hemostatic mechanism responsible for the life-saving blood clot sometimes assumes major pathologic importance when intravascular coagulation or **thrombosis** occurs. When formed, such thrombi sometimes break off from their initial point of formation to sail downstream as **emboli** to lodge in a smaller, distant vascular site. These intravascular coagula not only produce major local hemodynamic changes, but also can occlude the blood supply to vital tissues and produce **ischemic necrosis,** or **infarction.**

Such changes rarely qualify as diseases in their own right. More commonly they are **manifestations** of some underlying disease process. As such, the kinds of pathologic alterations to be discussed here are basic expressions of disease mechanisms that have broad application to a wide variety of clinical settings.

HYPEREMIA AND CONGESTION

Hyperemia literally means "too much blood." This refers to a volume and flow change, however, and should not be confused with **polycythemia,** too many red cells. The terms hyperemia and congestion are basically synonymous, although they often are used to imply different mechanistic and anatomical information. **Hyperemia** usually is used to imply an active, arteriolar-mediated engorgement of the vascular bed, whereas **congestion**

usually is used to indicate a passive, venous engorgement. Both terms, however, indicate an excess of blood in the vessels of a given tissue or tissue site. Our purpose here is to discuss the mechanisms of hyperemia, and therefore we will use passive hyperemia to indicate congestion. Our discussion is, therefore, predicated on the idea that hyperemia can basically only occur in two ways: either too much blood is being brought in via the arterioles (active hyperemia) or too little blood is being removed by the venules (passive hyperemia).

It is important to make a clear distinction between hyperemia and hemorrhage. While some hemorrhage can occur via a slow dribbling of a small number of red cells through the vessel walls into tissues **(hemorrhage by diapedesis)** during hyperemia, the two phenomena are, by definition, different in that hyperemia implies that the blood is still **within** the vascular system whereas hemorrhage implies that blood has escaped into extravascular sites.

Types of Hyperemia

Although all forms of hyperemia are basically similar in that there is vascular engorgement of the affected tissue, it is useful to dissect the various kinds of hyperemia into categories which have different pathophysiologic backgrounds.

Physiological Hyperemia

Not all hyperemia is pathological. The increase in blood flow to the stomach and intestines during digestion is a form of physiological hyperemia. The red faces on many members of Ithaca's jogging fraternity represent an increased blood flow to the skin in an effort to augment cutaneous heat loss by escalating the rate and volume of blood flow to exposed, cooler surface sites. Similar active increases in perfusion occur in the muscles of athletes during exercise. Blushing as a manifestation of acute embarrassment or nervousness is basically a form of neuro-vascular hyperemia. These and other physiologic forms of hyperemia are interesting, but are less germane to our focus than are the pathologic forms of hyperemia.

Pathologic Hyperemia.

Other than the types of physiological changes mentioned above, all forms of hyperemia are pathologic. In virtually all situations, hyperemia is only a **manifestation** of some alteration in blood flow characteristics. It is not the **cause,** but rather the **result** of some underlying pathologic process. It is useful in sorting out the various kinds of hyperemia to consider three factors: the **duration** of the hyperemia, the **extent** of hyperemia within the tissue or within the body as a whole, and the **mechanism** by which the hyperemia occurred (Table 3.1).

The duration of hyperemia can be sim-

Table 3.1
Classification of Hyperemia

Duration
Acute: abrupt onset, rapid development
Chronic: slowly developing, present for long time
Extent
General: generalized, systemic, or throughout an organ or system
Local: confined to a discrete area, localized, limited
Mechanism
Active: increased arteriolar inflow
Passive: engorgement of vascular bed, venous impedance
Examples in Use
Acute local active hyperemia: the hyperemia of inflammation
Acute local passive hyperemia: engorgement of bowel in a torsion
Chronic local passive hyperemia: engorgement behind progressive obstruction; tumor, abscess, etc.
Chronic general passive hyperemia: as in congestive heart failure

ply divided into **acute** and **chronic.** Acute hyperemia implies an abrupt onset and a fairly rapid development. Chronic hyperemia indicates that the lesion has been present for a longer time period or has been slow to develop, or both. It is similarly convenient to divide the hyperemias into **local** or **generalized** hyperemia based on the extent of tissue involvement. Local hyperemia implies that the change is confined to a discrete area and is localized or limited in extent. Generalized hyperemia implies a somewhat different picture. Usually it is used to indicate systemic changes (as in the generalized passive hyperemia of heart failure), but it also can mean that the hyperemia is generalized within an organ. For example, if the entire lung is hyperemic then there is generalized pulmonary hyperemia, even though the change may be restricted to the lungs.

A simple view of the mechanisms behind hyperemia already has been given. If the hyperemia is due to increased arteriolar flow, it is **active** hyperemia. If the hyperemia is due to impaired venous drainage, it is **passive** hyperemia. With this background, it is possible to construct an anatomical and mechanistic classification scheme for the hyperemias which can be useful clinically (Table 3.1). It should be noted that not all combinations and permutations theoretically possible based on this scheme occur in real life. For example, chronic generalized active hyperemia is an impossible situation. There is simply not enough blood in the vascular system to produce active arteriolar hyperemia at all sites simultaneously. Indeed, there are basically only four patterns of hyperemia that are sufficiently repeatable to warrant our attention.

ACUTE LOCAL ACTIVE HYPEREMIA. As the name implies, this is an engorgement of the vascular bed due to increased arteriolar blood flow into the area. As we will learn in the next chapter, **redness**

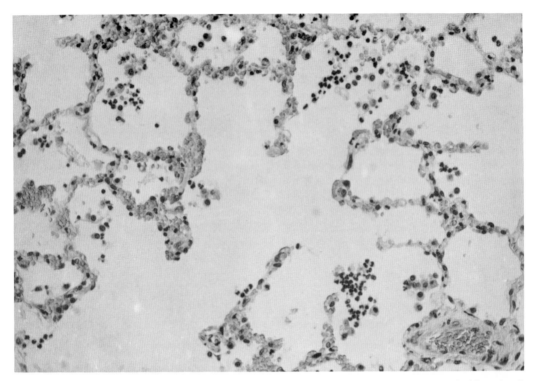

Figure 3.1.   Acute Hyperemia. The alveolar capillaries in this dog lung are engorged with red cells. A few leukocytes have emigrated into alveolar spaces.

(along with heat, swelling, and pain) is one of the cardinal signs of inflammation. Acute local active hyperemia is the **hyperemia of inflammation** (Fig. 3.1). The redness and heat we associate with acute inflammatory reactions is due to the active hyperemia that occurs. The increased rate of blood flow to the area and the increased **volume** of blood in the region at any one time form the basis for the redness and warmth. Increased arteriolar flow opens new capillary beds and the newly dilated small vessels extend the arteriolar blood pressure into smaller vascular radicals. It is sometimes even possible to feel a pulse over acutely inflamed areas because of the arteriolar dilatation and increased blood flow. Acute local active hyperemia is an event fairly specific to inflammation. It is a chemically mediated response of the microvasculature to histamine, bradykinin, and other vasoactive substances in acute inflammatory reactions.

ACUTE LOCAL PASSIVE HYPEREMIA. When local obstruction to venous drainage occurs, there is passive engorgement of the drainage area served by the obstructed vessel. Blood backs up into the microvascular bed, and local venous engorgement occurs. In contrast to the situation in acute local active hyperemia, the involved tissues here are dark red in color, rather than being bright red, as they are engorged with poorly oxygenated venous blood instead of well-oxygenated arterial blood. Additionally, it is unlikely that any pulse wave would be palpable because of the lower blood pressure in the venous system, and because the arteriolar flow here is normal. Such hyperemic changes may be seen in the service area of thrombosed or otherwise acutely obstructed veins. Acute local passive hyperemia may reach its maximal levels in situations where torsion of a viscus has occurred. In this situation, the venous drainage is seriously impaired but the thicker-walled arteries remain functional so that the interposed microvascular bed becomes extremely engorged with blood. Lesions such as this form the basis for one form of equine colic.

CHRONIC LOCAL PASSIVE HYPEREMIA. The only major difference between acute and chronic forms of local passive hyperemia is the time frame required for their development. Lesions such as extravascular tumors or abscesses, which slowly enlarge and eventually compress adjacent veins, can produce passive hyperemia. Because the development of the venous obstruction is slow, the vascular system often has an opportunity to adjust to the progressing obstruction, and channels of collateral flow gradually are opened to provide alternative routes of venous drainage. If this adaptive mechanism is successful, hyperemia may not develop at all.

Sometimes chronic local passive hyperemia can occur when organs or organ systems develop chronic inflammatory lesions that progress to fibrosis and hence to obstruction of that tissue's venous system. A reasonable example of this can be drawn from hepatic **cirrhosis** in which the progressive loss of hepatic lobular structural architecture by fibrosis eventually leads to portal hypertension. In addition to developing ascites (edema fluid in the peritoneal cavity), such patients often develop substantial collateral venous channels and intrahepatic arteriovenous anastomoses. The normal route of blood flow may be reversed in such situations so that portal blood is shunted to the esophageal veins and thence into the azygos system. The greatly heightened pressure in the esophageal plexus produces dilated tortuous vessels called **varices.** In man, where advanced cirrhosis is more common than in other animals, ap-

proximately two-thirds of all cirrhotic patients have esophageal varices which sometimes rupture and produce life-threatening episodes of hemorrhage. As in other forms of chronic local passive hyperemia, the clinical signs and the vascular engorgement itself are related to changes away from the actual causative lesion. In other words, the effects of local, passive hyperemia are always **upstream** from the location of the underlying lesion.

CHRONIC GENERALIZED PASSIVE HYPEREMIA. It is a useful rule of thumb that **all** generalized passive hyperemias (congestions) involve either the heart or the lungs as the major site of underlying pathologic change. If the heart is the source of the problem, the chronic generalized passive hyperemia that results is usually referred to as **congestive heart failure.** Most often the underlying lesion is a valvular one. Depending on the nature of the lesion and its location within the heart, the primary tissue target for chronic passive hyperemia may be either the liver or the lungs. This makes sense if you merely reconstruct the routes of blood flow through the heart (Fig. 3.2). In the case of **pulmonic stenosis** (narrowing of the pulmonary valve), insufficient right ventricular emptying during right ventricular systole backs blood up into the right atrium and the vena caval system, and the primary target for the venous engorgement would be the liver. The same situation would prevail in **tricuspid insufficiency** in which blood is ejected through the insufficient tricuspid valve during right ventricular systole and eventually backs up through the right atrium and vena caval system to the liver. Hence, pulmonic stenosis and tricuspid insufficiency produce chronic passive hyperemia of the liver as the initial vascular bed to experience the engorgement.

On the left side of the heart, **aortic stenosis** tends to produce chronic passive hyperemia that first involves the lungs, as blood is backed up through the left

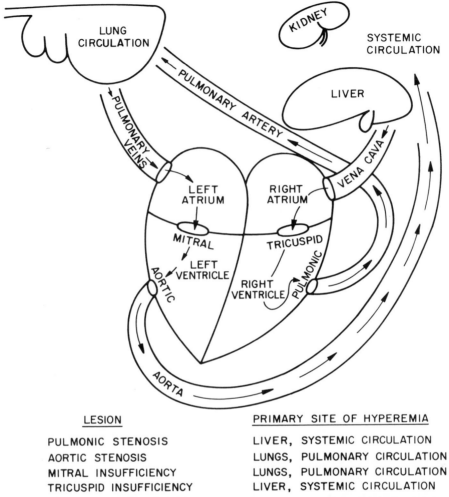

LESION	PRIMARY SITE OF HYPEREMIA
PULMONIC STENOSIS	LIVER, SYSTEMIC CIRCULATION
AORTIC STENOSIS	LUNGS, PULMONARY CIRCULATION
MITRAL INSUFFICIENCY	LUNGS, PULMONARY CIRCULATION
TRICUSPID INSUFFICIENCY	LIVER, SYSTEMIC CIRCULATION

Figure 3.2. Routes to Generalized Passive Hyperemia. The anatomic location of lesions involving cardiac valves is a major determinant of the primary site of passive hyperemia in other tissues.

atrium and pulmonary veins because of insufficient left ventricular ejection through the narrowed aortic orifice during left ventricular systole. By the same token, dogs with **mitral insufficiency,** a fairly common acquired valvular lesion, often first present with a chronic nonproductive cough that is related to chronic passive hyperemia and edema of the lungs. Here, the insufficient mitral valve allows blood to be ejected back into the left atrium and pulmonary veins during left ventricular systole. Congestive heart failure tends to be a progressive disorder, and, while

the organ distributions described above hold true initially, generalized hyperemia involving both the lungs and the liver eventually may be seen as the cardiac decompensation becomes more advanced.

Chronic generalized passive hyperemia also may accompany certain types of primary pulmonary disease in which there is progressive loss of the pulmonary vascular bed and consequent **pulmonary hypertension.** When heart failure occurs secondary to primary pulmonary disease, the syndrome is referred to as **cor pulmonale.** As pressure is greatly elevated in the normally low-pressure pulmonary arterial system, blood is backed up through the right side of the heart, and ascites and chronic passive hyperemia of the liver can result.

Appearance of Hyperemia

If a cut were made through a hyperemic tissue examined at necropsy, the cut surface would be excessively bloody. The reasons for this are obvious. It also is likely that edema would be encountered, as the congestion of capillary beds is closely allied with the development of edema. Hyperemia and edema are often found concurrently. This is particularly true in the case of the acute local active hyperemia of inflammation in which edema is almost always seen.

In chronic hyperemias, the engorgement of the tissues by poorly oxygenated venous blood often leads to a degree of chronic local hypoxia, which can produce degeneration or even necrosis of the relatively delicate cells of parenchymal organs. As the lungs and liver are the most common targets for chronic passive hyperemia, we will examine the characteristic changes in these tissues in more detail.

In chronic passive hyperemia of the **lungs,** the alveolar capillaries become engorged with blood, dilated, and sometimes tortuous. Many such small capillaries may rupture so that minute intra-alveolar hemorrhages occur. These extravascular red cells become the targets of the alveolar macrophages that phagocytize and break down the red cells, to eventually become laden with the hemoglobin breakdown pigment called **hemosiderin.** Indeed, the appearance of these hemosi-

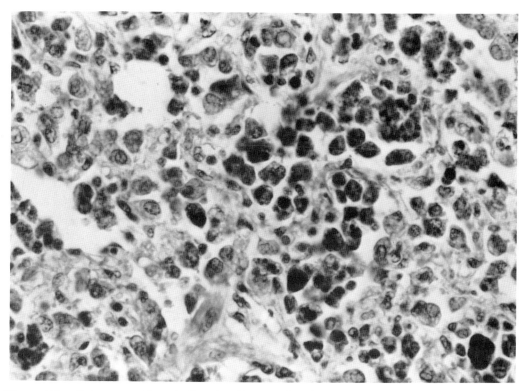

Figure 3.3. Pulmonary Chronic Passive Hyperemia. The persistent hyperemia and diapedesis of red cells leads to phagocytic degradation of the red cells to produce these dark-staining "heart-failure cells," or macrophages full of hemosiderin.

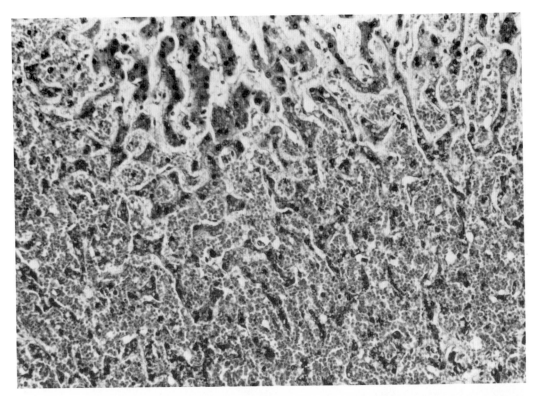

Figure 3.4. Hepatic Chronic Passive Hyperemia. The prolonged hyperemia and low-grade hypoxia has led to marked dilatation of hepatic sinusoids and atrophy of hepatic epithelial cells. Hepatic cords are reduced to thin wispy rows of cells.

derin-laden macrophages is so characteristic of chronic passive hyperemia of the lungs that they have become widely known as simply **"heart failure cells"** (Fig. 3.3). In severe forms of chronic passive pulmonary hyperemia, the alveolar walls themselves become widened both by edema fluid and by the dilated and engorged alveolar capillaries. Such edematous and hyperemic alveolar septa eventually can become fibrotic.

In chronic passive hyperemia of the **liver,** there is initially an overall increase in hepatic size owing to the volume and mass of added blood. Eventually, the chronic low-grade hypoxia and the pressure of the added blood in the widely dilated sinusoids will produce atrophy and loss of hepatic cord cells (Fig. 3.4). Such livers often exhibit a characteristically

mottled gross appearance referred to as **"nutmeg liver"** owing to the dark red appearance of the zones around the central veins and the yellow-brown appearance of the less affected parenchyma around the portal areas (Fig. 3.5). Hemosiderin-filled fixed macrophages (Kupffer cells) may be found in such livers for the same reasons that they are found in chronically hyperemic lungs. If sufficient time passes, there may be fibrous thickenings around the central veins in response to the increased blood pressure to which the area is being subjected. This fibrous tissue sometimes can extend even into the surrounding lobule creating a fairly distinctive pattern sometimes referred to as **"cardiac cirrhosis".**

It must again be stressed that in both the liver and the lung in chronic passive

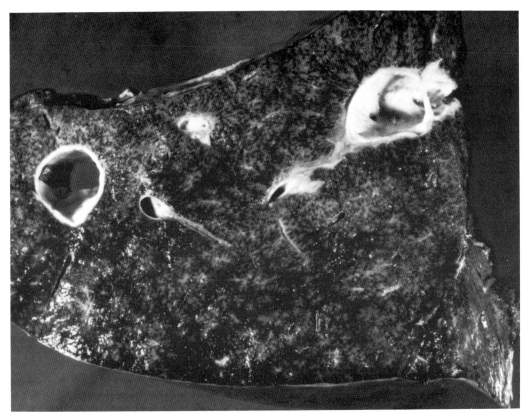

Figure 3.5. Hepatic Chronic Passive Hyperemia. Greatly dilated central vein regions and less involved portal areas give this cow's liver a distinctly mottled pattern called "nutmeg liver."

hyperemia, the real underlying lesion is not located in these tissues. Rather, the lung and liver end up expressing major pathologic changes because they bear the brunt of the pressure alterations created elsewhere, usually in the heart. The astute clinician or pathologist who encounters chronic passive hyperemia of the liver or lungs always conducts a thorough examination of the heart as the most likely underlying source of the problem.

HEMORRHAGE

The escape of blood from the cardiovascular system is known as **hemorrhage.** In the event that a substantial rent or tear is present in the blood vessel (or heart), then the flow of blood from the defect is substantial and is known as **hemorrhage by rhexis.** If only a small defect is present or if red cells merely pass through vascular structures in the process of, for example, hyperemia or inflammation, then the event is known as **hemorrhage by diapedesis.** Obviously, there are considerably different outcomes to these two events, and the clinical significance is similarly varied.

In either event, the escaped blood may accumulate within tissues or within tissue spaces to produce a three-dimensional extravascular clot known as a **hematoma** (Fig. 3.6). Small hematomas often result from simple venipuncture procedures and are especially common whenever blood is drawn from, or injections given into, the arteries. Hematomas are also frequently seen following trauma, where much of the visible lesion seen clinically is related to

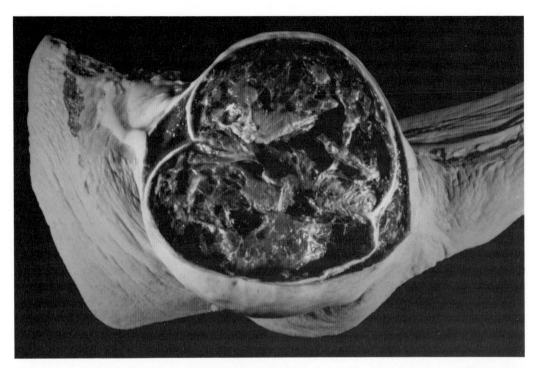

Figure 3.6.   Hematoma. The prominent three-dimensional mass of hemorrhage in this equine spleen is a hematoma. This hematoma is beginning to organize.

hemorrhage into tissue. The **significance** of this type of hemorrhage depends largely on the **site** of its accumulation, the **rate** of accumulation of the hemorrhage itself, and the total **volume** of blood lost, which will determine the size of the hematoma. A substantial subcutaneous or intramuscular hematoma may be awkward and painful, but it carries no great life-threatening significance. A much smaller subdural hematoma, on the other hand, may produce a comatose state due to the pressure it exerts on the brain within the bony anatomical confines of the calvaria.

The same processes which produce hematomas in tissue or in tissue spaces may lead to hemorrhage that is named differently in different anatomical locations. For example, if blood escapes into a serous cavity it is referred to as **hemopericardium, hemothorax,** or **hemoperitoneum.** Blood within the joint spaces is called **hemarthrosis,** and the coughing

up of blood clots from the trachea and bronchi is called **hemoptysis.** Bleeding from the nose is **epistaxis.** Most of these terms are really only regional derivatives useful to a particular organ or organ system. In all cases they basically represent hemorrhage, or **extravasation** of blood from vessels into extravascular sites.

Hemorrhages often are named by their size. For example, **petechial** hemorrhages (or petechiae) are minute, pin-point foci of hemorrhage up to 1 or 2 mm in size (Fig. 3.7). **Ecchymotic** hemorrhages (ecchymoses) are larger than petechiae and are usually blotchy or irregular areas up to 2 or 3 cm in size (Fig. 3.8). Extensive hemorrhage within the substance of a tissue is sometimes referred to as simply extravasation (Fig. 3.9). Sometimes hemorrhages are more linear or streaked in appearance, particularly on serosal or mucosal surfaces, and look at though a brush dipped in red paint was hastily

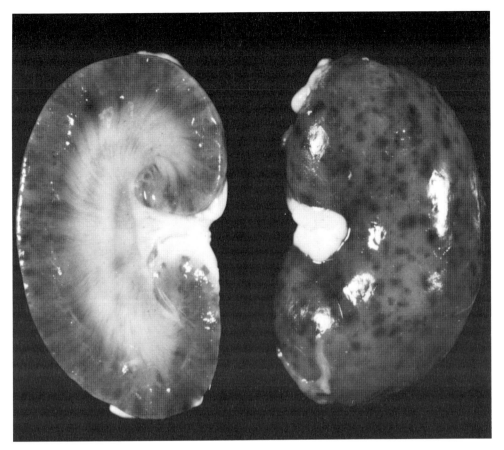

Figure 3.7. Petechiae. The multiple small hemorrhages on the kidney of this pup that died of *Herpesvirus* infection are petechial hemorrhages.

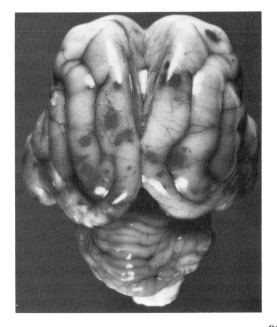

Figure 3.8. Ecchymoses. The blotchy hemorrhages on the brain of this cat are larger than petechiae and are called ecchymoses.

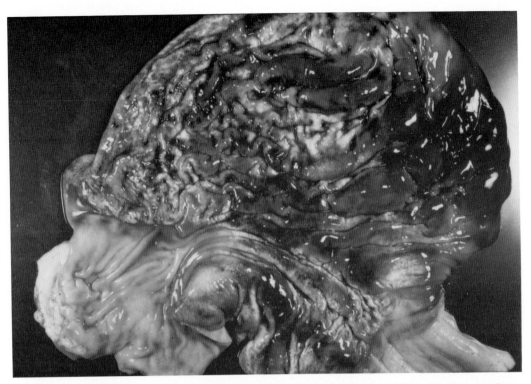

Figure 3.9. Hemorrhage. There has been considerable extravasation of blood in the gastric mucosa of this dog with renal failure (uremic gastritis).

splashed across the tissue. These hemorrhages are, appropriately, referred to as **paint brush** hemorrhages. When petechiae, ecchymoses, and even larger areas of hemorrhage are scattered on many body surfaces, the lesion is said to represent **purpura.** Many of these terms are useful for communication purposes if nothing else. When the pathologist tells the clinician that there were many petechiae and ecchymoses found on the capsular surfaces of the kidneys of a patient recently necropsied, the terms bring to mind a specific image of what the tissue looked like.

Causes of Hemorrhage

There are many kinds of disease backgrounds that can lead to hemorrhage. In domestic animals surely the most common cause is **trauma.** In general, hemorrhage is a nonspecific lesion; it suggests only that vascular injury of some kind has occurred. Despite its lack of specific-

ity, there are some useful and repeatable patterns that can be helpful to the practicing pathologist and clinician.

Widespread petechiae and ecchymoses often suggest a septicemic, viremic, or toxemic condition in which systemic damage to many small vascular radicals has occurred. Hemoperitoneum, on the other hand, would be caused by local blood loss into the abdominal cavity and the underlying cause most likely would be located in proximity to that cavity itself. Subcutaneous or intramuscular hemorrhage is often a manifestation of trauma.

Hemorrhage often is associated with a variety of disorders of the coagulation mechanism. Prothrombin deficiency may be encountered as an acquired condition in vitamin K deficiency or in some diffuse liver diseases. Several of the clotting factors are vitamin K–dependent. Synthesis by the liver of Christmas factor (factor IX), proconvertin (VII), Stuart-Prower factor (X) as well as prothrombin (II) depend upon the availability of vitamin K. Vitamin K is required for the transformation of protein precursors into the structure of these clotting factors. Cattle fed **dicoumarol** (which is abundant in lush sweet clover) can develop a devastating hemorrhagic disorder associated with prolongation of the clotting time, which is actually due to prothrombin (II) deficiency. Dicoumarol and the related **Warfarin** (a widely used rat poison) have structural similarities to vitamin K and presumably exert their effect by competitive inhibition.

Hereditary deficiencies of coagulation factors, such as **hemophilia,** often become clinically significant due to hemorrhage. Similarly, thrombocytopenia leads to abnormal bleeding tendencies because there are too few platelets to aggregate and form the initial hemostatic plug as a nidus for clot formation. In many of these situations, defects in the clotting mechanism predispose the patient to the development of substantial hemorrhage from relatively trivial traumatic damage to small vessels. This increased tendency toward hemorrhage in the clotting deficiency syndromes is responsible for their being grouped under the name **hemorrhagic diatheses.** Because the various specific etiologic factors related to hemorrhage are more properly the domain of special pathology, we will not detail them here. Of greater concern to us from the standpoint of disease mechanisms is developing an understanding of the potential significance of hemorrhage and the ways in which extravascular blood is handled by the body.

Clinical Significance and Outcome of Hemorrhage

As we mentioned above, the clinical significance of hemorrhage depends largely on three things: **where, how fast,** and **how much.**

The **location** of hemorrhage, by itself and independent of volume considerations, narrows our view to two critical sites: the central nervous system and the heart. Even a small amount of hemorrhage into the brain parenchyma can have a disastrous outcome if it interrupts or interferes with vital functions. This might be especially true of hemorrhage into the brain stem or medulla. The all too common **stroke** or **cerebrovascular accident** in man produces clinical signs not by virtue of the underlying vascular disease but because hemorrhage (and sometimes infarction) has occurred in the brain. Similarly, extracerebral but intracranial hemorrhage is always potentially dangerous because of the space limitations of the calvaria. **Subdural hematomas** thus can produce the same sort of clinical signs as might an abscess or a neoplasm that compresses the brain from without.

The heart is similarly vulnerable because intramyocardial hemorrhage may weaken or destroy vital cardiac muscle cells or may interrupt important conduction pathways. In like fashion, hemopericardium (which is the heart's answer to the brain's subdural hematoma) can be serious because of **pressure** on the heart from without, which impairs diastolic filling and therefore adversely affects cardiac output. **Cardiac tamponade** refers to a specific syndrome of acute cardiac failure which is caused by massive hemopericardium (Fig. 3.10).

In contrast to the situation in the central nervous system and the heart, most tissues can tolerate some hemorrhage without undue loss of function. When substantial hemorrhage occurs in any tissue, however, clinical disease may result. Thus, the **volume** of blood lost becomes important, not only to the potential effects on the tissues where the hemorrhage occurred, but to the body as a whole should sufficient blood be lost to lead to the syndrome of **hemorrhagic shock.** This form of shock occurs when blood loss has been sufficient to result in an impairment of peripheral perfusion. The critical volume of blood loss necessary to produce shock

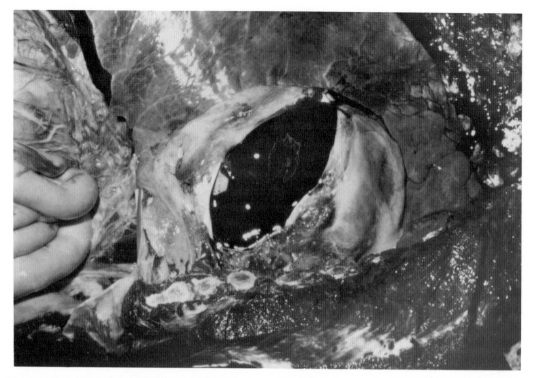

Figure 3.10.   Hemopericardium. Massive hemorrhage into the pericardial space. Such lesions compress the heart and produce "cardiac tamponade."

varies with the rate of hemorrhage, but it is generally in the neighborhood of 20–40% of the total blood volume. Because this syndrome is based on blood loss it is often referred to as **hypovolemic shock** to reflect the underlying problem. The more rapid the hemorrhage, the less will be the total volume of lost blood required to produce shock.

Shock has so many variable features and so many pathophysiologic implications and pathogenetic sequences that it is difficult to construct a meaningful brief definition. It is basically a clinical term meaning **peripheral circulatory failure.** This results in inadequate perfusion of tissue cells with a resultant imbalance between the available vascular supply and the metabolic needs of the cells and tissues. Cellular hypoxia results, which leads to a decline in aerobic glycolysis and an increase in anaerobic glycolysis. This in

turn leads to increased production of lactic acid, and the resultant metabolic acidosis further perpetuates cellular injury (*see also* Chapter 2). This vicious circle eventually leads to peripheral vascular collapse, visceral pooling of blood, and inadequate central perfusion, which ultimately can be fatal. It is beyond our scope here to discuss the fascinating subject of shock in detail. Readers seeking additional information should consult the reading list at the end of the chapter.

We have mentioned previously that the **rate** of hemorrhage may play an important role in determining the outcome of bleeding. Extremely slow blood loss, as might occur through a chronic inflammatory lesion in the stomach, is probably of less significance than the underlying lesion actually responsible for producing the hemorrhage. On the other hand, an acute gastric ulcer may hemorrhage profusely into the lumen of the stomach and intestinal tract, and the patient may in fact die of shock before a single indication of blood has appeared in the feces. In these two situations, the **amount** of blood lost may be similar. That is, over a period of months the chronic gastric inflammatory lesion may produce a volume of blood loss by diapedesis equal to that lost by rhexis in the acutely fatal gastric ulcer. The volume is the same, but the clinical significance is different because the **rate** of blood loss is clearly different.

It is also worth noting that in clinical settings where a small amount of blood is lost over a long period of time, such as the gastric inflammatory lesion mentioned above, the host has time to invoke different adaptive responses such as increased blood production (**hematopoiesis**). These adaptive responses usually take time to occur, which helps to further explain why different clinical outcomes attend different **rates** of blood loss.

Resolution of Hemorrhage

After hemorrhage has occurred, the problem for the patient is a simple one. What now happens to the blood? Assuming that the hemorrhage has not been fatal and that the bleeding has been arrested, there are really only two options open for the resolution of hemorrhage into tissue spaces. It is either **resorbed** or it must be **organized.** Which of these options actually occurs depends on several factors, and in many situations probably both apply.

Because extravascular blood tends to clot, the opportunity for resorption of fluid blood is usually limited. As the clot contracts, there may be local plasma, which has been expressed from the clot, to resorb. Usually, however, much of the blood lost to hemorrhage must be handled by the processes of phagocytosis and organization. In an **organizing hematoma** (Fig. 3.6), the mass of fibrin and red cells

is surrounded by vascular connective tissue that supplies the nutritive and supporting structures necessary to sustain the phagocytes that leave the blood stream and enter the hematoma. Here they phagocytose and degrade both the fibrin and the red cells themselves. Such phagocytes often become ladened with **hemosiderin,** a breakdown product of hemoglobin, which often is abundant in sites of old hemorrhage. The process of organization of a hematoma is very similar to the organization of a thrombus, which we will discuss in a later section.

THROMBOSIS

General Background

Blood is normally a flowing fluid within the vascular conduits of the cardiovascular system. When a solid mass is formed within the blood vessels or the heart from the constituents of the blood, the process is called **thrombosis,** and the resultant mass is called a **thrombus.** If several are formed they are called **thrombi.** If pieces of a thrombus break off from the original mass and sail downstream in the flowing bloodstream to lodge at a distant site, that process is called **embolism,** and the mass that broke off and lodged at the distant site is called an **embolus.** If several of these are present they are **emboli.**

It is difficult to make a clear definitional distinction between a **thrombus** and a **blood clot,** since the two are clearly related. A thrombus is essentially a pathologic type of blood clot which is formed **intravascularly,** that is, within the vascular system. A blood clot, on the other hand, differs from a thrombus since **blood coagulation** is a physiological necessity whereas **thrombosis** is a pathological manifestation of blood coagulation. The classical definition of a thrombus also states that it is attached to the vessel wall. Such attachments are not always easy to find. Perhaps the simplest way to solve this definitional problem is to consider thrombi as a special subset of blood clots, formed under pathologic conditions. The **chicken-fat clot** commonly seen at necropsy in horses is really a plasma clot that develops because of spontaneous erythrocyte **rouleaux** formation and the rapid sedimentation rate of red cells in equine blood; this type of postmortem clot therefore is gelatinous in appearance and contains relatively few red cells. Chicken-fat clots are intravascular, but they are not thrombi because they are not pathological.

Normal blood coagulation often takes place largely extravascularly, for example in the arrest of hemorrhage, and is often referred to as **hemostasis** to distinguish it from the process of **thrombosis,** or **thrombogenesis.** Both hemostasis and thrombosis involve **coagulation of the blood.** Hemostasis, or clotting of the blood, is a vital physiological process necessary to life; thrombosis is a pathologic event.

With the recent rapid advances in the field of coagulation and thrombosis research, it is difficult to present the subject in a relevant and contemporary factual manner without losing sight of the classical pathology of thrombosis, which is essential to an understanding of the process. We hope here to provide a contemporary synopsis of the pathogenesis of thrombosis, one which presents it as a dynamic process involving the interplay of many factors and forces present in the blood and the living blood vessels. In this context, thrombosis may be viewed as an abnormal or exaggerated expression of the hemostatic mechanism, and often involves underlying vascular damage. A good example of this is the thrombosis that can follow coronary artery disease in man. Thrombosis also often involves hemodynamic adjustments. Nonetheless, the cornerstone of the process of thrombosis is the coagulation of the blood, and we will begin our study of thrombosis by reviewing the mechanisms by which this fascinating biological phenomenon occurs.

Overview of Blood Coagulation

Scientists have long marvelled at the curious way in which fluid blood transforms into a solid coagulum when it leaves the vascular system. Indeed, curiosity about the coagulation of the blood can be traced to antiquity. Blood coagulation involves a delicate interplay between the vascular tissues themselves and the blood cells and plasma. After injury, the vessel walls have the unique ability to constrict and to provide a variety of platelet and plasma protein activators and inhibitors. The platelets, by the processes of adhesion and aggregation, provide the initial means of arresting blood loss. The plasma protein constituents of the coagulation process serve to provide local fibrin formation to impart structural solidity to the platelet plug at the site of injury and to ultimately contribute to the tissue repair process. As in many other complicated biological events, a variety of chemical signals, which initiate and terminate different stages of the process, serve to amplify and dampen the coagulation events with a built-in system of checks and balances. Many of these initiation and control events are carefully coordinated enzymatic reactions. Things which disturb this delicate balance disturb the entire system and the result is usually a pathological manifestation of the coagulation process: either too much at the wrong time and place (thrombosis), or too little when needed the most (hemorrhage). These abnormalities of the coagulation mechanism can be either localized or disseminated.

In order to appreciate abnormalities that can result from defective function of the coagulation mechanism, it is necessary for us to understand the various coagulation factor interactions which ultimately produce the fibrin clot. It is not our intention to review *ad nauseam* the incredible amount of biochemical detail available regarding blood coagulation. We do feel strongly, however, that students with a good grasp of the players in this drama and their various interactions have a much better chance to actually understand the process of thrombosis. Those seeking information beyond what is provided here are referred to the reading list at the end of this chapter.

Mechanisms of Blood Coagulation

An explanatory note regarding terminology seems an appropriate beginning to this discussion. Most clotting factors are enzymes (proteins) or coenzymes that are synthesized independently. They are gen-

Table 3.2
Coagulation Factors

Factor	Name	Properties and Functions
I	Fibrinogen	M_r 340,000; 6 disulfide-linked peptide chains; converted by thrombin to fibrin monomer
II	Prothrombin	M_r 72,500; single chain glycoprotein; circulating precursor converted to thrombin by factor Xa proteinase
III	Tissue thromboplastin	Several biochemical identities; markedly shortens clotting time; initiates extrinsic system; tissue factor
IV	Divalent calcium	Cofactor in several activation steps; forms molecular bridges
V	Proaccelerin	M_r 350,000; glycoprotein; participates with factor Xa in prothrombin activation
VI	(There is no factor VI in current terminology)	
VII	Proconvertin	M_r about 50,000; single polypeptide chain glycoprotein; precursor of proteinase that activates factor X
VIII	Antihemophiliac factor	Ambiguity in molecular weight; accessory protein with factor IXa in intrinsic activation of factor X
IX	Christmas factor	M_r 56,000; single polypeptide chain glycoprotein; participates in intrinsic activation of factor X
X	Stuart-Prower factor	M_r 56,000; two polypeptide chain glycoprotein, precursor of proteinase that converts prothrombin to thrombin
XI	Plasma thromboplastin antecedent	M_r 124,000 (bovine); two equal polypeptide chains in disulfide linkage; precursor of factor XIa which converts IX to IXa; Hageman factor substrate
XII	Hageman factor	M_r 80,000; single polypeptide chain glycoprotein; initiates intrinsic (contact) coagulation system
XIII	Fibrin stabilizing factor	M_r 320,000; four different peptide chains; precursor of transglutaminase which covalently crosslinks fibrin monomers to fibrin polymer
(None)	Prekallikrein (Fletcher factor)	M_r 88,000; single polypeptide chain; precursor of proteinase kallikrein; participates in cleavage of XII to form XIIa
(None)	High molecular weight kininogen (Fitzgerald factor)	M_r 76,000 (bovine); single polypeptide chain glycoprotein; accessory protein in factor XII–factor XI activation scheme

erally present in the plasma in an inactive **zymogen** form and must be "activated" to become biologically functional in the clotting mechanism. This activation is accomplished either by the activated form of the clotting factor's predecessor or, more often, by a complex composed of activated and nonactivated components. Much of the activation process takes place on surfaces of one kind or another. In the presently accepted nomenclature (Table 3.2), Roman numerals refer to the **inactive precursor** state (zymogen) of the various clotting factors, whereas the **active form** is designated by the letter "a" following the Roman numeral. The coagulation factors also have names. Indeed, they often have several names as a natural outgrowth of the sequence of discovery, and recent advances in our understanding of coagulation have lengthened the list of participating coagulation factors.

In our discussions here, we have tried to utilize the most commonly used names as well as their Roman numerals. Thus, we will refer to prothrombin (II), thrombin (IIa), plasma thromboplastin antecedent (XI), and activated Hageman factor (XIIa) by both name and numeral. You will note that not all of the coagulation factors have Roman numerals. For example, prekallikrein and high molecular weight kininogen are not numbered although they are important to the activation of Hageman factor (XII). von Willebrand factor and protein C also did not make the numbered list. In like fashion, the numbered list does not include platelets, although they are clearly of critical importance in coagulation. Other cofactors, such as divalent calcium (IV), however, are both named and numbered. To round things out, there is no factor VI. It is almost inevitable that some confusion will result from this complex terminology. In this regard, we can only suggest that "familiarity breeds contentment."

At a simplistic level, clot formation consists of the conversion of a soluble plasma protein called **fibrinogen** (I) into an insoluble polymer called **fibrin** by the action of an enzyme called **thrombin** (IIa). Accomplishing this involves the sequential interaction of a large number of plasma proteins as well as some derived from tissue cells, phospholipid membrane surfaces derived largely from platelets, divalent calcium (IV), a variety of other full-time and part-time reactants, and an equally complicated system of control mechanisms.

It must be stressed that much of our understanding of blood coagulation has been acquired primarily in the test tube and not in living animals. We must recall, however, that hemostasis in the living animal involves phenomena that take place on the surfaces of biological membranes, not the walls of test tubes, and that *in vitro* systems may only partly reflect the processes by which hemostasis and thrombosis are triggered in living tissues. There are few laboratory containers in which normal blood will *not* clot unless anticoagulants are added; thus there is a fundamental difference between the fluidity of the blood in clotting tubes and that in the circulation. The key issue, it seems to us, is not to explain why blood clots in a tube, but to understand why it does *not* clot *in vivo*. This issue is much easier to raise than to resolve. Nonetheless, the disease states in which one or more of the clotting proteins or regulatory molecules are deficient generally have confirmed or extended what was discerned based on test tube data. In addition, many of the coagulation proteins and regulatory molecules were, in fact, discovered through the study of living patients with hemostatic problems. These "experiments of nature" have proven to be invaluable in validating the scientific data from the laboratory. Examples are scattered throughout our discussion, and we will briefly highlight three examples here to illustrate the value of a contemporary biochemical understanding of disease **prior** to our discussion of coagulation in the hope of making the entire business more *real* for students.

1. It has long been known that fibrinogen is essential for platelet aggregation and that platelet aggregation is a crucial step in normal hemostasis. **Glanzmann's thrombasthenia** is a rare congenital hemorrhagic disorder in which the platelets have defective aggregation responses. Platelets from such patients do not bind fibrinogen, and two major platelet membrane glycoproteins, the **GP IIb-IIIa complex,** are markedly diminished or absent in such patients. As a result, these patients have bleeding tendencies and poor clot retraction. Glanzmann's patients have allowed the demonstration that the GP IIb-IIIA complex is in fact the platelet fibrinogen receptor, and the clotting defect in these patients has thus been explained in molecular terms. Beyond that, such patients have contributed much to our understanding of platelet function in normal hemostasis.

2. The **von Willebrand factor complex** is a noncovalent association of two biologically important proteins; one, antihemophilic factor (VIII), is a procoagulant cofactor that is deficient in **hemophilia A,** and the other, **von Willebrand factor** (vWF), is a large glycoprotein with an essential role in primary hemostasis and is deficient or dysfunctional in **von Willebrand disease.** Patients with this disease have recurrent episodes of mucocutaneous bleeding, bruising, epistaxis, and gingival hemorrhage. von Willebrand factor is essential for platelet adhesion to subendothelial collagen that is exposed by vessel wall damage. It is synthesized and secreted by endothelial cells, and it binds to subendothelial type I and type III collagen. When vascular damage occurs, the initial platelet adhesion to the damaged site is mediated by platelets binding to this collagen-bound von Willebrand factor *via* specific surface receptors on platelets. von Willebrand disease has been extensively studied in swine. Pigs homozygous for the defect have a hemophilia-like condition and exhibit the same impairments of primary hemostasis noted in the severe form of the disease in man: serious hemorrhagic tendencies, a prolonged bleeding time, reduced platelet adhesion, very low (3% of normal) levels of von Willebrand factor, and reduced levels of antihemophilic factor (VIII) coagulant activity. Such pigs have also stimulated investigations into the role of platelets in coronary atherosclerosis and thrombosis, since the absence of vWF may be responsible, in part, for the impaired platelet–arterial wall interactions and resistance to atherosclerosis and thrombosis found in these animals. Thus, the ability to define the defect in von Willebrand patients at a molecular level has greatly increased our understanding of both normal hemostatic mechanisms and thrombosis.

3. Unlike most of the coagulation factors, **protein C** was discovered and its basic biological functions determined by a combination of biochemical and physiological experiments before its clinical relevance was understood. Only recently has clinical information been obtained linking protein C to thrombotic disease. Protein C interacts with thrombin (IIa) bound to a specific endothelial cell receptor **(thrombomodulin),** which results in the activation of protein C (*see* Fig. 3.17). The activated protein C subsequently serves a regulatory role in hemostasis by inactivating proaccelerin (V) and antihemophilic factor (VIII). All of the biochemical data from the laboratory suggested that protein C was an important regulatory molecule and that a deficiency in protein C would be associated with thrombotic tendencies. A screening program was initiated, and such patients were subsequently identified. Protein C deficiency was found to be associated with recurrent thrombotic tendencies in the

heterozygote and early, lethal thrombosis in the homozygote. Once again, the biochemical and clinical data correlated well.

These few examples are taken from many and serve to collectively emphasize that an understanding of coagulation at the molecular level has very real clinical significance. We reiterate this point since students sometimes feel overwhelmed by the abundant detail inherent in blood coagulation. All complexity is, however, relative. Anyone who has survived calculus and organic chemistry, as many of our students have, should find the level of detail presented here to be absolutely refreshing.

For our purposes, we will divide the clotting process into four major steps of importance rather than paying specific attention to all of the intricacies of the coagulation scheme. We will consider (1) the activation process and the early steps in coagulation, (2) the formation of the enzyme-activated Stuart-Prower factor (Xa) as a central character around which the intrinsic and extrinsic coagulation systems meet, (3) the formation of the enzyme thrombin (IIa), and (4) the formation of fibrin.

Activation Process and Early Steps in Coagulation

Traditionally, the clotting system has been divided into two pathways (Fig. 3.11). The **intrinsic** pathway involves components normally present in the circulation, and the **extrinsic** pathway involves a "tissue factor" in addition to blood components. These alternate activation mechanisms are reflected in the main screening tests used in the clinical pathology laboratory to examine the coagulation cascade, **prothrombin time** (PT) and **activated partial thromboplastin time** (APTT); PT reflects extrinsic system activation, and APTT reflects intrinsic system activation. The two activation systems merge around the activation of Stuart-Prower factor (X) into a final com-

mon pathway leading to fibrin formation (Fig. 3.12).

In the **intrinsic** pathway or "contact" system, activation revolves around the cleavage of **Hageman factor** (XII). Hageman factor (XII) is a surface-sensitive single polypeptide chain protein with an M_r of about 80,000. Native Hageman factor (XII) is converted to activated Hageman factor (XIIa) by cleavage of one or more internal peptide bonds to yield two chains linked by disulfide bridges. The aminoterminal end of the heavy chain contains surface **binding** sites, while the carboxy-terminal end of the lighter chain contains the active **proteolytic** site. The cleavage of Hageman factor (XII) can occur in several ways and usually involves activation on a negatively charged surface. Collagen (particularly types I and III) exposed by vascular injury presumably forms the usual *in vivo* substrate upon which activation takes place, but other surfaces also suffice.

Factor XIIa becomes bound to the negatively charged surface *via* the surface binding sites on its heavy chain, and, once bound, has the ability to activate **prekallikrein** and **plasma thromboplastin antecedent** (PTA, XI), utilizing the proteolytic sites on its light chain. These activities are enhanced by **high molecular weight kininogen** (HMW kininogen), which acts as an important cofactor. This is not a simple affair. At least four proteins seem to be involved in this set of activation reactions; Hageman factor (XII) itself, prekallikrein, plasma thromboplastin antecedent (XI), and HMW kininogen, and the precise sequence of biochemical reactions that ultimately results in the cleavage of PTA (XI) is still not entirely clear. It appears that Hageman factor (XII), prekallikrein, and HMW kininogen are assembled when plasma contacts a negatively charged surface, and the resultant activity can cleave PTA (XI) to initiate the "waterfall cascade" of intrinsic coagulation.

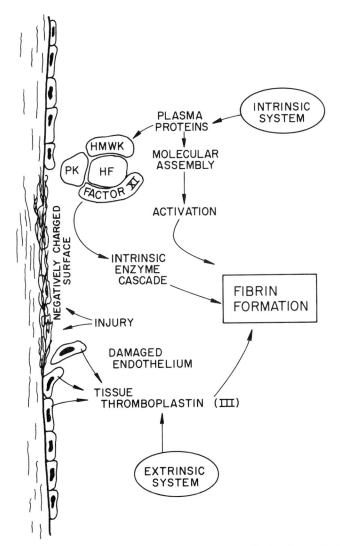

Figure 3.11.   Blood Coagulation. Vascular injury exposes negatively charged subendothelial structures upon which the contact activation (intrinsic) system can be assembled and activated, and extrinsic activation proceeds with expression of tissue thromboplastin (III) by injured endothelium. (*HF*, Hageman factor (XII); *PK*, prekallikrein; *HMWK*, high molecular weight kininogen).

The major regulator of this system appears to be the same molecule as the inhibitor of activated complement component C1 (C1 esterase inhibitor, **C1-INH**), the deficiency of which is not manifested in blood coagulation, but as **hereditary angioedema.** C1-INH contributes about 90% of the inhibitory activity in normal plasma toward activated Hageman factor (XIIa).

In the intrinsic system, most of the components exist in plasma in precursor form and become sequentially activated through cleavage by an active enzyme generated during the previous step (Fig. 3.11). Thus, activated Hageman factor (XIIa) cleaves PTA (XI) to produce a proteinase (XIa) that functions as a proteolytic enzyme to activate **Christmas factor** (IX). Activated Christmas factor (IXa)

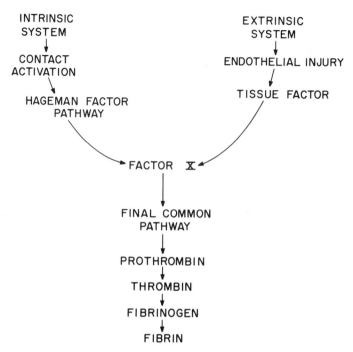

Figure 3.12. Pathways to Fibrin Formation. The extrinsic and intrinsic pathways join around factor X activation into a final common pathway leading to fibrin formation.

then combines with **antihemophilic factor** (VIII), which along with **proaccelerin** (V), phospholipids, and divalent calcium (IV) activate the **Stuart-Prower** factor (X).

The relative importance of the "contact" or intrinsic system to normal blood coagulation is unclear because patients with Hageman factor (XII), prekallikrein, or HMW kininogen deficiency do not exhibit bleeding tendencies or deficiencies in the inflammatory response. Only PTA (XI) deficiency is associated with a mild bleeding state. The Hageman factor (XII) pathways, however, may be more important in a broader setting in the inflammatory response, since they link together other plasma proteolytic pathways capable of generating inflammatory mediators like bradykinin as well as fibrinolytic activity (*see* Chapter 4). The relative importance of such basic processes as inflammation, blood coagulation, and fibrinolysis

is underscored by the extreme redundancy of available initiating pathways.

The **extrinsic** system is so named because its major initiator, "tissue factor", "thromboplastin" or the term we will use, **tissue thromboplastin** (III), is found in tissue rather than blood. Tissue thromboplastin (III) is an integral membrane glycoprotein which is found in most tissues and apparently comes largely from endothelial cells, with some coming apparently from fibroblasts, smooth muscle cells, or from injured cells of other types. Its structural identity is less secure than most of the other factors, and efforts to elucidate the molecular nature of "tissue factor" have spanned most of this century. It apparently exists as a membrane-bound glycoprotein that forms a stable complex with lipid and has a M_r of around 52,000. The structural similarities of many human and bovine coagulation proteins and the activity of human tissue thromboplastin (III) with bovine enzymes predict that the basic features of tissue thromboplastin (III) action will be similar in many species.

The extrinsic system begins with tissue thromboplastin (III) existing in a sort of protected state within the plasma membrane. Upon endothelial injury, it can be released into the circulation to form a complex with **proconvertin** (VII) in the presence of divalent calcium (IV). Proconvertin (VII) is a vitamin K–dependent protein. The activity of the complex of tissue thromboplastin (III) and proconvertin (VII) seems to be largely dependent on the concentration of tissue thromboplastin (III), although the subsequent enzymatic activity generated and the proteolytic activation of Stuart-Prower factor (X) *via* this extrinsic pathway resides in the activated proconvertin (VIIa) molecule. It is clear, however, that proconvertin (VII) and its activated form (VIIa)

have an obligate requirement for tissue thromboplastin (III) in order to interact with their substrate proteins.

Formation of Activated Stuart-Prower Factor (Xa)

As we have indicated above, the active enzyme Xa can be derived from the inactive glycoprotein precursor Stuart-Prower factor (X) *via* both the intrinsic and extrinsic coagulation pathways (Fig. 3.13). In the extrinsic pathway, released tissue thromboplastin (III) in a complex with proconvertin (VII) and in the presence of divalent calcium (IV) form a molecular complex that can generate the active enzyme Xa from native Stuart-Prower factor (X). Clot formation *via* the extrinsic system is remarkably more rapid than it is *via* the intrinsic pathway. Indeed, clotting tests, which may take several minutes in intrinsic system assays, are accelerated to about 10–15 sec when tissue

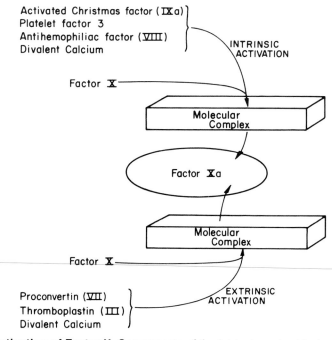

Figure 3.13. Activation of Factor X. Components of the intrinsic and extrinsic pathways each form a molecular complex with Stuart-Prower factor (X), which results in its cleavage to form activated Xa.

thromboplastin (III) is added to initiate activation of the extrinsic system. The reason for this is not entirely clear, but it appears to be due to the increased activation of Stuart-Prower factor (X) *via* the extrinsic system in a reaction catalyzed by proconvertin (VII). In short, this is essentially a single-step reaction in the extrinsic system, whereas several sequential steps are required to activate Stuart-Prower factor (X) via the intrinsic pathways (*see* Fig. 3.11). Recent evidence indicates that proconvertin (VII) can also attack Christmas factor (IX) to produce activated Christmas factor (IXa), thus providing yet another link between the extrinsic and intrinsic coagulation pathways. This story will no doubt continue to unfold.

The intrinsic pathway to Stuart-Prower factor (X) activation involves the participation of activated Christmas factor (IXa), antihemophilic factor (VIII), phospholipids (platelet factor 3), and divalent calcium (IV). These various factors again form a complex, and it is the complex that generates the enzyme Xa from native Stuart-Prower factor (X). In this reaction it is believed that antihemophilic factor (VIII) plays a regulatory role, while activated Christmas factor (IXa) serves as the cleaving enzyme. Indeed, activated Christmas factor (IXa) alone can cleave Stuart-Prower factor (X) to Xa, but the reaction is greatly accelerated in the presence of the other components. Antihemophilic factor (VIII) in this setting appears somehow altered, probably by thrombin, and this alteration seems to be required for its functioning in the complex. Activated Christmas factor (IXa) serves as the cleaving enzyme. Indeed, activated (VIII) for this purpose. Thus, intrinsic activation of Stuart-Prower factor (X) is greatly aided by prior cleavage of Stuart-Prower factor (X) *via* extrinsic activation to provide Xa, or by thrombin (II) generation in order to suitably "alter" antihemophilic factor (VIII) for its participa-

tion in the intrinsic activation of Stuart-Prower factor (X). Given these subtleties, it is not surprising that the extrinsic system is much more rapid.

The actual activation of Stuart-Prower factor (X) to Xa is a proteolytic process in which the native molecule is cleaved to release one or more polypeptide fragments, one of which becomes the active enzyme Xa, which figures prominently in the activation of prothrombin (II) to form the enzyme thrombin (IIa).

Formation of Thrombin

The active enzyme **thrombin** (IIa) is derived from its inactive precursor protein prothrombin (II). **Prothrombin** (II) is a constituent of normal plasma, where it circulates as a single polypeptide chain glycoprotein with a M_r about 70,000. Prothrombin (II) is a vitamin K–dependent factor synthesized in the liver. Thrombin (IIa) itself is about half the size of prothrombin (II) and usually has two polypeptide chains linked by a disulfide bridge.

The conversion of prothrombin (II) to thrombin (IIa) occurs in several steps. Activated Stuart-Prower factor (Xa) is the enzyme basically responsible for cleaving two essential peptide bonds in prothrombin (II) to produce thrombin (IIa). While factor Xa can cleave prothrombin (II) by itself, it functions optimally when linked with proaccelerin (V), divalent calcium (IV), and phospholipids derived primarily from platelets (platelet factor 3, phosphatidylinositol, and phosphatidyl-L-serine). Thus, a molecular complex of all five components is formed, and under these conditions optimal thrombin (IIa) generation occurs (Fig. 3.14). If any one of the five components that comprise the complex is reduced in concentration, there is a corresponding reduction in the rate and amount of thrombin (IIa) generation. Thus, despite the delicacy and complexity of the reaction, a precise quantitative relationship between the components seems to be essential. Thrombin (IIa) attacks only the

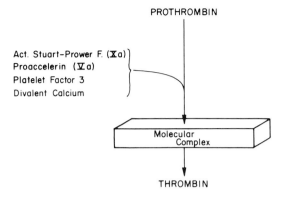

PROTHROMBIN

Act. Stuart–Prower F. (**X**a)
Proaccelerin (**V**a)
Platelet Factor 3
Divalent Calcium

Molecular
Complex

THROMBIN

Figure 3.14. Formation of Thrombin. The cleavage of prothrombin (II) requires phospholipids (platelet factor 3) as a surface upon which the enzyme Xa, the determiner (factor V), and the substrate (prothrombin II) interact in a complex mediated by divalent calcium (IV).

amino-terminal region of specific chains within the fibrinogen (I) molecule where it breaks specific arginyl-glycine peptide bonds. Its activity in the production of fibrin is explained more fully in the next section.

Formation of Fibrin

While we might consider the penultimate stage in the coagulation process to be the critical conversion of prothrombin (II) to thrombin (IIa), it is the formation of **fibrin** that is the visible end point of all of the preceding biochemical intricacies. It is easier to understand the events associated with fibrin formation if we dis-

sect the process into three distinct phases: (1) the proteolysis of fibrinogen (I), (2) the polymerization of fibrin monomers, and (3) the stabilization or cross-linking of fibrin (Fig. 3.15).

PROTEOLYSIS OF FIBRINOGEN. It will facilitate our understanding of this process if we first take a look at the fibrinogen (I) molecule (Fig. 3.16). It consists of three pairs of disulfide-linked polypeptide chains which are designated $(A_\alpha)_2$, $(B_\beta)_2$, and γ_2. In the proteolytic phase of fibrin formation, the enzyme thrombin (IIa) attacks the amino-terminal region of the A_α and B_β chains and splits specific arginyl-glycine peptide bonds to release a pair of

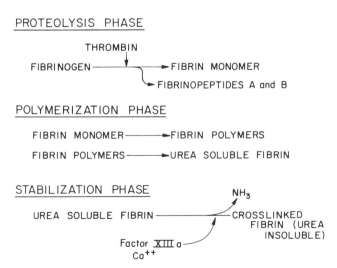

PROTEOLYSIS PHASE

THROMBIN

FIBRINOGEN ⟶ FIBRIN MONOMER
⟶ FIBRINOPEPTIDES A and B

POLYMERIZATION PHASE

FIBRIN MONOMER ⟶ FIBRIN POLYMERS

FIBRIN POLYMERS ⟶ UREA SOLUBLE FIBRIN

STABILIZATION PHASE

NH_3

UREA SOLUBLE FIBRIN ⟶ CROSSLINKED FIBRIN (UREA INSOLUBLE)

Factor **XIII** a
Ca^{++}

Figure 3.15.   Phases of Fibrin Formation. Fibrinogen is acted on by thrombin (IIa) to produce fibrin monomers, which are first spontaneously polymerized and then stabilized by factor XIIIa.

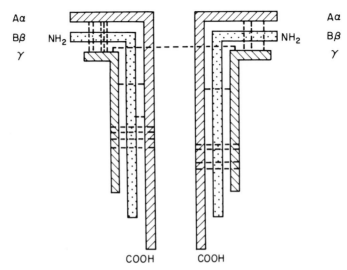

Aα
Bβ
γ   NH₂   NH₂   Aα
                                                                       Bβ
                                                                       γ

COOH   COOH

Figure 3.16. Fibrinogen Molecule. Three pairs of disulfide-linked peptide chains designated $(A_\alpha)_2$, $(B_\beta)_2$, and γ_2 make up the native molecule. This is a dimeric molecule as shown, and the dashed lines indicate the disulfide bonds. The cleavage site by thrombin (IIa) is located near the N-terminal end of both subunits of the A_α and B_β chains.

peptides from the native fibrinogen (I) molecule. These are called **fibrinopeptides** A and B. The γ chains of the native fibrinogen (I) molecule are not involved in this process, and the resultant molecule (consisting of fibrinogen minus the fibrinopeptides A and B) is called **fibrin monomer.** Because of the specificity of thrombin (IIa) for arginyl-glycine peptide bonds in the A_α and B_β chains of fibrinogen (I), the carboxy-terminal amino acid of the fibrinopeptides A and B is always arginine.

POLYMERIZATION OF FIBRIN MONOMERS.   During the polymerization phase of fibrin formation, various fibrin monomer molecules are assembled into a structure known as **fibrin polymer.** This is basically a spontaneous, nonenzymatic, self-assembly process whereby end-to-end and side-to-side aggregation of individual fibrin monomer molecules takes place. Although this is a self-assembly process, it is no mere casual gathering together of pieces of fibrinogen (I). The formation of fibrin polymers results from the exposure of sets of **polymerization domains** in

the fibrinogen (I) molecule, after thrombin (IIa) cleavage, which are responsible for the local conformational changes associated with fibrin polymer formation. One set of such domains appears to govern end-to-end assembly, while a second set is responsible for side-to-side assembly. The resulting aggregate (fibrin polymer) remains soluble in such solutions as 5 M urea and hence is sometimes referred to as **soluble fibrin polymer.** It is only after specific cross-linking of the polymerized fibrin network that the final end product, insoluble fibrin, is created.

STABILIZATION AND CROSS-LINKING OF FIBRIN.   The stabilization of fibrin occurs through the process of **cross-linking,** in which covalent bonds are introduced into the already polymerized fibrin network. This process is the result of the activity of activated **fibrin stabilizing factor** (XIIIa). This enzyme exists in plasma (and in platelets) as an inactive precursor (factor XIII), which is a tetramer of about M_r 320,000. It is activated to XIIIa by the enzymes thrombin (IIa) and activated Stuart-Prower factor (Xa) in a reaction that requires divalent calcium (IV). The active molecule, fibrin stabilizing factor (XIIIa), functions as a unique transpeptidase, which, in the presence of divalent calcium (IV), can introduce isopeptide bonds between the amino groups of lysine residues and the carboxyamide groups of glutamine residues.

The cross-linking process produces the kind of fibrin that forms in the normal plasma clot. It is structurally more solid than soluble fibrin polymers, more elastic, and less susceptible to lysis by various fibrinolytic agents. Interesting enough, plasminogen is also incorporated into the clot (see section on Fibrinolysis and Thrombolysis). Thus, through the series of reactions outlined above, the soluble molecule fibrinogen (I) is converted into the insoluble gel called fibrin.

Regulatory Mechanisms in Hemostasis and Thrombosis

One would expect that any system as complicated as blood coagulation would have equally complicated regulatory controls to keep the system in balance. This is, in fact, true. Living animals are continually subjected to various minor traumatic episodes that trigger local hemostasis, yet the clotting mechanism rarely proceeds uncontrolled. What are the mechanisms by which the body contains thrombosis and prevents the propagation of clots? It is beyond our scope to detail the biochemical intricacies of the various control mechanisms, but recent studies that have added to our understanding of the diversity of regulatory mechanisms involved in maintaining hemostatic balance are worthy of our attention. We will address three major regulatory mechanisms that control the activity of the coagulation system (Fig. 3.17): (1) the **antithrombin III system** in which the proteases of the coagulation cascade are directly inhibited by protease inhibitors, (2) the **protein C system** in which control involves regulation of the cofactors,

and (3) **fibrinolysis.** Each of these control systems acts on different aspects of the coagulation mechanism, and each appears essential for effective control of clot formation. That is, if any one of these three regulatory systems is faulty, the entire control system is faulty.

Antithrombin III. The large family of glycoprotein serine proteases include several important inhibitors such as the C1 esterase inhibitor, α-1-antitrypsin (also known as α-1-antiproteinase to better reflect its broad substrate activity), α-2-antiplasmin, and **antithrombin III (AT III).** Many of these inhibitors exhibit a considerable degree of functional cross-reactivity and even sequence homology. AT III is the major physiologic inhibitor of thrombin (IIa) as well as activated Stuart-Prower factor (Xa), two of the most important enzymes of the entire coagulation cascade, and it can inhibit several other coagulation factors.

Precisely how AT III interacts with thrombin (IIa) in the circulation is not yet clear, but it appears that neutralization of thrombin (IIa) actually occurs on the surfaces of endothelial cells (Fig. 3.17); thrombin (IIa) rapidly binds to the surfaces of endothelial cells and can be neutralized there by AT III. Heparin and heparin-like glycosaminoglycans (heparan sulfate) at the endothelial surface catalyze the inactivation of thrombin by antithrombin III. AT III serves as a substrate for thrombin (IIa) and Stuart-Prower factor (Xa), and the resultant cleavage of AT III forms very stable bonds between the substrate (AT III) and the enzyme, which resist denaturation. The enzyme thus is linked to AT III in a 1:1 molar complex, the active site of the enzyme is bound into the complex, and the enzyme is thus effectively neutralized. It seems likely that the AT III–enzyme complex does not remain bound to the endothelium but is released back into the circulation, where it is apparently eventually removed via specific receptors in the liver.

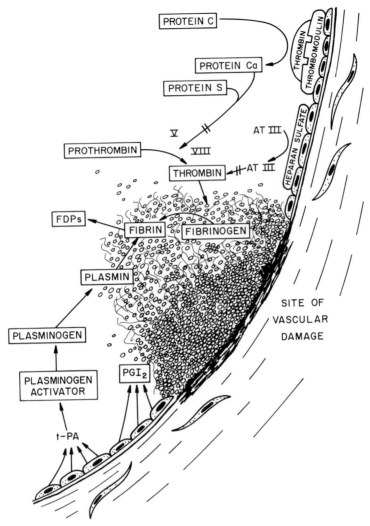

Figure 3.17. Regulatory Mechanisms in Thrombosis and Hemostasis. The actions of activated protein C (Ca), antithrombin III (AT III), and fibrinolysis obtained *via* tissue-type plasminogen activator (t-PA) assist in local regulation of the developing clot. Prostacyclin (PGI$_2$) from endothelial cells also contributes.

Patients with antithrombin III deficiency have an increased tendency for the development of thrombosis. There has been increasing interest in identifying such patients in veterinary clinical medicine in recent years.

Protein C. Current evidence strongly suggests that the protein C anticoagulation pathway is one of the major regulatory mechanisms responsible for the control of coagulation through the selective inactivation of the cofactors proaccelerin (V) and antihemophilic factor (VIII). Protein C is a vitamin K–dependent proenzyme that is normally present in plasma, and the activated form (protein Ca) actually degrades proaccelerin (V) and antihemophilic factor (VIII). Protein C activation is a unique process initially involving the interaction of thrombin (IIa) with an endothelial cell thrombin (IIa) surface receptor called **thrombomodu-**

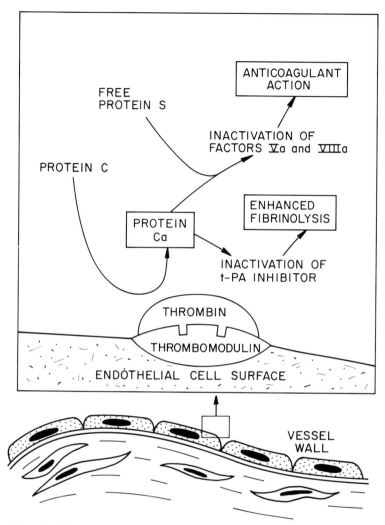

Figure 3.18.   Protein C System. Protein C is activated to protein Ca by the thrombin-thrombomodulin complex on the endothelial surface. Protein Ca with cofactor protein S inactivates Va and VIIIa, and neutralizes a circulating t-PA inhibitor.

lin. When thrombin (IIa) binds to thrombomodulin, a marked alteration in enzyme reactivity occurs; it can no longer either activate proaccelerin (V) or cleave fibrinogen (I), but the thrombin-thrombomodulin complex can rapidly activate protein C to protein Ca (Fig. 3.18). Once activated, protein Ca is released to the circulation where it expresses its considerable anticoagulant activity by selective proteolytic inactivation of proaccelerin (V) and antihemophilic factor (VIII). It should

be noted, however, that activated protein Ca has an almost total dependence on the availability of a cofactor called **protein S,** also a regulatory protein of the complement system, in order to express its anticoagulant activity.

Recent work additionally suggests that protein Ca also interfaces with the fibrinolytic system through its ability to neutralize a circulating inhibitor of tissue-type plasminogen activator (t-PA). By shifting the balance between t-PA and its inhibitor in the direction of increased activation of circulating t-PA, protein Ca accelerates the conversion of plasminogen to plasmin and hence facilitates fibrinolysis. These fibrinolytic reactions are more fully explained later.

Fibrinolysis. In addition to the regulatory coagulation controls available *via* the antithrombin III and protein C systems, fibrin deposition and clot removal is effected *via* the fibrinolytic systems. These are not really regulatory systems for hemostasis, since they function only after fibrin has been formed, but they are clearly linked to the overall control of blood coagulation. (*see* Fibrinolysis and Thrombolysis).

Perspectives on Coagulation

It is easy to get lost in the biochemical complexities of the coagulation pathways. The terminology and the numbering system for the various components seem awkward and difficult. The reactions are complicated, and we sometimes find ourselves falling prone to memorization for the sake of memorization and because routine cerebrations often fail to place things into proper perspective for us. These are the prices that we all, as students of disease, must pay for medical progress. How much simpler it must have been for Galen, who could only marvel at the way in which fluid blood transformed magically into a jelly-like mass. The payoff for us is that an understanding of the basic mechanisms behind the coagulation process allows us to appreciate how blood loss occurs, how thrombosis is achieved, and how we might be able to intervene in a therapeutic sense. Galen did not have such luxuries.

Pathogenesis of Thrombosis

A major turning point in our understanding of the pathogenesis of thrombosis came around 1845, when a young German pathologist delivered a lecture on his views of the mechanisms of thromboge-

nesis. In this lecture, Dr. Rudolf Virchow (who was then only 23 years old) presented a conceptual framework for the pathogenesis of thrombosis which has stood the test of time. Virchow envisioned that thrombosis basically involved three related but distinct mechanisms: (1) changes in the vessel wall or surface, (2) changes in the hemodynamics of blood flow or stasis, and (3) changes in the blood itself and its coagulability. This has become known as "Virchow's triad" (Fig. 3.19), and it remains an extremely useful way to approach an understanding of the pathogenesis of thrombosis.

Thrombosis is a common and often catastrophic complication of a wide variety of disease states, and as such it contributes to the natural history of many pathologic processes. It remains one of the central remaining enigmas of modern medicine, and many of the readers (and perhaps the authors) of this book will succumb to it. In spite of intensive study, its precise etiology remains obscure, its diagnosis difficult and often inaccurate, its prophylaxis of unproven efficacy, and its treatment largely empirical. The pathogenesis of this important process involves an interplay between vessel walls

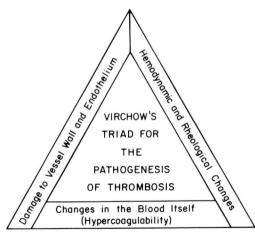

Figure 3.19. Virchow's Triad. The three major determinants in the pathogenesis of thrombosis are grouped as Virchow's triad.

and the blood-clotting system and cellular elements in blood. The initiation of thrombosis is still not well understood, but it appears to be triggered most often by an **injury** of some sort to the vessel wall and by alterations in the blood itself. The local characteristics of the thrombus that forms are determined, at least in part, by the character of local blood flow and greatly influenced by hemodynamic alterations.

Virchow's triad remains a useful approach to an understanding of the pathogenesis of thrombosis, and we will direct our attention here to (1) changes in the vessel wall or its surface, (2) changes in the hemodynamics of blood flow or stasis, and (3) changes in the blood itself.

Vascular Mechanisms in Thrombosis

Injury to the vessel wall in general and to the endothelial lining specifically may be the major event that precipitates the thrombotic process. It is known that platelets, white blood cells, and fibrin itself rarely adhere to normal intact endothelium. In direct opposition to the thromboresistant properties of the endothelial lining, however, are the thrombogenic properties of the deeper portions of the vessel wall, particularly the collagenous supporting structures. Much of this relates to type III collagen in the surrounding tissues; the basement membrane contains mostly type IV collagen, which is not particularly thrombogenic. If a vessel is injured, the injured vessel wall along with platelets, circulating coagulation factors, and, finally, fibrinolytic factors combine in a series of interlacing reactions resulting in vasoconstriction and the formation of a coagulum consisting of platelets and fibrin. These plugs form within the lumen of the vessel, and the thrombus tends to enlarge by additional coagulation occurring on its surface, propagating the thrombus in the direction of blood flow (Fig. 3.20).

Numerous studies have documented that

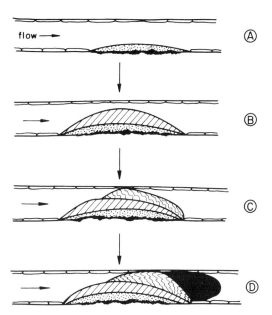

Figure 3.20. Thrombus Propagation. A thrombus grows by layering, particularly where blood flow is rapid. Intimal damage leads to deposition of a layer of platelets *(A)*, which is followed by the deposition of fibrin and white blood cells *(B)*, and later by further fibrin deposition *(C)*. A tail of clotted whole blood *(D)* may become attached in the area immediately downstream from the thrombus.

if the vessel wall is injured, platelet thrombi occur only where the endothelium is detached and the underlying connective tissue exposed. The earliest morphologic expressions of endothelial injury are generally visible only with the electron microscope and include a separation of endothelial cells from basement membrane, disappearance of certain organelles, and swelling of the mitochondria and endoplasmic reticulum. Vacuoles may appear in the cytoplasm, and the cells appear to "round up" or contact to expose underlying structures. Eventually, partial detachment leads to complete detachment as the injured endothelial cells are lost and swept downstream.

There are a large number of ways in which such thrombogenic endothelial injury can occur. One obvious method is by direct physical force (trauma); but electrical damage, chemical injury, infection, inflammation, drugs such as epinephrine, and even high doses of vitamin D can produce the endothelial injury necessary to initiate thrombogenesis. Bacterial endotoxins also have been shown to produce endothelial injury that may be widespread and of importance in the pathogenesis of the "consumption coagulopathy" or **disseminated intravascular coagulation** (DIC) syndrome that can accompany Gram-negative sepsis (*see* Chapter 7).

Inflammation of vessels certainly can produce the necessary endothelial injury. This may include **vasculitis** (inflammation of blood vessels) in a general sense or be restricted to **arteritis** (inflammation of the arteries) or **phlebitis** (inflammation of the veins). Phlebitis can be a particular problem, because the blood flow is slower in veins and hence favors interaction of the blood components with the injured endothelium.

As the propagating thrombus develops, leukocytes and platelets often become trapped in the fibrin mesh. On aggregation, platelets have been shown to release serotonin, acid hydrolases, ADP, an elastolytic factor, thromboxane A_2, permeability factors, and other reactive chemicals. The products released from platelets can additionally influence other cell types. Leukocytes, particularly the neutrophils, are similarly endowed with an impressive battery of chemicals that can be released locally. Thus, further endothelial damage may occur once the platelet and leukocyte release reactions have occurred. In addition, the disturbance to local blood flow may produce a local hypoxemia, which also is damaging to the endothelial cells.

Whatever the specific etiologic background, it is clear that in most clinical conditions in which thrombosis occurs, vascular injury with disruption of endothelial continuity occurs. Minor degrees of injury do not necessarily result in thrombosis, but, even here, the opportunity is enhanced over the situation in normal vessels. The more usual situation, however, is that before large vessel thrombosis can occur, areas of endothelial sloughing must occur to expose large zones of underlying basement membrane and supporting connective tissue. The bottom line in all of this is the need for **endothelial continuity** if normal blood flow is to be maintained. Because of this, the endothelial cells themselves are worthy of our consideration.

Role of the Endothelial Cell

One of the fundamental properties of normal, intact, nonactivated endothelial cells is that they promote neither activation of the extrinsic or intrinsic coagulation pathways nor adherence of unstimulated platelets and leukocytes. These nonthrombogenic properties of the lining of vessel walls have been known since the days of Virchow. For a long time, at least part of the reason for this phenomenon has been attributed to the carbohydrate-rich cell coat, or **glycocalyx.** Biochemically the glycocalyx is a composite of intrinsic membrane glycoproteins and glycolipids as well as membrane-associated polysaccharides and glycosaminoglycans. Heparan sulfate in the glycocalyx has similarities to the anticoagulant heparin. In addition, an α-2-macroglobulin that is a potent antiprotease is associated with the vascular lining and can serve to inhibit activation of some of the clotting factors.

It also is possible that the **surface negativity** of endothelial cells (and the leukocytes and platelets with which endothelium might interact) lead to a sort of mutual electrostatic repulsion between the two sets of negatively charged cells and that this repulsion in part prevents the platelets and leukocytes from adhering to the endothelial surface. This point recently has been challenged, however, by data that suggest that such thrombogenic substrates as collagen and elastin have charge densities similar to that of the endothelial surface. Both the "glycocalyx" theory and the "surface negativity" theory are still widely debated. Both concepts place the endothelial cell in a somewhat passive role; it just lies there, and its thromboresistant properties are related to surface modifications in charge and chemistry.

It is now clear that this limited view of the endothelium is far too restrictive. There is abundant evidence that the endothelial cell is *not* merely a passive lining for the blood vessels which lies there and lets things pass over it. Indeed, endothelial cells are emerging from their previous role as passive participants and are now known to be metabolically active cells that influence both the plasma coagulation system and platelet function. Endothelial cells have been shown to actively metabolize some of the prostaglandins, serotonin, adenine nucleotides, bradykinin, and angiotensin I, all of which promote platelet aggregation. They are rich sources of tissue thromboplastin (III). Endothelial cells also apparently can bind thrombin (IIa) and other coagulation components, and can secrete both the tissue-type and the urokinase-type of plasminogen activator for entry into the fibrinolytic schemes.

Because of their location and contact with the flowing blood stream, endothelial cells are perfectly positioned to modulate the various biological systems in blood, particularly the coagulation system. A contemporary view of these flattened cells lining our blood vessels must therefore recognize their active involvement in the coagulation process. In addition, these cells play both sides of the game; they have procoagulant and anticoagulant properties (Table 3.3).

Endothelial procoagulant properties. One of the first visible components of a developing thrombus is a layer of platelets deposited where endothelial damage has occurred to expose subendothelial structures. Platelets bind not to the endothelial cells themselves, but to

Table 3.3
Procoagulant and Anticoagulant Properties of the Endothelium

Procoagulant properties
  Synthesis, storage and release of von Willebrand factor/factor VIII
  Major tissue thromboplastin (III) source
  Plasminogen activator inhibitors
  Platelet-activating factor source
Anticoagulant properties
  Barrier between blood and thrombogenic subendothelium
  Endothelial cell surface properties (heparan sulfate, α-2-macroglobulin)
  Surface inactivation of thrombin (IIa) via antithrombin III
  Thrombin-thrombomodulin complex and protein Ca
  Prostacyclin (PGI$_2$)
  Conversion of ADP to nonaggregating nucleotides

subendothelial collagen, where they aggregate and release their constituents, including **thromboxane A$_2$ (TXA$_2$),** to promote further platelet aggregation. Adhesion of platelets to the subendothelium is dependent on **von Willebrand factor (vWF),** which is synthesized and stored in the so-called **Weibel-Palade bodies** of the endothelial cells for later secretion. Released vWF subsequently binds to subendothelial collagen. Platelets bind to the subendothelial collagen bound–vWF *via* membrane receptors for vWF (Fig. 3.22). Endothelial cells can express tissue thromboplastin (III) on their surface to promote proconvertin (VIIa)-mediated activation of cell-bound Christmas factor (IX) and Stuart-Power factor (X). They can also modulate certain "antithrombogenic" activities, for example, by producing plasminogen-activator inhibitors. Lastly, endothelial cells can release platelet-activating factor (PAF), a very potent platelet aggregating agent.

Endothelial anticoagulant properties. In addition to the surface properties of endothelial cells mentioned previously, normal endothelium contributes to the inhibition of thrombosis *via* the inactivation of thrombin, fibrinolysis, and the inhibition of platelet aggregation. As we have mentioned, endothelial cells can bind thrombin (IIa) and other coagulation factors. Heparin-like glycosaminoglycans (heparan sulfate) at the cell surface catalyze the inactivation of bound thrombin by antithrombin III. Thrombin also binds to thrombomodulin receptors, where it is involved in the cleavage of protein C to release the activated anticoagulant protein Ca (*see* section on Regulatory Mechanisms in Hemostasis, and Fig. 3.18). Endothelial cells are also rich sources of tissue-type plasminogen activator (t-PA) and hence assist in controlling thrombosis *via* local fibrinolysis.

Endothelial cells have the capacity to convert the strongly proaggregating substance ADP released from platelets to adenine nucleotide platelet inhibitors. Endothelial cells also down-regulate thrombotic events by inhibiting platelet aggregation in another way. A novel cyclo-oxygenase-produced derivative of membrane-esterified arachidonic acid, called **prostacyclin (PGI$_2$)**, is released at low levels even by resting endothelial cells, and increased release can be stimulated by a variety of agents including interleukin-1, thrombin (II), endotoxin, and cachectin (tumor necrosis factor, TNF). This discovery considerably altered thinking about endothelial cell and platelet physiology. Through the local release of adenosine diphosphate (ADP) and the generation of prostaglandin endoperoxides and thromboxane A$_2$ (TXA$_2$), adherent platelets form the initial primary hemostatic plug and promote local vasoconstriction.

Thromboxane A$_2$ is a potent platelet-aggregating agent and additionally promotes vasoconstriction. It seems reasonable, then, that if endothelial cells are to be truly thromboresistant, they should somehow be able to counteract the potent thrombogenic activities generated during the formation of the initial hemostatic platelet plug. This in fact occurs through the endothelial synthesis and release of PGI$_2$, which converts the released platelet endoperoxides and thromboxanes to unstable structures that can prevent or reverse platelet aggregation and relax several kinds of blood vessels. It has been suggested that the ability of the endothelial cells to produce PGI$_2$ is a basic thromboresistant mechanism characteristic of the lining of the vasculature. It is currently envisioned that when the endothelial cells are injured, there is a lack of PGI$_2$ synthesis and release, and local clot formation occurs. In other settings, an interplay presumably takes place between the TXA$_2$ in the platelets, with its strong platelet-aggregating and vasoconstrictive properties, and the PGI$_2$ in the endothelium, with its potent antiaggregating activity and vasodilator functions. A powerful set of checks and balances is thus visualized.

It is also interesting to note that the PGI$_2$ synthetic enzymes in the endothelial cells can apparently use platelet-derived endoperoxides as a substrate. Hence a novel surveillance system exists to prevent or counteract any overzealous platelet activation. It must, however, be stated that PGI$_2$-TXA$_2$ interaction is certainly not the only control mechanism available, since incubation of endothelial cells with cyclooxygenase inhibitors (preventing synthesis of PGI$_2$) does not completely remove the "nonthrombogenic" properties of endothelial cells. The discovery of these unstable but very active products of arachidonic acid metabolism has, however, allowed fresh insight into the control of hemostasis and possible prevention of thrombosis.

Rheological and Hemodynamic Mechanisms of Thrombosis

The thrombogenic contributions of decreased blood flow and vascular stasis have also been recognized since Virchow's time.

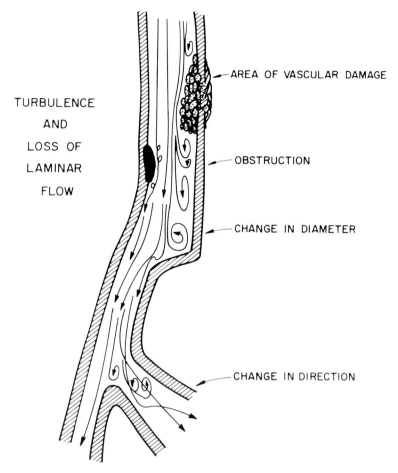

TURBULENCE
AND
LOSS OF
LAMINAR
FLOW

AREA OF VASCULAR DAMAGE

OBSTRUCTION

CHANGE IN DIAMETER

CHANGE IN DIRECTION

Figure 3.21. Turbulence and Loss of Laminar Flow. Schematic representation of how changes are produced in the normal axial streaming of flowing blood by vessel lesions, changes in lumen size, or flow direction. Such changes increase the opportunity for thrombi to form.

Venous stasis may occur in a wide variety of pathologic and physiologic conditions including immobilization, pregnancy, shock, heart failure, or even during anesthesia. The rheological properties of blood are such that a drop in flow rate results in increased viscosity. It appears that altered rheology augments the thrombotic process largely in two ways: by creating altered turbulence to accelerate the cellular and enzymatic reactions important in thrombogenesis, and also by producing further injury to the vessel wall itself.

Blood flow in arteries and veins is normally **laminar.** This means that the blood tends to flow as a series of concentric fluid cylinders with the innermost stream moving forward at the fastest rate and with each "layer" moving successively slower as one moves toward the wall of the blood vessel. Immediately adjacent to the endothelium is a thin layer of plasma. In areas of hydraulic stress such as sharp bends, valves, and branches, there is a natural tendency for turbulence to occur, which tends to disturb the laminar flow of the blood (Fig. 3.21). Indeed, such areas of turbulence are more prone to develop thrombi than other sites.

In areas where vascular injury has taken

place, the disruption of the endothelium and the local hemostatic plug that develops also create turbulence and disrupt laminar flow. A vicious circle can thus become established, where local platelet clumping at a site of endothelial discontinuity causes turbulence, and the turbulence thus created increases thrombus formation to accelerate and aggravate the process. Turbulence also occurs in the slower-flowing venous system, for example, around the venous valves.

In addition to turbulence, slowing of the blood flow and stasis increase the probability for thrombosis, although stasis alone probably does not cause thrombosis unless accompanied by endothelial damage or a hypercoagulable state of the plasma. Precisely how stasis contributes to thrombosis is not entirely clear. At a mechanistic level, the increased viscosity of the blood and the loss of laminar flow disturb the relationships of cellular and plasma elements in the blood and favor the interaction of coagulable proteins and platelets with the endothelium. It also may be that stasis reduces the removal of activated clotting factors by delaying their clearance in the liver and reticuloendothelial system. It would also presumably delay the dilution of activated clotting factors and slow their inactivation by naturally occurring inhibitors. It also has been suggested that the slowing of blood flow and stasis are sufficient to produce local hypoxemia, and that one endothelial response to hypoxemia is to release tissue thromboplastin (III) to initiate extrinsic coagulation.

Although the precise reasons why the rheological properties of blood are so important to thrombosis are as yet not clear, it would appear that at least certain hemodynamic alterations such as turbulence, loss of laminar flow characteristics, and increased blood viscosity increase the likelihood of thrombosis. The opportunity for thrombosis to occur in the face of any or all of these hemodynamic changes is greatly increased by damage to the endothelial lining of the blood vessels or by changes in the blood itself, which may lead to a hypercoagulable state.

Basic Mechanisms in the Blood Related to Thrombosis

There are three major biological contributions or functions of the blood that may become activated or altered to participate in the pathogenesis of thrombosis. There are the formation of the fibrin coagulum *via* the intrinsic and extrinsic coagulation pathways, the phenomenon of platelet aggregation and adhesion, and fibrinolysis. We have previously discussed the first two points, and the third is covered in some detail in a later section.

Most of the plasma clotting factors were discovered during investigations of clinical patients in whom abnormalities of coagulation were diagnosed. Many of these patients had bleeding tendencies or a hemorrhagic diathesis. It is still reasoned by some that if a deficiency of the coagulation factors leads to hemorrhagic tendencies, then thrombosis might be promoted if an increased concentration of the clotting factors was present. There is very little experimental proof for this concept, however, although increased concentrations of some clotting factors are found in certain thrombotic conditions. This situation is sometimes referred to as a **"hypercoagulable state"**, which we might define as an altered state of the circulating blood which requires a smaller quantity of clot-inducing substance to produce intravascular coagulation than is required to produce comparable thrombosis in a normal subject.

During pregnancy there are often elevated levels of fibrinogen (I), as well as antihemophilic factor (VIII), proconvertin (VII), and Stuart-Prower factor (X). In the immediate postpartum period and after some surgical operations, where the risk of deep vein thrombosis is elevated, increased plasma concentrations of coagulation factors can be demonstrated. It is equally possible, however, that hypercoagulability could result from deficiencies in control mechanisms; rather than more procoagulants, a decrease in inhibitors. For example, patients deficient in antithrombin III or protein C have an increased incidence of thrombosis.

There also seems to be an increased tendency for thrombosis associated with the nephrotic syndrome (protein-losing renal failure), diabetes mellitus, cardiac failure, valvular heart disease, severe trauma or burns, disseminated cancer, prolonged immobilization during severe illness or after surgery, and virtually all chronic debilitating diseases. Despite these situations, it has been very difficult to draw any solid conclusions about a definite cause and effect relationship. That is, while we are quite aware of the many situations that may predispose to thrombosis, we are still relatively unable to adequately **define** hypercoagulability and its relationship to thrombotic events. This is, in part, because thrombosis is usually studied after the fact since we lack truly useful diagnostic tests to identify patients at risk in a prospective way. Much current research is directed at this precise problem.

As in other areas of science, more attention has been directed to the forward activation phase of blood coagulation than to the inhibitory mechanisms that keep the system in check. It is reasonable at the outset, however, to consider that a disturbance in the levels of natural inhibitors of the coagulation process also might predispose to thrombosis. In short, a hypercoagulable state theoretically might result from either increased activation of the clotting system or from decreased inhibitory activity. Clinicians have identified patients that support both possibilities. With respect to blood coagulation, several major groups of inhibitors have been defined (*see* section on Regulatory Mechanisms in Hemostasis).

Although we have added many details since the times of Virchow, his triad remains the best overall explanation of the various factors that participate in the pathogenesis of thrombosis. It should hardly be necessary for us to point out that any predisposition to the development of thrombosis is magnified by any increase in the number or intensity of various predisposing influences in any one individual. Of Virchow's triad, probably only endothelial injury itself can stand alone in inducing thrombosis. When all three are present, the risk is clearly higher, but any two of the three corners of the triad may suffice. Thus, a patient with vessels roughened by arteriosclerosis or atherosclerosis who, because of persistent proteinuria due to the nephrotic syndrome, is deficient in antithrombin III, would be a prime candidate for the development of thrombosis.

Role and Properties of Platelets in Hemostasis and Thrombosis

The platelets are important components of blood, which circulate as anucleate bits of cellular cytoplasm derived from the megakaryocytes in the bone marrow and other hematopoietic tissues. The past two decades have given rise to remarkable advances in our understanding of blood platelets and their interactions with the vessel wall.

The physiological integrity of the circulation depends on continuous monitoring of the vessel wall by circulating platelets. This is quantitatively no small chore. During each minute of transit time within the circulation, 10^{12} platelets survey thousands of m^2 of capillary surface carpeted with 7×10^{11} endothelial cells. If the platelets detect a break in the continuity of the vessel wall, they immediately respond by contacting the area of injury, spreading out and adhering to the injured zone, and clumping. Such platelets become activated, and their surfaces are transformed into batteries of receptors.

Their interiors receive an influx of Ca^{2+} and become metabolic furnaces for the enzymatic oxidation of arachidonic acid into endoperoxides, which are subsequently converted to powerful thromboxanes, potent vasoconstrictors, and platelet aggregators. The storage granules of the platelets are discharged into the local environment where they are targeted toward other platelets as well as cells of the vessel wall such as smooth muscle. The platelets are remarkable, hair-trigger surveillance instruments; unfortunately they participate with equal fervor in covert pathologic operations such as thrombosis.

Although the platelets that circulate in the blood do not normally adhere to each other or to normal endothelium, a primary function of platelets is adhesion. **Adhesion** in this context refers to sticking to a nonplatelet surface, and is distinct from **aggregation,** which refers to the sticking of platelets to each other. When the endothelium is stripped from the inner aspect of the blood vessels, platelets adhere to the subendothelial extracellular matrix. When platelets are exposed to collagen (especially types I and III), microfibrils, elastin, smooth muscle cells, or fibroblasts, they adhere to these structures rapidly and become activated. Part of the activation process involves platelet aggregation, which leads to what is known as the **platelet release reaction.** This is a nonlytic, secretory reaction whereby platelets release their stores of active chemicals, form thromboxane A_2, participate in activation of the blood coagulation system, and cause further platelet aggregation.

The biological role of platelets in hemostasis and thrombosis is well established although probably not completely understood (Table 3.4). Primary arrest of bleeding in small vessels is achieved initially by the formation of a platelet plug at the severed end of the vessel. Platelets provide critical phospholipids such as

Table 3.4
Biological Properties of Platelets with Respect to Hemostasis and Thrombosis

Hemostasis
  Adhesion to subendothelium (collagen)
  Primary arrest of bleeding
  Formation of initial platelet plug
  Furnish phospholipids for coagulation
  Enhance blood coagulation
  Help cover areas of stripped endothelium
Thrombosis
  Respond to vascular injury
  Platelet factors accelerate thrombogenesis
  Platelet plug promotes turbulence
  Enzymes can further damage endothelium
  Generate thromboxane A_2
  Promote thrombus propagation

platelet factor 3 to promote clot formation. By restoring a covering over areas of vessels denuded of endothelium, they also assist in reducing the exposure of plasma to the clot-promoting subendothelial surfaces. They also participate in inflammatory reactions (*see* Chapter 4).

Unfortunately, the platelet properties of adhesion, aggregation, and secretion which make them so useful in the hemostatic mechanism also allow them to participate in thrombogenesis. We can perhaps best appreciate the functions of platelets in hemostasis and thrombosis if we briefly consider the three critical functions of platelets in these processes: adhesion, aggregation, and secretion, or the platelet release reaction.

PLATELET ADHESION. As we mentioned before, adhesion refers to the ability of platelets to stick to nonplatelet surfaces. With respect to the vascular system, a number of subendothelial surface components promote such adhesion: collagen, elastin, basement membrane, microfilaments, fibronectin, and even amorphous ground substances. Platelets have been observed microscopically to adhere to all of these substrates. Hence, in an injured blood vessel where endothelial cells have been lost, abundant opportunities for platelet adhesion are created by the exposure of subendothelial connective tissue components. Prominent among these is **collagen** (types I and III) because of its ability to bind von Willebrand factor, as previously discussed. Other formed elements of the blood seem to participate in this process. Erythrocytes, for example, may be important to the process of platelet adhesion both by virtue of their rheological properties and because they are an important source of ADP which can precipitate platelet aggregation and the release reaction. The adhesion of platelets to the subendothelium also seems to require divalent calcium (IV).

The biochemical and biophysical basis for platelet adhesion has been clarified in recent years. Factor VIII/von Willebrand factor appears to be the major adhesive cofactor for platelet adhesion to subendothelium (Fig. 3.22). Normally, vWF does not bind to circulating platelets, but it binds "on demand" when released from the Weibel-Palade bodies of injured endothelial cells, when platelets need to be anchored to the break in the continuity of the vessel wall. The binding of vWF to platelets is stimulated by ADP. A long list of other agents may activate platelets and promote their receptor-mediated interaction with the vessel wall including epinephrine, thrombin, certain prostaglandins (TXA_2), and platelet-activating factor (PAF). It is likely that, *in vivo,* many of these various stimuli can affect increased platelet adhesiveness, and the length of the list is only a reflection of the need for redundancy in a system so critical to the formation of the initial hemostatic plug.

PLATELET AGGREGATION. If collagen is added to a suspension of platelets in plasma, some of the platelets will stick to the collagen (adhesion); but after a short delay, the remaining platelets begin to swell, adopt considerable conformational changes, and stick to each other. This is platelet aggregation. Pseudopodia protrude from the platelet surface, the organelles are centralized within the platelet, and the overall shape changes from that of a somewhat flattened disc to a rotund sphere. Such conformational changes appear necessary in order to reorganize platelet surface membrane components to expose the clot-promoting phospholipids called platelet factor 3. A number of biological stimuli can induce platelet aggregation and thus can predispose to thrombus formation. This long list includes ADP, thrombin, collagen, arachidonic acid, TXA_2, epinephrine, immune complexes, and platelet-activating factor (PAF).

Recent studies have confirmed that certain components of plasma are essential to the platelet aggregation process. Platelet aggregation is diminished in patients with **congenital afibrinogenemia,** and *in vitro* studies have documented that fibrinogen (I) is an essential cofactor for platelet aggregation. Similar evidence can be cited for patients with antihemophilic factor (VIII) or von Willebrand factor deficiency. Platelet aggregation has been extensively studied, and the physiological basis for this important event can now be understood at a molecular level.

It is useful to break platelet aggregation down into two phases; a primary reversible phase, and a secondary irreversible phase. In primary **reversible** aggregation, platelets undergo shape change with pseudopod formation. In resting platelets, the GP IIb-IIIa membrane glycoprotein complex that constitutes the fibrinogen receptor is distributed uniformly over the platelet membrane. Following stimulation, however, large clusters of GP IIb-IIIa co-localize with fibrinogen on the developing pseudopods and between adherent platelets and initiate the secondary **irreversible** phase of aggregation with recruitment of additional platelets and the release of platelet granule proteins (Fig. 3.22).

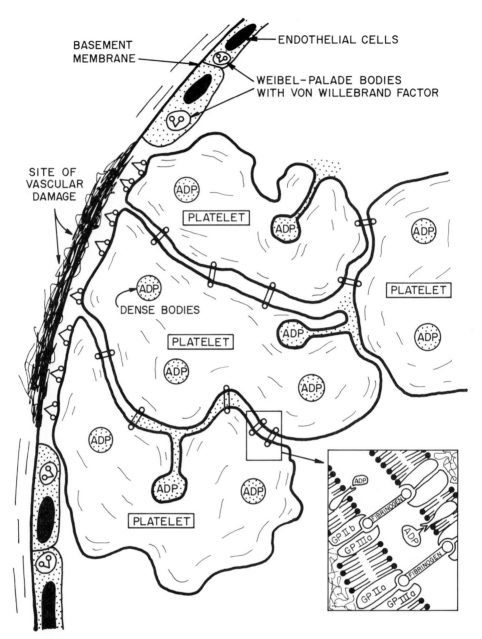

Figure 3.22.   Mechanisms of Platelet Adhesion and Aggregation. *Platelets* are anchored to sub-endothelium *via* receptors for collagen-bound von Willebrand factor (vWF). vWF is synthesized and stored in granules *(Weibel-Palade bodies)* in the *endothelial cell* and released upon injury. Platelets bind to each other *via fibrinogen,* linking at the *GP IIb-IIIa* receptor site in an ADP-catalyzed reaction. (adapted from: Hawiger, J.: Formation and regulation of platelet and fibrin hemostatic plug. *Human Pathology 18*:111–122, 1987).

The triggering event for platelets to form aggregates is ADP-catalyzed exposure of binding sites for fibrinogen on the platelet membrane. As a result, fibrino-gen links platelets together, which are rapidly joined by others through a "snow-ball effect" to produce a platelet aggregate. It is now felt that the primary role of agonists like ADP is to induce exposure of binding sites for fibrinogen. This is no small affair; ADP induces approximately 40,000 to 50,000 binding sites for fibrinogen on a single platelet. In addition to other constituents, the platelet α-granules contain four major adhesion proteins: fibrinogen, von Willebrand factor, thrombospondin, and fibronectin. **Thrombospondin** is secreted by platelet α-granules and binds to the activated platelet surface, where it interacts with bound fibrinogen and other components to function as a sort of agglutinin to stabilize platelet aggregates and support the conversion of microaggregates into macroaggregates. The release of these various granule contents during platelet aggregation allows them to achieve high local concentrations and play an important role in irreversible aggregation and the secretion phase of aggregation. Irrespective of the various contributory forces behind platelet aggregation, once it occurs the platelets change their shape radically, develop secretory channels to the outside, and progress through a series of events known as the platelet release reaction.

PLATELET SECRETORY EVENTS: THE PLATELET RELEASE REACTION. Platelets are secretory cells; as a consequence of aggregation, platelet constituents are released into the local environment. This release reaction has basically two stages (Fig. 3.23). At first, a variety of intense cytoplasmic activity can be detected, which culminates in the extrusion of the contents of the cytoplasmic dense bodies or storage granules into the surrounding medium. This phase places dense body contents such as adenine nucleotides and serotonin into the local environment. Sometimes, the reaction stops here, but if the stimulus for aggregation is strong enough, a second phase of release occurs in which the contents of the lysosomal granules are discharged. At this time, hydrolytic enzymes such as β-glucuronidase, acid cathepsins, and β-N-acetylglu-

cosaminidase are released. After the release reaction, most of the cytoplasmic organelles of the platelet are gone. The platelet itself usually is not lysed, as documented by the fact that cytoplasmic enzymes such as lactic dehydrogenase (LDH) are not released. The released ADP is a major stimulus for the formation of additional platelet aggregates. Platelets stimulated to aggregate also produce thromboxane A_2 (TXA$_2$), one of the most potent platelet-aggregating agent known. It may well be that the generation and release of TXA$_2$ is even more important than ADP in promoting additional platelet aggregation.

During the conformational changes that accompany platelet aggregation, platelet factor 3 (PF3) is made available on the platelet cell membrane, as mentioned previously. PF3 is an important procoagulant molecule that appears to participate in the formation of thrombin (IIa) in at least two reactions: the activation of factor VIII, and the cleavage of prothrombin (II). Precisely how it contributes is not yet totally understood. Platelets also release platelet factor 4, a basic polypeptide that can function to inhibit the prolongation of clotting time produced by heparin. It also can neutralize the anticoagulant properties of some of the fibrin degradation products (FDPs), may alter the surface properties of the platelet membranes to expose more PF3, and apparently can assist in the polymerization of soluble fibrin monomers.

The mechanism by which products stored in the secretory granules of platelets are released to the exterior has been the subject of considerable interest. In human platelets, an extensive **cytocavitary network** known as the **open canalicular system** (OCS) communicates directly with the surrounding medium *via* uninterrupted openings to the plasma membrane. Following platelet activation, the various secretory granules in human platelets become centrally concentrated within the platelets, and then fuse their

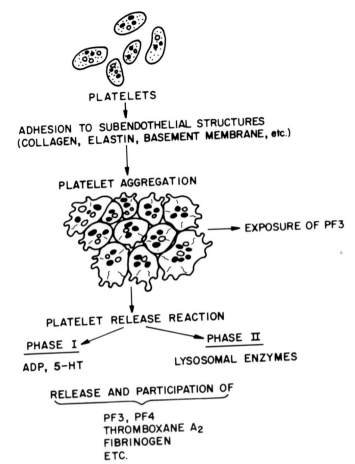

PLATELETS

↓

ADHESION TO SUBENDOTHELIAL STRUCTURES
(COLLAGEN, ELASTIN, BASEMENT MEMBRANE, etc.)

↓

PLATELET AGGREGATION

⟶ EXPOSURE OF PF3

↓

PLATELET RELEASE REACTION

PHASE I ⟵ ⟶ PHASE II

ADP, 5-HT   LYSOSOMAL ENZYMES

RELEASE AND PARTICIPATION OF

PF3, PF4
THROMBOXANE A₂
FIBRINOGEN
ETC.

Figure 3.23. Platelet Aggregation and Release. The exposure of platelets to appropriate stimuli produces platelet aggregation first and then the platelet release reaction with its two characteristic phases. *PF,* platelet factor; *ADP,* adenosine diphosphate; and *5-HT,* 5-hydroxytryptamine (serotonin).

membranes with the cytoplasmic OCS, which serves as a conduit for the release of secretory products to the exterior. Interestingly enough, **bovine platelets** lack the OCS found in human platelets and, following activation, secretory granules remain more peripheral within the cytoplasm, and secretion occurs by direct fusion of the granule membranes with the plasma membrane. The basis for these species variations in platelet structure which result in different routes for secretion of granule contents remains unknown.

It is increasingly clear that platelets are intimately linked to the hemostatic mechanism and to the pathogenesis of thrombosis. This is a two-way street: platelets promote blood coagulation and blood coagulation promotes platelet aggregation and its attendant effects.

Morphology and Morphogenesis of Thrombi

Thrombi can occur anywhere within the cardiovascular system. When they occur within the vascular system they are **vascular thrombi,** which can be in arteries **(arteriothrombosis)** or within veins **(phlebothrombosis).** They also can occur within the heart itself **(cardiac thrombosis)**, where they can involve either the cardiac valves **(valvular thrombosis)** or the walls of the chambers of the heart **(mural thrombosis)**. When thrombi build up on the cardiac valves, they are commonly referred to as **vegetations** or **vegetative valvular thromboses** because of their appearance.

Thrombi vary widely in their appearance and composition because of local factors that affect their formation. One of the most important determinants of the size and structure of a thrombus is the rate of blood flow in the area in which they are formed. Thrombi formed in a rapidly flowing blood stream (arterial thrombi) differ in appearance from thrombi arising in a sluggish blood flow (venous thrombi).

Arterial Thrombosis

In most of the arterial system, blood flows at a high rate under normal conditions. If endothelial injury occurs in an artery or arteriole, a fairly predictable type of thrombus will develop. The rapid blood flow and high pressure are sufficient to sweep away all but the most tenacious of the clotting contributors, and the typical arterial thrombus is a pale gray-tan mass that consists of nearly concentric layers of alternating bands of fibrin and platelets mixed with rather scanty amounts of darker red coagulated blood (Fig. 3.24). The laminated appear-

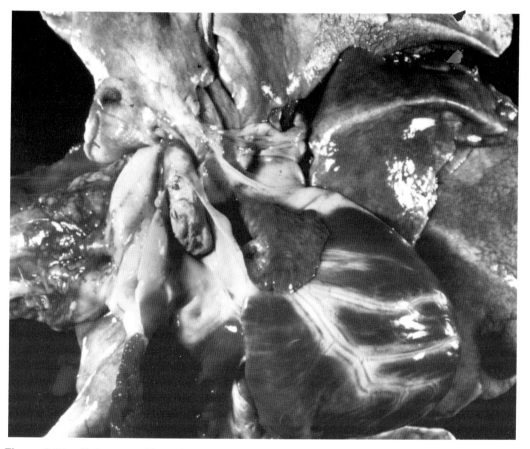

Figure 3.24.   Pulmonary Thrombosis. A large thrombus is present in the main branch pulmonary artery of this dog with renal amyloidosis and the nephrotic syndrome.

ance of such thrombi relates to their underlying pathogenesis. As the rapid flow sweeps away many of the components of blood, currents conducive to activation and accumulation of clotting factors are found only in the peripheral recesses of the developing low-profile thrombus. They are rarely **occlusive thrombi** at first, but require a slower build-up of components.

The flow of blood over the developing thrombus contributes to its gradual increase in size, a phenomenon referred to as **propagation** of the thrombus. A platelet layer that may be deposited first by adhesion to the damaged endothelium is followed by local platelet aggregation. Gradually fibrin forms to stabilize the platelet mass. The flow of blood deposits more platelets onto the growing mass, which is followed by more fibrin deposition. It is this layering effect, largely due to alternating zones of platelets and fibrin with scant amounts of blood, that produces the laminations known as the **lines of Zahn.** Because such thrombi are composed largely of platelets and fibrin, they are often called **"white"** or **"pale"** thrombi.

While the flow of blood in the arterial system usually prevents these thrombi from being occlusive initially, eventually the thrombus formed on the damaged arterial wall propagates to form an **"occlusive"** thrombus. In such situations, the **head** of the thrombus tends to receive accumulations of fibrin and platelets because of its exposure to the flowing blood stream and hence remains pale, while the **tail** of the thrombus accumulates coagulated blood from the stagnant downstream flow and the turbulence of the blood on the leeward side of the propagating thrombus. The tail of such thrombi thus tends to be dark red due to its accumulation of coagulated blood (*see* Fig. 3.20). Not all of the thrombus may be attached to the vessel wall. The distal or downstream segment may be more or less suspended in the flowing blood as a sort of undulating tail. Such segments often break off and as such are a common source of emboli (Fig. 3.25).

Venous Thrombosis

Blood flow in the venous system is often slow. This is especially true in larger distal veins in which gravity works against the system. Indeed, it has been shown that blood flow can virtually stop during prolonged periods of inactivity.

Much of the ability to move blood in the larger distal veins is tied to the pumping actions of the skeletal muscles through which the veins run. Hence, muscular activity is necessary to keep the venous system flowing properly and flow rates decline markedly during inactivity. Thrombi developing within the deep veins tend to resemble an intravascular clot of whole blood, much as one might expect if blood were drawn into a glass tube. They are dark red in color, more moist or gelatinous than arterial thrombi, and sometimes are referred to as **"red"** thrombi, **"stasis"** thrombi, or **"coagulation"** thrombi. Such thrombi can be difficult to distinguish from **postmortem thrombi,** which result from coagulation of the blood within vessels after death. They differ from postmortem thrombi by having a point of attachment to the vessel wall and by virtue of the fact that they usually have some tangled strands of fibrin mixed within their substance. They are easily separated by their appearance from the so-called **chicken-fat clot** so commonly seen as a postmortem event, particularly in horses. Here, the rapid sedimentation rate for equine red cells allows separation of the blood prior to postmortem coagulation, and the result is a moist golden-yellow plasma clot attached to a dark red blood clot.

Venous thrombi, unlike arterial thrombi, are rarely mural. The slow blood flow in the veins permits total blood coagulation so that all of the cellular elements become trapped in the thrombus

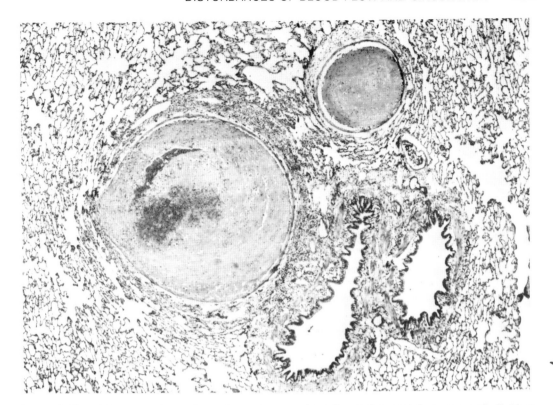

Figure 3.25. Pulmonary Embolism. Two pulmonary branch arteries contain recent emboli. Note that the surrounding lung tissue is normal (not infarcted) because of the rich collateral blood supply to the lung.

rather than being swept away as they are by the higher flow rates on the arterial side. Because of this, venous thrombi tend to be occlusive and often resemble nearly perfect casts of the lumen of the vessel in which they are found.

In a venous thrombus, the distribution of the formed elements of blood is more or less random, as it is in normal whole blood, so that few, if any, of the structural or architectural features of the arterial pale thrombus can be identified. An additional difference relates to the tenacity of the attachment to the underlying vessel wall. Since venous thrombi are formed in a slow-flowing system, they do not usually generate strong points of attachment to the vessel wall as do arterial thrombi. Therefore the venous thrombus is in many ways easier to dislodge, and some impressive emboli can result when this occurs.

Such emboli can be a serious clinical problem in man where sudden activity such as walking or merely standing up after prolonged bed rest or inactivity may be sufficient to dislodge a poorly attached venous thrombus in a deep leg vein and send it sailing toward the heart and lungs (pulmonary embolism), where the results can be catastrophic.

Fate of Thrombi

After a thrombus has formed, what then? Much of the answer to this question lies in the nature of the local collateral vascular supply to the tissue supplied by the thrombosed vessel. That is, if there is abundant collateral circulation, the service area of the thrombosed vessel may not be sufficiently altered to result in clinical signs.

There are basically only four different

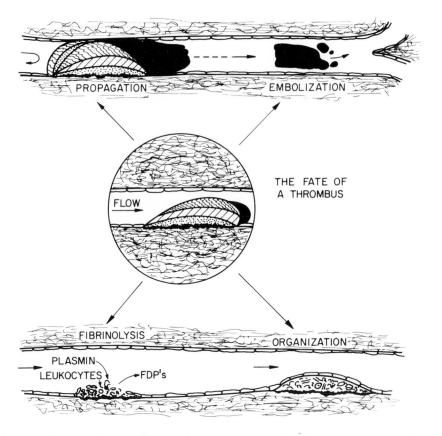

Figure 3.26. Fates of Thrombi. Schematic representation of what can happen to thrombi. Once formed, thrombi either propagate, embolize, undergo fibrinolysis, or organize. *FDP,* fibrin degradation products.

evolutionary pathways that a thrombus can follow (Fig. 3.26). Either the thrombus will be (1) **propagated,** become larger, and eventually produce obstruction, or it will be (2) fragmented to result in **embolism** of distal tissues, or it will be (3) removed by **fibrinolysis** (thrombolysis) *via* either the plasma-derived fibrinolytic systems or phagocytes, or it will be (4) **organized** into the vessel wall. There is a degree of mechanistic overlap in some of these options, but they do basically represent divergent outcomes.

Propagation of Thrombi

We already have touched briefly on the means by which thrombi are propagated. The basic outcome is an overall increase in the size of the thrombus itself. Because of the nature of blood flow in the arterial and venous divisions of the vascular system, propagation differs in much the same way that thrombus formation differs. Basically, thrombus propagation in both systems refers to the overall enlargement of the thrombotic mass due to progressive clot formation. Usually this elongates the mass in the direction of the heart. It is possible, particularly in the venous system, for such propagating thrombi to become extremely large. A thrombus originating, for example, in a branch of the femoral vein may become locally occlusive and subsequently propagate until it protrudes into the lumen of the femoral vein itself. Occasionally, further propagation occurs, and the thrombus may even extend into the iliac vein or caudal vena cava. Propagation of thrombi is one of the major events underlying embolism, since the growing, advancing tail of the thrombus is particularly susceptible to fragmentation and subsequent embolism. As the advancing tail of the thrombus reaches a bifurcation, rapidly flowing blood sweeps past the thrombus to cause dislodgement of part of the thrombus and give rise to an embolus.

Embolism

An **embolus** is a detached physical mass carried in the blood stream from its site of origin to a more distant site. As an embolus moves downstream, it eventually encounters a blood vessel smaller than the diameter of the embolus, and partial or complete occlusion of the vessel then occurs. While most emboli originate from thrombi, there are other, less common types of emboli including fat, air bubbles, tumor cell clumps, aggregates of bacteria or other parasites, and even amniotic fluid. Following extensive trauma with fractures, bone marrow embolism may even occur. Most commonly, however, emboli originate from intravascular thrombi. As such, they are most common at sites downstream from the most common sites for thrombosis.

In man, approximately 95% of all venous emboli arise from thrombi within the deep leg veins. While this can occur in animals, it is unusual because most animals are active and hence use their leg muscles constantly. As we have mentioned previously, activity of this kind tends to prevent venous thrombosis through the continual accessory pumping action of the skeletal muscles. In domestic animals, it is more common for thrombosis to occur in the heart and on its valves than anywhere else, hence emboli and their sites of arrest are determined by the specific location of the thrombi in the heart. Valvular thrombosis involving the left heart usually produces emboli in the systemic circulation, whereas right heart thrombosis more often produces pulmonary embolism. Cattle sometimes develop liver abscesses that can erode into the vena cava and initiate local thrombosis. Emboli arising from such caval thrombi usually are arrested in the lungs. Thrombosis of the vena cava is not, of course, limited to cattle and can in fact occur in any species (Fig. 3.27). Cats with primary cardiomyopathy often develop left atrial thrombi, and embolism of the iliac bifurcation is a common sequel. Such iliac emboli often lie directly at the bifurcation and extend into the right and left main branches. They are often referred to as "saddle emboli" (Fig. 3.28).

Once an embolus has arrived at an appropriately sized vessel, it usually becomes attached to the underlying vessel wall, and may begin to propagate locally much as would a thrombus forming at the same site. Indeed, it can be extremely difficult to discern, in many cases, whether one is dealing with an attached and propagating embolus or if the mass is in fact a thrombus that originated locally. For this reason, the term **thromboembolism** is sometimes used to avoid having to make an arbitrary distinction. From our standpoint, it is clear that the *processes* of thrombosis and embolism are different, and that the two terms describe quite different events.

The eventual outcome of embolism is much the same as thrombosis, for emboli also can propagate, form more emboli, undergo fibrinolysis, or become organized. They also can produce ischemic necrosis or infarction of the tissues served by the vessels they occlude, as we shall discuss shortly.

Fibrinolysis and Thrombolysis

The systems responsible for clot resolution and fibrinolysis form an integral part of the physiological mechanism by which any fibrin, formed extravascularly

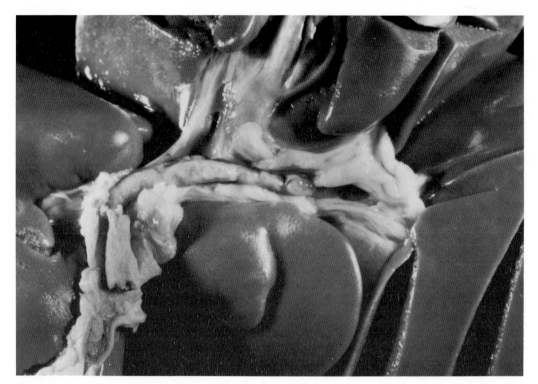

Figure 3.27. Vena Caval Thrombosis. Dog. A large thrombus is present in the vena cava and portal vein. Note that the liver here appears normal. This thrombus is paler than many caval thrombi.

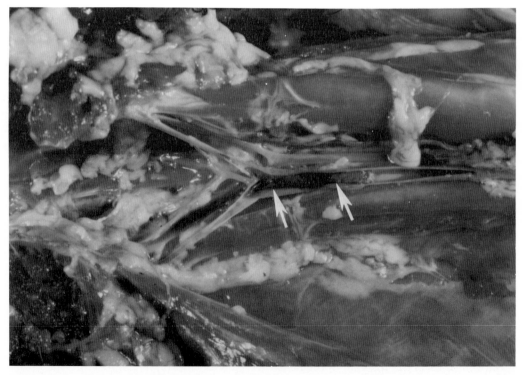

Figure 3.28. Iliac Embolism. The terminal aorta and iliac bifurcation *(arrows)* contain a "saddle embolus" in this cat with hypertrophic cardiomyopathy.

as well as intravascularly, is removed. As such, **fibrinolysis** functions not only in the resolution of thrombi, but also in the degradation of fibrin deposited in inflammatory reactions and in healing and repair processes (*see* Chapter 4). Fibrin that is formed at sites of thrombosis or tissue inflammation must be removed if normal tissue structure and function is to be restored. The fibrinolytic system is the principal effector of clot removal and controls the enzymatic degradation of fibrin. Its action is controlled by the coordinated interaction of inactive precursors (**zymogens**), their activators, specific inhibitors, and active enzymes to provide local control at sites of fibrin deposition.

The proteolytic degradation of fibrin clots (**fibrinolysis**) is mediated by the enzyme **plasmin,** a trypsin-like endopeptidase that can hydrolyze susceptible arginine and lysine bonds in fibrinogen and fibrin. Plasmin is formed from the inactive precursor **plasminogen,** a normal constituent protein of plasma as well as body fluids including saliva, tears, and milk. It is formed by cleavage of a single peptide bond through limited proteolytic action of **plasminogen activators,** serine proteases with a high specificity for their substrate plasminogen.

There are a number of different plasminogen activators, all apparently serine proteases, and some of them function in such diverse processes as ovulation and spermatogenesis, embryonic development, mammary gland involution, prohormone processing, and keratinocyte differentiation as well as fibrinolysis. Plasminogen-activator secretion thus appears to be a general cellular mechanism for inducing localized extracellular proteolysis. Like many other biologically relevant biochemical schemes, the activation of plasminogen is a complex process that is apparently regulated at several levels. Nonactive proactivators first require activation. In addition, the "active" activator can be bound by specific inhibitors and the substrate, plasminogen, is

itself modulated during the activation process. Fibrin itself can modulate the activity of some types of plasminogen activators. The active enzyme plasmin also creates a positive feedback mechanism through its ability to activate additional proactivator and convert plasminogen to plasmin. Plasmin itself is inhibitable by a variety of protease inhibitors. As is so often the case in biological responses, the outcome of any fibrinolytic process represents a functional summary of the relative contributions of different inhibitory and activation pathways.

It is also interesting to note that this is not strictly a host-derived defense system, as several activators of plasminogen have been described in microorganisms such as β-hemolytic streptococci (streptokinase), staphylococci (staphylokinase), and certain fungi (brinase). Since the activation of plasminogen is a key step in the production of fibrinolytic activity (and hence thrombolysis), we will briefly describe some of the means by which plasminogen activator generation can occur. Some of these are shown in Figure 3.29.

FIBRINOLYSIS: ACTIVATION OF PLASMINOGEN. Mammalian plasminogens can be identified and isolated from plasma and serum and are single-chain monomeric proteins with multiple molecular forms. Most forms have an M_r of about 85,000. The mechanism of activation of plasminogen to the active enzyme **plasmin** involves the cleavage of one or more specific peptide bonds in the native plasminogen molecule. Different methods of activation of plasminogen appear to involve slightly different bond cleavages, but by all pathways of plasminogen activation, the fibrinolytic product generated from the cleavage of plasminogen is an active enzyme called plasmin.

Plasmin has general proteolytic activity and is able to hydrolyze a wide variety of proteins. Plasmin resembles trypsin and thrombin in the sense that it splits only lysyl and arginyl bonds in proteins. As indicated in Figure 3.29, there are a num-

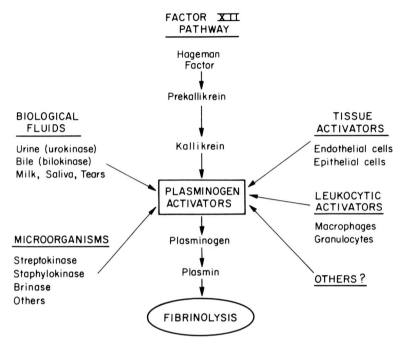

Figure 3.29. Plasminogen Activation. A variety of cellular and humoral sources of plasminogen activators provide multiple entry points to the fibrinolytic system.

ber of ways of generating plasminogen-cleaving activity (plasminogen activators) and hence gaining access to the biologically important fibrinolytic process. It is useful to divide the plasminogen activators into the **intrinsic** activators, derived from activation of the Hageman factor–dependent pathways, and the **extrinsic** activators, derived from most tissues and body fluids.

Hageman-Factor-Dependent Activity. Shortly after the discovery of coagulation factor XII (Hageman factor), it was found that the surface-dependent activation of Hageman factor (XII) also resulted in the generation of fibrinolytic activity (*see* Fig. 4.38). It is now known that at least four proteins participate in the generation of fibrinolytic activity in this system: Hageman factor (XII) itself, prekallikrein, high molecular weight kininogen, and plasminogen. The first three are the same molecules responsible for initiating intrinsic coagulation (Fig. 3.11). Activation

involves molecular assembly of the various components to result in limited proteolytic cleavage of the native molecule into one or more active fragments. These fragments then activate prekallikrein to kallikrein, which in turn activates plasminogen to plasmin.

Little or no plasmin generation occurs in plasma that is deficient in prekallikrein, high molecular weight kininogen, or Hageman factor, but the physiological importance of this fibrinolytic system remains uncertain. No clearly identifiable pathologic state due to impaired fibrinolysis has been identified in patients with profound defects in components of the Hageman factor system, although the original Hageman factor–deficient patient (Mr. John Hageman) died of pulmonary embolism. In addition, Hageman factor pathway–derived plasminogen activators appear to have one ten-thousandth to one forty-thousandth the plasminogen-activating activity of, for example, urokinase. It is interesting to note, however, that at least two products of this activation scheme, kallikrein and plasmin, can cleave additional native Hageman factor (XII), thus providing a means for cyclical activation of the system for continuing mediator production (*see* Fig. 4.38).

Fibrinolysis: Extrinsic Plasminogen Activators. The plasminogen activators important to fibrinolysis that are present in most tissues and fluids can be divided into two major types, one related to the activator found in tissues and referred to as **tissue-type plasminogen activator (t-PA),** and the other related to the activator found in urine **(urokinase)** and referred to as **urokinase-type plasminogen activator (u-PA).**

These two types of plasminogen activators have somewhat different biochemical and functional characteristics. The **t-PAs** consist of a single polypeptide chain and have the properties of binding avidly to fibrin and expressing greater enzymatic activity in the presence of fibrin. Molecular sites responsible for the affinity of t-PA for fibrin reside in the so-called "kringle" structures of t-PA, which are similar to the fibrin-binding "finger" domains of **fibronectin,** the important extracellular matrix glycoprotein and cell-adhesion molecule. The t-PA binds to lysine residues in fibrin which are not exposed in the native fibrinogen molecule. Thus, the binding of t-PA to fibrin is specific. In addition, native plasminogen binds to the same lysine residues in fibrin and, as a result, becomes both localized and rendered 10-fold more susceptible to conversion to plasmin by t-PA. There are many inhibitors of t-PA, but so long as t-PA remains bound to fibrin, it is resistant to inhibition, because the inhibitors also utilize the lysine binding site of t-PA as their own binding site.

The production of fibrin therefore has built-in mechanisms for inducing its own degradation in a localized manner. Fibrin binds t-PA as well as plasminogen and thereby greatly increases the local production of plasmin. Plasmin degrades the fibrin and in so doing is eventually released. The freed enzymes are then susceptible to rapid inhibition by inhibitors. These unique characteristics both localize t-PA activity and enhance its fibrinolytic activity at sites of fibrin deposition.

Because **thrombosis** represents intravascular coagulation, it stands to reason that **vascular** sites for fibrinolysis would be important. Indeed, the vascular endothelium is a rich source of plasminogen activator (t-PA type), which probably mediates much of the clot removal within the circulation *via* local vascular fibrinolysis. The activity of t-PA is down-regulated by plasma plasminogen activator–inhibitors, which form stable covalent complexes with t-PA to provide a viable local control mechanism.

The structure and properties of **u-PAs** are different from T-PAs in that they generally contain two polypeptide chains, apparently lack the fibronectin-like "finger" domains for high-affinity binding to fibrin, and do not exhibit enhanced plasminogen-activator activity in the presence of fibrin. Very small amounts of u-PA activity can be detected in plasma, and certain molecular forms of u-PA (single-chain urokinase-type plasminogen activator, **scu-PA**) may also be involved with t-PA in intravascular thrombolysis, although they are not as important in this regard as t-PA. However, u-PA may be very important to certain types of **tissue fibrinolysis.**

Whereas t-PA is secreted primarily by endothelial cells to provide enzymatic activity largely restricted to the circulation, the biochemically and functionally distinct u-PA is secreted by many cell and tissue types, including tissue macrophages. Urokinase has the unique property of functioning in a cell-associated form and of being less reactive to the protease inhibitors of plasma. This has considerable implications for active tissue fibrinolysis since the inhibitor-activator balance would be shifted towards activation. As an example of the importance of u-PA in tissue fibrinolysis, fibrin-rich alveolar exudates in the lung are handled primarily by u-PA of alveolar macrophage origin rather than t-PA of vascular origin. Investigations of pulmonary fibrinolytic activity in lung lavage fluids has shown that the bulk of the plasminogen activation is associated with u-PA of macrophage origin.

Macrophages have unique capabilities relative to coagulation and fibrinolysis. They can degrade fibrin through secretion of soluble u-PA or by direct contact of plasminogen incorporated in the fibrin clot with macrophage membrane-bound u-PA, the latter having the unique advantage of being relatively protected from soluble proteinase-inhibitors. Macrophage production of uPA, modulated by specific plasminogen activator-inhibitors, may play a key role in macrophage migration through inflamed tissue and in the removal of fibrinous deposits from sites of inflammation. Macrophages apparently have considerable procoagulant activity as well, and can synthesize and express the coagulation factors VII and III as well as others on their cell surface. It thus appears that macrophage-mediated formation and degradation of fibrin results from the coordinated expression of procoagulant and fibrinolytic functions.

At the present time, it is thus envisioned that two quite distinct fibrinolytic schemes exist; the **t-PA** system, which functions largely within the circulation, and the **u-PA** system, which functions largely at tissue sites. It is also probable that some interaction between these two systems occurs. Finally, for students of disease, it is worth noting that these advances in the molecular definition of plasminogen activation are *not* merely exercises in biochemical verbosity, but hold

very real promise for direct clinical application. Indeed, the first clinical trials with recombinant t-PA indicate that effective thrombolysis can be obtained under certain conditions. Further developments in this field can be expected.

Fibrinolysis: Degradation of Fibrinogen/Fibrin Clots. The biochemistry of the action of plasmin on fibrinogen/fibrin substrates has been extensively detailed, and interested readers are referred to the reading list at the end of this chapter. We will only briefly review the essential features of the process here. The proteolysis of fibrin (or fibrinogen) by plasmin involves essentially the same steps (Fig. 3.30). The initial cleavage liberates the carboxy-terminal polar appendage of the A_α chain and also a peptide from the N-terminal portion of the B_β chain producing a fragment termed **fragment X,** which has an M_r of about 240,000. Fibrinogen itself, we must recall, is the plasma precursor of insoluble fibrin and circulates as a plasma protein with an M_r of around 340,000.

After initial cleavage by plasmin, subsequent proteolysis of fragment X results in the formation of **fragment Y,** which has an M_r of around 155,000, and a smaller piece (called **fragment D**), which has an M_r of about 83,000. The final stage of fibrinogen/fibrin fragmentation involves the breakdown of fragment Y into a second fragment D and another piece of smaller size (M_r 50,000), called **fragment E.** Plasmin degradation of non-cross-linked fibrin is essentially identical to that of fibrinogen in both the kinetics of the reaction and the structure of the derivative fragments. This supports the concept that there is little structural change in the fibrin monomer unit during polymerization. On the other hand, cross-linked fibrin is degraded more slowly by plasmin and the derivative fragments released during solubilization are distinct. These unique degradation products are the re-

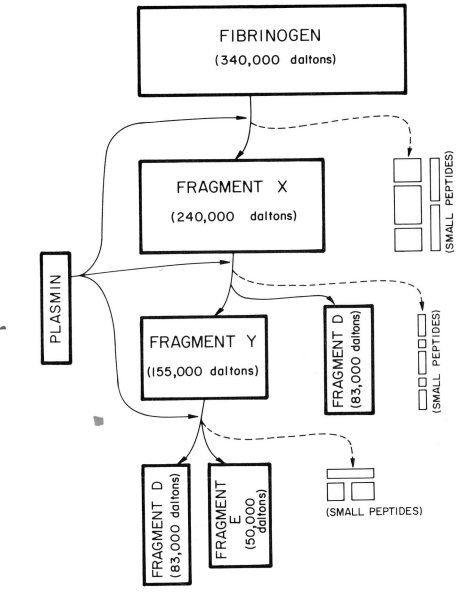

Figure 3.30. Plasmin-mediated Fibrinolysis. Schematic view of the sequential breakdown of fibrin-fibrinogen by plasmin to yield the FDPs (fibrin degradation products, fragments X, Y, D and E).

sult of prior cross linking of fibrin monomer *via* factor XIII, not of a unique proteolytic attack by plasmin.

The details of the proteolytic attack of plasmin on fibrin clots are not just an impractical recitation on the making of biological alphabet soup (fragments X, Y,

D, E, *etc.*), for the breakdown products of fibrinogen/fibrin (called **fibrin degradation products, FDPs**) have considerable relevance to our focus on the pathogenetic mechanisms of disease. The most pronounced biological activity of the FDPs is their anticoagulant action through competitive inhibition of the clotting action of thrombin on fibrinogen substrates. In addition, the smaller FDPs impair platelet adhesiveness, aggregation, and release reactions, while the larger ones may have an opposite effect. Some of the fragments also can cause smooth muscle contraction, increase capillary permeability, and induce the chemotaxis of granulocytes.

Because of their biological importance, it is common in clinical medicine to measure the circulating levels of FDPs. Elevated levels of FDPs in the circulation are used as an indication of clinically important states of elevated fibrinolysis such as disseminated intravascular coagulation (DIC) which may follow Gram-negative sepsis, surgical trauma, shock, and different infectious and neoplastic disease states (see also Chapter 7). Lastly, we should not fail to mention that while enzymatic degradation of fibrin/fibrinogen by plasmin constitutes an important means of fibrinolysis and thrombolysis, phagocytic degradation also occurs, with intracellular digestion of the coagulum taking place within neutrophils and macrophages. This is of particular importance to the process of organization.

Organization of Thrombi

Many thrombi are dissolved by the actions of the plasma-derived fibrinolytic scheme just described. This system is so efficient that it is often difficult, in experimental settings, to preserve an intravascular clot long enough to properly study it. Thrombi of clinical significance, however, are usually large enough to produce a delay in resolution via the plasmin system. In addition, the local hemodynamic alterations caused by the thrombus and the potential local hypoxia often lead to additional damage to the vessel wall, so that a kind of inflammatory reaction ensues. It can, in fact, become rather difficult to differentiate between an inflamed vessel in which thrombosis has occurred

and a thrombosed vessel in which inflammation has occurred. In time, thrombi not resolved via the plasma fibrinolytic system undergo a process called **organization** (Fig. 3.32). This basically refers to a sequence of events in which the thrombus is reduced in size and becomes ultimately converted into a fibrous connective tissue thickening within the wall of the vessel itself.

Thrombi become organized by processes that are remarkably similar to those that occur in wound healing and repair. The adjacent endothelium begins to grow over the surfaces of the thrombus, insulating it from the circulating blood and hence diminishing the possibility of continued propagation of the thrombus. Sometimes the thrombus itself becomes vascularized in order to restore blood flow via the process of **recanalization** (Fig. 3.31). It seems clear that both the regrowth of endothelium over the surface of a thrombus and the growth through the thrombus of restored vascular channels originate from preexisting endothelium at the margins of the thrombus itself as its attachment point to the vessel wall. Neither reendothelialization of the surface of the thrombus or recanalization of its mass can occur unless the thrombus is attached. Hence, in order for organization of a thrombus to occur, attachment to the vessel wall is an absolute prerequisite.

As the surface of the thrombus is being covered by endothelium, growth of small capillaries into the thrombotic mass occurs from the base at its attachment point to the denuded vessel wall. These capillaries provide the nutrient supply for the phagocytic cells that soon emerge from the neocapillaries to enter the thrombus itself. Their job is to phagocytose, degrade, and remove the clotted blood (Fig. 3.33). This is primarily a job for the macrophages, but granulocytes also contribute in the clearing of debris from the organizing thrombus. Macrophages ingest the fragments of red cells and plate-

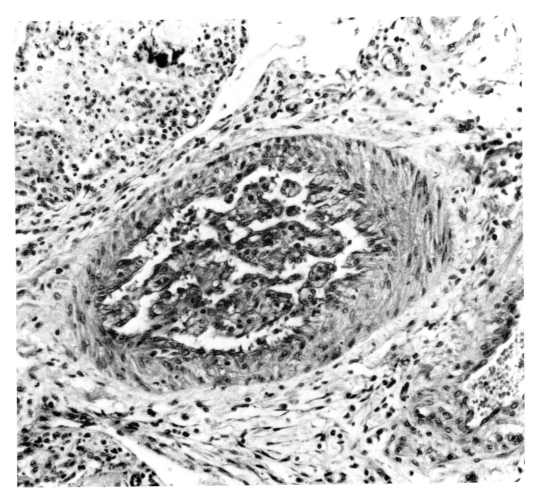

Figure 3.31.   Recanalized Thrombus. This pulmonary arteriole from a dog with dirofilariasis was thrombosed some time ago, and the thrombus has now been invested with endothelial-lined channels to permit some blood flow through the area.

lets present in the thrombus and assist in the fibrinolytic breakdown of the fibrin meshwork that the cellular elements have invaded (Fig. 3.33). Ultimately, fibroblasts invest the area and lay down collagen so that the thrombus eventually can become completely converted into fibrous connective tissue and incorporated into the wall of the preexisting vessel. Such structures may produce a narrowing of the lumen of the vessel, but either *via* circumferential flow or *via* recanalization, it often is possible for an adequate nutritive blood supply to become reestablished. The success of this process often is ser-endipitously confirmed when old organized or recanalized thrombi are discovered as totally incidental findings at necropsy. Such events suggest that organization and recanalization can be highly useful biological means of dealing with thrombi.

INFARCTION

An **infarct** is a localized area of ischemic necrosis in a tissue or organ. It can be produced by occlusion of either the arterial supply or the venous drainage of the tissue, but by far the most common cause is occlusive arterial obstruction. The

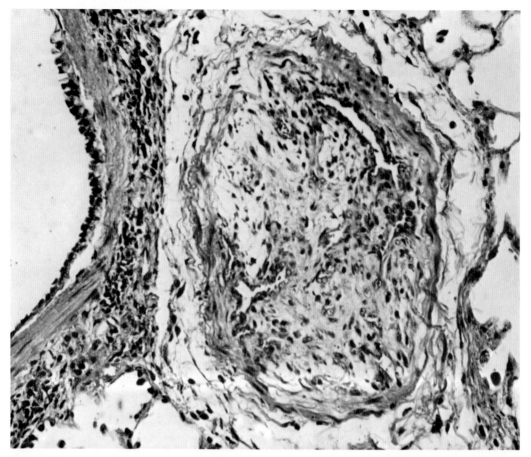

Figure 3.32. Organization of a Thrombus. This pulmonary thrombus shows infiltration by phagocytic cells, several areas of firm attachment to the vessel wall, and peripheral recanalization.

all too common "heart attack," which awaits many members of civilized western society, is, in fact, acute myocardial infarction due to occlusive coronary arterial thrombosis. Emboli can, of course, produce the same effect, although there are often mechanistic differences that relate to the processes whereby thrombi form in arteries and veins. Venous infarction usually is related to direct intravascular venous thrombosis without embolization. Arterial infarction, on the other hand, is more often embolic in nature, although direct thrombotic infarction certainly can occur.

We must again stress that arterial in-

farction is far more common than venous infarction. The reasons for this are largely anatomical. There are greater numbers of vascular collaterals on the venous side so that occlusion may produce only sufficient stasis and back pressure to open anastomotic channels. Infarcts vary somewhat in appearance depending on their pathogenesis and the time after infarction when the tissue is examined. Venous infarcts are usually intensely hemorrhagic as blood backs up into the affected tissue behind the obstruction. Arterial infarcts vary in appearance but are often initially hemorrhagic and later become pale as the area of coagulation necrosis becomes ev-

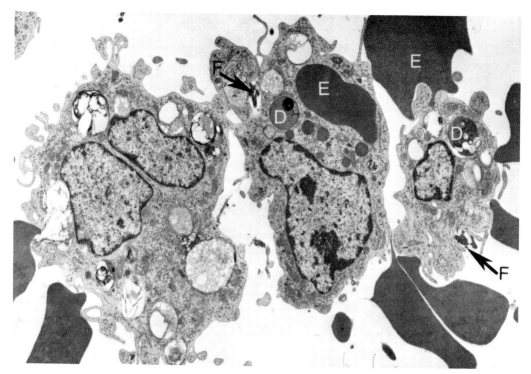

Figure 3.33.   Phagocytic Cells in a Thrombus. These macrophages are ingesting fibrin *(F)* and erythrocytes *(E)* in a thrombus. Several degraded red cells also are seen in the cells *(D)*. (Micrograph courtesy of Dr. W. L. Castleman.)

ident. There may be later hemorrhage into the necrotic tissue, however (Fig. 3.34).

There are also some variations depending on the tissue involved. Solid parenchymatous organs such as the heart and kidneys tend to have pale infarcts. The spleen also sometimes has pale infarcts, but they clearly can be hemorrhagic (Fig. 3.34). Arterial infarcts in "loose" tissues such as the lung are usually hemorrhagic, however. All infarcts tend to be shaped according to the service area of the vessel whose occlusion was responsible for the development of infarction. Hence, many infarcts are wedge shaped with the apex directed toward the area of vascular occlusion (*see* Fig. 2.22).

The typical histologic appearance of infarcted tissues is that of **ischemic coagulation necrosis** of the affected cells. The morphologic and biochemical alterations that characterize coagulation necrosis have been detailed in Chapter 2 and will not be reiterated here. We will instead focus on certain characteristics of various tissues which are important in determining the outcome of an episode of occlusive thrombosis or embolism. These include features related to the cardiovascular system as a whole as well as the specific vascular anatomy of a tissue and its general vulnerability to ischemia.

Determinants of Infarction

Ischemic Susceptibility

Not all tissues respond equally to ischemia. Since ischemic injury is basically anoxic injury, another way to state the problem is to note that there are wide variations in the tissue responses to an-

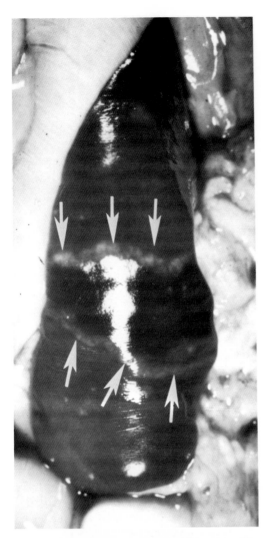

Figure 3.34. Splenic Infarct. The area of infarction *(arrows)* is well delineated from the surrounding parenchyma in this spleen from a cat with calcivirus infection. A pale border of leukocytes is present.

oxia. Possibly the most sensitive are the cells of the central nervous system, which will tolerate total anoxia for only a few minutes before undergoing irreversible degenerative changes and necrosis. Renal tubular epithelium is also extremely sensitive to anoxia. Most parenchymal cells and tissues are, in fact, quite susceptible to ischemic necrosis because of their intolerance of anoxia. Indeed, renal tubular

epithelial cells do not even like hypoxia, much less anoxia. The metabolically and physiologically active myocardial cells also are susceptible to ischemia, and usually respond by dying.

It is not coincidental, therefore, that the brain, the kidneys, and the heart are rather common sites for infarction. An additional reason for this lies in the nature of the blood supply to these tissues, as we shall see presently. In contrast to the situation in the brain, the heart, the kidneys, and most parenchymal tissues, mesenchymal cells such as fibroblasts are relatively resistant to anoxic injury. This is an extremely useful distinction, as the preservation of these stromal supporting elements often allows survival of the **framework** of a tissue even though the more sensitive parenchymal elements have succumbed. As we shall see in Chapter 4, the maintenance of the stromal supporting framework is an essential prerequisite for the reconstruction of injured tissue, by regeneration, in those tissues composed of labile or stable cell populations capable of controlled cell proliferation as a repair mechanism.

Anatomy of the Vasculature

Most tissues of the body have one of three basic patterns of vascular supply. Many tissues and organs are limited to a blood supply that arrives *via* a **single vessel,** which then ramifies into smaller and smaller radicals within the tissue or organ. Vessels of this type often are referred to as "functional end arteries," and are typified by the kind of vasculature that serves the spleen and the kidneys. Thrombotic or embolic occlusion of such end arteries almost invariably leads to infarction unless the occluded vessel is an extremely small one. To a large extent the cerebral and coronary vessels are also functional end arteries.

Some organs and tissues receive their blood supply through separate but functionally **parallel systems,** which often have substantial numbers of functional and/or anatomic anastomotic channels. Thrombosis rarely produces infarction of skeletal muscles for this reason. Similarly, the arterial supply to the tubular viscera includes many plexiform anastomotic networks near the mesenteric border of the intestines. When such vessels are occluded by thrombi or emboli, infarction rarely results because the circulation at the level of the tissue cells may be largely unaffected. We should point out, however, that if one of the larger mesenteric vessels becomes occluded near its origin at the abdominal aorta, infarction certainly can occur. This forms the basis for what is known clinically as "thromboembolic colic" in horses. In this disease, verminous arteritis and thrombotic occlusion of the cranial mesenteric artery and embolism of smaller vessels follows vascular damage caused by larval stages of the helminth *Strongylus vulgaris* (Fig. 3.35).

Only a few tissues have a truly **dual blood supply.** The lungs are perfused by both the pulmonary arterial system and the bronchial arterial system. The liver also receives blood through two distinct circulatory systems, the portal vein and the hepatic artery. In most instances, occlusion of one of these blood supplies is without significant effect because tissue remains perfused *via* the other. Thus, hepatic and pulmonary infarction is an uncommon event provided that the overall cardiovascular function of the host is normal. If, however, such changes as severe anemia or chronic passive congestion from cardiac failure are present, infarction can occur in the liver or lungs because the dual blood supply system is compromised. It is a useful rule of thumb for clinicians and pathologists alike that

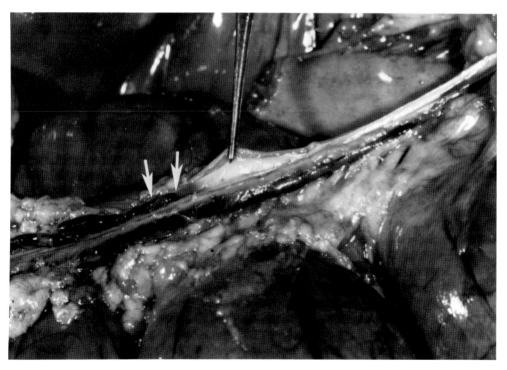

Figure 3.35. Thromboembolic Colic. The colonic artery in this horse contains a large embolus *(arrows)* that originated from a thrombus at the cranial mesenteric artery where verminous arteritis was present.

pulmonary infarction is unusual unless the lung already has chronic passive congestion. The same might be said for the liver.

Overall Cardiovascular Function

As we have suggested in the preceding paragraphs, the overall cardiovascular and hematologic health of the individual can play a deciding role in determining the outcome of an episode of occlusive thrombosis. Anything that reduces the oxygen-carrying capacity of the blood predisposes to infarction as a sequel to thrombosis. Similarly, significant alterations in the velocity of blood flow or blood volume actually can favor the development of ischemic infarction. Severe anemia, by virtue of the overall reduction in blood oxygenation, predisposes to thrombosis. It has been shown experimentally that even partial coronary occlusion leads to myocardial infarction in severely anemic subjects, while control subjects with normal red blood cell counts rarely develop myocardial infarction. It is also a well known clinical observation that aged humans with severe coronary arteriosclerosis may develop myocardial infarction following episodes of anemia or acute blood loss. It stands to reason that generalized circulatory conditions such as shock or congestive heart failure impair the circulation and hence the oxygenation of all tissues, and therefore predispose to the development of infarction should thrombosis or embolism occur.

Clinical Significance of Infarction

As a cause of tissue destruction and acute clinical disease with considerable morbidity and mortality, infarction ranks equally with the various infectious diseases and malignancies as a major pathologic process in man. It is a grim statistical prospect indeed to realize that some 20% of *all* human deaths from *all* causes in the United States are due to myocar-

dial infarction. When the reaper comes, he may well arrive disguised as a thrombus designed with malice aforethought to steal in and occlude our coronary arteries (Fig. 3.36).

The situation in most other animal species is, happily, not quite so bad. Infarction of the heart or the brain or even the lungs are occasional causes of death in any species, but there is no one single syndrome in any species that assumes the importance that myocardial infarction does in man. Often, infarcts may be associated with other underlying disease problems such as vegetative valvular endocarditis with embolism of a variety of distant sites. The clinical significance of infarction depends upon **where** it occurs and upon the **size** of the infarct. In this regard it is somewhat similar to hemorrhage as a pathologic event. A small cerebral infarct may have considerable clinical importance and be a much more ominous development than would be, for example, an infarct twice as large in the spleen. Myocardial infarcts similarly are usually serious pathological changes. Fatality from infarction thus depends to a large extent on the site where the infarction occurred, with the brain and the heart being the least tolerant. Substantial infarcts of any tissue can be serious, and certainly pulmonary infarction can lead to fatality.

In many tissues, and particularly in the case of smaller infarcts, only transient clinical signs or none at all may be apparent. The frequency with which healed infarcts are discovered as incidental findings in routine necropsy specimens bears this out. Usually such infarcts have healed by fibrosis, but the compensatory functional capacity of the affected tissues is often sufficient to circumvent lasting clinical effects. This in no way should be construed to indicate that ischemic necrosis secondary to infarction is not an important pathologic process. Virtually all pathologists and clinicians have seen in-

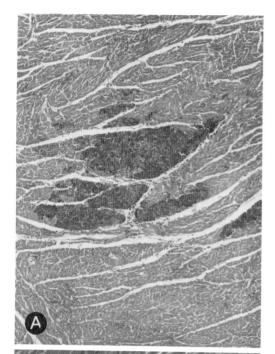

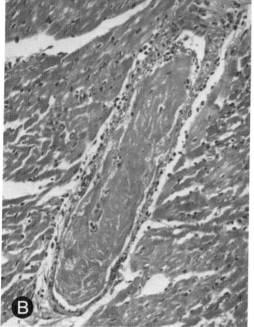

Figure 3.36. *A,* **Myocardial Infarction.** The area of acute ischemic necrosis and hemorrhage is clearly visible in this section of heart. *B,* **Coronary Thrombosis.** This section is from an area adjacent to the infarct in *A.* The small coronary arteriole contains a recent thrombus.

farction cause death often enough to hold it in considerable respect as significant mechanism of disease.

EDEMA

Edema is the accumulation of excessive amounts of extracellular water in the interstitial fluid space, that is, outside the vascular fluid compartment and outside the cellular fluid compartment. It does not imply anything about the plasma volume or about the volume of cells themselves. Indeed, the plasma volume may or may not be increased at all, and cellular fluid volumes are usually normal. It is possible, however, to get an increase in the fluid volume of cells. This usually produces cell swelling and is often a reflection of cellular injury with sufficient damage to the cell membrane and its functions that alterations in water and electrolyte fluxes across that membrane are produced. Cell swelling also can occur as a consequence of decreased osmolality of the extracellular water or increased osmolality of the intracellular water. Such changes are more properly discussed as functions of cellular injury (*see* Chapter 2), and we will direct our attention here to **tissue edema,** or the accumulation of excessive interstitial or extracellular fluid. To understand the pathogenesis of edema, it will be helpful to briefly review the structure and physiology of the terminal vascular bed, the interstitial space, and the extracellular matrix.

Interstitium and Extracellular Matrix

What is the **interstitium?** This is a reasonable question and a reasonable place to begin. The interstitium is the space between tissue compartments, and it binds most cellular and structural elements into discrete organs and tissues. At a simplistic level, it is what is left over after you remove all of the blood and lymphatic vessels, nerves, and parenchymal cells from a tissue. It is the place where tissue

Table 3.5
Composition of the Extracellular Matrix

Component	Structure	Features
Collagens	Triple helix, fibrils, fibers	Several types, present in all tissues
Elastic fibers	Cross-linked network of elastin	Can stretch and recoil
Fibronectin	Large fiber-forming glyco-protein	Promotes cell adhesion, *etc.*
Laminin	Large glycoprotein, two subunits	Found in all basal laminae, diverse functions
Glycosaminoglycans (GAGs)	Unbranched chains of polysaccharides	Bound to protein in ECM, attract water
Proteoglycans	Protein spine with attached GAGs	Form hydrated gels, large ag-gregates with link proteins

edema fluid accumulates. The intersti-tium is not acellular, but contains both cellular and extracellular elements. It consists mainly of various fibers and fi-brils and connective tissue cells like fi-broblasts, but it is the **extracellular ma-trix (ECM)** itself that is of particular interest (Table 3.5). Until recently, the ECM was thought to be largely a rela-tively inert structural scaffolding that stabilized the physical structure of tis-sues. It is now clear that the ECM plays a far more active and complex role in regulating the behavior of the cells that contact it, and the water-attracting prop-erty of glycosaminoglycans is particularly germane to our discussion of edema.

The ECM consists of various glycopro-teins, proteoglycans, and glycosamino-glycans that are secreted by cells and assembled locally into an organized net-work. The metabolism of the cells embed-ded in the ECM, such as fibroblasts, is particularly concerned with the biosyn-thesis and secretion of matrix material. For convenience, the ECM may be viewed as consisting of an **insoluble** fibrous phase containing proteins like collagen, tissue fibronectin, elastin, and other structural glycoproteins, and a **soluble** gel phase, largely protein polysaccharides, or pro-

teoglycans, which fills the space between the insoluble fibers and fibrils. Thus, the ECM consists primarily of fibrous pro-teins embedded in a hydrated proteogly-can gel. Connective tissue cells are com-pletely surrounded by the ECM, while other types of epithelial, endothelial, and muscle cells are separated from it by a specialized sheet of ECM known as the **basal lamina** (basement membrane) (*see also* Chapter 2).

The biochemical composition of the ECM varies among tissues, but the two main classes of extracellular macromolecules are the **collagens** and the polysaccharide **glycosaminoglycans (GAGs),** which are usually covalently linked to protein to form **proteoglycans.** The GAGs and pro-teoglycan molecules form a highly hy-drated, gel-like "ground substance" in which the collagen fibers are embedded. In many areas, fibers of **elastin** are also present and contribute to the resiliency of the ECM. In addition, two high molec-ular weight glycoproteins are among the major components of the ECM: tissue **fi-bronectin,** which is widely distributed in connective tissues, and **laminin,** which is found largely in basement membranes.

The **collagens** are the most abundant of the ECM components, and are so abundant that they constitute about 33% of the total protein mass of most animals. A central feature of all collagens is their stiff, triple-stranded helical structure. Three collagen polypeptide chains are wound around each other in a regular helix to form the rope-like collagen molecule. After being secreted into the extracellular space, the collagen molecules are assembled into ordered polymers, called collagen **fibrils,** which are usually grouped together into larger bundles, called collagen **fibers,** which can be seen in the light microscope. A number of different types of **collagen** have been identified, which vary in the composition of the chains in the triple helix and in tissue distribution. Type I collagen, for example, is widely distributed in skin, tendon, and bone, whereas type IV collagen is the main type in basement membranes. The collagens serve a wide variety of structural and mechanical functions.

Certain tissues that require greater elasticity (skin, blood vessels, lung) have an extensive network of **elastic fibers.** The main component of elastic fibers is **elastin,** an M_r 70,000 protein, which is secreted into the ECM where filaments and broad sheets are formed in which the individual elastin molecules are highly cross-linked to each other to form an extensive network. These unique molecules remain unfolded, so that random coils are formed. This cross-linked, random-coil structure of the elastic fiber network allows it to stretch and recoil like a rubber band. Collagen fibers interwoven with the elastic fibers limit the extent of stretching and prevent tissue tearing.

The noncollagen glycoproteins of the ECM have been relatively ignored until recent years. **Fibronectin** first attracted attention when it was found to be present in greatly reduced amounts on the surface of malignant fibroblasts as compared to normal fibroblasts. Fibronectin is now known to be a member of a growing family of ECM glycoproteins with dramatic effects on cell migration, differentiation, morphology, and metabolic activities. It is probably the best characterized of the ECM **cell adhesion molecules,** and it has the ability to interact specifically with a large number of other biologically important molecules. Fibronectin is a large, fiber-forming glycoprotein composed of two disulfide-bonded subunits of about M_r 250,000 each, which exists in the ECM as large filaments and aggregates. It functions in a wide variety of ways, many of which are associated with cell-to-substrate adhesion and migration, and it has been recently implicated in embryonic differentiation. Fibronectin is perhaps best viewed as a multifunctional molecule with a series of specialized binding sites that mediate its functions. In addition to binding to the surfaces of most eukaryotic cells, fibronectin binds to collagen, fibrin and fibrinogen, heparin and heparan sulfate, actin, DNA, and the Clq component of complement. The potential range of functions mediated by this molecule is thus as long as the list of its major binding activities.

The **basal lamina** (basement membranes) are the thin sheets of specialized ECM that underlie all epithelial cell sheets and tubes and surround certain individual cells such as muscle cells and Schwann cells, separating them from the underlying or surrounding connective tissue matrix. There is increasing evidence, however, that the basal laminae serve more than a simple structural and filtering role; they can induce cell differentiation, influence cell metabolism, and direct specific cell migration. The basal lamina is synthesized by the cells that rest on it, and hence it has a somewhat different chemical composition at different sites. In addition to type IV collagen, the basal lamina contains proteoglycans, fibronectin, hyaluronic acid molecules, and the large glycoprotein **laminin,** which has been shown to be a major component of all basal laminae studied to date. Laminin consists of at least two large subunits (M_r 220,000 and 440,000), which are disulfide-bonded.

It is interesting to note that recent sequencing data have shown considerable homology in the cell surface receptors for fibronectin, laminin, the platelet membrane glycoproteins GP IIb-GP IIIa, and the leukocyte adhesion molecule complex LFA-1/Mac-1/p150,95. Many of these receptors recognize sites that include the tripeptide arg-gly-asp **(the RGD sequence),** suggesting a common genetic background. This family of cell surface receptors has been called the **integrins,** and participates in a variety of cell-matrix and cell-cell adhesion events important to embryological development, wound healing, immune and nonimmune host defenses, as well as hemostasis and thrombosis.

Glycosaminoglycans (GAGs), formerly known as mucopolysaccharides, are long, unbranched polysaccharide chains with repeating disaccharide units. They are perhaps the most important constituents of the ECM with respect to their potential role in edema. The name glycosaminoglycans comes from the fact that one of the two sugar residues in the repeating disaccharide unit is always an amino sugar, (either N-acetylglucosamine or N-acetylgalatosamine). Like the collagens, there are several different types of GAGs (dermatan sulfate, chondroitin sulfate, heparan sulfate, *etc.*), which differ chemically and in tissue location.

All of the GAGs are covalently linked to a protein core to form a **proteoglycan.** Sometimes giant aggregates of proteoglycans are formed in which many proteoglycan monomers are noncovalently bound to a central core through special **link proteins.** These large molecules are folded and refolded every few hundred Angstroms, so that instead of a long linear fibril, they actually form jumbled, folded, random coils. In the interstitial space, there are literally millions of these coiled springlike molecules. They entangle and compress each other and restrict each other's movement. They also can interact with dissolved substances in the interstitial fluid and can hold other molecules by electrostatic charges. It is this tangled mass of proteoglycans that gives the interstitium its gel-like characteristic. The GAG chains thus form extended, random-coil conformations, which occupy a huge volume relative to their mass. They effectively *fill* the extracellular space even though by weight the GAGs constitute less than 10% of the contribution of the fibrous proteins like collagen and elastin. The proteoglycans attract large amounts of water and are **hydrated gels** even at low concentrations, a tendency markedly enhanced by their high density of negative charges. Their porous and hydrated organization allows them to participate in the diffusion of water and water-soluble molecules in the extracellular space, and it is likewise responsible for the pressure (turgor) of the ECM.

Most of the interstitial fluid is water. Since molecular coils of the proteoglycans are of appropriate molecular dimensions, they offer tremendous viscous resistance to the flow of water molecules through their substance. Water thus moves through the interstitial space largely by diffusion rather than by convectional flow. The gelled interstitial fluid exhibits the phenomenon of **thixotropy.** This means that if the interstitial fluids are somehow stirred up, so that the entangled proteoglycan coils become separated, the interstitium takes on more fluid characteristics. An additional example of this phenomenon comes from the fluids of the synovial, pleural, pericardial, and peritoneal cavities, which all contain similar molecules to the interstitial fluid. However, these fluids are constantly "stirred up" by the motions of the tissues they bathe, and hence they have a much more fluid state than does normal interstitial fluid. Even so, such fluids are highly viscous, almost like an oil in the case of synovial fluid, and perform an important lubricating function in their respective cavities.

The proteoglycans and GAGs in the interstitium behave as giant polyelectrolytes in that they can undergo sensitive changes in conformation with changes in the local environment; when the ionic strength is lowered, as might be expected with the addition of low protein-content edema fluid, the polysaccharide backbone structures have a greater tendency to repel one another and the molecules take on an extended conformation. There is also evidence that the polymer chain formations are affected in concentrated solutions; when concentration increases, as might be expected with the addition of protein-rich edema fluid, the molecules collapse into more compact coils.

It is currently envisioned that this molecular compression is an osmotic effect of competition between neighboring molecules for water, with the result that water is withdrawn from the hydrated domain of the molecules. Thus, the old explanation that "connective tissue substances bind edema fluid" has been given a potentially useful molecular definition. It has been theorized that a two-phase system exists, consisting of a gel-like phase composed of proteoglycans associated with a fluid volume from which the protein content of the fluid is excluded and, between the proteoglycans, a free fluid phase containing the plasma proteins. Fluxes of fluid between these two phases would depend on the relative concentrations of protein and polysaccharide in the various compartments. With increased molecular definition of the composition and function of the ECM, particularly the proteoglycans and GAGs, a better understanding of edematous states can be envisioned for the future.

Our consideration of the interstitial space where edema fluid accumulates would not be complete without a consideration of **interstitial fluid pressure.** Interstitial pressure is important in the determination of edema since it can determine in part where and to what extent fluid can move. It is made up of several components including interstitial osmotic pressure, interstitial hydrostatic pressure, and pressure exerted by the elasticity of the gel matrix itself. Interstitial pressure helps to determine whether fluids can leak from the vascular to the interstitial compartment and helps the movement of fluid from the interstitial compartment into lymphatics. It will play an important role in our discussion of the physiology of fluid movements at the terminal vascular bed and their functions in the pathogenesis of edema.

Microvascular Physiology

The details of capillary exchange and tissue fluid convection are fascinating subjects in their own right, which have attracted and stimulated a large number of physiologists. Our interest is more directed, and we will be concerned here only with those features of the structure and function of the terminal vascular bed that relate to body fluid homeostasis and its alteration in the edematous state. In short, we will deal only with those factors (forces) that control the net balance between the outward and inward movement of fluid at the capillary membrane.

In a typical capillary bed, an arteriole gives rise to numerous capillaries, which then coalesce to form venules. True capillaries arise from either a **terminal arteriole** or a **meta-arteriole,** which is a sort of structural intermediary between arterioles and capillaries. At the point where the capillaries emerge, there is usually a smooth muscle fiber, wrapped around the mouth of the capillary, called the **precapillary sphincter.** This structure helps control flow conditions within the capillary network. The structure of a typical terminal vascular bed is shown in Fig. 3.37.

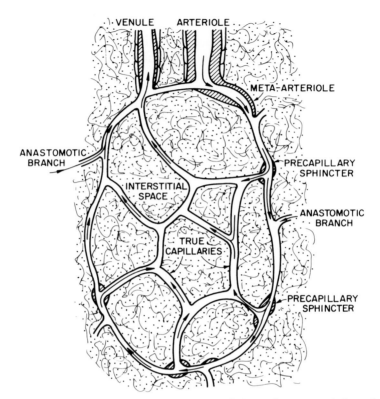

Figure 3.37. Microcirculatory Bed and Interstitium. Schematic representation of a typical capillary bed lying between the terminal arteriole and the collecting venule. The interstitial space lies between the anastomotic branches of the capillary bed.

It is across the capillary wall itself that filtration actually takes place. If we examined a typical capillary, we would find an endothelial lining resting on a thin basement membrane and little else (*see* Fig. 4.12). The interendothelial junctions are not true tight junctions, and they can open to allow communication between the intravascular and extravascular fluid compartments.

There are basically three major physical factors that normally are operative in regulating the exchange of water and electrolytes between the vascular compartment and the interstitial compartment. These are (1) an intact, functioning circulatory system, (2) a normal, functioning lymphatic system, and (3) the concentration of albumin in the serum. If one or more of these factors is significantly altered, water and electrolytes may escape from the circulation faster than they return, and edema results.

To understand edema it is necessary to review the **Starling equilibrium,** which describes the relationships between the various forces at work at the level of the microcirculatory bed (Fig. 3.38). Starling equilibrium is achieved by the balance of filtration pressures and absorption pressures exerted across the filtering membranes of the terminal vascular bed. The **net filtration pressure** is represented by the differences in hydrostatic and colloidal osmotic pressures between the plasma and tissue interstitial compartment at the arterial end of the capillary vascular bed, and the **net absorption pressure** is determined by differences in hydrostatic and colloidal osmotic pressures between the

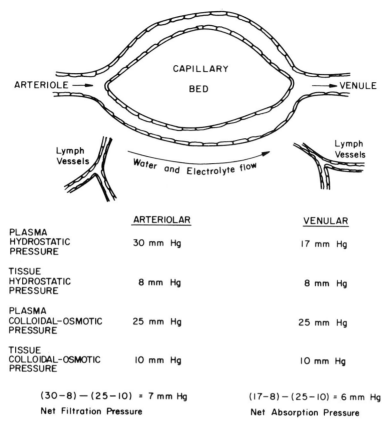

	ARTERIOLAR	VENULAR
PLASMA HYDROSTATIC PRESSURE	30 mm Hg	17 mm Hg
TISSUE HYDROSTATIC PRESSURE	8 mm Hg	8 mm Hg
PLASMA COLLOIDAL–OSMOTIC PRESSURE	25 mm Hg	25 mm Hg
TISSUE COLLOIDAL–OSMOTIC PRESSURE	10 mm Hg	10 mm Hg
	$(30-8)-(25-10) = 7$ mm Hg	$(17-8)-(25-10) = 6$ mm Hg
	Net Filtration Pressure	Net Absorption Pressure

Figure 3.38. Starling Equilibrium. Schematic drawing to show the interplay of plasma and tissue colloidal-osmotic and hydrostatic forces, which determine filtration and absorption across the microvascular bed.

plasma and tissue interstitial compartment at the venous end of the capillary vascular bed. Basically, at the **arteriolar end** of the microvascular bed there is a plasma hydrostatic pressure of about 30 mm Hg, which is offset by a tissue hydrostatic pressure of about 8 mm Hg, leaving a balance of 22 mm Hg pressure (30 minus 8), which favors filtration. Operating against the hydrostatic pressure favoring filtration at the arterial end of the bed is the colloidal osmotic pressure of plasma, which acts as a force to keep fluid within the vascular lumen. This colloidal osmotic pressure of plasma (about 25 mm Hg) must work against a tissue colloidal osmotic pressure of about 10 mm Hg, which tends to "pull" fluid towards the intersti-

tium. Hence an osmotic pressure differential of 15 mm Hg (25 minus 10) results, which basically is the difference between the osmotic pressure of plasma and that of tissue, and which acts to keep fluid in the cardiovascular compartment. The net filtration pressure at the arteriolar end of the microvascular bed then is about 7 mm Hg, and represents the difference between the hydrostatic pressure difference (22 mm Hg) favoring filtration and the osmotic pressure difference (15 mm Hg) working to keep fluid in the vascular compartment.

At the **venular end** of the system, the plasma hydrostatic pressure is lower (about 17 mm Hg), but the other pressure relationships remain similar to those encountered at the arteriolar end. Hence, a plasma-tissue hydrostatic pressure difference of 9 mm Hg (17 minus 8) favoring filtration is offset by a plasma-tissue colloidal osmotic pressure difference of 15 mm Hg (25 minus 10) which leaves a net absorption pressure at the venular end of about 6 mm Hg. As you will recall, the net filtration pressure at the arteriolar end was about 7 mm Hg. With an arteriolar input to the interstitial space of 7 mm Hg and a net absorption pressure of only 6 mm Hg, edema would gradually develop. What happens to the extra 1 mm of pressure? This is where the lymphatics enter the picture. The lymphatics are basically a very low pressure system that can operate to maintain fluid homeostasis at the level of the microvascular bed by taking care of this 1 mm of pressure *via* absorption. With the lymphatic system functioning normally, the system is then in equilibrium.

It is likely that the Starling equilibrium hypothesis is a gross oversimplification even though it is widely accepted as the explanation for water and small molecule transfer in the terminal vascular bed. Certainly it is reasonable not to attach too much specific significance to the actual numbers associated with the various forces at work (Fig. 3.38). These undoubtedly vary from species to species and from region to region within the body. For our purposes, however, Starling equilibrium provides an extremely useful way to look at the pathogenesis of edema. Indeed, **virtually all clinical forms of edema can be traced to some alteration in Starling equilibrium or to increased vascular permeability that disturbs Starling equilibrium.**

Pathophysiology of Edema

Most animals are about 60% water by mass, divided into intracellular and extracellular compartments, the latter consisting of plasma water and interstitial water. In the final analysis, edema basically is nothing more than an expansion of the interstitial fluid compartment. As we have discussed above, the interchange of water between the vascular and interstitial compartments is governed by the forces responsible for Starling equilibrium, the plasma and tissue hydrostatic and osmotic pressures and the contribution of interstitial lymphatics. While not actively a part of the forces at play in Starling equilibrium, it should be obvious that the entire system is ultimately dependent upon the normal integrity of the endothelial barrier lining the vascular bed in which the fluid exchange takes place. In the normal animal, there is almost certainly a continual balancing of these various factors in order to maintain fluid homeostasis. Edema results only when the balancing ability of the various forces at play is disturbed to the point where equilibrium is lost in favor of accumulation of fluid in the interstitial compartment.

Theoretically, any disturbance of Starling equilibrium could lead to edema, but from a practical standpoint, there are basically only four dynamic mechanisms that can underlie the development of edema: (1) decreased plasma colloidal-osmotic pressure, (2) increased blood hydrostatic pressure, (3) lymphatic obstruction, and (4) increased vascular permeability. The location and extent of edema formation depends in part on which of these mechanisms is operative. For example, a decrease in plasma colloidal-osmotic pressure would tend to produce a generalized effect, increased plasma hydrostatic pressure might induce either local or systemic effects depending on the pathogenesis of the increase, whereas lymphatic obstruction and vascular permeability increases are almost always localized effects producing localized edema. Let us examine these four major mechanisms of edema in somewhat more detail.

Decreased Plasma Colloidal-Osmotic Pressure

Colloid osmotic pressure refers to the effect of colloidal solutes on the chemical potential of water molecules. The largest and most important group of colloids in body fluids such as plasma are the proteins. In plasma, proteins function as giant "polyelectrolytes" because they are generally negatively charged, and the pH of most body fluids is well off the isoelectric point of the proteins. Proteins normally are present in plasma in concentrations of 60 to 70 g/liter, and they exert their full effective osmotic pressure across the capillary membrane to oppose the flow of liquid to the interstitial compartment under the force of hydrostatic pressure in the capillary bed. As the most abundant of the plasma proteins, with a relatively low M_r (68,000), albumin is the most important of the plasma proteins to edema formation, as it exerts the major portion of the plasma colloid osmotic effect. Hence, decreases in plasma colloid osmotic pressure reflect a decrease in total plasma proteins, but this is largely due to decreases in albumin concentration, since globulins are only about 25% as effective in maintaining colloid osmotic pressure as albumin. Therefore, edema due to a decrease in plasma colloid osmotic pressure usually has its basis in hypoalbuminemia.

Returning to the Starling equilibrium (*see* Figure 3.38), a 50% drop in the albumin concentration in plasma would produce a corresponding decline in the plasma colloid osmotic pressure to a value, to use our previous numbers, of about 12.5 mm Hg. This would so disturb the system that the net filtration pressure on the arteriolar side would be about 19.5 mm Hg. Although the decline in plasma colloid osmotic pressure also would affect the venular side of the equation, the change would be less dramatic because of the lower plasma hydrostatic pressure on the venous side. Nonetheless, if you work through the numbers, you will find that rather than having a net absorption pressure on the venous side, a decline in albumin levels of this magnitude would in fact produce a net positive filtration pressure of about 6.5 mm Hg, even on the absorptive end of the capillary bed. In such a situation, lymphatic flow would no doubt be increased, but the net result would be the accumulation of fluid in the interstitial space, as the lymphatics could not effectively deal with a total net filtration pressure across the vascular bed of some 26 mm Hg. Edema would result (Fig. 3.39).

Decreases in the albumin concentration can, at a simplistic level, result from basically only two mechanisms: either not enough albumin is being synthesized to keep up with its normal rate of catabolism, or albumin is being normally synthesized and delivered to the plasma but is being lost at a rate greatly exceeding normal. Decreases in albumin synthesis can occur in starvation syndromes where a protein-deficient diet fails to provide sufficient material for albumin synthesis. As albumin is synthesized in the liver, some forms of liver disease also are accompanied by hypoalbuminemia due to a decrease in hepatic albumin synthesis. Albumin can be lost from the body largely *via* two routes; renal and gastrointestinal. For example, the dog described in the case study in Chapter 5 was losing protein through damage to the glomerular ultrafiltration system because of diffuse glomerulonephritis. This is one form of protein-losing renal disease, and edema is often a part of the clinical picture. Gastrointestinal loss can occur in various infectious enteric diseases, in the various protein-losing enteropathy syndromes, and when whole blood is lost *via* the gastrointestinal tract in some kinds of parasitism such as haemonchosis. Regardless of the

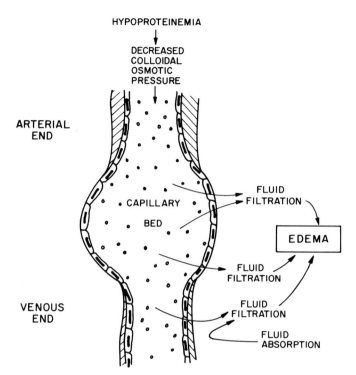

Figure 3.39.   Edema—Decreased Osmotic Pressure. Decline in plasma protein levels *(small open circles)* decreases the colloidal-osmotic pressure of plasma and upsets Starling equilibrium to result in edema.

specific etiological background, all of these forms of clinical edema have their basis in decreased plasma colloid osmotic pressure due to hypoalbuminemia.

Increased Blood Hydrostatic Pressure

The hydrostatic pressure of the blood is the force that acts to overcome the colloid osmotic pressure of the plasma and acts normally to allow the passage of nutritive fluids into the tissues. If it is increased, edema can result. We must recall that the pressure at the level of the capillary bed is influenced mostly by the venous pressure and not the arterial pressure. Thus, while arterial hypertension might seem to be a likely background for the development of edema, this is in fact a rather unusual occurrence. A far more important group of causes are those that

increase capillary pressure by raising the venous pressure. To return to our model of Starling equilibrium, envision what might occur if the blood hydrostatic pressure were raised to about 30 mm Hg, or the same as it is at the arterial end of the microvascular bed. This would be an approximate doubling of the hydrostatic pressure at the venous end of the capillary bed. Now, if you do the arithmetic, you will discover that rather than having a net absorption pressure of 6 mm Hg at the venous end of the capillary bed, you have a net filtration pressure of some 7 mm Hg. Thus, the increase in venous back pressure negates the absorptive function of the venous bed and, in fact, fluid filtered at the arterial end fails to return to the circulation. The result is edema (Fig. 3.40).

This process can occur at both localized and generalized levels. At a local level,

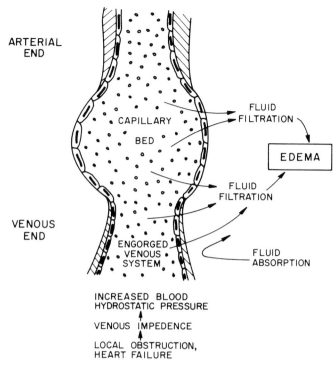

Figure 3.40.   Edema—Increased Blood Hydrostatic Pressure. Venous engorgement from raised hydrostatic pressure dilates the venules (passive hyperemia) and disturbs Starling equilibrium to result in edema. (Protein, *small open circles*).

the most common backgrounds to increased hydrostatic pressure involve **local obstructions** to venous flow, which, naturally enough, raise pressure behind the obstruction. This can be related to occlusion of a vein by an intravascular thrombus or a tumor, or can occur if the vessel becomes obstructed from without as might occur with pressure on a vessel by a tumor or an abscess. The gravid uterus sometimes can exert enough pressure on iliac veins to cause increased venous pressure and edema in the posterior limbs. An additional example of this phenomenon can be drawn from equine medicine and surgery where a 180° or 360° rotational torsion of the abdominal viscera sometimes occurs around the root of the mesenteric vasculature. In this situation, the more easily collapsed veins become totally obstructed while the thicker-walled arteries remain at least partially

operative. The result is an extremely edematous and congested intestine, which often produces severe colic and death.

Cardiac failure is the most important cause of a generalized increase in venous pressure. Because the anatomic cause of the problem here is such that a generalized elevation in blood pressure occurs at the venous end of the capillary bed, the edema also tends to be more generalized than would result from a locally obstructive lesion. In cardiac failure, the venous pressure rises markedly, and the stretching and dilatation of the venules and capillaries may render them more permeable as well. This excessive venous pressure that occurs in cardiac failure is by no means the only mechanism by which heart failure causes edema. An increase in aldosterone production leading to increased sodium retention also contributes to the process.

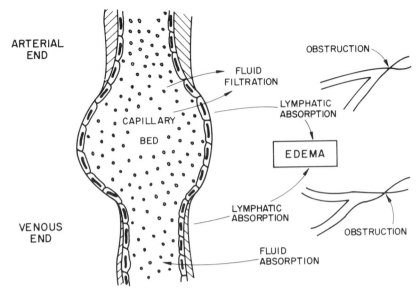

Figure 3.41.   Edema—Lymphatic Blockade. Failure of lymphatic vessels to absorb filtered fluid causes accumulation of that fluid in the interstitial space and edema results. (Protein, *small open circles*).

Lymphatic Obstruction

If we return to our model of Starling equilibrium once again, the effects of a functional removal of lymphatic drainage should be clear. Recall that in the normal state, the difference between the 7 mm Hg net filtration pressure and the 6 mm Hg net absorption pressure is made up by lymphatic absorption. When the lymphatics are obstructed by any lesion that impedes normal lymph flow or absorption, excess tissue fluid accumulates in the interstitial space and edema results (Fig. 3.41). The lesion need not be within the lymphatic channels themselves, as lesions at the level of the lymph nodes which impede lymphatic flow also may cause edema. Thus, damage to or obstruction of the lymphatics by trauma, surgical intervention, or inflammatory or neoplastic disease can result in edema. This form of edema is particularly common in association with certain kinds of malignant tumors which grow into and obstruct lymphatic drainage. A striking cause of this

form of edema is the inflammatory obstruction of lymphatics that occurs in certain filarial infections of man, such as that caused by *Wuchereria bancrofti* (elephantiasis). Here, massive lymphatic obstruction and striking local edema are clinical highlights.

In lymphatic obstruction, the edema that results almost always is localized because the lesion almost always is localized. There are virtually no acquired forms of generalized lymphatic edema, and even in elephantiasis the edema is usually localized.

Increased Vascular Permeability

As mentioned previously, the success of Starling equilibrium depends on the structural integrity of the microvascular bed. When endothelial integrity is compromised, edema results. This can occur in a generalized way with certain potent toxins or chemicals, but, for the most part, the edema resulting from increased capillary permeability is a localized phenomenon. This, in fact, is the **edema of in-**

flammation. A critical feature of the evolving inflammatory reaction is the opening of interendothelial gaps to permit plasma proteins and circulating leukocytes to enter the tissue to perform their critical defensive functions (*see* Chapter 4). Anyone who has experienced a bee sting has experienced this form of edema. In this example, part of the edema is probably a direct result of damage to the endothelium from toxins in the bee venom, and part of the edema is a result of chemically mediated increases in local vascular permeability due to local histamine release from tissue mast cells. We will explore this phenomenon in greater detail in the next chapter.

An additional feature of inflammatory edema, which sets it apart from most other forms of edema, is the **high protein content** of the fluid leaving the vasculature and entering the tissues. In most forms of edema, the fluid itself remains an ultrafiltrate of plasma, consisting largely of water and dissolved electrolytes. In inflammatory edema, however, the integ-

rity of the microfilter is lost due to endothelial damage and chemically mediated permeability alterations so that, in addition to water and dissolved electrolytes, significant amounts of protein are found in the fluid (Fig. 3.42).

Appearance of Edema

It should be obvious that the changes produced by edema in the tissues will reflect the severity, rapidity of onset, extent, anatomic location of the edema, and the underlying cause. In generalized edema, fluid tends to collect in the lowermost portions of the body such as the ventral abdomen and the limbs, a pattern referred to as **dependent edema.** When such edema is severe and generalized, it produces a diffuse marked swelling of the subcutaneous tissues. Because the swelling represents an expansion of the interstitial fluid space, it often is possible to push a finger against such edematous tissues and actually produce a dent in the tissue. Such edematous changes are known as **pitting edema.** When edema is severe

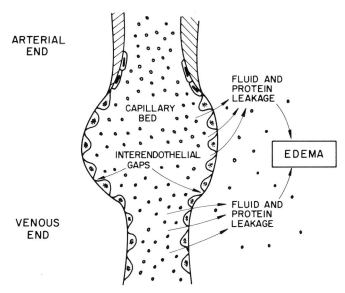

Figure 3.42. Edema—Increased Vascular Permeability. The edema of inflammation involves changes in endothelial cells, which permit not only water and electrolytes but also protein **(small open circles)** to accumulate as edema fluid.

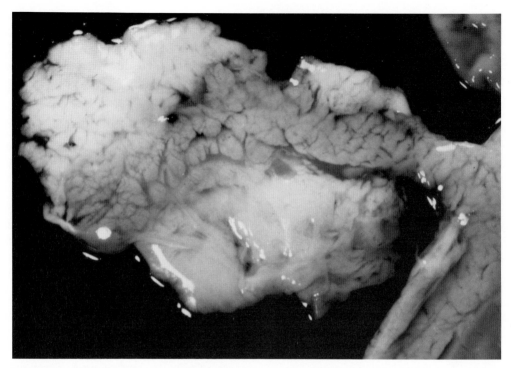

Figure 3.43.   Edema. The wet, glassy appearance of this edematous dog pancreas is due to edema fluid. Note that the fluid has dissected the pancreas into visible lobulations and arborizations not normally seen.

and generalized and causes diffuse swelling of all tissues and organs in the body, particularly noticeable in the subcutaneous tissues, it is called **anasarca.**

While edema fluid often accumulates in tissue interstitial compartments, it may be prominent in body cavities as well. The collection of edema fluid in the peritoneal cavity is known as **ascites,** in the pleural cavity as **hydrothorax,** and in the pericardial sac as **hydropericardium** or **pericardial effusion.**

Edema is often easier to detect grossly than microscopically. At the gross level, the accumulation of edema fluid can be recognized by the excess clear fluid within a body cavity or a tissue. This is most easily visualized in a loosely organized tissue with much interstitium where the edema fluid physically pushes apart the normal tissue structures (Fig. 3.43). The

tissues are wet, shiny or glistening, and heavy due to the added component of water. It is sometimes more difficult to detect edema in a solid parenchymatous organ such as the liver or kidney, where the only visible manifestation may be an overall increase in size and weight.

Edema fluid varies in its microscopic appearance. If the fluid is largely composed of water and electrolytes (a transudate), there is nothing to take up a stain and the presence of edema may be detected only by its **dilutional effect** on normal tissue components. Water is invisible microscopically, hence its presence must be assumed by the spreading apart of normal tissue components and the **dilatation of lymphatics** in the tissue. If inflammatory edema is present, the protein content of the fluid will allow easier visualization of the lesion, as the protein

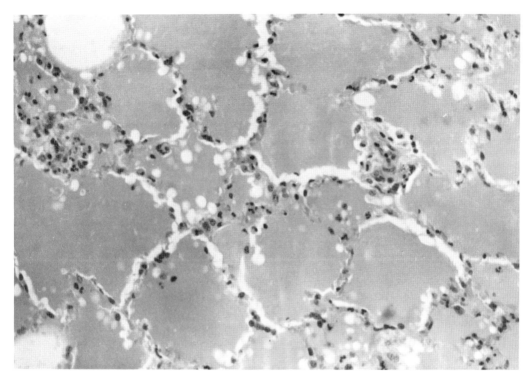

Figure 3.44.   Pulmonary Edema. The protein-rich edema fluid in alveolar spaces here is visible because of the staining properties of the protein present in the fluid.

will stain **pink** in hematoxylin and eosin preparations making it easily visible (Fig. 3.44).

Clinical Significance of Edema

The significance to clinical medicine of edema depends largely on its extent, its location, and its duration. In the brain and lungs, for example, edema may have serious or fatal consequences, whereas edema of the subcutis may have little functional significance. Cerebral edema is a justifiably feared consequence of various forms of brain injury, and it can have a fatal outcome. In addition to the violent headaches, projectile vomiting, and convulsive seizures that may accompany cerebral edema, herniation of the brain stem or cerebellar tonsils into the foramen magnum can occur as a result of the greatly raised intracranial pressure. In pulmonary edema, we are presented with the unique situation of "drowning from within." As fluid fills the alveoli and terminal bronchioles, the gas-exchange function of the lungs can become so compromised that it produces sufficient hypoxia to be fatal. In addition, the accumulation of fluid in the lungs is accompanied by an increased opportunity for secondary infections to become established. With the possible exceptions of cerebral and pulmonary edema, where direct intervention may be needed to prevent a fatality, edema usually is approached by attempting to sort out the ultimate **cause** and pathogenesis and then treating it accordingly. This is as it should be, and an understanding of the basic mechanisms underlying the development of edema make the process of therapy a good deal easier.

Table 3.6
Mechanistic View of Seven Clinical Forms of Edema

Name	Clinical Feature	Basic Problem	Disturbance of Starling Equilibrium
Renal edema	Proteinuria	Hypoproteinemia	Decreased plasma colloidal osmotic pressure
Cardiac edema	Generalized edema	Venous impedance	Increased blood hydrostatic pressure
Nutritional edema	Decreased protein intake	Hypoproteinemia	Decreased plasma colloidal osmotic pressure
Parasitic edema	Loss of whole blood in gastrointestinal tract	Hypoproteinemia	Decreased plasma colloidal osmotic pressure
Hepatic edema	Loss of hepatic albumin synthesis	Hypoproteinemia	Decreased plasma colloidal osmotic pressure
Inflammatory edema	Direct or indirect microvascular injury	Leaky vessels	Increased vascular permeability
Lymphatic edema	Lymphatic obstruction	Raise lymphatic pressure	Increased tissue hydrostatic pressure

From a clinical standpoint, edema often is classified according to the nature of the disease that produced the edema. Hence, you will read about "renal edema," "cardiac edema," "nutritional edema," "parasitic edema," and so on. Implicit in such terms is an understanding of the basic mechanisms which underlie the development of edema in these various disease states. It is beyond our scope to enter into a detailed discussion of clinical edema, but Table 3.6 should help in documenting that most common clinical forms of edema obey the rules we have set out here. They all involve a disturbance of one or more of the critical variables responsible for maintaining homeostasis *via* Starling equilibrium at the level of the microcirculation.

Reference Material

Albelda, S.M., Karnovsky, M.J., and Fishman, A.P.: Perspectives in endothelial cell biology. *J. Appl. Physiol. 62*:1345–1348, 1987.

Andersson, B.: Regulation of body fluids. *Ann. Rev. Physiol. 39*:185–200, 1977.

Beilke, M.A.: Vascular endothelium in immunology and infectious disease. *Rev. Infect. Dis. 11*:273–283, 1989.

Blasi, F., Vassalli, J-D., and Dano, K.: Urokinase-type plasminogen activator: proenzyme, receptor, and inhibitors. *J. Cell Biol. 104*:801–804, 1987.

Brandt, J.T.: Current concepts of coagulation. *Clin. Obstet. Gynecol. 28*:3–14, 1985.

Bruijn, J.A., Hogendoorn, P.C.W., Hoedemaeker, P.J., and Fleuren, G.J.: The extracellular matrix in pathology. *J. Lab. Clin. Med. 111*:140–149, 1988.

Carson, S.D.: Tissue factor-initiated blood coagulation. *Progr. Clin. Pathol. 9*:1–14, 1984.

Clouse, L.H., and Comp, P.C.: The regulation of hemostasis: The protein C system. *New Engl. J. Med. 314*:1298–1304, 1986.

Cokelet, G.R.: Rheology and hemodynamics. *Ann. Rev. Physiol. 42*:311–324, 1980.

Collen, D., Stump, D.C., and Gold, H.K.: Thrombolytic therapy. *Ann. Rev. Med. 39*:405–424, 1988.

Colman, R.W.: Surface-mediated defense reactions: The plasma contact activation system. *J. Clin. Invest. 73*:1249–1253, 1984.

Comp, P.C.: Hereditary disorders predisposing to thrombosis. *Progr. Hemostas. Thromb. 8*:71–102, 1986.

Doolittle, R.F.: Fibrinogen and fibrin. *Ann. Rev. Biochem. 53*:195–229, 1984.

Erickson, L.A., Schleff, R.R., Ny, T., and Loskutoff, D.J.: The fibrinolytic system of the vascular wall. *Clinics in Hematology 14*:513–530, 1985.

Esmon, C.T.: The regulation of natural anticoagulant pathways. *Science 235*:1348–1352, 1987.

Esmon, C.T.: The roles of protein C and thrombomodulin in the regulation of blood coagulation. *J. Biol. Chem. 264*:4743–4746, 1989.

Francis, C.W., and Marder, V.J.: Physiologic regulation and pathologic disorders of fibrinolysis. *Human Pathol. 18*::263–274, 1987.

Francis, C.W., and Marder, V.J.: Concepts of clot lysis. *Ann. Rev. Med. 37*:187–204, 1986.

Furie, B., and Furie, B.C.: The molecular basis of blood coagulation. *Cell 53*:505–518, 1988.

Fuster, V., and Griggs, T.R.: Porcine von Willebrand disease: Implications for the pathophysiology of atherosclerosis and thrombosis. *Progr. Thromb. Hemostas. 8*:159–184, 1986.

Gerard, R.D. and Meidell, R.S.: Regulation of tissue plasminogen activator expression. *Ann. Rev. Physiol. 51*:245–262, 1989.

Green, R.A.: Clinical implications of antithrombin III deficiency in animal diseases. *Compend. Cont. Educ. 6*:537–545, 1984.

Hawiger, J.: Formation and regulation of platelet and fibrin hemostatic plug. *Human Pathol. 18*:111–122, 1987.

Hormia, M., and Virtanen, I.: Endothelium: An organized monolayer of highly specialized cells. *Med. Biol. 64*:247–266, 1986.

Jaffe, E.A.: Cell biology of endothelial cells. *Human Pathol. 18*:234–239, 1987.

Kane, K.K.: Fibrinolysis—a review. *Ann. Clin. Lab. Sci. 14*:443–449, 1984.

Kaplan, A.P., and Silverberg, M.: The coagulation-kinin pathway of human plasma. *Blood 70*:1–15, 1987.

Kluft, C., Dooijewaard, G., and Emeis, J.: Role of the contact system in fibrinolysis. *Sem. Thromb. Hemostas. 13*:50–68, 1987.

Lämme, B., and Griffin, J.H.: Formation of the fibrin clot: the balance of procoagulant and inhibitory factors. *Clin. Haematol. 14*:281–341, 1985.

Leung, L., and Nachman, R.N.: Molecular mechanisms of platelet aggregation. *Ann. Rev. Med. 37*:179–186, 1986.

Lijnen, H.R., and Collen, D.: Mechanisms of plasminogen activation by mammalian plasminogen activators. *Enzyme 40*:90–96, 1988.

Longenecker, G.L.: *The Platelets: Physiology and Pharmacology.* Academic Press, New York, 1985.

Mann, K.G.: Membrane-bound enzyme complexes in blood coagulation. *Progr. Hemostas. Thromb. 7*:1–24, 1984.

Mayne, R.: Collagenous proteins of blood vessels. *Arteriosclerosis 6*:585–593, 1986.

Meyer, D., and Baumgartner, H.R.: Interactions of platelets with the vessel wall. *Adv. Inflamm. Res. 10*:85–98, 1986.

Meyers, K.M.: Pathobiology of animal platelets. *Adv. Vet. Sci. Comp. Med. 30*:131–166, 1985.

Moroose, R., and Hoyer, L.W.: von Willebrand factor and platelet function. *Ann. Rev. Med. 37*:157–164, 1986.

Mosler, D.F.: Physiology of fibronectin. *Ann. Rev. Med. 35*:561–576, 1984.

Müller-Berghaus, G.: Pathophysiologic and biochemical events in disseminated intravascular coagulation: dysregulation of procoagulant and anticoagulant pathways. *Semin. Thromb. Hemostas. 15*:58–87, 1989.

Nawroth, P.P., and Stern, D.M.: Endothelial cell procoagulant properties and the host response. *Sem. Thromb. Hemostas. 13*:391–397, 1987.

Oates, J.A., Hawiger, J., and Ross, R.: *Interaction of Platelets With the Vessel Wall.* American Physiological Society, Bethesda, MD, 1985.

Ogletree, M.L.: Overview of physiological and pathophysiological effects of thromboxane A_2. *Fed. Proc. 46*:133–138, 1987.

Packard, M.A., and Mustard, J.F.: Platelet adhesion. *Progr. Hemostas. Thromb. 7*:211–288, 1984.

Phillips, D.R., Charo, I.F., Parise, L.V., and Fitzgerald, L.A.: The platelet membrane glycoprotein IIb-IIIa complex. *Blood 71*:831–843, 1988.

Pietra, G.G.: Biology of disease: new insights into mechanisms of pulmonary edema. *Lab. Invest. 51*:489–494, 1984.

Pober, J.S.: Cytokine-mediated activation of vascular endothelium: physiology and pathology. *Am. J. Pathol. 133*:425–433, 1988.

Robbins, K.C., Barlow, G.H., Nguyen, G., and Samara, M.M.: Comparison of plasminogen activators. *Sem. Thromb. Hemostas. 13*:131–138, 1987.

Rosenberg, R.D.: The biochemistry and pathophysiology of the prethrombotic state. *Ann. Rev. Med. 38*:493–508, 1987.

Rosenberg, R.D., and Rosenberg, J.S.: Natural anticoagulant mechanisms. *J. Clin. Invest. 76*:1–5, 1984.

Runge, M.S., Quertermous, T., and Haber, E.: Plasminogen activators: the old and the new. *Circulation 79*:217–224, 1989.

Ryan, U.: The endothelial surface and responses to injury. *Fed. Proc. 45*:101–108, 1986.

Saito, H.: Contact factors in health and disease. *Semin. Thromb. Hemostas. 13*:36–49, 1987.

Saksela, O.: Plasminogen activation and regulation of pericellular proteolysis. *Biochim. Biophys. Acta 823*:35–65, 1985.

Saksela, O., and Rifkin, D.B.: Cell-associated plasminogen activation: Regulation, and physiological functions. *Ann. Rev. Cell Biol. 4*:93–126, 1988.

Schafer, A.I.: Focussing of the clot: Normal and

pathologic mechanisms. *Ann. Rev. Med. 38*:211–220, 1987.

Schaub, R.G., Simmons, C.A., Koets, M.H., Romano, P.J. II, and Stewart, G.J.: Early events in the formation of a venous thrombus following local trauma and stasis. *Lab. Invest. 51*:218–224, 1984.

Simeonescu, M., and Simionescu, N.: Functions of the endothelial cell surface. *Ann. Rev. Physiol. 48*:279–293, 1986.

Staub, N.C., and Taylor, A.E.: *Edema.* Raven Press, New York, 1984.

Steen, V.M., and Holmsen, H.: Current aspects on human platelet activation and responses. *Eur. J. Haematol. 38*:383–399, 1987.

Stemerman, M.B., Colton, C.K., and Morell, E.M.: Perturbations of the endothelium. *Progr. Hemostas. Thromb. 7*:289–324, 1984.

Stern, D.M., Carpenter, B., and Nawroth, P.P.: Endothelium and the regulation of coagulation. *Pathol. Immunopathol. Res. 5*:29–36, 1986.

Thomas, D.P.: Venous thrombogenesis. *Ann. Rev. Med. 36*:39–50, 1985.

Wallis, W.J., and Harlan, J.M.: Effector functions of endothelium in inflammatory and immunologic reactions. *Pathol. Immunopathol. Res. 5*:73–103, 1986.

White, J.G.: The secretory pathway of bovine platelets. *Blood 69*:878–885, 1987.

Zucker-Franklin, D., Benson, K.A., and Myers, K.M.: Absence of a surface-connected canalicular system in bovine platelets. *Blood 65*:241–249, 1985.

4

Inflammation and Repair

Inflammation in General
  Ten Generalities about Inflammation
Types of Inflammation
  Classifying Inflammatory Reactions
    Degree of Severity
    Duration
    Distribution of Inflammatory Lesions
  Types of Inflammatory Exudate
    Suppurative Exudation
    Fibrinous Exudation
    Serous Exudation
    Other Types of Exudates
Manifestations of Acute Inflammation
  Vascular Events in Inflammation
    Hemodynamic Changes
    Permeability Changes
Cells of the Inflammatory Exudate
  Granulocytes: Red, White, and Blue
    Neutrophils
    Eosinophils
    Basophils (and Mast Cells)
  Mononuclear Phagocytes: Macrophages
  Lymphocytes and Plasma Cells
  Platelets as Inflammatory Cells
  Endothelial Cells and Fibroblasts
Cellular Events in Inflammation
  Margination and Pavementing
  Emigration
  Chemotaxis
    Mechanisms of Chemotaxis
  Cell Accumulation
  Phagocytosis
    Microbicidal Mechanisms
      Oxygen-Dependent Killing Mechanisms
      Oxygen-Independent Killing Mechanisms
Importance of Leukocytes as Secretory Cells in
  Inflammation
Release of Lysosomal Enzymes and Tissue In-
  jury
  Lysosomal Suicide
  Regurgitation during Feeding
  Frustrated Phagocytosis
Leukocyte Activation: Stimulus-Response Cou-
  pling

Receptor Definition and Function
Role of Membrane Lipid Remodeling in Cell
  Activation
Transmembrane Signaling and Second Mes-
  sengers
Chemical Mediators of Inflammation
  General Features of Mediators
  Vasoactive Amines: Histamine and Serotonin
  Kinins
  Complement Fragments as Mediators
  Arachidonic Acid Metabolites
  Lymphokines
    Inflammatory Lymphokines
    Interferons
    Interleukins
  Tumor Necrosis Factor
  Platelet-Activating Factor
  Products of Blood Coagulation
  Lysosomal Enzymes as Mediators
Humoral Amplification Systems in Inflammation
  Hageman Factor-Dependent Pathways
  Complement System and Inflammation
  Complement Activation
  Complement Functions in Inflammation and
    Host Defense
Perspectives on the Inflammatory Response
Healing and Repair
  Healing by Parenchymal Regeneration
    Cellular Regenerative Capability
      Labile Cells
      Stable Cells
      Permanent Cells
Healing by Connective Tissue Replacement
  Morphology of Granulation Tissue Formation
    Macrophages
    Fibroblasts
      Elaboration of Extracellular Matrix Com-
        ponents
      Extracellular Matrix Remodeling
      Wound Contraction and the Myofibroblast
    Endothelial Cells
Role of Growth Factors in Healing and Repair
Wound Healing
Healing and Repair in Perspective
Reference Material

It is difficult to put inflammation into proper perspective. It is simultaneously the most important and most useful of our host defense mechanisms and the most common means by which tissues become injured. More animals have died of inflammatory diseases than all other causes combined, yet without an adequate inflammatory response, none of us would be living. It is the most important of the various types of changes which the body undergoes as a result of disease. Inflammation is among the oldest of recognized pathological phenomena and has been studied since ancient times. The history of medicine itself is closely paralleled by the history of inflammation, and the last chapter has by no means been written. As in many other fields, knowledge of inflammation grew through the careful observations of curious individuals (Table 4.1).

The inflammatory process is closely interdigitated with the responses that constitute **healing** and **repair.** Inflammation acts fundamentally as a host defense mechanism, but there is no distinct line between where inflammation leaves off and repair begins. Indeed, it is best to view **inflammation** and **repair** as a continuum, and much evidence has accumulated to indicate that repair processes begin even during the early phases of inflammation. The **vascular** and **cellular** events that highlight **acute inflammation** are aimed at mobilization of host defenses in order to neutralize whatever the offending agent might be, while the **repair** phase is aimed at the reconstitution of tissue structural and functional integrity *via* either parenchymal regeneration or by filling the defect with less specialized fibroblastic connective tissue.

The word **inflammation** itself takes us back a long way in the history of medicine. Literally it means "a burning." Inflammation was studied for hundreds of years before any true insight was obtained into the mechanisms by which it occurred. In the first century A.D., observations of clinical patients had allowed the Roman **Cornelius Celsus** to formulate his famous "cardinal signs" of inflammation: *calor, rubor, tumor,* and *dolor.* These are still true today: "Now the characteristics of inflammation are four; heat and redness with swelling and pain" (Table 4.2). To this classic list of four signs must be added *functio laesa* or loss of function. This fifth sign is often attributed to **Galen** (A.D. 130–200), but it really originated with **Rudolf Virchow** (1821–1905) (the father of modern pathology). It is now clear that most of these clinical signs relate to vascular phenomena. By the middle of the 19th century, one of Virchow's students, **Julius Cohnheim** (1839–1884), had described in considerable detail the vascular changes in inflammation. He observed injured blood vessels in thin membranes such as frog mesentery and detailed the vasodilation, augmented blood flow, and increased vascular permeability that occurred.

Despite their obvious importance, these vascular changes are not the sum total of inflammation. It remained for the Russian zoologist **Elie Metchnikoff** (1845–

Table 4.1
Giants in the Early History of Inflammation

Name	Time	Contribution
Cornelius Celsus	1st century A.D.	*Calor, rubor, tumor, dolor*
Rudolf Virchow	1821–1905	Father of modern pathology, *functio laesa*
Julius Cohnheim	1839–1884	Vascular phenomena
Elie Metchnikoff	1845–1916	Importance of leukocytes, phagocytosis
Louis Pasteur	1822–1895	Microbial causation
Robert Koch	1843–1910	Koch's postulates
Paul Ehrlich	1845–1915	Humoral theory of host defense

Table 4.2
Classical Clinical Signs of Inflammation

Sign	Originator	Translation
Calor	Celsus	Heat
Rubor	Celsus	Redness
Tumor	Celsus	Swelling
Dolor	Celsus	Pain
Functio laesa	Virchow	Loss of function

1916), in his still highly readable book on the comparative pathology of inflammation, to draw our attention to the central theme of inflammation as the activities of the "wandering mesodermal cells" (leukocytes) against an irritant. Metchnikoff discovered the process of phagocytosis by observing the ingestion of rose thorns by amebocytes of starfish larvae, and concluded that the purpose of inflammation was to bring phagocytic cells to the injured area such that they could engulf invaders. It was at about this same time that sweeping changes in medicine were taking place related to the discoveries of **Louis Pasteur** (1822–1895) and **Robert Koch** (1843–1910) that microorganisms like bacteria were important in the etiology of disease. Thus, the phenomenology of inflammation was fairly well described almost a century ago; it had become clear that the vascular phenomena detailed by Cohnheim set the stage for the cellular events of Metchnikoff.

Although both the vascular and cellular aspects of the inflammatory response are closely interdigitated, a substantial argument regarding which part was more important occupied early investigators for some time. The same type of argument followed the discovery that blood serum could have a protective effect against microorganisms which was equal to or even greater than phagocytosis. It was somehow fitting, then, that **Paul Ehrlich** (1854–1915) who developed the "humoral theory" of host defense (antibodies) and Metchnikoff shared the Nobel Prize in

1908. For the first time, both cellular (phagocytosis) and serum factors (antibodies) were jointly recognized for their importance to host defense.

We should also point out that neither Cohnheim, Metchnikoff, nor Ehrlich considered the role of chemical mediators in inflammation. **Sir Thomas Lewis,** in a series of beautifully simple experiments with skin reactions published in 1927, established that locally produced chemical substances mediate the vascular changes in inflammation. The "triple response" of Lewis can be elicited by firmly stroking the forearm with a blunt instrument like a pencil or the edge of a ruler. Within seconds, a dull red line forms along the line of the stroke, followed by a bright red halo around the stroke mark. The third feature, swelling of the stroke mark accompanied by its blanching, follows soon thereafter. Lewis postulated that these vascular phenomena were due to a chemical he called "H-substance" (histamine), and he thus ushered in the modern era of biochemical and molecular approaches to the study of inflammation.

The history of inflammation, healing, and repair is a fascinating one, but it is not our purpose to provide the details here. Interested readers would greatly profit from Dr. Guido Majno's excellent book, cited in the reference list. Dr. Henry Movat's book also provides interesting historical information on the subject.

INFLAMMATION IN GENERAL

What is inflammation? Inflammation has long been considered simply as the reaction of tissues to an irritant. More properly, it is the **reaction of vascularized living tissues to local injury,** which comprises a series of changes in the terminal vascular bed, in the blood, and in the connective tissues, which are designed to eliminate the offending irritant and to repair the damaged tissue. Because it is such a complex series of events,

Table 4.3
Ten Generalities about the Inflammatory Response

1. It is a process involving multiple participants.
2. It occurs only in living tissue.
3. It is a series of events overlapping into a continuum.
4. It is an evoked response that requires initiation by a stimulus.
5. It can be more harmful than the initiating stimulus.
6. It is fundamentally a defense reaction.
7. It is fairly stereotyped irrespective of the initiating stimulus.
8. It has most of its reactive components in the blood.
9. It is highly redundant with many promoters and regulators.
10. It is largely a surface-oriented phenomenon.

and because it is difficult to define usefully, some generalities about inflammation may help to place it in perspective (Table 4.3).

Ten Generalities About Inflammation

1. **Inflammation is a process.** An understanding of the complexity of the inflammatory response can be facilitated by first noting that it is a **process** involving multiple cellular, humoral, and tissue participants. It comprises a complex series of events, some sequential, others virtually simultaneous, but all overlapping and interdependent. Inflammation begins with or is preceded by cell or tissue injury, which leads to the hemodynamic and permeability adjustments that follow. Affected vessels readily exude fluids, plasma proteins, and white blood cells. The machinery activating such events includes a constellation of chemical mediators. Once gathered in a focus of injury, the various types of white blood cells contribute to the defense reaction by virtue of their ability to migrate, release enzymes, and phagocytose particulate matter.

In inflammatory reactions that evoke systemic responses, there is often an increase in circulating leukocytes **(leukocytosis),** and the lymphoreticular system throughout the body sometimes becomes involved. Although all inflammatory responses tend to be alike in their early phases, many factors relating to both the inciting agent and to the host modify the evolving reaction. Other modifiers include the nature of the exudate, the specific cause of the inflammation, and the location of the reaction.

2. **Inflammation occurs only in living tissue.** Cells can die in the living organism (necrosis), or they can die after the entire organism has ceased living (postmortem autolysis). Intravascular blood clots can form in the living animal (thrombosis), or they can form in the dead animal (postmortem thrombi). In both of these situations, some experience may be necessary before one can discern whether the events took place before or after death. Students should be pleased, then, to note that **postmortem inflammation does not occur.** The inflammatory process, with its many vascular and cellular subsets, depends wholly on viable tissue. Inflammation cannot occur in a dead organism. If one were examining a histologic section of kidney in which thrombi filled the vessels, the tubular epithelium was dead, and numerous neutrophils were present in the interstitium, one might wonder about the authenticity of the thrombi (ante- or postmortem?), and of the dead tubular epithelial cells (necrosis or autolysis?), but one would not have to worry about the inflammatory aspects of the lesion. The neutrophils present in our example migrated into the inflamed kidney while the animal was still alive. This is **always** the case. Inflammation cannot occur in a dead organism.

3. **Inflammation is an overlapping series of events that form a continuum.** The terms acute, subacute, and chronic, as applied to disease in general

and to inflammation in particular, have survived over the years because they are practical. We can assume they are here to stay. It is easy to use such terms, but more difficult to define their significance in the light of the modern biology of inflammation. While such terms are useful to pathologists and clinicians alike, it is more correct to envision inflammation as a single continuum that cannot truly be split on the basis of its course in time. It is a well-planned mechanism of defense, with multiple overlapping pathways leading to similar effects, no matter what the cause. The inflammatory response has two themes, inflammation and repair, but the two processes are so closely interdigitated that they really represent different parts of a single continuing process. Inflammation begins with injury to tissue and ends with permanent destruction of tissue or with complete healing. This response serves to defend against the injurious stimulus and to repair or replace injured tissue cells.

4. **Inflammation is a response.** Inflammation does not just occur. It is always an **evoked** response set into motion by some kind of a stimulus, usually one which injures tissue. It is therefore appropriate to think of inflammation in terms of a cause and effect relationship. Bacteria, viruses, mycoplasma, fungi, protozoans, chemicals, physical injury, immunologic injury, and a variety of other kinds of stimuli can all evoke an inflammatory response. In addition, the products of injured tissue (dead cells, and so on) can themselves serve as an inflammatory stimulus. Thus the inflammatory response, once set into motion by a variety of kinds of stimuli, can become self-perpetuating by virtue of its ability for cyclic self-stimulation. It is important to conceptualize inflammation as an evoked response that **always** requires an initiating stimulus.

5. **Inflammation can be harmful.** In many situations, the host may suffer more

tissue damage as a result of an inflammatory reaction than would have been caused by the initiating stimulus had there been no inflammatory response at all. Some of the best examples of this phenomenon come from immunopathology (see Chapter 5). Horse serum, for example, is by itself nonpathogenic when injected into an animal, but repeated injections can lead to the production of a violent, destructive, and sometimes fatal localized or generalized inflammatory response (Arthus reaction, anaphylaxis, or serum sickness) in which the reaction of the host is considerably more damaging than the horse serum itself. Thus, within certain limits, the inflammatory reaction is rather stereotyped or programmed and cannot distinguish readily between those instances in which it is called into play to protect the host and those instances in which the host is unnecessarily harmed. Indeed, it is probably true that **all** inflammatory reactions, no matter how useful to host survival, produce some damage to host tissue.

Inflammation is, therefore, like certain other vital life processes that may become harmful. **Hemostasis** is a vital process in the arrest of bleeding, yet the same coagulation pathways can produce fatal thrombosis. Insulin is necessary for life, but its excessive production by a neoplasm of the pancreatic islet cells can result in death. Many diseases such as rheumatoid arthritis, asthma, and glomerulonephritis are associated with inflammatory reactions that provide the host no obvious benefit but rather inflict considerable harm. In addition, the end result of many localized inflammatory reactions, **scarring,** can lead to significant undesirable sequelae; adhesions of lung to pleura, fibrous constrictions of the intestine, joint immobility, renal fibrosis, excessive wound contraction, and the formation of exuberant **granulation tissue.** These are common clinical problems that must be dealt with on a regular basis. It is for this reason that our pharmacies are loaded with such an increasingly wide variety of "anti-inflammatory" drugs, which we employ in towering quantities in attempts to limit, control, or otherwise modify inflammation. The inflammatory response is a crucial host defense mechanism, but it has a destructive, harmful side as well.

6. **Inflammation is fundamentally a defensive reaction.** Our ability to recover from various infectious and noninfectious injuries is related to the fact that the inflammatory response is a survival-oriented process. It has been shown to be the most fundamentally important host defense system in virtually all living things; mammals, birds, reptiles and amphibians, fish, even invertebrates and plants all have their own responses to local injury. Without effective inflammatory responses, bacterial infections are difficult to contain, wounds do not heal well, and damaged tissues are not repaired.

The end result of inflammatory activity usually includes **repair,** which begins during the active phases of inflammation but reaches completion only after the initiating stimulus has been removed. The damaged cells and tissues are either replaced by vital cells (**repair by regeneration**) or by less-specialized fibroblasts (repair by connective tissue replacement, **scarring**). A prompt and effective response destroys or neutralizes most injurious agents before much cell and tissue destruction takes place, and the need for repair is minimized with little or no scarring. If, on the other hand, the injury is severe and repair by regeneration cannot occur, scarring will result. The inflammatory process itself is aimed at maximizing normalcy as an end point. Ideally, this can be accomplished *via* removal of the initiating stimulus and regenerative repair of the injured tissue. Scarring, however, is at least a part of the end result of many inflammatory responses,

even when the initiating stimulus is as clean and closely controlled as, for example, a surgical incision. Nonetheless, both inflammation and repair generally serve useful purposes.

Perhaps some of the best examples of the importance of inflammation as a survival-oriented defense mechanism come from patients in whom the inflammatory response is defective because of disorders of phagocyte function. A syndrome in man of severe recurrent infections is known as **chronic granulomatous disease** because of the persistent infections of skin, lymph nodes, lung, liver, gastrointestinal tract, genitourinary tract, and bones. Such patients have a profound impairment in leukocyte oxidative metabolism leading to defective microbicidal function. The **Chediak-Higashi syndrome** (CHS) has been described in man, Aleutian mink, beige mice, partial albino Hereford cattle, albino whales, and cats. CHS is a genetically determined autosomal-recessive disease characterized by neutropenia and recurrent pyogenic infections associated with abnormal, giant phagocyte lysosomal granules and defective microbicidal activity. A syndrome called **canine granulocytopathy syndrome** has been described in which the neutrophils have a defect in the ability to kill phagocytized bacteria. Dogs with this disease usually have a clinical history of recurrent life-threatening bacterial infections. All of these clinical examples represent naturally occurring illustrations of situations in which a defective cellular inflammatory response exists, and serve to document the importance of inflammation as a vital defense mechanism (*see also* Chapter 7).

7. **Inflammation is fairly stereotyped.** The long list of potential causes of tissue injury is **not** paralleled by an equally long list of types of inflammatory responses. Indeed, the basic character and progression of events in the inflammatory response is quite stereotyped. We nor-

mally think of bacteria or other microorganisms as the cause of inflammation, but many nonliving agents such as heat, cold, radiation, electrical or chemical injury, and simple mechanical trauma also may act as destructive influences and evoke inflammatory reactions. In addition, the products of dead tissue released during the reaction can also serve as inflammatory stimuli.

While the basic pattern is stereotyped, variations in the reaction are determined by both the nature and severity of the injurious stimulus and the inflammatory responsiveness of the host. The intensity and duration of inflammatory reactions may be viewed as a delicate balance between attacker and host. Slight infection may produce a serious and sustained response in a compromised host, such as a dog with canine granulocytopathy syndrome, but even the strongest of individuals in any species can succumb to inflammation. Depending on the severity of the injury and the adequacy of the defense, inflammation may remain localized to its site of origin and evoke no systemic reactions, or may involve dramatic systemic responses.

Despite these variables, the inflammatory response is fairly stereotyped, and basically similar reactions develop almost irrespective of the nature of the initiating stimulus. Local increases in blood flow (**hyperemia**) develop. Increased vascular permeability occurs. Leukocytes leave the blood stream and enter the inflamed tissues. The reaction usually differs only in timing and magnitude. The chronic form often represents persistence of the causative agent and an immune response; that is, a response to an antigenic substance. In these cases, the nature of the leukocytic infiltrate may differ; lymphocytes and plasma cells may predominate. When the irritant is nonantigenic and difficult to degrade, such as a lipid or an insoluble foreign body, macrophages may predominate, with or without giant cells. An acute response does not necessarily evolve into a typical chronic response with a full complement of all types of mononuclear cells. A typical example is the acute allergic reaction, where the acute response may resolve without any chronic consequences.

8. **Inflammation is critically tied to the blood.** Most of the components of an inflammatory response are normally found in the blood, whereas injury is usually in the tissues. If we examine a typical acute inflammatory reaction, certain features are apparent. When we look closely at the tissue microscopically, protein-rich edema fluid, fibrin, leukocytes, and injured tissue are visible. With the exception of the injured tissue itself, all of these typical components of the acute reaction are blood derived, largely white blood cells and serum proteins (Fig. 4.1). Indeed, you will see as we further dissect the inflammatory process that almost all of the participants in this vital host defense mechanism are blood derived: the white blood cells, the platelets, the coagulation factors, the fibrinolytic enzymes, the complement system, antibody, the kinins, and so on.

It should also be clear that a very important barrier exists between the **tissue** where injury takes place and the **blood** where the defenses are marshalled. The barrier is the wall of the terminal vascular bed across which the blood-borne defenses must move in order to gain access to the injured tissue itself. This places the **vascular endothelium** in a unique position as the only continuous cellular layer between the leukocytes and plasma proteins and the tissue sites of injury. It is not surprising, then, that the terminal microvascular bed and the endothelial cells play a vitally important role in the development of inflammatory reactions.

9. **Inflammation is highly redundant.** The inflammatory response is a beautifully orchestrated defense mechanism essential to life. Because of its im-

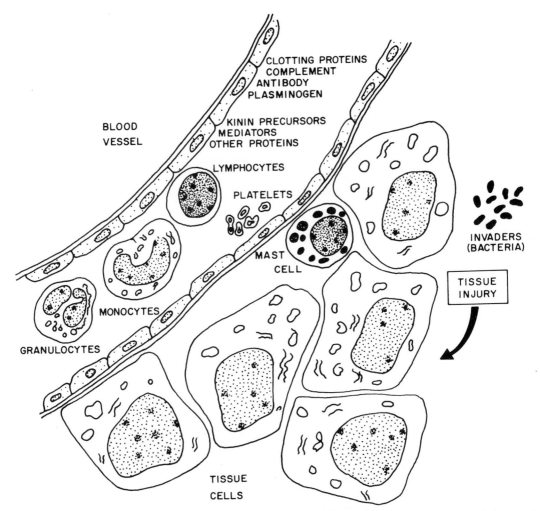

Figure 4.1. Cellular and Humoral Participants in Inflammation. With the exception of the mast cells, most of the host defenses that are involved in inflammation are blood borne. Therefore, the blood vessel walls become critical barriers across which the defenders must pass.

portance, it makes sense that there are usually multiple ways to get any one aspect of it initiated as well as complicated feedback loops and control mechanisms. It would make no biological sense for neutrophils to exhibit directed migration (**chemotaxis**) toward only one specific chemical signal; indeed, they will respond to many such chemotactic stimuli. This is in keeping with their importance to the inflammatory response and the survival dependence of their successful employment. There are two major pathways for

initiating blood coagulation, each with interconnecting loops, and several routes by which fibrin removal can be achieved. The list of stimuli that will cause lysosomal enzyme release from leukocytes is a long one. Collagen, thrombin, epinephrine, and ADP, among other stimuli, will cause platelets to aggregate at inflammatory foci. The more refined and detailed our ability to look at inflammatory mechanisms becomes, the more we discover the complicity of molecular and cellular interactions and the redundancy of initiation and control signals. This will become a recurrent theme in our discussion of inflammation.

If all of the interlacing activation and control pathways involved in inflammation could be drawn on a single piece of paper, it would make those giant intermediary metabolism charts that used to hang in every college biochemistry laboratory look like child's play. The cascades of closely interdigitated events which constitute the reaction of tissues to injury over a variable time scale involve a large cast of cellular participants, each with numerous functions that are mediated, modulated, and orchestrated by a multiplicity of chemical messengers that influence and determine the vascular, extravascular, and cellular sequelae of inflammation. It is easy to get lost in the labyrinthine interlacings of the inflammatory pathways and to lose sight of the forest for the trees, to forget that inflammation is a vital host defense mechanism and a healing response.

It may be that increased microcirculatory permeability, which is a primary event in the inflammatory process, is designed to bring plasma defense systems such as complement and antibody from the circulation into the extravascular space as a major first line of defense against infection. It is now well established that **complement** is a complex collection of proenzymes that, upon activation, release a number of chemical messengers directed largely toward the attraction of polymorphonuclear leukocytes (and eventually macrophages) into the area. Thus chemical messengers bring the second line of defense (white cells from the blood) into the site of injury. Messengers also are capable of degranulating mast cells to release histamine and thereby increase the permeability of the microcirculation to further augment this response. Interspersed among the extravascular connective tissues are mast cells which function by degranulation to release histamine

which increases the permeability of the microcirculation, heparin which inhibits clotting in the area of injury, and a number of proteases that can further alter the ground substance and increase the diffusion of various other chemical components of the serum into the injured area.

The chemical messengers of inflammation center largely around the issue of increased permeability of the microcirculation and the attraction, proliferation, activation, and movement of various cellular elements. It is also clear that many interrelated events follow the initial microvascular permeability adjustment. It is these various interdigitated events and their mediation that make inflammation fascinating.

10. **Inflammation is a surface phenomenon.** It is important to note how much of inflammation is "surface oriented." Bacteria become opsonized to make them more readily available (*via* surface receptors) for phagocytosis. Leukocytes crawl on surfaces, they do not swim in fluids; their locomotor activities involve reversible adherence of the leukocyte exterior to the surface over which they move. Mast cell activation and degranulation involve stimulation *via* surface-related membrane events. Platelets adhere to subendothelial collagen *via* surface receptors for von Willebrand factor, which is bound to the collagen. The Hageman factor–dependent pathways are initiated by contact activation on negatively charged surfaces. The leukocytes basically respond to membrane events related to perturbation of surface membrane receptors.

These surface-related phenomena, particularly as they relate to cells, are manifestations of the basic "irritability" of the responding cells. Since inflammatory cells can neither hear nor see, their membranes act as their eyes and ears. It may be helpful in contemplating the complicity of the inflammatory response to consider that the many overlapping signals really only represent different communication systems. By perceiving various signals in the immediate microenvironment, the leukocytes "read" the messages and act accordingly. The stimulus, whether it be a phagocytic stimulus, chemotactic attraction, movement along a surface, interaction with immune reagents, or whatever, involves specific surface membrane receptor interaction, which can then subsequently activate the signals for the intracellular events necessary for specific cellular functions. In such a fashion, smooth muscle cells relax and contract, platelets aggregate and release, lymphocytes transform and proliferate, macrophages activate, endothelial cells contract to open interendothelial gaps, mast cells and basophils degranulate, and neutrophils adhere, crawl, phagocytose, and release enzymes, The messages responsible for this intense cellular activity are all received at the cell surface for translation into functional activity by the events of intracellular biochemistry. Viewed as such, the biology of inflammation becomes only a special subset of cell biology in general. This is as it should be.

Inflammation: Are These Things Real?

In the pages that follow, we will dissect the inflammatory response into its component parts and attempt to explain how the various vascular, cellular, and humoral ingredients function and relate to each other. In so doing, there is a decided risk that one can lose sight of the "big picture," a risk that, for example, the molecular events in leukocyte activation and the biochemistry of phagocytosis somehow become more important than knowing what **pus** is. The newer knowledge about inflammation is a wonderful thing, for it allows us to begin to understand **how** and **why** things happen in a certain way. The greater our level of understanding, the more likely we are to be able to **interpret** clinical signs and to

approach inflammatory lesions with rational, specific therapy. We must constantly remind ourselves, however, that all of the world's molecular prose is not worth the paper it's printed on if it seduces us in any way into forgetting the overall nature of inflammation as it occurs in living animals. It is also worth noting that while the **details** of inflammation can be rather challenging to students, those investigators who work most intimately with it are quick to admit that what we have learned so far has actually only allowed us to realize how much it is that we do **not** know.

> . . . each level of scientific understanding reveals equally new displays of ignorance.
> Gerald Weissmann

Some of the "new biology" of inflammation is complicated, but no more so than is an inflammatory reaction occurring in a living animal. The laboratory scientist has the advantage of being able to examine in detail one discrete part of the inflammatory puzzle in an isolated, controlled way. The clinician must deal with the entire response occurring all at once, and the pathologist must deal with the aftermath. Both are greatly aided by an increased level of biological understanding, but when a severe inflammatory reaction with all of its vascular, cellular, and chemical components explodes simultaneously in a tissue, the result can be just as devastating now as it was 50 years ago. Inflammation is a contemporary **real-life** phenomenon, and it is commonly encountered in many very practical, real-life situations. We will examine inflammation of the lungs (**pneumonia**) in cattle as an example.

Although the estimates of losses to the cattle industries from respiratory diseases vary, the assessment of their importance does not. With losses running around $300–$500 million a year, bovine respiratory diseases continue to hold top priority among problems needing research. They are among the most economically devastating diseases of any species. It is now being recognized that much of the actual tissue injury in pneumonia is in fact "self-inflicted" through an excessive response on the part of the host's inflammatory defense mechanisms. Unraveling the specific infectious etiology of such diverse syndromes as enzootic pneumonia of calves, atypical interstitial pneumonia, and the fibrinous pneumonia–shipping fever complex so prominent in both beef and dairy cattle is a complicated affair. This is highlighted by the fact that many years of research activity directed at the causes of these diseases has yet to be translated into any truly effective preventive, control, or therapeutic measures. These diseases remain genuine problems costing millions of dollars annually.

Given the immense environmental variables of housing, nutrition, management, and disease prophylaxis plus a probable mixed etiology consisting of several viruses (IBR, PI3, etc.) plus bacterial species like *Pasteurella haemolytica,* perhaps mycoplasma, and varying states of host immunity, the opportunities to establish realistic cause-and-effect relationships for any agent or combination of agents are difficult. Researchers are now focusing on the basic injury process, its manifestations in the lung, and the critical interface between levels of injury and the levels of host response. Certainly microorganisms are initiative, but irrespective of specific etiologic considerations, what actually transpires in the injured lung is an intense inflammatory response **provided by the host,** which leads to massive exudation of leukocytes and fibrin, edema, and other defensive efforts that are equally threatening and perhaps more damaging than the initial insult provoking the inflammatory response.

It has recently been shown, for example, that neutrophil depletion in calves with experimental pneumonic pasteurellosis protects against the development of hypoxemia, hypercarbia, bradycardia, tachypnea, and the development of characteristic pneumonic lesions. These changes, therefore, appear to be **neutrophil mediated** rather than being due to the direct effects of the causative agent, *Pasteurella haemolytica.* Hence, a thorough understanding of the nature and control of the pulmonary inflammatory response may, in the long run, translate into better means of therapeutic intervention more quickly than will further attempts at the unraveling of specific etiologic factors. We may then have the opportunity to utilize information about the nature of the tissue injury process and host repair responses which could tell us how best to proceed after the injury.

In short, regardless of the various infectious agents and combinations of agents associated with pneumonia in cattle, the basic problem for the affected animal is the development of an intense inflammatory reaction in the lung in which the tissue-damaging contributions of the host defense mechanism (leukocytes, fibrin, *etc.*) often seem to outweigh the tissue-damaging contributions of the original infectious agents (Fig. 4.2). An inappropriately excessive level of host inflammatory reaction develops, which becomes a major contributor to the ongoing disease process rather than fulfilling its function as a defensive maneuver. A thorough understanding of the inflammatory process will assist in providing the necessary tools for a greater appreciation of what is actually occurring in the tissues of patients with such inflammatory lesions.

TYPES OF INFLAMMATION

While all types of inflammatory responses have similar mechanistic backgrounds as far as the cells participating, the vascular phenomena, and the chemical mediators involved, the result in tis-

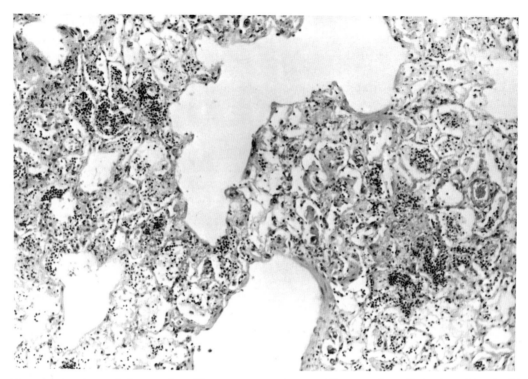

Figure 4.2.   Acute Inflammation. There are many neutrophils as well as fibrin deposition in this acutely inflamed dog lung. These typical hallmarks of inflammation are host-derived contributors to the inflammatory process.

sue does not always look the same. Many factors, relating to both the inciting agent and the host, modify the evolution and appearance of the reaction, the nature of the local exudate, the distribution in tissue, the time course of the reaction, and its severity. It is beyond our scope and needs to discuss all of these variables in detail. Rather, we will focus on features of inflammation that are useful to the clinician and the pathologist in the interpretation of inflammatory lesions in disease settings. We will direct our attention here to the various appearances of inflamed tissues that reflect differences in severity, time frame, distribution, and exudation as fundamental manifestations of inflammation in tissue. In later sections, we will explore the fascinating **biology** of the cells involved and the **mechanisms** by which inflammatory reactions develop.

Classifying Inflammatory Reactions

Throughout medicine, we become accustomed to the use of precise terminology to designate imprecise biological matters. Nowhere is this more true than in the naming and classification of inflammatory reactions. We attempt to be thorough in our descriptions of gross and histologic lesions, but what winds up on the bottom line too often reflects a general rather than a specific designation. A lengthy and detailed examination of an inflamed lung deserves a better inscription than just "pneumonia." What was the distribution of the lesion? How severe was the process? How long had the process been underway? What type of exudate or injury pattern characterized this particular inflammatory response? Did the pneumonia largely involve airways and contiguous parenchyma or was it predominately interstitial? This type of information possibly can be extracted from the pathologist's description of the lesion, but it is far preferable to include it as part of the **morphologic diagnosis.** It is not only more complete, but it also forces one to think in terms of the process rather than the end point. It provides a language that both clinicians and pathologists can understand. Descriptions designating the severity, duration, distribution, pattern of exudate or injury, useful anatomic modifiers, and the principle organ involvement can be combined to provide a more complete overall appreciation of the lesions at hand (Table 4.4). Thorough designation of the character of inflammatory lesions as they are reflected in tissue reactions allows a far better understanding of the processes that underlie the lesion.

Degree of Severity

Inflammation can be mild, as in the reaction to a wood splinter in one's finger, or it can be severe and life threatening, as in a severe bronchopneumonia. In between lies a grey zone in which moderate (but perhaps significant) inflammation occurs. Much of this reflects a value judgment on the part of the individual making the assessment as to mild, moderate, or severe, but certain guidelines are useful. **Mild** reactions might include little or no tissue destruction, slight evidence for vascular involvement (hyperemia and edema), and little in the way of exudation. **Moderate** reactions usually contain some damage to host tissue and an easily visible host reaction to the injury, manifest by leukocytic accumulation and vascular phenomena. **Severe** reactions are an extension of moderate reactions, in which considerable tissue damage is present along with abundant exudation. Such designations are only as useful as they are made to be by the individual making the assessment. They can be helpful in communicating such value judgments among clinicians, among pathologists, or between pathologists and clinicians.

Table 4.4
Classification of Inflammatory Lesions

Extent	Duration	Distribution	Exudate	Anatomic Modifiers	Organ
Minimal Mild Moderate	Peracute Acute Subacute	Focal Multifocal Diffuse	Suppurative Nonsuppurative Serofibrinous	Interstitial Broncho- Glomerulo-	Nephritis Hepatitis Enteritis, etc.
Severe	Chronic	Locally extensive	Fibrinopurulent	Submandibular, etc.	
Extensive	Chronic active		Necrotizing Granulomatous, etc.		

Examples in Use

Mild acute diffuse serous submandibular lymphadenitis
Severe chronic diffuse membranoproliferative glomerulonephritis
Moderate chronic-active multifocal granulomatous segmental bronchitis
Severe acute locally extensive fibrinopurulent bronchopneumonia
Severe chronic focal caseous submandibular lymphadenitis

Duration

All inflammatory reactions have a beginning, and most have an end. In between lies a variable span of time in which the character of the evolving reaction can change. **Peracute** inflammation is manifest very soon after its initiation, perhaps only a few hours, and usually is caused by a potent stimulus. There may be little evidence at this point in time of host contributions in terms of exudation. Rather, tissue damage, with perhaps some of the vascular events of inflammation, is often all that is visible. Hence, slight edema, hyperemia, hemorrhage, and a few leukocytes beginning to infiltrate the damaged tissue may be the only visible markers. This type of lesion is less commonly seen than are acute responses.

Acute inflammation usually begins within 4–6 hours and can remain fairly constant in appearance, depending on the initiator, for several days. Here, the evidence of vascular involvement is readily visible. Vessels are engorged with blood, dilated, and occasionally even contain thrombi. Local hemorrhage and edema may be present. Fibrin is often visible. Clinically, the involved tissues are warm, reddened, swollen, and painful (calor, rubor, tumor, dolor). The leukocytic contribution here is variable and may be sparse early but usually is well developed within a day or two. Neutrophils usually are predominant, although in some cases mononuclear cells can be present in large numbers in acute inflammation. Edema and hyperemia are prominent in acute inflammation. This is the picture we usually think of when imagining what an inflammatory reaction looks like (Fig. 4.2). The lymphatics play a major role in transporting away the various components of an acute inflammatory exudate. This function of the lymphatic system begins early in an acute inflammatory reaction, and the transportation of the inflammatory flotsam may lead to an acute regional **lymphadenitis;** astute clinicians know to look in the drainage field "upstream" for a primary lesion when they encounter an acutely inflamed lymph node.

The distinction between acute inflammation and subacute inflammation is not an abrupt one, but rather there is a gradual change in character. **Subacute** inflammation usually is characterized by a decline in the magnitude of the vascular contribution (edema and hyperemia) and often by a change in the character of the infiltrating leukocytes. The declining evidence of edema and hyperemia can be explained both by gradually moderating vascular contributions and by the lymphatic drainage that occurred during the more acute phases. Although subacute inflammation still may be predominately neutrophilic, the infiltrate becomes mixed, with mononuclear cells (lymphocytes, macrophages, and maybe a few plasma cells) visible in reasonable numbers along with the neutrophils (Fig. 4.3). Subacute inflammation may cover a considerable time span between truly acute reactions and those in which evidence of chronicity is apparent. It is an intermediate time frame that can vary from a few days to a few weeks, depending on the nature of the inciting stimulus. The designation of subacute often is used for such inflammatory reactions until evidence of host tissue reparative responses (angiogenesis, fibroplasia, and so on) are manifest, at which time the lesions begin to grade into what is usually called chronic inflammation.

Although **chronic** inflammation is primarily a clinical concept pertaining to prolonged duration of an inflammatory lesion, it has some sufficiently unique characteristics to warrant our special attention. It is really more than just a time frame. It represents a rather specific, if vaguely defined, entity in which ongoing inflammation is often accompanied by evidence of host tissue reparative responses (Fig. 4.4). Although the transi-

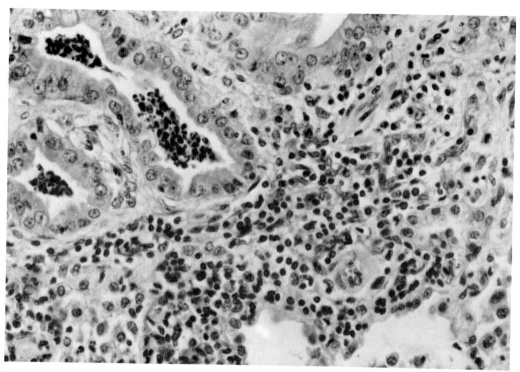

Figure 4.3.   Subacute Inflammation. Mixed populations of inflammatory cells are present here including many mononuclear cells (lymphocytes and macrophages) although the glandular lumens still contain acute phase debris and neutrophils. No hyperemia is visible.

tion from acute to subacute to chronic is often hard to define precisely, we can nonetheless pinpoint certain key features of chronicity: (1) it often is caused by persistent inflammatory stimuli in which the host has failed to completely rid the tissue of the invader; (2) the inflammatory response usually is accompanied by an immune response, due in part to the duration of the insult and in part to the persistence of the invader; (3) it is usually highlighted by evidence of host tissue contribution in terms of reparative responses. This may be by parenchymal regeneration, but **fibrosis** (scarring) remains the most reliable criterion of chronicity; and (4) it is characterized histologically by both mononuclear cell infiltrates and by connective tissue cells such as fibroblasts. Proliferation of small blood vessels (angiogenesis) also may be present.

Chronic inflammation usually develops in one of two forms; it may follow an acute inflammatory phase, or it may develop as an insidious, low-grade, subclinical process in which there is no history of a prior acute episode. Furthermore, both pathways to chronicity can develop in the same tissue. An acute glomerulonephritis may develop into a chronic glomerulonephritis, but the latter is more commonly seen as a slowly progressive, insidious, initially subclinical process. This is particularly true in veterinary medicine since we often do not see patients until they are sick enough to get the attention of the owner; acute lesions that are not too severe are thus often missed.

The interrelationships between the various cellular and humoral components of the inflammatory response and their contributions to the subsequent events that occur during chronic inflammation

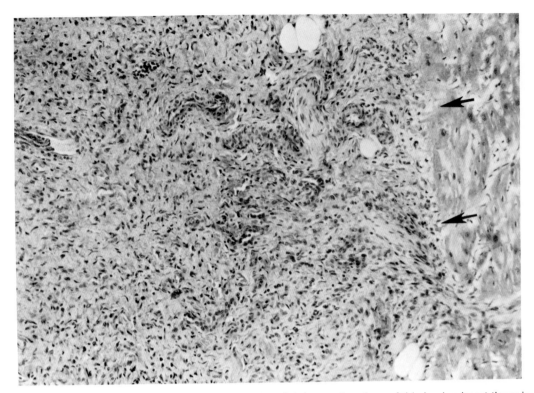

Figure 4.4.   Chronic Inflammation. On the epicardial *(arrows)* surface of this bovine heart there is active fibrovascular connective tissue (scarring) as well as scattered numbers of inflammatory cells. Fibrosis is the single best indicator of chronicity.

and fibrogenesis are as yet poorly understood. It has long been observed that inflammation represents a fairly reproducible sequence of events in terms of the chronology of appearance of cells derived from the blood and their link to ultimate repair of the injury. Neutrophils can elaborate substances chemotactic for macrophages, and the macrophages play a role in wound repair. This predictable sequence of events may be necessary for the ultimate stimulation of fibroblasts and capillaries.

Macrophages at sites of inflammation and wound repair consist of two populations, both having their origin in the bone marrow. The first, a minor component in most tissues, is the "resident" tissue macrophage. It appears to be present in tissues at all times, and under suitable stimuli is capable of entering the mitotic cycle

and undergoing cell division. The other, the major component at most sites of chronic inflammation, is directly recruited from hematogenous precursor cells, the monocytes, which themselves are derived from a rapidly dividing pool of cells in the bone marrow, the promonocytes. Most macrophages in sites of inflammation are derived from the monocytes in the blood. The role of the blood monocyte in chronicity and wound repair has been very difficult to define. Its activity as a phagocyte has been recognized since the early work of Metchnikoff, and its relationship to other cells in the reparative response has been the subject of numerous investigations. The mononuclear phagocyte is the cell principally responsible for phagocytosis and tissue debridement in a chronic lesion.

The ultimate causes of chronicity remain largely an enigma, although a few significant clues exist. The use of a wide variety of radiolabeled irritants has failed to reveal any instance where a chronic reaction is not accompanied by tissue persistence of the irritant, or where disappearance of the irritant is not accompanied by disappearance of the reaction. In the clinical situation, a similar condition exists in diseases such as tuberculosis or in foreign-body reactions. In other less well defined diseases of obscure etiology, no irritant can be seen or recovered with certainty. However, since a small amount of irritant, especially microbiological, still can provoke a chronic response, the persistent stimulus may nevertheless be present, even in these cases.

Persistence of an irritant within cells or tissues may be caused by survival of living organisms but also may follow the failure of macrophages to degrade dead organisms to diffusible products. This has been demonstrated by quantitative analysis of the degradation by macrophages of various kinds of bacteria. Breakdown of bacteria is initially rapid, proceeding to completion for simple organisms, but ceasing at 48–72 hours in the case of bacteria that induce chronicity. The reason for this cessation of degradation by macrophages is still not clear, but it appears to be due in part to the protective chemical nature of the cell coat on certain microorganisms as well as to more complicated intracellular dysfunctions such as inhibition of phagosome-lysosome fusion and failure of degranulation mechanisms.

Hypersensitivity often is invoked as a cause of chronicity, but hard evidence is lacking. An excess of antibody over antigen in the formation of immune complexes can lead to chronic rather than transient inflammation. The balance of evidence indicates that delayed-type hypersensitivity may accompany chronic inflammation and may cause it, but that it is not a requirement. The chronic inflam-

mation that results from certain foreign-body reactions clearly does not have a hypersensitivity basis.

Macrophages **always** play an essential role in the pathogenesis of chronic inflammatory lesions. The macrophage may fulfill its role in chronic inflammation by its capacity to secrete a variety of biologically active macromolecules. Macrophages usually are thought of as phagocytic cells, with ingested materials being degraded by hydrolytic enzymes maintained in a latent form within the large number of lysosomes present in the cells. It has become clear in recent years, however, that these enzymes may be released from macrophages in a selective manner by certain stimuli in much the same way as enzyme release occurs from neutrophils. Available evidence suggests that many of these stimuli are capable of contributing to chronic inflammation. More recently it also has become apparent that macrophages can secrete large quantities of two other types of hydrolytic enzymes, namely neutral proteinases and lysozyme. The former are only secreted after an appropriate stimulus but lysozyme seems to be constantly secreted as a constitutive product of the macrophage.

Macrophages also secrete other biologically active products, but the chemical nature and function of some of them is still poorly defined. Thus, although it is clear that macrophages always are present at sites of chronic inflammation, their contribution to the evolution of these lesions is still not precisely understood in molecular terms. We will explore the biology of the all-important macrophage in greater detail later.

Chronic inflammation may be accompanied by acute exacerbations in which the tissues exhibit all of the usual features of chronicity, with features of acuteness superimposed. That is, it is not unusual to find acute suppurative inflammation side by side with fibrosis and tissue regeneration. Such lesions are usually designated as **chronic-active** inflammation and imply that either repeated episodes of inflammation have occurred and overlapped in their evolutionary cycles, or that failure of host defenses to adequately contain the invaders has led to episodes of local reappearance to elicit new acute responses. Such lesions are not at all uncommon.

Before leaving the subject of chronic inflammation, we should note that the line between chronic inflammation and repair (or healing) is often a blurred one. Many of the features of chronicity also are found in healing wounds.

Distribution of Inflammatory Lesions

It often is useful to evaluate the inflammatory response on the basis of its distribution within the involved tissue. Such designations generally are used for gross descriptions of lesions, but they can be useful histologically as well. Lesions may be focal, multifocal, locally extensive, or diffuse (Fig. 4.5). **Focal** lesions are usually a single abnormality or inflamed area within the tissue. Such an area is called a **focus** of inflammation. These can be very small lesions of 1 mm or less, or they can be up to a centimeter or more in diameter. They are surrounded by relatively normal tissue. **Multifocal** lesions

represent several or many scattered **foci** of inflammation within the tissue. Again, the size can be variable, but each focus of inflammation is separated from other inflamed foci by an intervening zone of relatively normal tissue. Such lesions often have a vascular basis for their distribution, such as a shower of septic emboli from an inflamed heart valve.

Locally extensive lesions involve all of a considerable zone of tissue within the inflamed organ. They may arise from severe local reactions that spread into adjacent normal tissue, or may evolve by the coalescence of foci in a multifocal reaction. A good example of inflammation having this type of distribution is the pulmonary lesion of pneumonic pasteurellosis in cattle, in which the cranioventral aspect of the lungs are involved while dorsal portions usually are spared. Lesions with this distribution often have a bacterial etiology. **Diffuse** lesions involve all of the tissue or organ in which they are found. There may be variations in severity within the diffusely inflamed tissue, but all of the tissue exhibits inflammation. An example to contrast with the locally extensive distribution of pneumonic pasteurellosis is the diffuse distribution of many of the interstitial pneumonias. Lesions of such distribution are often viral in etiology, but certain toxicants can produce a similar pattern.

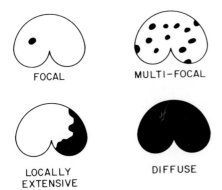

Figure 4.5.   Distribution of Lesions. Lesions usually are described as either *focal, multifocal, locally extensive,* or *diffuse.*

Types of Inflammatory Exudate

As inflammation can be variable, so can the nature of the exudate that characterizes inflammation. The variations in fluid, plasma protein content, and cellular composition are generally reflections of the duration and severity of the inflammatory process, although variations related to the causative agent are also notable. While a long list of kinds of exudate could be generated, in real life there are certain repetitive patterns that warrant our attention.

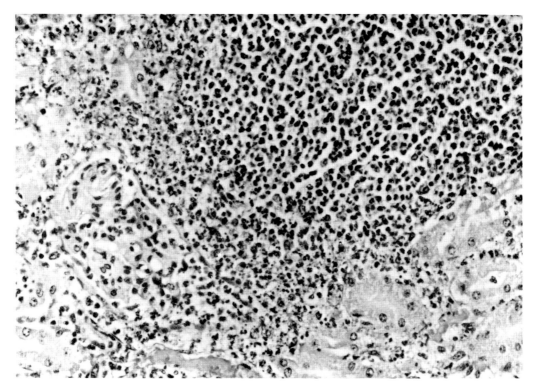

Figure 4.6.   Suppurative Exudate. Almost all of the inflammatory cells in this focus of inflammation are neutrophils. This makes the lesion suppurative, or purulent, and the exudate is called pus.

Suppurative Exudation

Suppurative exudates are composed largely of neutrophils along with dead cells including both dead host tissue cells and dead inflammatory cells (Fig. 4.6). A synonym for suppurative is **purulent,** which means that the predominant feature of the exudate is the formation of **pus.** The process by which pus is formed is called **suppuration,** and, in general, it implies that neutrophils and their proteolytic enzymes are present and that necrosis of host tissue cells has occurred. Pus itself is composed largely of accumulated dead cells, both tissue cells and inflammatory cells, and contains a variable number of viable leukocytes as well as fluids added by the inflammatory edema-forming process. **Abcesses** are a localized form of suppurative inflammation. Suppurative lesions are often bacterial in origin.

Fibrinous Exudation

The increased vascular permeability accompanying acute inflammation permits the egress of large amounts of plasma protein, including fibrinogen, and the formation of large fibrin coagula in the inflamed tissue is characteristic of some kinds of inflammation (Fig. 4.7). An example is the "shipping-fever" type of pneumonia in beef cattle, which often is decidedly fibrinous in character (Fig. 4.8). Fibrinous pericarditis occurs in cattle in which foreign bodies penetrate the pericardial sac from the retriculum (traumatic reticulopericarditis). Fibrin formation is an acute phenomenon. It takes only seconds for fibrin to form under normal circumstances. One must be careful not to mentally or visually confuse **fibrin** with **fibrosis,** the latter being a decidedly chronic event. Fibrin on a surface can be

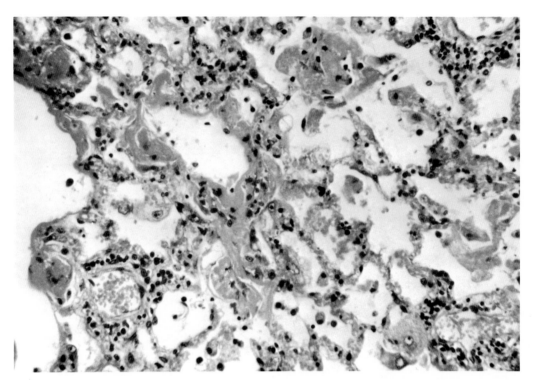

Figure 4.7.   Fibrinous Exudate. The strands and accumulations of pale-staining debris here consist largely of fibrin deposits in this acutely inflamed bovine lung.

identified by the ease with which it can be broken down. Histologically, it is a thread-like eosinophilic meshwork that sometimes forms masses of solid amorphous eosinophilic coagulum. Fibrin provides a meshwork for the ingrowth of fibroblasts and neocapillaries, which can transform the fibrinous exudate into well-vascularized connective tissue, a process known as **organization** of the exudate. This can be a harmful sequel, as obliterative scarring may be the end result. Much fibrin in acute exudates is, however, removed by enzymatic fibrinolysis or by phagocytosis by macrophages before organization can occur. When many neutrophils are present along with fibrin, the exudate is properly termed **fibrinopurulent.**

Serous Exudation

When lesions are characterized by the outpouring largely of fluid relatively rich in protein, the lesion is said to represent serous inflammation. The blisters that result from burns are good examples of serous inflammation. Within the blister is a volume of fluid derived partly from the blood stream and partly from the locally injured cells. This type of exudate can be characteristic of the very early aspects of many kinds of evolving inflammatory responses. It may be the dominant pattern of exudation for a wide variety of mild inflammatory injuries.

Other Types of Exudates

There are probably as many types of exudates as there are types of inflammation, and it is beyond our scope to more than highlight some of these variations on the theme. **Necrotic** inflammation is characterized largely by necrosis, with only scant evidence of vascular or leukocytic contributions. When this occurs on an epithelial surface (*e.g.*, trachea, intestine,

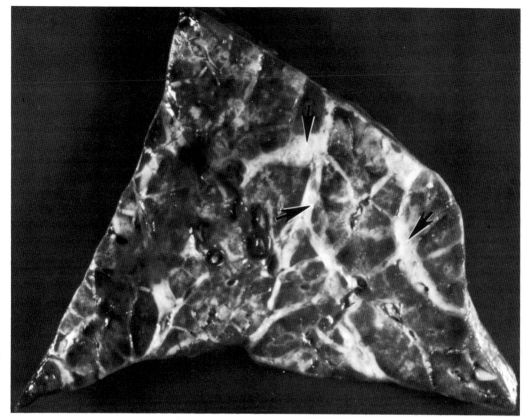

Figure 4.8.   Bovine Fibrinous Pneumonia. The interlobular deposition of fibrin *(arrows)* is a typical finding in the acute infectious "shipping-fever" pneumonias of cattle.

nasal passages) that is well vascularized, serum often oozes out to produce fibrin formation, and **fibrinonecrotic exudation** results. Such exudates sometimes form **pseudomembranes** over their damaged surfaces, which are often called **diphtheritic** membranes. Infectious bovine rhinotracheitis often is characterized by a fibrinonecrotic or diphtheritic tracheitis (Fig. 4.9). If hemorrhage is the predominant feature of an inflammatory lesion, the designation **hemorrhagic** inflammation is used. Such lesions are usually acute or peracute and often include necrosis of blood vessels. **Mucoid** exudate consists largely of mucus, but often is mixed with neutrophil infiltrates, in which case the lesion becomes **mucopurulent.** Such lesions can occur only on

mucous membranes, where the appropriate secretory cells are present. A synonym for mucopurulent is **catarrhal.** Lesions often are designated by the cellular nature of the exudate, just as "suppurative" exudate is used to designate a largely neutrophilic accumulation. An acute serous inflammatory reaction with neutrophil infiltrates in subcutaneous tissues is referred to as **cellulitis.** If the lesion in question is composed largely of eosinophils, as can occur with many kinds of parasitic lesions, then **eosinophilic** inflammation is present. Salt poisoning in swine is often characterized by an eosinophilic encephalitis. By the same token, **basophilic** dermatitis sometimes is seen at reaction sites from tick infestations.

Lesions in which mononuclear cells

predominate usually are referred to as **nonsuppurative,** to differentiate them from suppurative lesions in which neutrophils predominate. The virus of canine

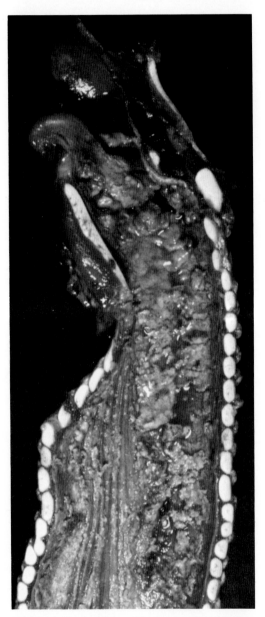

Figure 4.9. Fibrinonecrotic Tracheitis. Necrosis and fibrin deposition on the damaged tracheal mucosa occurs quite commonly in infectious bovine rhinotracheitis. Such lesions also are called "pseudo-membranous" or "diphtheritic" tracheitis.

distemper, for example, produces a nonsuppurative encephalitis. If the lymphocyte predominates, then **lymphocytic** exudate is present. The viral disease lymphocytic choriomeningitis is named for its characteristic lymphoid infiltrate, as is lymphocytic thyroiditis.

Granulomatous inflammation is a category that warrants our special attention. It is always chronic and may have a wide range of histologic appearances and inflammatory cell types involved, but central to granulomatous inflammation is the macrophage. Granulomatous inflammation also is almost impossible to define. Originally the term **granuloma** defined the tiny, white, granular bodies that could be seen in tissues as a result of systemic (hematogenous) spread of the tuberculosis organism and the peculiar local inflammatory reaction to the mycobacterium. The term was later redefined according to certain microscopic criteria. At the present time, granulomatous inflammation usually refers to an inflammatory response characterized by the presence of lymphocytes, macrophages, and plasma cells, with the predominant cell being the macrophage. Macrophages are clustered in a characteristic elliptical formation around the causative agent, or around a central necrotic area, or simply as organized nodules. Large macrophage-like cells with abundant cytoplasm are sometimes referred to as **epithelioid cells,** and it seems more than likely that they are derived from local tissue macrophages that are, in turn, derived from blood monocytes. It also is common to see multinucleate **giant cells** associated with granulomas. In addition, fibroplasia often is seen. The relative amounts of these various components can vary considerably in different lesions, hence granulomatous inflammation can have a wide range of histologic forms and still qualify as granulomatous (Fig. 4.10). Some would claim that a lesion is not truly a granuloma (or granulomatous) unless it contains epithe-

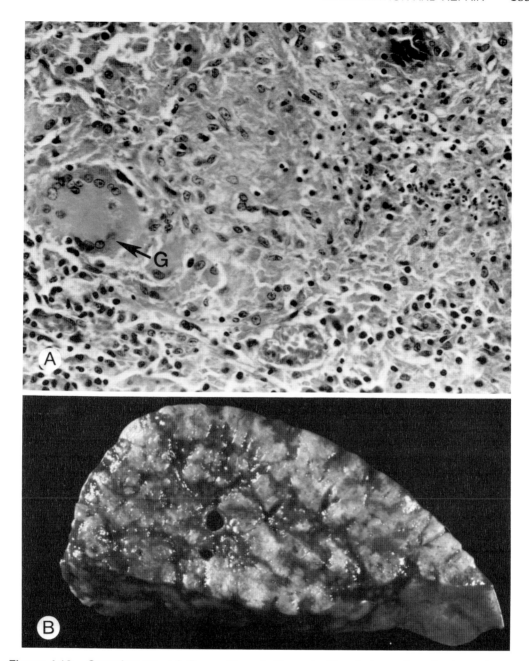

Figure 4.10.   Granulomatous Inflammation. *A,* Necrosis, fibroplasia, and a mixed population of inflammatory cells including lymphocytes and many macrophages are seen in this section of lung from a tuberculous monkey. Giant cells *(G)* are commonly seen in granulomatous inflammation. *B,* This lung from a case of canine blastomycosis shows numerous irregular pale zones, which represent areas of granulomatous inflammation. The unitized nature of the lesions here and their separation from each other by relatively normal tissue is typical, and each inflamed focus represents a discrete granuloma.

lioid cells, but most would favor a broader definition. Central to this form of inflammation is the presence of some indigestible organism or particle which serves as a chronic inflammatory stimulus.

There is some evidence that granulomas are potentiated by, or even require, delayed-type hypersensitivity for their full expression. This is perhaps true for some of the infectious granulomas (such as tuberculosis), but it becomes difficult to accept for those lesions caused by foreign bodies. While the nature of these lesions remains somewhat questionable, they are perhaps best thought of as a special form of persistent chronic inflammation characterized by either nodular or diffuse accumulations of mononuclear cells, principally macrophages and modified macrophages (epithelioid cells and giant cells). This type of inflammation characterizes the tissue response to certain kinds of microorganisms *(Mycobacterium, Actinomyces, Blastomyces, Coccidioides, etc.)* as well as noninfectious agents such as mineral oil, complex polysaccharides, polymers, and even simple foreign bodies.

MANIFESTATIONS OF ACUTE INFLAMMATION

Acute inflammation may produce clinical signs localized to the site of injury or may be accompanied by profound systemic changes. For example, an infected cut on the digit usually causes only local signs, whereas bronchopneumonia may produce not only local signs but also a significant systemic reaction, including leukocytosis and fever. The local clinical signs of inflammation have been mentioned previously, and classically have been characterized as heat, redness, swelling, pain, and loss of function (Table 4.2). The local heat and redness are apparently the result of dilatation of the microcirculation in the local environment of the injury. The swelling is largely produced by the escape of fluid (inflamma-

tory edema) containing plasma proteins and other solutes from the blood to the perivascular tissues. Leukocytes also escape, and the two processes together are known as **transudation** and **exudation.** The origin of the pain is more difficult to pin down, but can be attributed either to the pressure of extravascular fluid on nerve endings or to direct irritation of local nerves by chemical mediators, or to both. We know very little about the causes of loss of function, but since function is usually a result of physiologic normalcy of the various cells and tissues, it seems reasonable to conclude that damaged and inflamed tissues should exhibit functional as well as structural deficits.

We mentioned previously the terms exudate and transudate (Table 4.5). An **exudate** is an inflammatory, extravascular fluid with a specific gravity usually above 1.018, resulting from its high content of proteins, cellular debris, and leukocytes. The white blood cells and cellular debris within it impart the yellow-white appearance of pus, more properly termed a purulent or suppurative exudate. When plasma proteins leak to the extravascular space, it implies significant alteration in the normal permeability of the microcirculation in the area of injury. In contrast, a **transudate** is a low-protein fluid with a specific gravity of less than 1.015. It is essentially an ultrafiltrate of the blood

Table 4.5
Exudates and Transudates

Characteristic	Exudate	Transudate
Definition	Inflammatory	Noninflammatory
Etiology	Inflammation, infection	Noninflammatory edema
Specific gravity	Above 1.018	Below 1.015
Protein content	Over 4.0%	Below 3.0%
Clottable	Often	Rarely
Inflammatory cells	Usually	Rarely
Bacteria	Often	Almost never

plasma, consisting primarily of water and dissolved electrolytes. The origin and role of transudates and exudates in inflammation will become more clear as our discussion progresses.

There is some correlation between the severity of the injury and the composition of the inflammatory fluid. Even very mild injuries can produce a protein-poor watery transudate. With progressively more potent injurious stimuli, the inflammatory fluid will acquire higher and higher concentrations of plasma proteins, red blood cells, and white blood cells and will become an exudate. These various local manifestations of acute inflammation collectively highlight the **three major parts of the inflammatory response:** (1) hemodynamic changes, (2) permeability changes, and (3) events involving leukocytes. Each of these will be discussed separately but we must emphasize that such a separation is strictly arbitrary. The hemodynamic changes that first signal the inflammatory response are followed very soon thereafter by alterations in the permeability of the affected vessels and by reactions involving white blood cells. There is much overlap in these three major aspects of the reaction, which actually form a continuum. Since the structural and functional elements that lie behind these three major aspects of inflammation are sufficiently distinct, it is useful to consider them separately.

Vascular Events in Inflammation

Hemodynamic Changes

Most of the local signs of inflammation arise from changes in the microcirculatory bed in the area of the injury. The hemodynamic alterations are an integrated chain of events activated by chemical mediators (Fig. 4.15) but perhaps transiently initiated by neurogenic mechanisms. These vascular events are usually manifested in the following order (*see* Table 4.6):

1. Arteriolar dilatation, sometimes preceded by transient vasoconstriction;
2. Increased rate of blood flow through the arterioles;
3. Opening of additional capillary and venular beds in the area;
4. Congestion of the venous efflux;
5. Increased permeability of the microvasculature with the outpouring of inflammatory fluid into the extravascular tissues;
6. Concentration of red cells in the capillaries and venules;
7. Slowing or stasis of flow in these small vessels sometimes leading to complete stagnation;
8. Peripheral margination of white blood cells in the capillaries; and
9. A sequence of subsequent white blood cell events (chemotaxis, phagocytosis, *etc.*) to be discussed in a later section.

Many of these changes begin at the same time but develop at varying rates depending on the severity of the injury. In virtually all inflammatory reactions, dilatation of arterioles associated with increased blood flow through the capillaries and venules occurs (Fig. 4.11). This is the **acute, local, active hyperemia of inflammation** associated with the opening of precapillary sphincters and the active perfusion of previously inactive capillaries and venules. It also may result from the dilatation of these small vessels. The overload of the venous drainage leads to passive congestion of these vessels, which contributes to the vasodilation. By this time, the permeability of the microcirculation usually has been altered, and fluid begins to leak out of the vessels. This leakage may at first be strictly a watery transudate but, in significant inflammatory responses, the progressive increase in permeability permits the escape of larger macromolecules, forming a protein-rich exudate. The loss of plasma fluid causes local hemoconcentration, and the small vessels become packed with eryth-

Table 4.6
Sequence of Events in Acute Inflammation

Event	Pathogenesis[a]
Transient vasoconstriction (lasts a few seconds to 5 min)	Possibly due to epinephrine or neurogenic
Vasodilatation (begins by 5 min and lasts 15–30 min)	Immediate histamine reaction; arteriolar dilatation; increased vascular leakage is primarily in venules; also caused by the kinins, serotonin, complement, fibrinopeptides and fibrin degradation products, prostaglandins, leukotrienes, and many other endogenous mediators of inflammation
Increased blood flow	More blood flow from vasodilatation
Increased vascular permeability	First and most severely in the postcapillary venules; due to "contraction" of endothelial cells of venules; passage of protein-rich fluids from plasma into tissues.
Slowing of flow or stasis	Due to blood sludging from fluid loss (increased viscosity through exudation; hemoconcentration and congestion)
Margination (pavementing, sticking to endothelium)	Probably relates to up-regulation of Leu-CAMs; WBC and endothelium both contribute to stickiness
Emigration and exudation	Between endothelial cell gaps; first and most severe in postcapillary venules; also noncellular elements: water, electrolytes, proteins, fibrinogen; RBC exit by a more passive mechanism classically called diapedesis.

[a] Abbreviations used are: Leu-CAMs, leukocyte cell adhesion molecules; WBC, white blood cell; and RBC, red blood cell.

rocytes that form agglutinated clumps of red cells. Such red cell sludging also contributes to the decrease in blood flow and occasionally leads to intravascular blood clotting.

Along with the slowing of blood flow, the clumped red cells collect in the central part of the blood stream, while the white cells assume a peripheral orientation along the endothelial surfaces of the affected vessels. The **venules** are the principal actors in the early phases of this evolving acute inflammatory drama. Capillaries play a larger role in the latter phases, particularly in more severe injuries.

Permeability Changes

The leakage of fluid occurring as a consequence of changes in the permeability of the microvasculature with resultant edema, is a major characteristic of virtually all acute inflammatory reactions. The fluid is at first a watery transudate or plasma ultrafiltrate, but the permeability changes within the venules and capillaries soon permit the escape of plasma proteins, leukocytes, and sometimes red cells. This protein-rich, cell-containing exudate appears in all but the most trivial of inflammatory responses. Transudation also can attend noninflammatory congestion of vessels, such as in the edema accompanying congestive heart failure, but exudation **always** indicates inflammation.

Understanding the pathogenesis of inflammatory exudation requires an understanding of the normal permeability of

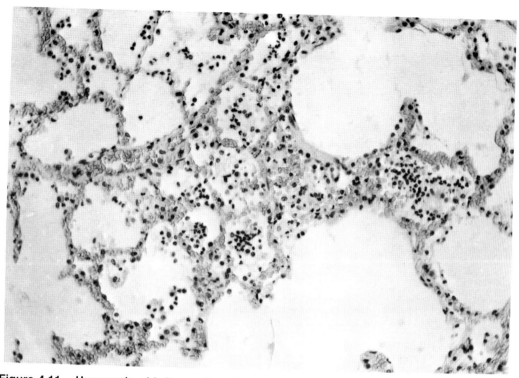

Figure 4.11. Hyperemia of Inflammation. The alveolar capillaries in this acutely inflamed bovine lung are engorged with blood. This is the acute, local, active hyperemia typical of inflammation.

the microcirculation. It once was thought that the plasma membranes of adjacent endothelial cells actually produce a tight junction. We now know, however, that although the cell junctions are narrow, a space or potential space does exist between contiguous cells (Fig. 4.12). This varies depending on the type of endothelium. Using particles of known molecular size visible in electron micrographs, investigators have been able to demonstrate filtration of small proteins through the normal intercellular junctions, while larger molecules are withheld.

Passage of fluid between the endothelial cells implies a passive role for the endothelium in the exchange of fluids. This is not entirely true. Endothelial cells have, on their luminal surfaces, small invaginations that become pinched off to create small endocytotic **vesicles** containing plasma. Transport of these vesicles across the endothelial cell, with dis-

charge of the contents on the other side, can comprise an active protein-transport mechanism. This pathway is probably not a significant transport pathway in a quantitative sense, but it is possible that it contributes to the limited passage of the large protein macromulecules characteristic of normal interstitial fluid.

Two major mechanisms appear to be operative in the development of edema at sites of acute inflammation. The first is purely hydrostatic, and the second involves alterations in permeability effected by the chemical mediators of inflammation. Remember that arteriolar dilatation leads to an increased blood flow in inflamed tissues. Accompanied by congestion of the venous drainage and increased hydrostatic pressures, this forces fluid, essentially an ultrafiltrate of plasma relatively free of protein, out of the vessels. Some protein may escape, but not enough to produce a characteristic exu-

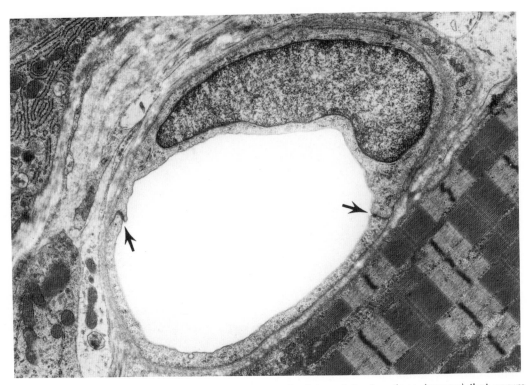

Figure 4.12. Capillary Endothelium. It is through the intercellular junctions *(arrows)* that serum proteins and leukocytes pass to gain entry to inflamed tissue.

date. Exudation soon follows transudation, however, as the permeability of the microcirculation increases. Using specialized techniques with intravascular tracers, investigators have been able to demonstrate varying patterns in the rise and ebb of increased permeability. These responses have been classified into different phases of altered permeability (Fig. 4.13). While much of this research work has been best demonstrated by fairly specific levels of thermal injury in the skin of the guinea pig and may not actually be evoked by chemical or other forms of injury, these variations are still distinctive and serve to illustrate certain points.

The first phase of increased vascular permeability appears to be mediated by **histamine,** since suitable chemical antagonists of histamine will completely prevent this change. As several investigators have pointed out, this histamine-

dependent phase is usually transient, lasting less than 1 hour. Within 2–4 hours a prolonged and quite different phase occurs. In contrast to the histamine-dependent phase, the secondary phase is prolonged, lasting over the next 3–4 hours. It is during this period that leukocytes begin to migrate out of blood vessels. The mediator of this secondary phase has not been identified, but it clearly is not histamine or serotonin, as antagonists of these amines are not effective in preventing the second wave of permeability change. It seems likely that no single mediator is responsible for this second, more prolonged phase of permeability increase. A large number of different chemical mediators of inflammation can invoke increased vascular permeability (Table 4.7), as we will discuss in greater detail later (*see* Chemical Mediators of Inflammation). It is also now clear that the **leu-**

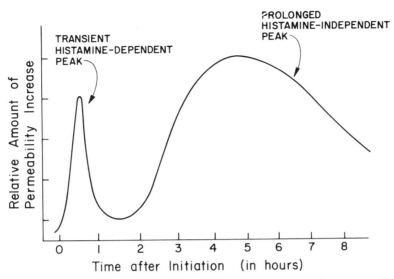

Figure 4.13.   Phases of Vascular Permeability. Antihistamines can eliminate or diminish the first peak of increased permeability but have no apparent effect on the second, more prolonged, phase of vascular leakage.

kocytes themselves participate in the mediation of vascular permeability and may be largely responsible for the second wave of permeability change.

The various phases of increased vascu- lar permeability are associated with the migration of fluids, not through endothe- lial cells, but **between** endothelial cells. Electron microscopic studies with tracer molecules have elegantly documented how

Table 4.7
Mediators of Vascular Permeability

Mediator	Special Characteristics[a]
Vasoactive amines	Histamine, serotonin; stored in granules of mast cells, baso- phils and platelets
Plasma kinins	Generated from plasma zymogens by enzymatic cleavage
Leukokinins	Derived from action of leukocytic lysosomal enzymes
Anaphylatoxins	C3a, C5a; peptides derived from complement activation. C5a works through the PMN
Leukotrienes	Some work independent of PMN (LTC_4, LTD_4, LTE_4) while some provoke PMN-dependent permeability changes (LTB_4)
Prostaglandins	Fatty acid derivatives of wide variety; many biological activi- ties; PGE_2 and PGI_2 cause vasodilation and potentiate vas- cular leakage
Lymphokines	Permeability factors from sensitized lymphocytes (lymph node permeability factor)
Neutrophil peptides	Preformed, basic peptides in lysosomal granules
Platelet-activating factor	Actions on endothelium and on PMN
Activated Hageman factor	Cleavage product; formerly PF-dil

[a] Abbreviations used are LT, leukotriene; PG, prostaglandin; PMN, neutrophil; PF-dil, permeability factor-dilute.

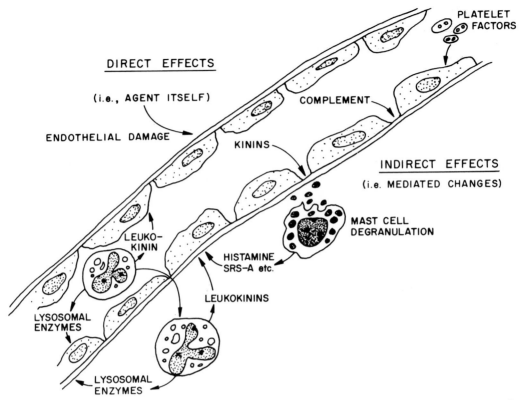

Figure 4.14. Mediation of Vascular Permeability. Changes in the microvascular bed can be brought about directly *via* injury to the endothelium, or indirectly *via* mediators generated from both cellular and plasma sources. Some mediators work directly on the endothelium, while others employ neutrophils as a cellular intermediary.

proteins, electrolytes, and water percolate through the junctional zones between endothelial cells, through the basement membrane of the vessel, and into the area around the blood vessel.

It is essential at this point to realize that vascular leakage after local injury can occur by at least two distinct mechanisms: (1) **directly,** as an effect of any kind of structural injury to the microvasculature or (2) **indirectly,** as an effect of chemical substances that appear in and around the site of injury (Fig. 4.14). In most well-developed inflammatory reactions, both mechanisms are probably operative. Vascular labeling techniques show that direct injury can affect all types of vessels (arterioles, capillaries, and venules), whereas indirect (chemically me-

diated) injury shows a high degree of specificity for the venules. The difference between these two patterns can be strikingly demonstrated by means of experimental burns of the skin: if the injury is appropriately calibrated, the underlying muscle will show a central patch in which only the venules are labeled.

The distinction between direct and indirect injury is of practical importance because the pharmacologic or therapeutic means to affect one or the other may not be the same. This distinction is not, however, always a sharp one. In the so-called delayed form of vascular leakage it was long debated whether the mechanism was direct or indirect. Furthermore, it is becoming increasingly obvious that bacteria can produce substances similar or identical in their effects to chemical mediators of inflammation produced by injured tissues. Hence, it is conceivable that a directly injurious agent, such as a bacterium, may induce inflammation by using its own "indirect" pathways. The very name of "pyogenic" bacteria indicates that some bacteria can produce substances chemotactic for polymorphonuclear leukocytes. Filtrates of cultures of various bacteria do indeed have chemotactic activity for neutrophils, and supernatants of *Escherichia coli* and other bacterial cultures contain a variety of other biologically active molecules. Permeability-increasing products of the histamine type, as far as we know, have not yet been described. They would be of no known help to the bacteria; indeed, they would have negative survival value by promoting inflammation. But then, the bacterial chemotactic factors also have a negative impact from the point of view of the bacteria, as they call in phagocytic cells programmed to destroy the organism that produces them. Host-parasite interactions are discussed more fully in Chapter 7.

Lastly, it has become increasingly clear in recent years that some of the differences in the effects of various mediators on vascular permeability can be attributed to whether or not they involve neutrophils as an intermediate (Fig. 4.14). For example, histamine seems to produce its vascular permeability adjustments *via* direct effects on the endothelial cell, independent of neutrophils. The same can be said for bradykinin. Other mediators such as the anaphylatoxin C5a and the leukotriene B_4 (LTB_4) appear to cause increased vascular permeability by inducing stickiness and pavementing of neutrophils in the venular part of the microvasculature, which is followed by neutrophil-mediated local extravasation of fluids and plasma proteins. This latter type of permeability adjustment seems to require neutrophils since, in their ab-

sence, increased permeability does not occur. Thus, chemical mediators of vascular permeability in acute inflammation can exert their effects either *via* direct effects on the microvasculature (histamine and bradykinin) or *via* use of the neutrophil as an intermediary (C5a and LTB_4) (*see* Fig. 4.14, 4.15). Again, the redundancy of ways to increase vascular permeability reiterates its importance to an evolving inflammatory reaction.

CELLS OF THE INFLAMMATORY EXUDATE

The three basic types of white blood cells that take part in inflammatory reactions are polymorphonuclear leukocytes or granulocytes (neutrophils, eosinophils, basophils), monocytes and macrophages, and lymphocytes and plasma cells. All of these leukocytes, save the plasma cells, are normal inhabitants of the circulating blood. The total leukocyte count in peripheral blood and the relative proportions of the different white blood cells may be greatly modified in systemic responses to inflammation. Each cell type plays a fairly distinctive role and enters into the inflammatory response in a definite sequence, as we have indicated previously. The discussion that follows is concerned principally with the major characteristics of these different types of leukocytes. We have not focused on the mast cell here as it is not really part of the inflammatory exudate, but rather it serves to promote the vascular permeability by which the blood-borne cells gain access to injured tissue. More information on mast cells is presented in Chapter 5.

Granulocytes: Red, White, and Blue

The term granulocyte derives from the fact that these cells have recognizable granules in their cytoplasm. The **eosinophil** has eosinophilic granules, the **basophil** has basophilic granules, and the **neutrophil** has granules that take nei-

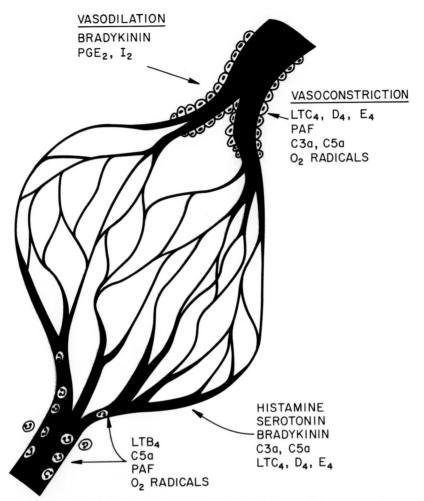

Figure 4.15. Influence of Mediators on The Microvascular Bed. The various inflammatory mediators work at different levels to influence both vascular dilatation and constriction as well as permeability and may function *via* different mechanisms. PGE_2 can potentiate vascular leakage by causing vasodilation. The vasoactive amines and others can cause increased permeability directly, while some mediators (LTB_4, C5a) promote leukocyte-dependent increased permeability. (Adapted from: Smedegard, G.: Mediators of vascular permeability in inflammation. *Progress in Applied Microcirculation* 7:96–112, 1985).

ther type of dye well and hence are "neutral." These cells also are sometimes referred to as **polymorphonuclear** leukocytes, as their nuclei are multilobed, as opposed to those of the mononuclear lymphocytes, monocytes, and plasma cells. In practical usage, the term polymorphonuclear leukocyte or simply "polymorph," "poly," or "PMN" generally refers to neutrophils.

Neutrophils

These cells are usually the first leukocytes to gather at sites of acute inflammation, where they play a key role. Neutrophils are fairly short-lived cells and are highly specialized. Like all of the granulocytes, neutrophils develop in the bone marrow, arising from a population of hematopoietic stem cells. Maturation proceeds through stages, beginning with myeloblasts and proceeding to promyelocyte, myelocyte, metamyelocyte, juvenile or band forms, and eventually mature neutrophils. This maturation process usually takes about 2 weeks, but can be speeded up when the demand for circulating neutrophils is high, and sometimes even immature neutrophils are released to the peripheral blood in stress situations. Once released from the bone marrow, mature neutrophils remain in the circulation for only a short time and then migrate into tissues, where they may survive for 1–2 days. Radiolabeling studies have shown that once neutrophils leave the vasculature to enter tissue, they do not return to the circulation.

There are two distinct pools of neutrophils in the blood, a **marginated** pool consisting of cells within blood vessels but lying out of the flow or "marginated" against the walls, and a **circulating** pool. It appears that neutrophils (and other leukocytes) may exchange freely between these two pools in response to various kinds of signals. Neutrophils in the circulating pool have a half-life in the blood of only about 4–6 hours and are quickly replaced. The circulating and marginated pools are of approximately equal size, and the neutrophils in the marginated pool can be mobilized very quickly. It is generally believed that once neutrophils leave the circulation to enter tissue, they do not return. The two major sources of reserve neutrophils, therefore, are those in the marginated pool and the bone marrow compartments.

The morphologic features of neutrophils suggest their major functions. They range from 10–12 microns in diameter, have polymorphonuclear characteristics, and contain abundant cytoplasmic granules. Ultrastructurally, neutrophils are characterized by a scarcity of organelles, except for the granules (fig. 4.16). The mature neutrophil contains no endo-

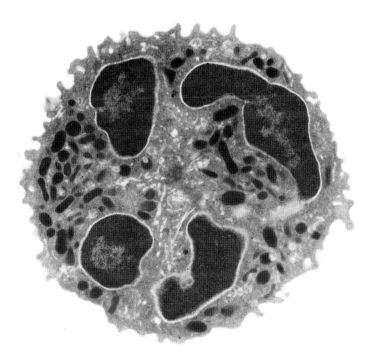

Figure 4.16. Neutrophil. The segmented nucleus and numerous lysosomal granules in the cytoplasm of this sheep neutrophil are typical of this kind of granulocyte.

Table 4.8
Neutrophil Granule Constituents

Specific Granules	Azurophil Granules	Type of Constituent
Lysozyme	Lysozyme Myeloperoxidase Phagocytin	Microbicidal enzymes
Collagenase	Collagenase Elastase	Neutral proteinases
	Cathepsins Proteinases	Proteolysis
	β-Glucuronidase α-Mannosidase N-Acetyl-β-glucosaminidase α-Glycerophosphatase (many others)	Acid hydrolases
Lactoferrin B$_{12}$-binding proteins		Miscellaneous

plasmic reticulum, a small Golgi apparatus, and a few small mitochondria. Two major classes of granules have been identified, each of which has a relatively distinctive profile of enzymes (Table 4.8). The **azurophil,** or primary, granules are large, oval, and electron dense. They contain neutral proteases, lysozyme, a variety of acid hydrolases, and **myeloperoxidase,** which is commonly used to identify these granules. The **specific,** or secondary, granules are smaller, less dense, and more numerous. They contain additional lysozyme, collagenase, and lactoferrin as well as other materials. Bovine neutrophils have a distinct third type of granule, which is less well characterized but apparently has potent microbicidal activity. All of the enzymes are essentially hydrolytic, and so all of the granules might be said to represent forms of lysosomes. Extracts of the lysosomes of neutrophils derived from inflammatory responses also have been shown to contain cationic proteins that include permeability factors and possibly pyrogens.

Neutrophils constitute the major cellular defense system of all higher organisms against bacteria. They are well equipped for their job by virtue of their motility, responsiveness to chemotactic stimuli, phagocytic abilities, and bactericidal activities. The major function of neutrophils in the inflammatory response involves their participation in phagocytosis, the release of their lytic lysosomal enzymes, and the formation of chemotactic factors (Table 4.9). Certain complement components can be activated by neutrophil enzymes to yield an attractant for neutrophils, thus providing for a cyclic

Table 4.9
Important Characteristics of Neutrophils

Important cell in host defense
Actively motile and actively phagocytic
Surface receptors for C3b and Fc opsonins
Contain neutral proteinases active against extra-
cellular substrates
Lysosomal (not cytoplasmic) enzymes can be
released during phagocytosis
Respond to variety of chemotaxins
Potent microbicidal systems
Secretory cell
Mediate vascular permeability (C5a, LTB$_4$)

Table 4.10
Partial List of Enzymes and Other
Substances in Leukocyte Lysosomes

Enzymes Acting on Carbohydrates
β-Acetyl galactosaminidase
α-Acetyl glucosaminidase
α-Galactosidase
β-Galactosidase
α-Glucosidase
β-Glucosidase
β-Glucuronidase
α-L-Fucosidase
β-D-Fucosidase
Hyaluronidase
Lysozyme
α-Mannosidase
Neuraminidase

Enzymes Acting on Proteins
Arylamidase
Cathepsin A, B, C, D, E
Chemotactic factor generating protease
Collagenase
Elastase-like enzyme
Histonase
Chymotrypsin-like enzyme
Renin
Plasminogen activator

Enzymes Acting on Lipids
Acid lipase
Cholesterol esterase
Glucocerebrosidase
Galactocerebrosidase
Phospholipase A_1
Phospholipase A_2
Organophosphate-resistant esterase

Enzymes Acting on Nucleic Acids
Acid deoxyribonuclease
Acid ribonuclease

Miscellany
Acid phosphatase
Anticoagulants
Arylsulfatase
Cationic proteins
Endogenous pyrogen
Mucopolysaccharides
Myeloperoxidase
Peroxidase
Phosphodiesterase
Phosphoprotein phosphatase

reaction. In addition, mononuclear cells respond to lysates of neutrophils, possibly to the liberated cationic peptides of lysosomal origin. The neutrophil with its granules is therefore crucial to the entire inflammatory process.

The main function of the neutrophil is phagocytosis. The purpose of phagocytosis is to ingest, neutralize, and, whenever possible, destroy the ingested particle. These functions are accomplished with the aid of intracellular enzymes located within the granules of the neutrophil. The enzymes and other substances in neutrophil lysosomes are many (Table 4.10). When neutrophils ingest bacteria or other particulate material, they form **phagosomes,** which fuse with the lysosomes to form **phagolysosomes,** and in this process they become degranulated.

The participation of the neutrophil granules in phagocytosis has been well documented. It can be shown that during phagocytosis, fusion of the granule membranes with the phagosome membrane takes place. By specialized electron microscopic techniques that allow demonstration of the lysosomal enzymes, discharge of the granule contents into the phagosome can be visualized. It is also now clear that while the fusion of the lysosomes with the phagosomes is an important neutrophil activity, many of the lysosomal enzymes do not actually participate in bacterial killing, but rather serve as digestive enzymes to degrade bacteria that have already been killed *via* both oxygen-dependent and oxygen-independent mechanisms in which relatively few of the granule enzymes actually participate. We will discuss phagocytosis and the mechanisms of bacterial killing in a later section (*see* section on Phagocytosis).

Eosinophils

Eosinophils are particularly abundant at sites of inflammation in diseases of immunologic or allergic origin, but they can be part of any exudate. They also are prominent inflammatory cells in reactions caused by parasites. Their significance in such tissue reactions is related to their unique functions as effector cells for killing helminths and their propensity for both causing and assisting in the regulation of tissue damage in hypersensitivity diseases. The eosinophil is distinguished from the neutrophil by the affinity of its coarse cytoplasmic granules for the acid dye eosin. The full spectrum of functional capabilities of the eosinophil is still a matter of dispute, although considerable recent progress has been made. There is general agreement that the eosinophil is phagocytic, but they are certainly less active phagocytes than neutrophils.

The eosinophil responds to many of the same influences as the neutrophil including soluble bacterial factors and activated components of complement, and eosinophil-specific chemotaxins have been defined. They are also responsive to antigen-antibody complexes and have membrane receptors for both IgG and C3 fragments. The lysosomal granules of the eosinophil contain a wide variety of catalytic enzymes similar to those in neutrophils, except that they lack lysozyme and phagocytin. Eosinophil granules also contain several specific granule proteins such as major basic protein and eosinophil cationic protein.

These cells have a shape and nuclear morphology similar to those of neutrophils, but are slightly larger than the latter cells. The granules vary considerably from species to species, but virtually all contain crystalloid structures (Fig. 4.17). The eosinophil leukocytes of the horse contain 25–50 granules, each approximately 1 micron in diameter, whereas those of the rat have up to 400 granules, measuring only about 0.2 microns. Histochemical studies indicate that the granules show a positive reaction with protein and lipid stains, and they contain large quantities of a stable peroxidase. As we have already pointed out, most enzymes demonstrable in neutrophils are found also in eosinophils. Thus, the eosinophil granules are true lysosomes.

The eosinophils make up a variable percentage (1–5%) of the total circulating leukocytes. They are produced in the bone marrow, and their differentiation and maturation are similar to those of neutrophil granulocytes, but slightly more rapid. Like neutrophils, they have a short lifespan. The ratio of eosinophils in blood, bone marrow, and tissue is 1:200:500. In tissues, they are found mainly in the intestinal wall, lungs, skin, and external genitalia. The circulating eosinophils are under the influence of adrenocortical hormones, and increased secretion of these hormones or their therapeutic administration results in a decrease in the number of eosinophils in the blood. Our evolving understanding of the tissue distribution and cellular characteristics of the eosinophil and the recognition of the range of diseases associated with eosinophilia provide compelling evidence that the eosinophil fulfills unique roles in host defense by modulating hypersensitivity reactions, especially those of the immediate type, and by helping to defend against helminthic infestations.

While eosinophils are derived from myeloid precursors and share diverse morphologic and functional characteristics with other leukocytes of the polymorphonuclear series, a variety of distinctive traits are notable (Table 4.11). The most remarkable ultrastructural feature of the eosinophil is a class of large cytoplasmic granules composed of a crystalloid core surrounded by a less dense matrix. The predominant protein of the core, termed **major basic protein,** constitutes about 50% of the granule protein content and is strongly cationic due to its high content of arginine. It has a M_r of about 9,000–11,000, depending on the species from which the eosinophils are obtained, and interacts with numerous other molecules by virtue of its strongly positive charge

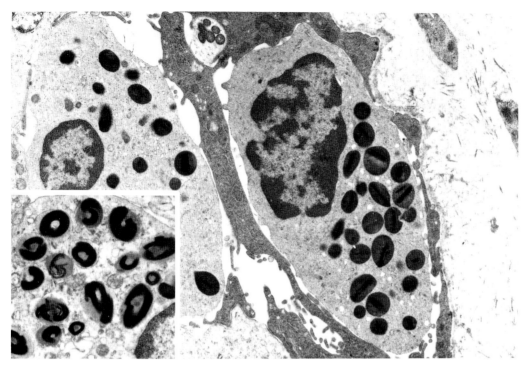

Figure 4.17.   Eosinophils. The hallmark of the eosinophil is the structure of the characteristic cytoplasmic granules, which have a dense central core. This dense core is the source of "major basic protein," an important eosinophil constituent. These eosinophils are from a rhesus monkey. To show the variation in granules between species, feline eosinophil granules are shown in the *inset.* (Micrographs courtesy of Drs. W. L. Castelman and J. M. Ward.)

and ready involvement in disulfide exchange reactions. Major basic protein is strongly toxic to parasites as well as other kinds of cells, and can additionally cause

Table 4.11
Distinctive Characteristics of Eosinophils

Constituent or Product	Function
Major basic protein	Neutralize heparin
	Parasite killing
	Histamine release
Eosinophil cationic protein	Parasite killing
	Shorten coagulation time
	Alter fibrinolysis
Arylsulfatase B	Inactive leukotrienes
Histaminase	Inactivate histamine
Phospholipase D	Inactivate PAF[a]

[a] Abbreviation used is: PAF, platelet-activating factor.

histamine release from mast cells and basophils as well as neutralize heparin. An additional unique eosinophil granule protein, **eosinophil cationic protein,** contributes to parasite killing and also shortens coagulation time and alters fibrinolysis.

While eosinophils respond chemotactically to fragments and complexes of certain complement components and to some lymphocyte products, migration-enhancing factors with preferential activity for eosinophils are derived largely from immediate-type hypersensitivity reactions. IgE-dependent activation of mast cells leads to the elaboration of a wide array of chemical mediators including both those released from preformed stores, such as histamine, heparin, and diverse peptides, and those generated *de novo,* which are lipids, such as the leukotrienes (slow-reacting substance of anaphylaxis, SRS-A), platelet-activating factor (PAF), hydroxy-fatty acids, and prostaglandins. The eosinophil chemotactic factor of anaphylaxis (ECF-A), which is the major chemical attractant for eosinophils, is also a preformed mediator that has been specifically associated with the mast cell and the basophil by its extraction from essentially pure populations of these cell types.

Eosinophils arrive at sites of immediate-type hypersensitivity reactions after the humoral phase has been established, and are capable of inactivating some of the mast cell–derived mediators by nonenzymatic and enzymatic mechanisms. The major basic protein neutralizes heparin, presumably by virtue of a charge interaction. Eosinophil **histaminase,** like that of the neutrophil, inactivates histamine with a pH optimum of 6–8. Eosinophil **arylsulfatase B** inactivates leukotrienes LTC_4, LTD_4, and LTE_4 (SRS-A) in a time- and pH-dependent reaction. **Phospholipase D,** like arylsulfatase B, is found in greater quantities in eosinophils than in other leukocytes, and specifically inactivates PAF. While the eosinophil is predominantly devoted to the degradation of mediators released from mast cells, the generation of prostaglandins of the E series by eosinophils exposed to IgE-containing immune complexes and the phagocytosis of extruded mast cell granules by eosinophils also constitute regulatory pathways directed at the limitation of the reactions that elaborate the mediators.

Eosinophils also have proinflammatory properties and can function as effector cells in causing tissue damage. Some of this can be explained by the fact that eosinophils can bind IgE and are activated by antigen-IgE complexes. Such eosinophil activation is thought to contribute to the tissue damage that occurs in certain forms of asthma as well as in allergic skin diseases. Eosinophils have also been associated with certain kinds of

endomyocardial disease, but their role in the pathogenesis of the lesions is largely unknown.

The antibody-dependent destruction of helminths by eosinophils has been demonstrated *in vitro* and *in vivo*. The eosinophils are attracted to sites of helminthic invasion in sensitized hosts by chemotactic factors elaborated predominantly as a result of the immune response to products of the parasite. The unique ability of eosinophils to adhere to and damage helminths has been confirmed by detailed morphological studies. Eosinophils have been shown to adhere to helminths and to degranulate against them, thus bringing the helminthotoxic major basic protein into play (Fig. 4.18). While the precise mechanisms underlying the helminthicidal activity of eosinophils have not been elucidated fully, it is clear that major basic protein is involved. Even rather low concentrations of eosinophil major basic protein can mimic the destructive effects of intact eosinophils on the helminths. The eosinophil thus is emerging from its past residence in obscurity and now is known to function broadly as both a "regulator" and "effector" cell in acute inflammatory and hypersensitivity reactions, as well as serving as a potential "killer cell" in helminthiasis.

Basophils (and Mast Cells)

These two cell types have been of interest to biomedical scientists for over a century since they were first described by Paul Ehrlich. Mast cells are found principally in perivascular sites in tissues while basophils are rare circulating granulocytes. Basophils and mast cells are very closely related functionally and have many similarities, such as cytoplasm that is literally loaded with coarse granules that appear blue-black with the usual blood stains. The granules are also metachromatic (that is, they stain pink to blue with such stains as toluidine blue) be-

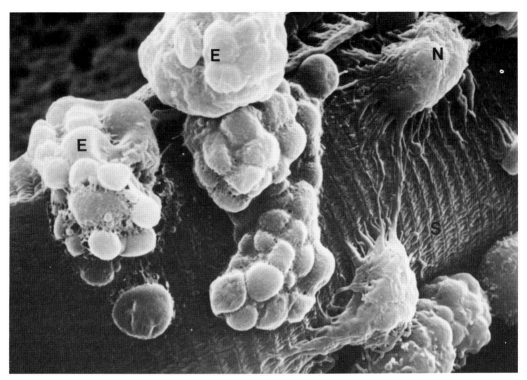

Figure 4.18.   Eosinophil Helminthotoxicity. These equine eosinophils *(E)* with their large granules are degranulating against the surface of a strongyle *(S)*. Such activity releases major basic protein and other toxic agents against the parasite. A few neutrophils *(N)* are also adherent to the parasite. (Micrograph courtesy of Dr. Thomas R. Klei.)

cause of their rich content of sulfated mucopolysaccharides, principally heparin. They also contain histamine, proteases, and other potent biologically active mediators. Both cell types are also characterized by receptors that bind the Fc portion of IgE antibody with high affinity. An explosive degranulation with release of histamine and other mediators occurs when basophils and mast cells are appropriately stimulated, as when specific antigen binds to cell-bound IgE molecules. Mast cells in particular are major cellular sources of the vasoactive amines so important to the vascular phenomena of acute inflammation. Despite their similarities, mast cells and basophils are also distinctly different, and there remains no convincing evidence that the mature circulating basophil represents a precursor of mature tissue mast cells.

Mast cells are granular connective tissue cells found throughout the connective tissues in virtually every organ (Fig. 4.19). They are most numerous at sites of "contact" with the external environment such as skin, respiratory tract, and gastrointestinal tract. Mast cells are most numerous about small blood vessels. They have mononuclear nuclei, are slightly larger, and have somewhat more abundant cytoplasm than the basophil. Their granules contain heparin, histamine, and other proteolytic enzymes. After the release of these products, the cells become degranulated. In some animals they also are rich in serotonin. These cells are intimately involved in the pathogenesis of acute inflammation, since it is their release of histamine which triggers many of the manifestations arising from smooth muscle contraction and edema formation.

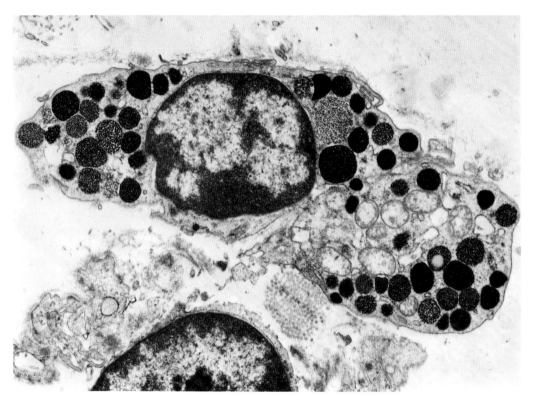

Figure 4.19.   Mast Cell. Equine subcutis. The mononuclear mast cell is strikingly similar ultrastructurally to the basophil. Note that the variation in granule morphology is similar to that of the basophil. These granules also contain potent mediators of inflammation. (Micrograph courtesy of Dr. John F. Cummings.)

Considerable evidence has accumulated in recent years on the heterogeneity of mast cells and the likelihood of subclasses. It is generally recognized that at least two populations of mast cells exist: the **mucosal** mast cells, found principally in the gastrointestinal and respiratory tracts, and the **connective tissue** mast cells, found in the skin. There are apparent species differences in the distribution of the mast cell types, and the specific origin of each type remains unclear.

The basophil (Fig. 4.20) is a granulocyte of bone marrow origin and is a rare member of the white cell population of the blood, where they constitute less than 1% of the circulating leukocytes. In the size and shape of their nuclei they closely resemble neutrophils. Bone marrow–derived blood basophils are recruited into the tissues of immune mechanisms in a variety of delayed time-course hypersensitivity responses. In the skin these are called **cutaneous basophil hypersensitivity** (CBH) reactions, and are elicited by certain ectoparasites. In guinea pigs, it is now established that the elicitation of CBH is dependent on T cell–triggered mechanisms. Both are subject to modulation. After basophils arrive at a CBH reaction they can be triggered by antigen to immediately release mediators such as histamine. Thus, one consequence of the arrival and accumulation of basophils at delayed hypersensitivity reactions is to augment the anaphylactic potential of a given tissue site. In reactions to parasites, release of mediators by tissue basophils seems to aid in the expulsion of these multicellular organisms. In addition, his-

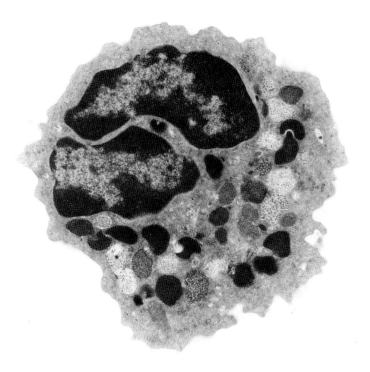

Figure 4.20.   Basophil. Sheep blood. The granules of the basophil vary from dense structures to more loosely associated aggregates of smaller, electron-dense granules sometimes organized into tubular or chainlike arrays. The granules contain potent inflammatory mediators.

tamine released by recruited basophils, or by locally resident mast cells, may modulate some delayed reactions through stimulation of type 2 histamine receptors on cells such as T lymphocytes. Basophil leukocytes and mast cells release histamine in a variety of immunologic and nonimmunologic settings. Degranulation of these cells usually does not lead to cell death. Rather, the mediator release process is a carefully controlled secretory event in which cell viability is maintained. Thus, basophils and mast cells and the release of mediators, such as vasoactive amines, are involved in the onset, development, and function of various tissue inflammatory responses.

Mononuclear Phagocytes: Macrophages

There is virtually unanimous agreement that the macrophages so prominent in inflammatory reactions are derived from circulating blood monocytes of bone marrow origin. A smaller proportion may originate from immature, resident, "fixed" mononuclear phagocytes in the tissues, but these are ultimately of bone marrow origin as well. The macrophages are larger than neutrophils, and, in routine blood stains, possess a gray-blue cytoplasm filled with very fine granules. Their nuclei are large, usually central, and may be folded or bean-shaped. The macrophage contains many lysosomes, and often has one or two nucleoli and cytoplasmic extensions called pseudopodia. The major function of the macrophage is phagocytosis, and they are the major scavenger cells in the inflammatory response (Fig. 4.21). Within inflamed tissues, the macrophages almost invariably contain phagocytic inclusions (phagosomes) that enclose bacteria and cell debris as well as lipid residues from

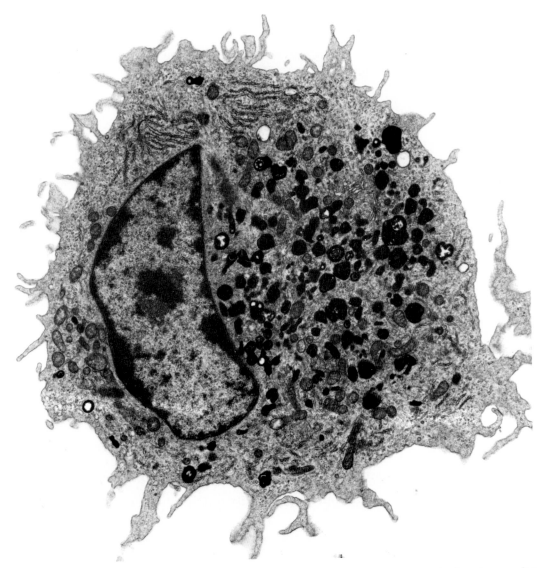

Figure 4.21. Macrophage. This rabbit alveolar macrophage shows abundant cytoplasmic granules many of which represent phagocytosed debris. Note the numerous cytoplasmic processes at the cell surface. (Micrograph courtesy of Jan Henson and Dr. Peter Henson).

dead cell membranes. In the course of such phagocytic orgies, these cells become swollen and ballooned.

Macrophages are sluggishly motile but are responsive to chemotactic influences. Both neutrophils and monocytes can emigrate simultaneously, but the migration of the former occurs more quickly, and so macrophages dominate the inflammatory white cell population in the later phases of many inflammatory reactions. They also have a longer life span than do neutrophils and may actually proliferate at sites of protracted inflammation, accounting for their large numbers in long-standing reactions.

Macrophages are the sources of the multinucleated **giant cells** present in some chronic inflammatory reactions (Fig. 4.10) in which the stimulus for giant cell formation is usually some rather indigestible object (foreign bodies, certain kinds of microorganisms). Giant cells are generally believed to be formed by the coalescence of single macrophages. Another type of macrophage seen in some kinds of chronic inflammatory reactions is the **epithelioid cell.** These are large, pale-staining macrophages that have an ovoid nucleus and an angular shape resembling epithelial cells. Their paleness is due to diffusely distributed lipid and other phagocytosed debris in their cytoplasm.

Circulating monocytes develop in the bone marrow. After the committed stem-cell stages, this cell line has two successive proliferating stages, the monoblast and the promonocyte. The monocytes arise from dividing promonocytes and emerge in the circulation. Unlike the neutrophils, the monocytes do not have a large reserve pool in the bone marrow, but they remain longer in the circulation, their half-life being 24–72 hours. Like circulating neutrophils, the blood monocytes are functional cells, but they require further "activation" under the influence of various chemical mediators before they can achieve their maximal functional competence as macrophages. Thus, one major difference between a **monocyte** and a **macrophage** relates to the state of activation. In addition, it has been traditional to divide these cells into two camps based on a definitional separation; once monocytes have migrated into tissues, they have usually been referred to as macrophages. Unlike neutrophils, such cells may have a life span of several months. This definition of a macrophage, however, is probably too restrictive. For example, in the category of **fixed mononuclear phagocytes,** the hepatic Kupffer cells clearly are in contact with the blood stream yet are not monocytes.

Additionally, the very interesting and recently described **pulmonary intravascular macrophages** (PIMs) are a unique category of fixed mononuclear phagocytes. They are found in ruminants (calves, goats, sheep), cats, and pigs, but not in dogs, most laboratory animals, or man. Located adherent to the capillary endothelium of the lung, they are morphologically similar to hepatic Kupffer cells and apparently serve similar functions in those species that have them, possibly being even more important than Kupffer cells in the removal of blood-borne particulates. Unfortunately, these cells are also highly responsive to bacterial endotoxins, and the pulmonary removal of circulating endotoxin by PIMs results in acute lung injury. The sensitivity of certain species to endotoxin-induced lung injury may be based in part on whether or not they possess PIMs.

Macrophages in tissues differ from monocytes by being larger (15–80 microns) and by having a variable number of azurophil granules and remnants of ingested material. Their nuclei vary in size and shape, and multinucleated forms are not uncommon. Ultrastructurally, macrophages have condensed peripheral nuclear chromatin and one or more nucleoli. They have a well-developed Golgi apparatus, composed of flattened sacks, small vesicles, and a few granules. In addition, the cytoplasm contains a moderate amount of endoplastic reticulum, a varying number of electron-dense bodies corresponding to the azurophil granules seen in stained smears, free ribosomes, mitochondria, and innumerable small vesicles (Fig. 4.21). Their structure depends in part on the state of activation. In the stimulated macrophage, there is considerable ruffled membrane activity and the Golgi apparatus is more complex and highly developed. Dense cytoplasmic granules are usually very prominent and numerous, and are believed to be secondary lysosomes.

The primary function of the macrophages, like the neutrophil, is to phagocytose and degrade ingested material. Macrophages also play a central role in the regulation of the immune response and are important effector cells in certain delayed-type hypersensitivity responses (*see* Chapter 5). Unlike neutrophils, which function mainly to dispose of bacteria, macrophages also are active against fungi, protozoa, viruses, cell debris, and whole dead or altered cells.

In addition to the enzyme release that is induced by the phagocytosis of a number of substances, the production and release of hydrolases from macrophages also can be induced by lymphokines derived from sensitized peripheral blood lymphocytes. Macrophages are very important cells in the host defense mechanism, but by virtue of their enzyme content they can contribute to the evolving inflammatory process in much the same fashion as neutrophils. Macrophages, for example, are the major sources of **IL-1** and **tumor necrosis factor** (*see* section on Mediators). Thus, both neutrophils and macrophages must be regarded as "secretory" cells.

Lymphocytes and Plasma Cells

Both of these cell types are principally involved in immune reactions and are the key cellular mediators of both the immediate antibody response and the delayed cellular hypersensitivity response. (Readers needing a brief review of the various types of lymphocytes and their participation in the immune system may wish to consult the appropriate section at the beginning of Chapter 5). The precise role of lymphocytes in nonimmunologic injuries and inflammation remains somewhat less clear, although they often are present in such lesions. They usually appear somewhat later than neutrophils in most inflammatory reactions, and may be prominent cellular features of the exudate in the subacute and chronic phase of many types of inflammatory lesions. Interestingly, however, certain infectious agents seem to provoke a lymphocytic response almost from the beginning. The

renal lesions of acute leptospirosis in dogs, for example, are often decidedly lymphocytic.

Lymphocytes (Fig. 4.22) are less motile than are neutrophils and monocytes. Certain types of lymphocytes (B cells) and their differentiated end stages, the plasma cells, can synthesize and elaborate antibody (Fig. 4.23). The responsiveness of lymphocytes to chemotactic agents has been more difficult to assess than similar responses of neutrophils, but they are clearly motile cells that can respond to several different chemotactic signals. Little is known of plasma cell chemotactic responses, and their presence in inflammatory lesions is generally presumed to result from local differentiation from B lymphocytes. It can appear that the appearance of lymphocytes and plasma cells in chronic inflammation may reflect some local immunologic reaction that has evolved over the course of an inflammatory response. At one time, it was thought that the presence of plasma cells in lesions always indicated infection, since sterile wounds rarely contain many plasma cells. We now know that this is an oversimplification, but the principle that lymphocyte and plasma cell infiltrates usually indicate a local immune reaction in response to some agent is still valid.

Lymphocytes are produced by the primary lymphoid organs at a rather high rate and migrate *via* the circulation to secondary lymphoid tissues such as the spleen and lymph nodes. It is also clear that lymphocytes recirculate among and between various lymphoid tissues through the blood and lymphatics. Some lymphocytes may normally leave the blood stream through non-specialized venules, but the majority exit through a highly specialized portion of the postcapillary venules known as **high endothelial venules (HEV)**. This appears to be a highly specific and probably receptor-directed event, since lymphocyte migration, at least within the lymphoid tissues, is not random. That is,

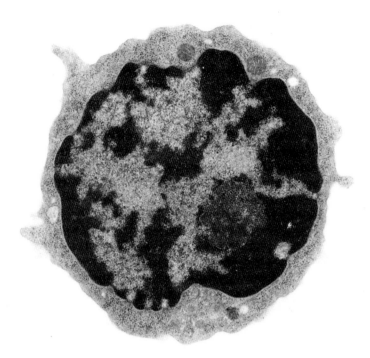

Figure 4.22.   Lymphocyte. This typical sheep lymphocyte has only scanty amounts of cytoplasm containing abundant polyribosomes, a few profiles of endoplasmic reticulum, mitochondria, and a Golgi zone. The nucleus has the usual pattern of peripheral heterochromatin.

lymphocytes that home to the gut are selectively transported across gut-specific HEV. The adherence of lymphocytes to endothelium may be related, at least in part, to interaction of **endothelial adhesion molecules** such as the recently described **ICAM-1** with certain leukocyte adhesion molecules like **LFA-1** (lymphocyte function-associated antigen 1), which is known to promote lymphocyte adherence. The relevance of these recent findings to lymphocyte migration into inflammatory lesions remains unknown, and it can be assumed for now that lymphocytes that enter inflamed tissues do so largely *via* the same interendothelial migration routes as do other leukocytes.

In a conventional blood smear, lymphocytes are heterogeneous in both size and morphology, but are generally smaller than neutrophils and have a densely staining nucleus and a scant amount of cytoplasm. In addition to the traditional division of lymphocytes into T cells and B cells, studies in the past decade have shown tremendous functional heterogeneity among different lymphocyte subclasses. These subclasses of lymphocytes express different cell surface proteins, which act as "markers." For example, among T lymphocytes, antibodies directed against these markers have allowed the identification of both helper T cells and suppressor T cells, which function differently in the immune response. We will discuss the role of the various functional lymphocyte types in immunologic reactions at greater length in Chapter 5.

Beyond their obvious importance in the generation of immune responses, lymphocytes are also consequential to the inflammatory response in several ways. By virtue of their terminal differentiation into

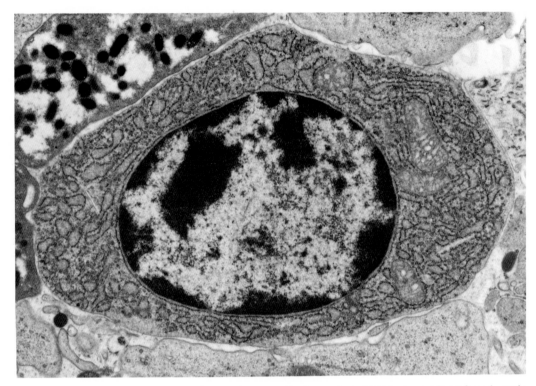

Figure 4.23. Plasma Cell. This sheep plasma cell shows the abundant, rough-surfaced, endoplasmic reticulum (RER) that fills the cytoplasm of most plasma cells. It is on these profiles of RER that immunoglobulins are synthesized and assembled.

plasma cells, B lymphocytes are of conspicuous importance in the production of antibody-forming cells. Antibody constitutes one of the major **opsonins,** and thus interfaces directly with the cellular, phagocytic arm of the host defense mechanism. In addition, T lymphocytes represent the cellular sources of the potent **inflammatory lymphokines,** which can modulate and expand local inflammatory reactions (*see* section on Mediators). Lastly, certain types of lymphocytes function as cytotoxic cells that can injure host tissue cells in both antibody-directed and antibody-independent ways.

Platelets as Inflammatory Cells

The blood platelets tend to be ignored by histopathologists because they are too small to be readily seen in routine histologic slides of inflamed tissue. When we think of platelets, we do not associate them with inflammatory processes other than to admit that they play a role in coagulation phenomena. This underestimate of platelet function requires reevaluation. In a local inflammatory reaction, damaged vessels or vessels altered by mediators leave subendothelial structures exposed to the circulating blood cells and plasma.

One of the earliest steps in the primary hemostatic defense mechanism involves the adhesion of circulating platelets to subendothelial structures such as collagen, basement membrane, and microfibrils in the vicinity of a damaged endothelial surface. Platelets activated by collagen release intracellular constituents including adenosine diphosphate (ADP), serotonin, platelet factor 4 (PF4), fibrinogen, various hydrolytic enzymes,

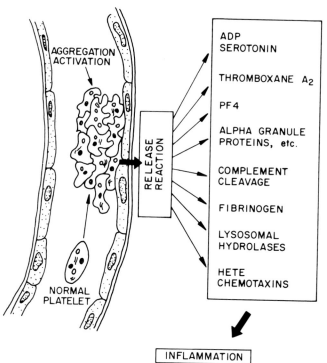

Figure 4.24. Platelet Release of Inflammatory Mediators. When platelets are activated and aggregated, the ensuing platelet release reaction causes the secretion of many chemical mediators of importance to inflammation. (*ADP*, adenosine diphosphate; *PF*, platelet factor.)

and products of the arachidonate transformation pathway (Fig. 4.24). The released ADP, thromboxane A_2, and prostaglandin endoperoxides formed from arachidonate lead to the formation of a platelet aggregate, which eventually plugs and seals off the disrupted vessel. Platelets contain intracellular granules similar to the classical lysosomes of polymorphonuclear leukocytes (Fig. 4.25). They can contribute to the inflammatory response accompanying tissue injury by releasing constituents that may provide local amplification (Table 4.12). Platelets accumulate in vessels adjacent to inflammatory sites and interact with bacteria, viruses, and antigen-antibody complexes.

Platelets have the same primitive phylogenetic ancestor as neutrophils and perform similar inflammatory functions in the intravascular compartment, while the neutrophil performs its major functions in extravascular spaces. In this regard, it is useful to consider primary hemostasis as a part of the inflammatory response. The platelet thus can be thought of as a special form of inflammatory "leukocyte" (Table 4.13).

It has been demonstrated that platelets contribute to the inflammatory response accompanying tissue injury by releasing constituents that increase vascular permeability. The fact that platelets contain an intracellular permeability-enhancing protein system further strengthens the analogy of these cells to exudative neutrophils. One important difference should be stressed when comparing the platelet inflammatory system to the leukocyte inflammatory system. Some of the leukocyte intracellular cationic protein mediators of inflammatory responses have been detected only in exudative cells. In contrast these same activities appear to

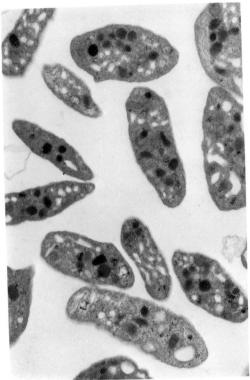

Figure 4.25. Platelets. Rabbit blood. These typically anucleate platelets show the cytoplasmic granules and dense bodies as well as the open cytocavitary network typical of most platelets, and through which granule constituents are secreted to the exterior. (Micrograph courtesy of Jan Henson and Dr. Peter Henson).

Table 4.12
Secretory Constituents of Platelets Related to Inflammation

Component	Location
Acid hydrolases	Lysosomes
Platelet factor 4	α-granules
Thromboglobulin	α-granules
Fibrinogen	α-granules
Cold-insoluble globulin	α-granules
Factor VIII	α-granules
Factor V	α-granules
Cationic permeability factors	α-granules
Antiplasmin	α-granules
Antibacterial factors	α-granules
Fibroblast-activating peptide	α-granules
Serotonin (and histamine)	Dense granules
ADP, ATP[a]	Dense granules
Ca^{2+} cations	Dense granules
Pyrophosphate	Dense granules
Arachidonic acid	Membranes
Complement-cleaving protease	Lysosomes
Platelet-activating factor	Precursor molecule

[a] Abbreviations used are: ADP, adenosine diphosphate; and ATP, adenosine triphosphate.

reside preformed in circulating platelets. Thus the platelets have a precommitted exudative function. Whether this function represents a phylogenetic vestige of little physiologic importance or is, in fact, the role of the platelets in mediating early blood vessel responses to local inflammatory stimuli remains to be determined.

There is more direct evidence suggesting that platelets participate in inflammatory responses. Platelets accumulate in blood vessels adjacent to areas of inflammation and tissue damage. Kidney transplant rejections may be associated with the formation of platelet aggregates in renal vessels. A similar phenomenon may characterize the kidney changes seen in the generalized Shwartzman reaction (*see* Chapter 7). Various stimuli including circulating antigen-antibody complexes, bacteria, and endotoxin, as well as endothelial disruption, may lead to platelet aggregation, degranulation, and release of cationic inflammatory mediators. Other released platelet constituents, such as cathepsins, prostaglandin (PG) endoperoxides, thromboxanes, and a connective tissue–activating peptide, also contribute to the propagation of the inflammatory response. This is particularly true for the various prostaglandin-like products of arachidonic acid metabolism.

In addition to their leukocyte-like functions, it has become evident in recent years that platelets also may participate in inflammatory responses by interacting with the complement system. Thus plate-

Table 4.13
Platelets as Inflammatory Cells

Lysosomal-like granule constituents
Release reaction is a secretory degranulation
Respond to vascular injury
Accumulate in vessels adjacent to inflamed areas
Interact with immune-complexes as well as
  microorganisms
Initiate intravascular inflammation
Enzymes can further damage endothelium
Adhesion to subendothelium (collagen)
Enhance blood coagulation and fibrin deposition
Promote local microvascular thrombosis

let aggregation and release can be initiated by stimuli that have activated the alternate pathway of complement activation. Conversely, platelets, on aggregation, release enzymes that can directly activate the fifth component of complement, producing chemotactic activity for leukocytes. A clotting abnormality related to abnormal platelet function has been reported in rabbits congenitally deficient in C6. C5b-C9 complexes have been demonstrated on the human platelet membrane following the incubation of platelets in fresh human serum. In addition, retraction and lysis of thrombin-induced blood clots can be inhibited by antiserum to C3 and C4.

It also has been reported that complement-dependent ultrastructural lesions can be visualized on the platelet surface subsequent to their incubation with thrombin and complement. Platelets also are reactive in several different ways to antigen-antibody complexes and to complement activation. These phenomena can cause platelets to release their constituents. In addition, platelets are highly responsive to platelet-activating factor (PAF), which produces platelet aggregation and mediator release. Thus the platelet can no longer be ignored as an inconsequential blood constituent useful only in coagulation. Its functions as a proinflammatory cell are becoming increasingly clear.

Endothelial Cells and Fibroblasts

For completeness, it is necessary to include endothelial cells and fibroblasts as part of the cast of cellular participants in inflammation. In order to leave the blood stream and enter tissue sites of inflammatory reactivity, the leukocytes must first adhere to and then migrate through the microvasculature. As we shall see, the endothelium is an active participant in these leukocyte-endothelial cell interactions. In addition, the endothelial cells have high proliferative potential, and play a critical role in healing and repair responses (*see* section on Healing and Repair). Fibroblasts are also important cells in the healing and repair of injured tissues by virtue of their ability to synthesize and lay down collagen. In addition, many of the important extracellular matrix proteins (*see* Chapter 3) are fibroblast products, and many of these are important to leukocyte activation and locomotion. Thus, while the endothelial cells and fibroblasts are clearly not leukocytes, they are vital tissue participants in inflammation. Their role in healing and repair responses is discussed in greater detail later in this chapter.

CELLULAR EVENTS IN INFLAMMATION

The appearance of leukocytes, principally neutrophils and macrophages, and the means by which they can accumulate at sites of inflammation may well constitute the prime defensive feature of the inflammatory response. Bringing leukocytes into play is the response's reason for being. Enzyme-rich phagocytic cells release powerful enzymes and engulf foreign intruders, usually destroying, or at least decreasing, the effectiveness of the invaders. Lysosomes, particularly those of neutrophil origin, harbor a host of factors that play pivotal roles. Leukocytes thus constitute the third leg (along with the hemodynamic and permeability changes) of the tripod on which the in-

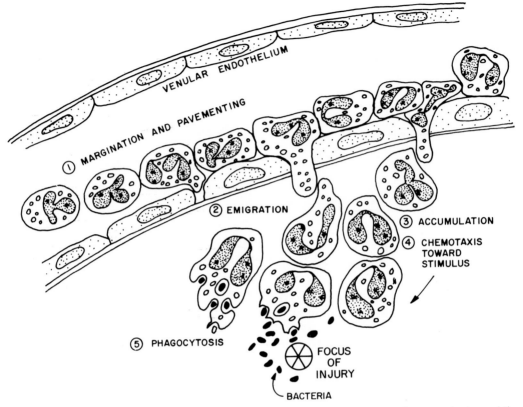

Figure 4.26. Leukocytic Events in Inflammation. The white blood cells first marginate and then literally pave the endothelium before emigrating between endothelial cells to accumulate in tissue, where they undergo chemotactic attraction toward the injurious stimulus. A major leukocytic function at the site of inflammation is phagocytosis.

flammatory process stands. An important question is: how do these cells get to the precise focus of injury and what do they do there once they arrive? The sequence of leukocytic events can be divided into (1) margination and pavementing, (2) emigration, (3) chemotaxis, (4) accumulation, and (5) phagocytosis (Fig. 4.26). Many of these events involve complicated biochemical and functional changes in the leukocytes themselves as they become converted from resting cells into **activated** cells.

Margination and Pavementing

The adhesion to and migration through the vascular endothelium is a prerequisite for the extravasation of leukocytes

from the blood to tissue sites of inflammation. The endothelium and leukocyte-endothelial interaction is therefore of central importance to the entire inflammatory drama. We already have mentioned briefly margination, or peripheral orientation of leukocytes from the moving blood stream, in our discussion of the hemodynamic changes in inflammation. Red and white cells in the normally flowing blood move within the microvessels in the central column, leaving a relatively cell-free layer of plasma in contact with the endothelial lining of the vessel wall. With the slowing of blood flow resulting from the hemodynamic changes in inflammation, this laminar pattern of blood flow changes. The leukocytes appear to fall out of the central column of flow to assume positions in contact with the endothelium. This phenomenon is known as **margination.** The cells appear to tumble slowly along the walls of the capillaries and venules to come to rest finally at some point. As the response accelerates, leukocytes stick not only to the endothelium (**adhesion**) but to each other as well, a phenomenon known as leukocyte **aggregation.**

Aggregation and increased stickiness (adhesiveness) can be induced in leukocyte populations exposed to various chemical mediators of inflammation. Initially, the leukocytes only appear to stick to the endothelium for rather short periods of time and are then washed away by the flowing bloodstream (acute local active hyperemia). With time and an appropriate inflammatory insult, they tend to stick longer and longer, but still some are pushed by the bloodstream along the vessel wall. Once leukocytes have passed the injured area, they appear to no longer stick to the endothelium but assume normal positions in the flowing blood stream. It has been observed repeatedly that leukocytes tend to stick to the side of the vessel wall nearest to the injury. Eventually, some leukocytes adhere firmly to the endothelium and can no longer be dislodged by the bloodstream. When numerous cells adhere to and virtually line the endothelium, the process is referred to as **pavementing.**

There are several theoretical explanations for the adherence of leukocytes to the walls of the vessels at sites of inflammation. Either the endothelium in some way becomes sticky, or the white blood cells develop increased adhesiveness, or both the leukocytes and the endothelium become altered, or some substance extraneous to both serves as a sort of cellular glue. Numerous studies on this particular problem have lead to observations in support of all of these theoretical possibilities, and perhaps all are indeed valid.

There is good evidence now that specific leukocyte cell surface molecules are involved in cellular adhesion. The availability of specific monoclonal antibodies has allowed the identification and characterization of a family of leukocyte surface glycoproteins (**leukocyte cell adhesion molecules, Leu-CAMs, CDW18 complex**) made up of three different heterodimers called **Mo1, LFA-1,** and **Leu M5,** each consisting of a common β-subunit of about M_r 95,000 and a unique α-subunit which varies in size (M_r 150–170,000) for each of the Leu-CAM molecules. Although the α-subunits are unique, the amino acid sequences of the different α-subunits show 33 to 50% homology, and for this reason the molecules are considered a protein family that most likely evolved through primordial gene duplication.

The plasma membrane expression of these glycoproteins depends on the state of cellular activation and appears to be separately regulated despite sharing a common β-subunit. The Mo1, LFA-1, and Leu M5 glycoproteins have different functions in leukocyte adhesion. Mo-1 (gp 155,95) has complement receptor (CR3) activity that binds the ligand C3bi; certain monoclonal antibodies to Mo1 inhibit binding and phagocytosis of C3bi-opsonized particles. Mo1 plays a role in myeloid cell adhesion, aggregation, and chemotactic phenomena and can mediate Mg^{2+}-dependent neutrophil adhesion to endothelial cells and a variety of substrates, but apparently does so *via* a distinct binding site on the Mo1 molecule independent of the C3bi binding site. LFA-1 (lymphocyte function-associated antigen 1; gp 170,95) is expressed on phagocytes and lymphocytes and promotes lymphoid cell adhesion interactions that include lymphocyte proliferation and cytotoxic effector cell activity and other types of immunologic reactions involving lymphocytes. The functional role of the Leu M5 (gp 150,95) molecule is less well characterized, but it appears to be a lectin-like surface molecule important in leukocyte adhesion to surfaces. Mo1 and Leu M5 are present in intracellular vesicles as well as on the cell surface in unstimulated leukocytes. It is also becoming apparent that lysosomal granule membranes also contain Leu-CAMs, and that the degranulation occurring in inflammation may be one way to ensure a renewable supply of these important molecules at the cell surface.

The binding of inflammatory mediators (such as C5a) to surface receptors triggers an increase in Mo1 and Leu M5 (but not LFA-1) expression on the leukocyte surface, resulting in increased adhesiveness to endothelium. This up-regulation occurs rapidly following stimulation and is not impeded by inihibitors of protein synthesis; thus, the molecules are preformed in the cell. Recently, canine (as well as human) patients have been identified who are genetically deficient in these leukocyte cell adhesion molecules as an apparent result of defective biosynthesis of the β-chain shared by all of the molecules. Such patients experience life-threatening recurrent bacterial infections, often without pus formation, and their leukocytes exhibit decreased adhesiveness and aggregation responses as well as other functional deficits.

It is also clear that the endothelial cells themselves participate in leukocyte adherence. Neutrophils preferentially adhere to endothelial cells when compared to other cell types such as smooth muscle cells and fibroblasts; such adherence occurs shortly after leukocyte contact with the endothelium and is cation (particularly Ca^{2+}) dependent. Endothelial injury augments this adhesive interaction with leukocytes. Recent work also suggests that endothelial cells can bind chemotactic factors, although the evidence is still circumstantial. Chemotactic factors such as the complement fragment C5a and the leukotriene LTB_4 are well-known leukocyte activators that increase adherence in a dynamic interaction that may be both dose- and time-dependent. Binding of these and other chemotactic factors to endothelium would provide a plausible explanation for increased leukocyte adherence at foci of inflammation.

It has also been shown that stimulated endothelial cells themselves can express surface factors that augment leukocyte adherence. Leading this group of molecules is the potent lipid mediator **platelet activating factor** (PAF), which is known to produce increased stickiness and aggregation of leukocytes. Endothelium-derived PAF activity is rapidly inducible by inflammatory stimuli and remains bound to the endothelial cell surface without alterations in endothelial cell morphology. Thus, one can envision stimulated endothelium in an inflammatory site binding chemotactic factors and expressing surface PAF, either of which would increase leukocyte adherence to the endothelium. Thrombin also acts on endothelium to result in increased subsequent adherence of leukocytes.

Once in the inflamed area, leukocytes also apparently contribute to increased endothelial adhesiveness by releasing cytokines such as **interleukin-1** (IL-1) and **tumor necrosis factor** (TNF), which induce proadhesive determinants at the endothelial cell surface. Bacterial **endotoxin** (LPS) also induces increased endothelial adhesivensss analogous to that observed with IL-1 and TNF. While the precise mechanism through which IL-1, TNF, and LPS induce increased endothelial stickiness is not fully elucidated, there is evidence that *de novo* protein synthesis by the endothelium is required for the increased adherence, and that the mechanism may involve increased surface expression of certain recently identified **endothelial adhesion molecules** (such as **ELAM-1** and **ICAM-1**), which are apparently endothelial cell analogues to the Leu-CAM–related surface adhesion molecules of leukocytes.

Attempts also have been made to implicate altered electrochemical forces in the adhesion of leukocytes to endothelium and to each other. The adhesive properties of leukocytes cannot be simply attributed to opposite surface charge, but they may be augmented by calcium bridging between the cells. Both leukocytes and red cells have only anions on their surfaces, and at physiologic pH levels, the surface charge density of the two types of cells is very similar. However, when leukocytes and red cells are suspended in a common protein pool, in the presence of the same mono- and divalent cations, and at a common pH, the two cell types behave differently. Only the leukocytes are adhesive and phagocytic, the erythrocytes remaining dispersed. It has been suggested that this difference might be attributed to different ionic species on the surface. Therefore, although red cells and white cells may have the same charge density, the anions contributing to the charge could be different and therefore would have different solubility products with a divalent cation, such as calcium. Injury of individual leukocytes by micropuncture also renders them more adhesive. Calcium may similarly play some role in this adherence, serving as a bridge between the negative charges on the endothelial cell and the white blood cell. Treatment with ethylenediamine-tetraacetic acid (EDTA), a chelator of calcium, has been shown to block the gathering of leukocytes at sites of injury.

The fact that leukocytes tend to adhere to the side of the vessel closest to the site of injury strongly suggests that the collective alterations that would explain increased adhesiveness are fairly specific and remain quite localized. It is also clear that well-characterized specific surface biochemical alterations take place in both leukocyte and endothelial populations in inflammation. In any event, early in all acute inflammatory reactions, the leukocytes can be observed to first marginate and then virtually pave the local endothelial surfaces. It must be stressed that this is almost entirely a microcirculatory phenomenon, with virtually all leukocyte margination, pavementing, and emigration in inflammation occurring especially within the postcapillary **venules** and small veins, but also in the capillaries.

Emigration

Emigration refers to the process by which leukocytes escape from their location in the blood to reach the perivascular tissues. Neutrophils, eosinophils, basophils, monocytes, and lymphocytes all appear to use similar pathways **between** the endothelial cells in moving from the blood stream into tissue. We will discuss each of these cell types individually later. It is interesting to note how correct Cohnheim's early descriptions of the morphodynamics of the emigration process were; we know much more now about mechanisms but little has been added to his descriptions.

Once in contact with the endothelium in an inflammatory reaction, the leukocytes put out large cytoplasmic extensions **(pseudopodia).** The motile leukocytes then force their pseudopodia into gaps between adjacent endothelial cells. These gaps are created through the actions of histamine and other chemical mediators on endothelium, and they can apparently be created by the leukocytes themselves. Once the pseudopod has passed, the entire cell follows through the widened interendothelial junctions. The leukocyte may then pass quickly through the basement membrane and between pericytes into the perivascular connective tissues and beyond. It is more often observed, however, that the leukocytes are held up for a while in a position between

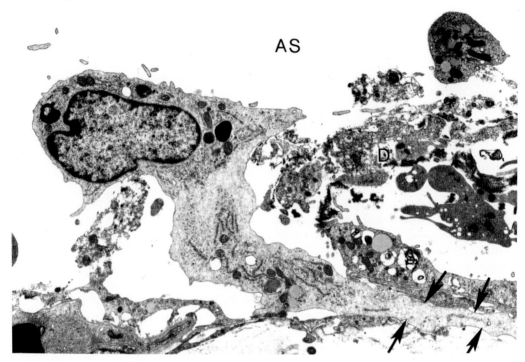

Figure 4.27.   Macrophage Penetrating the Basement Membrane. This macrophage has inserted a long pseudopod *(arrows)* through the basement membrane in this inflamed lung. Debris *(D)* consisting of red cells, fibrin, and cell fragments is in the alveolar space *(AS).* (Micrograph courtesy of Dr. W. L. Castleman.)

endothelial cell and basement membrane. The reason for this is not known. They then penetrate the seemingly impermeable barrier of the basement membrane to achieve an extravascular position (Fig. 4.27).

The precise manner in which leukocytes pass through basement membranes is also not known. Electron microscopic observations have shown the incredible plasticity of the relatively bulky white cells as they crawl through the narrow serpentine pathways opened by the contracted endothelial cells (Fig. 4.28). The process is one of active locomotion rather than of passive extrusion by the hydrostatic pressure of the blood.

It has now been clearly established that the pathway of the migrating cells is intercellular (Fig. 4.28). The earlier contention that lymphocytes could have an intracellular pathway has been shown to be

wrong. The occasional appearance of cells as apparently intracellular was a misconception caused by the plane of section of the material examined by transmission electron microscopy. The plasma membrane of the leukocyte forms a pseudopod that penetrates into the intercellular space. It is remarkable to note that the whole migrating cell changes its shape and even the nucleus elongates itself to an extreme. When circulating, neutrophils have a diameter of approximately 10 microns, but they are capable of reducing their width to less than 1 micron when migrating. Monocytes and macrophages seem no less athletic (Fig. 4.27).

It is no longer reasonable to speak of endothelial cells as a homogeneous cell population. It has become clear in recent years that there are important structural and functional differences in endothelial cells along the terminal arborizations of

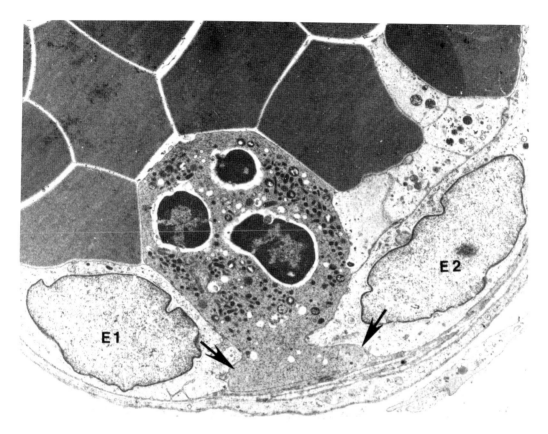

Figure 4.28.   Leukocyte Emigration. The neutrophil shown here has inserted a pseudopod *(arrows)* into the interendothelial space between two adjacent endothelial cells *(E1* and *E2).*

the microvascular tree. Segmental differences in, for example, the number of types of interendothelial junctions and attachment devices may be of considerable importance to leukocyte emigration. The venules, which are so important to inflammation, have a combination of open and loose junctional complexes, which renders them uniquely susceptible to the development of interendothelial gaps under the influence of histamine. It is also now apparent that venular endothelium contains more histamine-specific receptors on the luminal endothelial cell surface than other types of endothelia. The histamine receptors are preferentially expressed in regions close to the endothelial junctions in regions rich in microfilaments. This may also help to substantiate

the phenomenon of endothelial cell contractility.

The rounded appearance of venular endothelial cells and the occurrence of interendothelial gaps after local application of histamine has been widely cited as evidence of endothelial cell contractility. Convincing proof, however, has been difficult to obtain. Our understanding of the biochemical basis of the observed morphologic changes has been greatly enhanced by the recent finding that endothelial cells contain actin and myosin much like muscle fibers. Although the contribution of these emerging definitions of endothelial cell function may be important to leukocyte migration, their role in regulating the opening of the intercellular space is still under discussion. In the postcapillary venules, where most of the leukocyte emigration important to inflammation takes place, tight junctions or desmosomes are normally absent or rare, whereas in capillaries they are prominent. Migration of leukocytes is, however, observed in both segments. Endothelial contraction undoubtedly plays an important role in this process, but the theory that contraction of the endothelial cells is the sole factor responsible for the creation of a passage is not completely convincing. In a capillary segment, where gap junctions are normally present, these junctions are no longer visible when leukocytes are migrating. After passage, junctional complexes seem to reappear. If such a disappearance and reappearance of junctional complexes occurs during the migration of leukocytes, one could assume that the migrating cells secrete enzymes capable of disjoining adjacent endothelial cells. Although evidence is beginning to accumulate, this suggestion also awaits definitive proof.

When leukocytes and monocytes reach the basement membrane, the membrane may be opened by collagenase-type enzymes. The "lysed" segment of the basement membrane rarely exceeds 1 micron in length, permitting only the passage of the elongated migrating cell. There is no longer any doubt that neutrophils and monocytes **actively** migrate through the vascular wall, using their pseudopodic and enzymatic properties. It also appears that lymphocytes possess the same properties, although morphologically they do not have pseudopods and have a poorly developed lysosomal system. The massive migration of neutrophils allows the **passive** extravasation of red blood cells. These microhemorrhages are always observed in acute inflammation. The fate of these red blood cells varies. Some are phagocytosed and completely degraded by local macrophages. Others are carried through the lymphatics to the corresponding lymph nodes where they are phagocytosed and

degraded by the macrophages normally present in the sinusoidal system of the lymph nodes. The presence of red cells at sites of inflammation, as we have noted above, is often regarded as a sort of bland, passive accident occurring secondary to the more dynamic, active leukocytic events. Such a view, however, may underestimate the truth. It is entirely possible that these scattered extravascular red cells serve as phagocytic stimuli for the emigrating monocytes, thus helping to transform them into actively functioning macrophages. Anything that assists in the enhancement of phagocytosis at inflamed sites should not be disregarded.

Two separate waves of leukocytic emigrational activity are apparent in most kinds of acute inflammation. An immediate wave reaches massive proportions in the venules in 30–40 min; the delayed wave occurs in both capillaries and venules some hours later. Neutrophils and monocytes both leave during the early wave, although the neutrophil is predominant, but in the delayed phase the continued recruitment of monocytes outpaces the neutrophils. The interdependence of cells is well illustrated by the fact that the emigration of monocytes is apparently at least partially dependant on neutrophils. A fraction derived from neutrophils has been shown to induce the emigration of monocytes. If animals are depleted of neutrophils, monocyte emigration also is inhibited. To date, few agents have been identified that will induce specific lymphocyte chemotaxis and emigration, although their presence in inflammatory reactions certainly suggests that it occurs.

The number of cells migrating into inflammatory exudates can be measured after the injection of inflammatory agents into the peritoneal cavity, the pleural cavity, or into small chambers placed over minor skin abrasions. The findings show that, with relatively mild irritants, neutrophil accumulation reaches peak at about

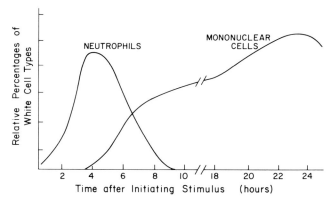

Figure 4.29. Leukocyte Accumulation. In many typical inflammatory reactions, the neutrophils arrive first and are followed by a more prolonged phase of mononuclear cell accumulation.

4–6 hours and then declines rapidly, whereas the total number of mononuclear cells begins to rise only after 4 hours and reaches a sustained peak at 18–24 hours (Fig. 4.29). The height of the neutrophil peak shows great variation with different stimuli, whereas less variation is found in the mononuclear peak. When living microorganisms are injected intrapleurally, massive numbers of neutrophils accumulate progressively throughout the first 24 h; no mononuclear response can be detected in this period. It previously was suggested that neutrophils and mononuclear phagocytes migrate simultaneously into inflammatory exudates, and that the neutrophils rapidly disappear, thus exposing the less numerous, but more long-lived, mononuclear cells at the later stages. This was supported, at the time, by the belief that neutrophils and monocytes showed no differences in chemotactic reactivity to various stimuli. Most current evidence suggests, however, that the entry of monocytes into the exudates starts as neutrophil emigration declines and continues for a considerably longer period.

Chemotaxis

It has been clear since the time of Metchnikoff that activated leukocytes are highly motile and seem to possess direction sense; that is, their wanderings in tissue are not random, but directed. The phenomenon of **chemotaxis,** or directional migration in response to a chemical gradient of chemoattractant, explains this phenomenon. Chemotaxis implies directed locomotion, and it must be distinguished from enhanced random movement called **chemokinesis.** Leukocytes are not the only cells that display chemotaxis. Bacteria, cellular slime molds, tumor cells, fibroblasts, endothelial cells, and smooth muscle cells also exhibit varying degrees of chemotactic responsiveness. As in bacteria, chemotaxis in leukocytes is a receptor-mediated process.

Much of what we now know of leukocyte chemotaxis has come from *in vitro* studies using a micropore filter that separates leukocytes on the one side from the chemotactic substance on the other side of the membrane. It has been convincingly shown that granulocytes will migrate only if the chemotactic factor is present at a distance from the cell (that is, in the opposite compartment). When various concentrations of the chemotactic factor on the two sides of the membrane are used, the cells respond to a concentration gradient. Neutrophils are very sensitive and can detect a 1% gradient across their dimensions. It thus became possible to obtain precise quantitative data for leukocyte chemotaxis, and the micropore filter technique and the related under-agarose assay have become popular methods for studying chemotaxis.

All leukocyte types exhibit chemotaxis, but neutrophils and macrophages have been best studied. Neutrophilic granulocytes respond to chemotactic signals quickly, which is reminiscent of their behavior *in vivo*. These cells require only about 90 min to complete their response in the chemotactic chamber. This is in sharp contrast to the time course of response for mononuclear cells, which may take several hours. Eosinophils are somewhat intermediate in chemotactic responsiveness, and less is known about lymphocyte chemotaxis than for the other major cell types.

At the site of a well-developed, acute inflammatory reaction, there is a veritable chemical soup of potential chemoattractants, and a large number of these different chemotactic factors have been studied (Table 4.14). Both endogenous and exogenous chemotaxins have been described. The most important of the plasma-derived endogenous chemotaxins are the complement fragments **C5a** and **C5a des Arg.** C5a is about 10-fold more potent as a chemoattractant than C5a des Arg in most *in vitro* systems, but we must recall that the C-terminal arginine of C5a is rapidly cleaved *in vivo* by a serum carboxypeptidase. Therefore C5a des Arg is the molecule more likely to be responsible for chemotaxis *in vivo*. **Kallikrein** (an enzyme responsible for plasma kinin and plasmin generation) has been reported to be chemotactic for neutrophils, although this has recently been challenged. Breakdown products of collagen also are reported to have this biological activity. **Fibrinogen** is another likely source of chemotactic activity, since both fibrinopeptide B and the plasmin-generated degradation products of fibrinogen and fibrin are chemotactic.

Many of the other chemotaxins, such

Table 4.14
Factors That are Chemotactic for Leukocytes

Plasma-derived
C5a, C5a des Arg
Fibrinopeptides
Fibrin degradation products
Kallikrein (?)
Plasminogen activator (?)
Fibronectin (?)

Inflammatory cell-derived
LTB$_4$[a]
HETEs
Platelet-activating factor
Interleukin-1
Lymphokines
ECF-A

Other origins
Bacterial chemotaxins
Formol peptides
Dead cells (necrotaxis)

[a] Abbreviations used are: LT, leukotriene; HETE, hydroxyeicosatetraenoic acid; ECF-A, eosinophil chemotactic factor of anaphylaxis.

as the arachidonic acid metabolite **LTB$_4$** and **platelet activating factor,** are cell-derived. Some of the products of activated lymphocytes, **lymphokines,** have been shown to be chemotactic. The growing length of the list of identified endogenous chemoattractants for leukocytes illustrates once again the enormous redundancy built into the inflammatory response. While there are many chemotactic factors, it is perhaps worth noting that not everything is chemotactic; proteolytic cleavage of most serum proteins fails to give rise to chemotactic fragments.

Of the exogenous chemoattractants, the **bacterial chemotaxins** are the most important. Many kinds of bacteria produce chemoattractants. These are of no known advantage to the bacteria since by calling leukocytes into play, they invite their own demise. Biochemical studies of different bacterial chemoattractants led to the development of the structurally similar synthetic **N-formylated oligopeptides,** of which N-formyl-methionyl-leucyl-pheny-lalanine (fMet-Leu-Phe, or simply **fMLP**) has been the most widely studied. Much of our present knowledge of the cell biology of leukocyte chemotaxis is based on observations made with synthetic oligopeptides like fMLP. The recent availability of recombinant C5a will provide another well-defined stimulus. Unfortunately, most domestic animal leukocytes respond poorly or not at all to fMLP, but C5a (and/or C5a des Arg) are good chemotaxins in virtually all species.

It is tempting to conclude that the production of chemotactic factors by bacteria in tissues accounts for the ability of most of these microorganisms to induce an acute inflammatory response characterized by massive accumulation of granulocytes. The fact that the complement system appears to be closely involved in the generation of chemotactic factors suggests that it consists of a series of substrates involved in the production of mediators capable of initiating the acute inflammatory response. It should be pointed out that, in addition to the chemotactic factors, the anaphylatoxins are generated also by sequential interaction of the complement system or by direct action of enzymes on C3 or C5. These factors increase the permeability of blood vessels. Thus, it is now well substantiated that many bioactive products can be derived from the complement system; one set of factors causes the soluble contents of plasma to leak out through permeability changes, while the others bring about chemotactic emigration of leukocytes. Taken altogether, the stage is set for the acute inflammatory response. Precisely which factors are involved in a given inflammatory reaction is a difficult question to answer because of the very short lifespan of these mediators *in vivo*. As for the multiplicity of factors that can produce increased vascular permeability, it seems likely that several different chemoattrac-

tants would be brought into play at any inflammatory site in tissue.

Mechanisms of Chemotaxis

It is not difficult to imagine the assorted chemical attractants oozing out of inflammatory foci to serve as "come hither" signals for the various leukocytes. To elucidate precisely **how** this takes place is an entirely different matter. As a starting point, let's look at the phenomenon morphologically. Based on a large number of careful ultrastructural and cinemicrographic studies, several general conclusions can be reached:

(1) Leukocytes crawl; unlike bacteria they do not swim. Proper locomotion requires reversible adhesiveness to a surface;

(2) The cells undergo characteristic morphologic changes, which begin with increased surface membrane ruffling within 30 seconds of stimulation (Fig. 4.30);

(3) Transient dose-dependent leukocyte aggregation may occur within the first few minutes of stimulation;

(4) Responding leukocytes assume a characteristic polarized orientation during locomotion, with broad, spreading lamellipodia at the leading edge which, when assessed by phase microscopy, are fairly free of organelles. A narrow, blunt tail (uropod) is at the rear of the cell;

(5) In a gradient of chemoattractant, the population of cells migrate toward the source of chemotactic factor; and

(6) Leukocytes appear to easily deform as they migrate through narrow places.

These morphologic observations contribute important clues about chemotactic mechanisms but do not provide a clear picture of the underlying cellular events. Various ways of looking at the biology of chemotaxis have produced some interesting ideas, some based on hard data, some based on speculation, but all of tremen-

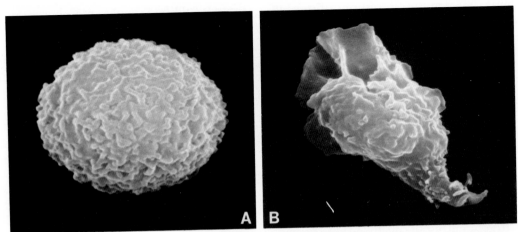

Figure 4.30.   Bovine Neutrophil Response to Chemoattractant C5a. The resting cells *(A)* shown by scanning electron microscopy exhibit only normal small surface membrane projections; 30 seconds after exposure to C5a the stimulated cells *(B)* exhibit marked ruffled membrane activity with the formation of large surface lamellipodia.

dous value in attempting to understand this vital biological phenomenon. The best models for understanding the mechanisms of chemotaxis seem based on the idea that chemotaxis requires careful integration of adherence, secretion, and locomotion. The first component of the model, the primed cell, would have increased adhesiveness, an increased tendency to aggregate, and an increased availability of chemoattractant receptors. Evidence for cell priming has come from studies indicating that C5a generated *in vivo* promotes neutrophil adhesion and aggregation and related margination. Purified C5a is also a potent secretagogue of neutrophil specific granules.

The initial event in chemotaxis is binding of the chemoattractant to the cell surface; this is a receptor-mediated event. What happens next is complicated and occurs very rapidly (Fig. 4.31). A number of biochemical processes have been described that develop within 5 seconds or so after ligand-receptor interaction. It remains somewhat unclear just which event occurs first and which are subsequently triggered, since many things occur almost simultaneously. One of the early consequences of chemoattractant binding to the cell seems to be a release of calcium from intracellular stores and membrane translocation of calcium. This leads to a measurable rise in cytosolic Ca^{2+}, which is apparently necessary for triggering both degranulation and changes in membrane polarity. An initial membrane depolarization is followed by a hyperpolarization within 1 min of stimulation. The physiological significance of the hyperpolarization remains unclear.

Increased intracellular Ca^{2+} also would be expected to influence the submembranous actin-myosin network. The reported increased local accumulation of submembranous calcium could neutralize inner membrane negative charge, facilitate granule membrane–plasma membrane fusion during exocytosis, and modulate membrane deformability. A possible role of methylation of carboxyl groups in modulating intracellular calcium and membrane charge as well as receptor expression has been proposed. As a consequence of the increase in intracellular calcium, cell recovery must involve the sequestration of calcium intracellularly and/or the extrusion of calcium from the cell. Chemotaxis is optimal in the presence of not only Ca^{2+}, but also Na^+, K^+, and Mg^{2+}.

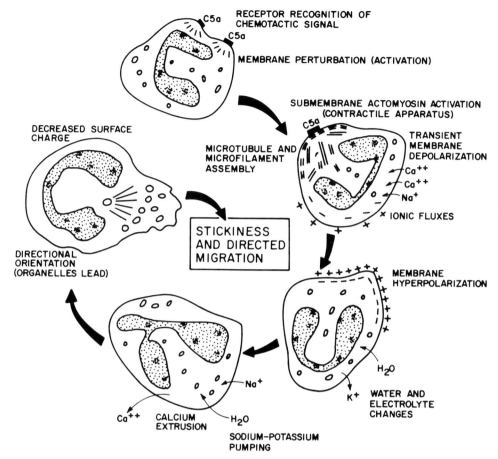

RECEPTOR RECOGNITION OF CHEMOTACTIC SIGNAL

MEMBRANE PERTURBATION (ACTIVATION)

SUBMEMBRANE ACTOMYOSIN ACTIVATION (CONTRACTILE APPARATUS)

DECREASED SURFACE CHARGE

MICROTUBULE AND MICROFILAMENT ASSEMBLY

TRANSIENT MEMBRANE DEPOLARIZATION

IONIC FLUXES

STICKINESS AND DIRECTED MIGRATION

DIRECTIONAL ORIENTATION (ORGANELLES LEAD)

MEMBRANE HYPERPOLARIZATION

WATER AND ELECTROLYTE CHANGES

CALCIUM EXTRUSION

SODIUM–POTASSIUM PUMPING

Figure 4.31.   Mechanisms of Chemotaxis. Binding of the chemotactic signal to specific membrane receptors causes membrane perturbation and activation of the cellular contractile apparatus. Microtubule and microfilament assembly allow cell motility and directed migration. A series of ionic fluxes and membrane electrical changes also are involved, and the end result is an actively motile cell, which exhibits specifically directional movement.

Cells exposed to chemotaxins undergo rapid changes in monovalent cation fluxes, and activation of a membrane-bound Na^+,K^+-ATPase may function as a cation pump.

It is also apparent that alterations in the intracellular levels of cyclic nucleotides can contribute to the regulation of chemotactic responses. A rise in cyclic AMP (cAMP) occurs within 5–15 seconds after ligand-receptor interaction and probably follows the rise in cytosolic Ca^{2+}. Cyclic nucleotides play important roles as "second messengers"; agents that stimulate cAMP formation inhibit chemotaxis, while agents stimulating increases in cyclic GMP (cGMP) enhance the chemotactic response.

Several important reactions occur that involve changes in membrane phospholipids. Following receptor-ligand interaction (with fMLP or C5a), activation of a membrane **phospholipase A_2** occurs as a Ca^{2+}-dependent step, which correlates well with the release of arachidonic acid from its esterified position in membrane phospholipids such as phosphatidylcholine. Arachidonate liberated from stimulated cells triggers the energy-producing hexose monophosphate shunt, and its subsequent metabolism generates a number of other powerful mediators such as LTB_4 which is also a potent chemoattractant (see Arachidonic Acid Metabolites in the Mediators section). The discovery of this phospholipase A_2 pathway has helped to explain the well-known antiinflammatory effects of **glucocorticoids,** since they induce the synthesis in many cells, including neutrophils, of a M_r 40,000 inhibitor of phospholipase A_2 known as **lipomodulin.** These various activation events involving receptor-ligand interaction, membrane polarity changes, cation fluxes, and arachidonic acid metabolism are not, however, the essence of chemotaxis because they do not explain sustained, directed locomotion.

It is important to note that there are two quite different but equally important aspects to chemotaxis, **orientation** and **locomotion.** We have already mentioned how increased locomotor activity can occur in stimulated cells without migration (chemokinesis). This is not chemotaxis, which requires both movement and direction sense. In a gradient of chemoattractant, orientation seems to occur before movement. That is, the cells become polarized before they start to move, with their leading edge in the direction of the highest concentration of chemoattractant. Indeed, it has been shown that if the gradient is suddenly reversed, neutrophils will stop and reorient themselves in the correct direction before they again start to move.

Studies over the past several years have clarified the role of different parts of the cell in orientation and locomotion. The ability of cells to properly orient in a chemotactic gradient is a function of the **microtubules,** while locomotion itself is tied to the **microfilaments.** Agents such as **cytochalasin B,** which disrupts microfilaments, prevent locomotion even though the cells remain oriented in the gradient. **Colchicine,** on the other hand, disrupts microtubules and produces disorienta-

Table 4.15
Some Proteins Important to Leukocyte Movement

Name	Characteristics
G-actin	Globular monomeric actin
F-actin	Polymerized filamentous actin
Actin-binding protein	Cross-links F-actin into dimensional networks
Profilin	Binds G-actin to prevent F-actin formation
Acumentin	Binds to F-actin to shorten filaments
Gelsolin	Maintains shortened F-actin filament length
Myosin	Reversibly binds F-actin to "move" actin

tion, while not interfering with locomotion. In a properly responding cell, coordinate microtubule and microfilament activity permits both movement and direction sense.

The biological basis for this complicated activity remains incompletely understood, but appears to involve the complex interaction of actin and myosin with several other important regulatory and modulating proteins (Table 4.15). Orientation and sustained locomotion must require that these events not be diffuse but occur in a restricted location within the cell. Degranulation at the leading edge of the cell would provide new membrane with chemoattractant receptors, which are known to be present on the granule membranes. Occupied receptors may be swept to the rear of the cell where they could be digested, shed, or internalized and reprocessed and made available again.

As far as actual locomotion is concerned, the leading edge of peripheral cytoplasm is apparently the most important region. This zone contains the highest concentrations of polymerized **actin** microfilaments, which are produced under the influence of a number of actin-modulating proteins such as **actin-binding protein,** which cross-links individual actin molecules into two- or three-dimensional networks in close contact with the plasma membrane. The importance of locomotion in leukocytes is emphasized by the fact that actin constitutes 10–20% of the total neutrophil protein content. Other proteins modulate the polymerized and cross-linked actin and influence cell contractility in Ca^{2+}-dependent ways. Most of the actin in resting neutrophils is of the nonfilamentous G-actin type (globular actin), implying that some mechanism must normally exist which inhibits G-actin from assembling into filamentous F-actin. A molecule called **profilin** seems to perform precisely this function; the profilin-actin complex is a sort of storage form of actin, which can be relocated within the cell. Under conditions of cell activation, actin dissociates from profilin and instead binds to the actin-shortening molecules acumentin and gelsolin. **Acumentin** is a globular protein that binds to one end of actin and functions to shorten actin filaments. **Gelsolin** is the name given to another protein, which affects actin filament length by binding to the end of actin opposite to that bound by acumentin. The interaction of profilin, acumentin, and gelsolin with actin serves to control actin filament length and contraction, events that appear to depend on the local Ca^{2+} concentration.

Although assembly and modification of the actin mocrofilament network may account for extension of the peripheral cytoplasm, actual pulling of the cell body forward would likely require more "muscle" than could be accounted for by simple actin reassembly. **Myosin** is present in leukocytes in much lower concentrations than actin (1% of total protein) and has two distinct domains, one of which is cell bound and one of which binds to the actin filaments. In the presence of increased ATP and Ca^{2+} levels in an activated leukocyte, myosin first dissociates from ac-

tin, then binds to a new site further along the filament, thus causing movement of the actin. Myosin in this setting seems to work under conditions analogous to two persons pulling on a rope, one in a boat and the other on land.

Movement toward a chemotactic stimulus is a very complex process requiring forward movement of the lamellipodia and subsequent attachment of this anterior portion of the cell to a substrate. This forward movement implies contraction within the lamellipodia, and contraction must also occur to draw the trailing sections of the cell toward the cranial region. The trailing portion of the cell must also detach from the substrate, possibly by recycling or interiorization of surface receptors with bound ligand. Directed locomotion presumably occurs because of increased receptor density at the leading edge, where the higher concentration of chemoattractant is detected. Extension of the lamellipodia is followed by myosin-based contraction, which serves to draw the cell toward the chemotactic gradient.

Obviously, considerable work remains to be done before a clear picture of the events of chemotaxis can emerge, but it is at least possible now to postulate several phases (Fig. 4.31) in the chemotactic response: (1) recognition of the chemoattractant followed by (2) transduction of the recognition of the chemoattractant signal into locomotion, which implies (3) an activation of the locomotor apparatus, which probably is not so very different from the contractile apparatus of muscle cells, (4) ionic fluxes to maintain membrane and submembrane organelle irritability, (5) changes in membrane charge and polarity, which may assist in maintaining adherence, and (6) sustained locomotion with its implicit reversible adhesion and renewable facility for gradient detection.

How do leukocytes know when they have "arrived?" In short, what turns this system off? The answer to this question is not entirely clear, but there are several intriguing suggestions. First, it is known that high concentrations of chemoattractant can **deactivate** the responding cells so that they do not migrate further. Since the highest concentrations of chemoattractant are presumably at the center of the site where injury and inflammation is underway, arriving cells might be expected to follow the chemical gradient until they reach this high concentration of chemoattractant and then become deactivated for further movement. Having "arrived," they need go no further. The exact mechanism of deactivation is not known, but it is most likely related to down-regulation of surface chemotaxin receptors. Since virtually all leukocyte activities are receptor-directed, this explanation makes a lot of sense. Even in the face of high concentrations of the chemotactic signal, if the receptors were down-regulated, the cells could not "read" the message. In addition, chemotactic-factor inhibitors have been identified in plasma, at least for the complement-derived chemotactic factors, and may serve to modulate local concentrations of chemotactic signals.

Our view of the biology of chemotaxis will no doubt be clarified in the future. Since many of the membrane and intracellular events central to chemotaxis are similar to those occurring in phagocytosis and granule extrusion (degranulation), it is likely that they represent fundamental phenomena in leukocyte physiology, which deserve intense study.

Cell Accumulation

The accumulation of white blood cells at an inflammatory focus follows a quite predictable pattern and comprises a major morphologic hallmark of inflammation. Most bacterial agents as well as thermal, chemical, and radiation injury will evoke an initial neutrophil response in the acute phase of the inflammatory reaction. In the later, chronic stage of the same response, macrophages and lymphocytes come to predominate (Fig. 4.29). There are a number of reasons for the fairly predictable sequence of leukocytic aggregation at the site of inflammation. While neutrophils and macrophages may emigrate simultaneously, the neutrophil is more motile and so may arrive at the inflammatory site first. In addition, these cells are present in greater numbers in the circulating blood in most species. They also emigrate over a shorter time than do the mononuclear cells. Thus the rate of arrival of neutrophils diminishes after the first few days, while the influx of mononuclear cells may remain constant for several weeks. In addition, the death of neutrophils releases enzymes that activate factors chemotactic for mononuclear cells. As a final note, it also has been shown that mononuclear cells outnumber neutrophils in the later phases of the inflammatory reaction in part because some can persist in a functional state for months without dividing, and others, that are more short lived, are capable of local proliferation.

Phagocytosis

Cellular endocytic activity traditionally has been divided into two categories: **phagocytosis,** or "eating," and **pinocytosis,** or "drinking" (*see also* Chapter 2). Most pathologists use the term phagocytosis to describe the active cellular uptake of larger particulate matter, such as bacteria, while pinocytosis is used to describe the vesicular uptake of virtually everything else, particularly soluble macromolecules, but also small particles. Hence the terms phagocytosis and pinocytosis have some empirical definitions, but it remains to be determined whether or not these two processes differ at the biochemical level. We will focus our attention here on phagocytosis.

This fascinating biological phenomenon has interested scientists for a long time. Nearly a century ago Metchnikoff stated that phagocytic cells were responsible for protecting the host from invasion by the innumerable microorganisms in the internal and external environment, and he was among the first to propose that phagocytosis was the basis for survival against infection. Time has proven Metchnikoff to have been right. We now know that phagocytic cells cooperate with a variety of humoral factors collectively called **opsonins** in improving the efficiency of the process. George Bernard Shaw focused scientists and nonscientists alike on this concept in *The Doctor's Dilemma:*

> The phagocytes won't eat the microbes unless the microbes are nicely buttered for them. Well, the patient manufactures the butter for himself all right; but my discovery is that the manufacture of that butter, which I call opsonin, goes on in the system by ups and downs; there is at the bottom only one genuinely scientific treatment for all diseases, and that is to stimulate the phagocytes.

Phagocytosis and the subsequent or concomitant release of enzymes by neutrophils and macrophages are two of the major functions associated with the accumulation of leukocytes at a focus of inflammation. The lysosomal granules of neutrophils and macrophages are rich in a wide variety of enzymes as well as in less well characterized products that can participate in the degradation of foreign materials (Table 4.10). These enzymes and antibacterial products are central to the effectiveness of the phagocytic capacity of these cells.

The phagocytic process involves specific membrane recognition events, surface attachment of the leukocyte to the particle, engulfment, formation of a phagocytic vacuole, or phagosome, and fusion of that vacuole with lysosomes, exposing the imprisoned object to the action of the lysosomal contents (Fig. 4.32). This sequence is particularly important in the defense against bacterial invasion. In the course

of this action, the neutrophils and the monocytes become progressively degranulated. A number of influences modify the vulnerability of bacteria to engulfment. Perhaps the most important is the phenomenon of **opsonization. Opsonins** are naturally occurring or acquired substances that coat bacteria and render them more susceptible to phagocytosis. While several different potentially useful opsonins have been characterized, by far the most important ones are antibody (which interacts with the Fc receptor on phagocytic cells) and the complement fragment C3b, for which phagocytes also possess receptors. **Fibronectin** is a large dimeric glycoprotein which can bind to a number of surfaces and may influence phagocytosis both as an opsonin and by increasing cell adhesiveness. Phagocytosis is favored by higher body temperatures. Febrile reactions in inflammation thus favor this phenomenon.

The morphology of phagocytosis has been well documented. Engulfment begins with a recognition event at the cell membrane. This is obviously favored if the stimulus has been opsonized, but may proceed anyway through nonspecific recognition systems. Upon contact, the cell extends small cytoplasmic extensions or pseudopods which become closely applied to the surface of the attached particle; these seem to flow around the particle until it is engulfed. The cytoplasmic processes pinch together, meet, and fuse around the particle, and the resulting phagosome is drawn into the cell. This is accompanied by the movement of the lysosomal granules toward the developing phagosome. By means of cinemicrophotography and electron microscopy, it has been demonstrated that the lysosomal granules converge on the forming phagosome, fuse with it to form the **phagolysosome,** and discharge their contents into the vacuolar lumen around the particle. This process is called phagocyte **degranulation.** In neutrophils, it appears

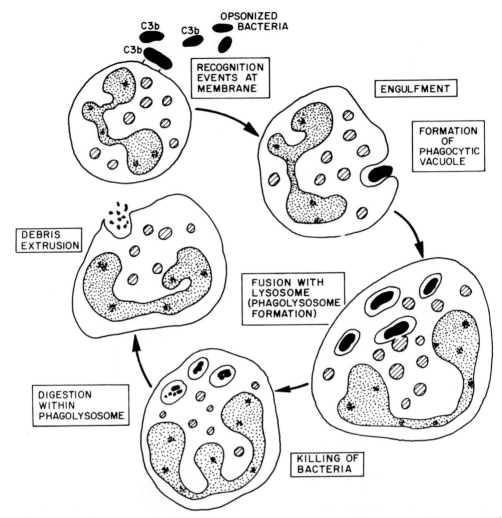

Figure 4.32. Phagocytosis. The initial event involves membrane receptor recognition events that trigger the formation of the phagocytic vacuole. Phagolysosome formation exposes the imprisoned object to the hydrolytic enzymes in the lysosome. After digestion, the residual debris often is extruded.

that the specific granules fuse with the phagosome slightly before the azurophil granules. This sequential fusion may relate to pH changes inside the vacuole.

The cellular mechanisms by which phagocytosis occurs seem to involve many of the same processes that are central to chemotaxis. Activation of the engulfment sequence is a response to receptor-ligand interaction, and the factors involved in formation of the pseudopods rest in activation of the leukocyte "motor" *via* the interaction of actin with other actin-mod-

ulating proteins in a Ca^{2+}-dependent way. The proteins that control actin filament length are the same as those involved in chemotaxis; actin, actin-binding protein, profilin, acumentin, and gelsolin (Table 4.15). These assembled cytoskeletal networks control the shape and development of the pseudopods and are apparently of importance in the distribution of organelles and the consistency of the cytoplasm. It has been well documented that actin-rich microfilaments are numerous in submembrane locations in the portions of the pseudopods which are in contact with phagocytosable particles. Ca^{2+} acts as a second messenger here to help convert the recognition events at the membrane into ingestion.

As in chemotaxis, the propelling movements of the cytoplasm during phagocytosis can result from assembly and activation of the actin network, but contraction and retraction probably require myosin. This is thought to be important for the actual internalization of the phagocytosed object and may be involved in the movement of the lysosomes toward the developing phagosomes. This latter phenomenon, movement of the lysosome toward the phagosome, is also thought to be under microtubular control.

Microbicidal Mechanisms

Phagocytosis is the major cellular mechanism of microbicidal activity. It is reasonable to assume that the ultimate purpose of bacterial phagocytosis is to kill and degrade bacteria. Two somewhat different oxygen-dependent killing systems, an **oxygen radical system** and the **H_2O_2-myeloperoxidase-halide system,** as well as oxygen-independent bactericidal mechanisms have been identified.

OXYGEN-DEPENDENT KILLING MECHANISMS. During phagocytosis neutrophils show a burst of metabolic activity, characterized by a 2- to 3-fold increase in oxygen consumption, an increase in superoxide anion (O_2^-) generation and hydrogen peroxide (H_2O_2) formation, and an increase in the amount of glucose metabolized *via* the hexose monophosphate shunt (HMPS). This collectively, has been called the **respiratory burst of phagocytosis** (Table 4.16). While data are still accumulating, it appears that much of this biochemical activity in phagocytes is due to a unique membrane-bound **NADPH-oxidase.** This oxidase is low or nonexistent in resting cells, but during phagocytosis it is transformed from a latent to an expressed activity. The acti-

Table 4.16
Major Features of the "Respiratory Burst" of Phagocytosis

Increased oxygen utilization by the cell
Increased glucose oxidation *via* HMPS[a]
Increased production of hydrogen peroxide (H_2O_2)
Generation of superoxide anion (O_2^-)

[a] Abbreviation used is HMPS, hexose monophosphate shunt.

vated NADPH-oxidase reduces molecular oxygen by electron transfer from NADPH, and in so doing forms O_2^- and NADP, the latter being required for operation of the HMPS. Most of the superoxide generated reacts rapidly with itself, spontaneously dismutating to produce oxygen and H_2O_2. The NADP-activated HMPS metabolizes glucose to regenerate NADPH which was consumed in the initial reaction with NADPH-oxidase.

The production of superoxide anion (O_2^-) and hydrogen peroxide (H_2O_2) during the respiratory burst is important, as they provide a direct link to the oxygen radical- and myeloperoxidase-based systems of phagocyte microbicidal and cytotoxic activities. Neither superoxide anion nor hydrogen peroxide are potent microbicidal molecules themselves. Superoxide anion, however, forms toxic oxyradicals such as singlet oxygen ($^1O_2$) and particularly hydroxyl radical ($\cdot OH$), which are the active principles in the **oxygen radical system.** The precise bacterial-killing mechanism remains unclear, but it presumably is related to oxidant damage and peroxidation of membrane lipids to which bacteria seem uniquely susceptible. It is also worth noting that much of the superoxide is generated on the outside of the cell membrane, but when phagocytosis occurs it ends up on the inside of the phagolysosome. Without this mechanism, these reactions would occur internally and could damage the phagocyte. It is likely, however, that the effective cytosolic molecular "scavengers" of oxyradicals exist largely to prevent such internal injuries.

The hydrogen peroxide produced in these reactions combines with the azurophil granule enzyme **myeloperoxidase** within the phagolysosome and, along with a **halide ion** such as iodide, bromide, or chloride (the latter being the usual physiologically relevant halide), form a potent bactericidal blend known, for obvious reasons, as the **H_2O_2-myeloperoxidase-halide system.** The molecular combination of these components produces a bactericidal consequence many times stronger than the effect that might be produced by any one of the molecules acting singly. In fact, it is now thought that the final reactive "killer" molecule in this system may be hypochlorite (HOCl), a powerful oxidant and antimicrobial agent. Again, this activity takes place within the phagolysosome in order to not kill the phagocyte.

OXYGEN-INDEPENDENT KILLING MECHANISMS. Bactericidal mechanisms not dependent on oxygen metabolic events have also been identified. The cationic enzyme **lysozyme** attacks bacterial cell walls, especially Gram-positive cocci, and hydrolyzes the muramic acid-N-acetylglucosamine bond found in the glycopeptide coat of most bacteria. **Lactoferrin** is an iron-binding glycoprotein found in the specific granules which is microbicidal at an acid pH *via* a mechanism related to its iron-binding capacity (*see* Chapter 7). **Cathepsin G** is a protease of azurophil granules, which has antimicrobial properties for both Gram-positive and Gram-negative bacteria as well as some fungi. Interestingly, the bactericidal activity of cathepsin G appears independent of enzymatic activity, since heat-inactivated cathepsin G retains its antimicrobial activity. Some of the cationic granule proteins such as **phagocytin** can also lyse bacterial cell membranes. A group of related arginine- and cysteine-rich peptides known as **defensins** are major constitu-

ents of azurophil granules and have broad-spectrum antimicrobial properties against both Gram-negative and Gram-positive bacteria, fungi, and even certain enveloped viruses.

Some of these non-oxygen-dependent systems appear less efficient than the oxygen-dependent killing pathways, and they may function largely as **bacteriostatic** mechanisms (loss of ability to multiply) rather than being truly bactericidal. It also seems clear that the oxygen-dependent systems attack all bacterial cell walls nonspecifically, whereas the oxygen-independent mechanisms often are more selective for certain species of bacteria. Fortunately, in a properly functioning phagocyte, both systems are operational, and the most effective microbicidal activity rests on this combined action.

What then of all of those lysosomal hydrolases (Table 4.10)? Most of the lysosomal enzymes do not have direct bactericidal activity, but are **digestive.** That is, following killing, the acid hydrolases and other lysosomal enzymes degrade and digest the bacteria within the phagolysosomes prior to subsequent extrusion of the debris from the cell. The pH of the phagolysosome drops to about 4–5 after phagocytosis, which is the optimum pH for the action of such enzymes. Thus, most of the acid hydrolases serve only a terminal degradatory role after the killing systems have completed their task.

Despite the fact that these phagocytic and bactericidal systems are usually highly successful, they are not always so. There are numerous examples in clinical medicine of diseases in which the primary problem is a failure of the phagocytic killing systems. Some organisms are sufficiently virulent to simply destroy the phagocytes. Others, like the tubercle bacillus, seem to happily survive within the phagocytes that engulf them, while some organisms seem to be able to escape from the phagosome and replicate in the cytoplasm or to somehow interfere with phagosome-lysosome fusion. Various "escape mechanisms" are discussed in greater detail in Chapter 7. These microorganisms within the phagocyte are protected against the action of antibacterial drugs as well as other defense mechanisms. When phagocytic cells containing microorganisms migrate through lymphatic or vascular channels, infections may be spread. The significance of phagocytosis in the body's defense against bacterial infections is perhaps best illustrated by the vulnerability of patients who suffer from a deficiency of circulating white blood cells or from defects in the phagocytic or enzymatic degradation process itself. Infections often cause the death of these predisposed individuals.

IMPORTANCE OF LEUKOCYTES AS SECRETORY CELLS IN INFLAMMATION

It has been known for over 100 years, since Metchnikoff pointed out that phagocytic cells contained lysosomal enzymes, that these enzymes are responsible not only for digesting material taken into the phagocytic vacuoles, but also for eliciting inflammation and degrading host tissues. At least three different broad categories of materials are released from phagocytic cells in response to a phagocytic stimulus: (1) lysosomal enzymes, especially neutral proteases such as collagenase, elastase, and plasminogen activator; (2) products of oxygen metabolism such as hydrogen peroxide (H_2O_2) and superoxide anion (O_2); and (3) products derived from the metabolism of membrane arachidonic acid such as prostaglandins, thromboxanes, and leukotrienes.

This release of materials from leukocytes has been subject to considerable research. When cells phagocytize, the ensuing events usually are tied to membrane-related activities. The plasma membrane invaginates to take in the phagocytic stimulus and ultimately to form the phagocytic vacuole, which is drawn toward the cell interior for fusion with the membrane-bound lysosome to form the phagolysosome. Lysosomal enzymes sometimes escape into tissue during this process, where they may contribute to inflammatory injury. The activity is also accompanied by a burst of oxidative metabolism related to the production of hydrogen peroxide, superoxide anion, and other oxyradicals useful in the killing of bacteria. In addition, plasma membrane fatty acids such as arachidonic acid are changed into hydroperoxides, endoperoxides, prostaglandins, and thromboxanes in a series of reactions initiated by phospholipases.

The series of events that lead up to final release of materials from leukocytes are worthy of note. The entire process has been referred to as **"stimulus-response coupling,"** a designation that highlights the mechanistic sequence of events set into motion by a phagocytic **stimulus** and ending with a secretory **response** (Fig. 4.36). The initial event, as you might suspect, involves binding of the phagocytic stimulus to the surface receptors on the leukocyte membrane. This is rapidly followed by changes in membrane polarity and alterations in intracellular calcium concentrations. The biochemical changes collectively referred to as the **respiratory burst of phagocytosis** (Table 4.16) ensue with generation of superoxide anion and hydrogen peroxide. The respiratory burst is accompanied by or followed by the generation of thromboxanes, prostaglandins, and leukotrienes from membrane arachidonate. If one examines these events morphologically, it is possible to document a subplasmalemmal concentration of microfilaments and an increase in microtubule assembly. This is presumably related to the intracellular movement required to join the phagosome to the lysosome. As we have stated before, many of these events central to cell secretion are highly reminiscent of those occurring in chemotaxis and phagocytosis.

The biochemical mechanisms regulating release or secretion require energy and are active processes that resemble in some ways the release of chemical mediators from mast cells and basophils during anaphylaxis (*see* Chapter 5). Calcium, a common requirement for most secretory processes, is essential for the release of enzymes from neutrophils. Calcium influx into the neutrophil enhances enzyme release. The function of the microtubular system is well illustrated by the fact that agents that promote disassembly of microtubules reduce enzyme release, whereas agents that promote microtubule assembly enhance it.

It must be recalled that the primary role of the leukocytes in inflammation is to ingest, kill, and degrade harmful microorganisms. In many inflammatory reactions, however, the phagocytic activities of neutrophils and macrophages can elicit tissue damage by virtue of the release of potentially damaging materials from those phagocytic cells.

RELEASE OF LYSOSOMAL ENZYMES AND TISSUE INJURY

Three basic mechanisms have been recognized whereby phagocytic cells can release their potent chemicals into the tissues at sites of imflammation and thus contribute to tissue injury. These have been variously referred to by the colorful designations of (1) "lysosomal suicide," (2) "regurgitation during feeding" or "premature ejaculation," and (3) "frustrated phagocytosis." We will briefly consider each of these.

Lysosomal Suicide

When a phagocyte interiorizes pathogenic bacteria, the potential exists for the bacteria to overwhelm the leukocyte rather

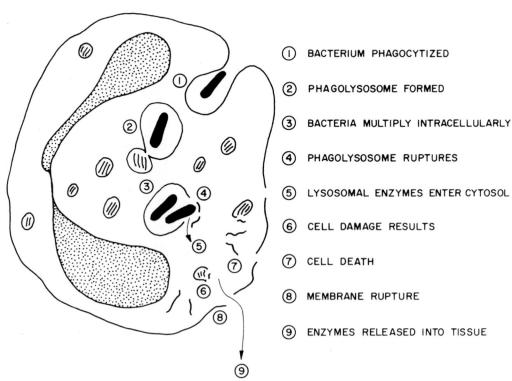

1. BACTERIUM PHAGOCYTIZED
2. PHAGOLYSOSOME FORMED
3. BACTERIA MULTIPLY INTRACELLULARLY
4. PHAGOLYSOSOME RUPTURES
5. LYSOSOMAL ENZYMES ENTER CYTOSOL
6. CELL DAMAGE RESULTS
7. CELL DEATH
8. MEMBRANE RUPTURE
9. ENZYMES RELEASED INTO TISSUE

Figure 4.33. Lysosomal Suicide. If the lysosome ruptures within the cell, powerful hydrolytic enzymes are released, which ultimately can cause death of the cell itself. Rupture of the cell membrane releases lysosomal contents into tissue sites.

than *vice versa*. When this occurs, the phagolysosome may rupture into the cytoplasm, spilling out potent hydrolytic lysosomal enzymes, which can then kill the leukocyte (Fig. 4.33). When the leukocyte dies, its stores of lysosomal enzymes are released into the local environment following lysis or rupture of the limiting cell membranes. Thus, the leukocyte actually can commit suicide after a fashion by turning its own lysosomal hydrolases loose on itself. The end result is escape of the lysosomal contents into tissue.

Regurgitation during Feeding (or Premature Ejaculation)

In the face of large numbers of bacteria (or some other phagocytic stimulus), the leukocytes sometimes make critical errors of timing, which no doubt have their basis in the membrane and microtubule-microfilament events associated with internalization of the phagocytic stimulus and lysosomal granule movement. During a serious phagocytic feeding orgy in which large numbers of bacteria are present, fusion of the lysosome with the developing phagosome may occur prior to the complete internalization of the bacterium. That is, fusion of lysosome to phagosome takes place before the plasma membrane has completely surrounded the bacterium (Fig. 4.34). In such an event, it is not difficult to imagine that the lytic enzymes present in the lysosome have direct access to the extracellular environment. The result is enzymatic damage to host tissues.

Frustrated Phagocytosis

Sometimes phagocytes encounter phagocytic stimuli that are simply too large to be internalized. Examples are bacteria immobilized against a fibrin meshwork or complexes of antigen and antibody fixed against a basement membrane or joint surface. Here, the cell responds appropriately to the phagocytic

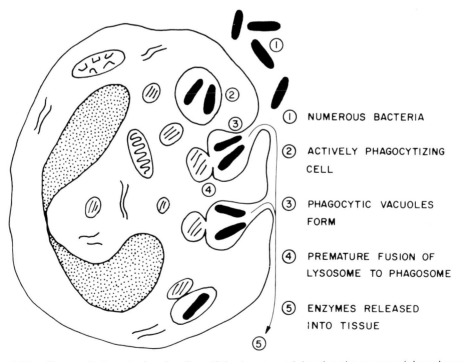

① NUMEROUS BACTERIA

② ACTIVELY PHAGOCYTIZING CELL

③ PHAGOCYTIC VACUOLES FORM

④ PREMATURE FUSION OF LYSOSOME TO PHAGOSOME

⑤ ENZYMES RELEASED INTO TISSUE

Figure 4.34.   Regurgitation during feeding. If the lysosome joins the phagosome (phagolysosome formation) prior to the complete closure of the cell membrane around the phagocytic stimulus, enzymes escape into the surrounding tissues.

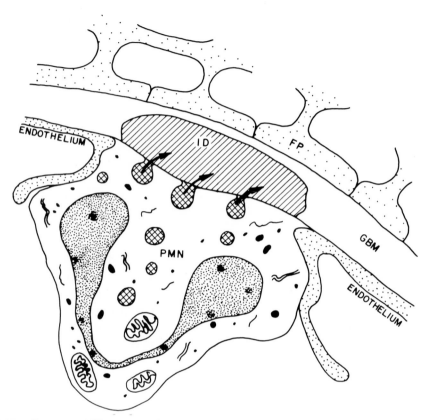

Figure 4.35. Frustrated Phagocytosis. The neutrophil *(PMN)* here has encountered a phagocytic stimulus (immune deposit, *ID*) too large to internalize because it is fixed against the glomerular basement membrane *(GBM)*. Fusion of the lysosome to the surface occurs and enzymes are discharged. (*FP,* foot processes of epithelial cells).

stimulus by attempting to internalize it, but as the stimulus is too large, formation of a phagosome does not take place. Rather, the membrane events associated with phagosome formation occur and set into play the intracellular mechanisms responsible for fusion of the lysosome with the developing phagosome (Fig. 4.35). Since the phagosome really never develops due to the size of the nonphagocytosable stimulus, union of the lysosome with the membrane results in discharge of the lysosomal contents against the nonphagocytosable stimulus, almost as though the leukocyte were frustrated or angry at its inability to internalize the bulky stimulus. If this occurs where the stimulus is adjacent to or integrated into host tissue, the enzymes released ultimately damage that tissue substrate adding to the injury process. Such a mechanism is believed to be operative in some of the immune-mediated diseases such as glomerulonephritis and rheumatoid arthritis (*see* Chapter 5).

LEUKOCYTE ACTIVATION: STIMULUS-RESPONSE COUPLING

As we have stated repeatedly, much of the leukocytic activity associated with inflammation occurs after these cells are stimulated *via* specific membrane receptor-ligand interactions. This linking of a "stimulus" at the cell membrane with some functional "response" has become known as **stimulus-response coupling.** Normal

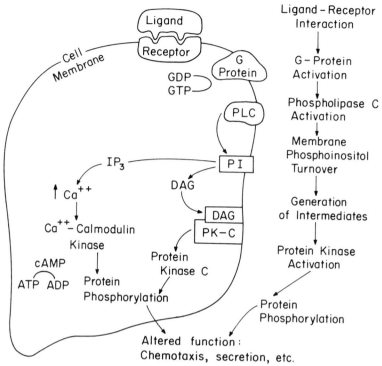

Figure 4.36.   Leukocyte Activation and Stimulus-Response Coupling. The sequence of events by which membrane-ligand interaction at the surface is translated into functional activity involves several important intermediate steps and the generation of second messengers. Receptor occupancy alters receptor affinity for the ligand and changes its conformation to activate G-proteins, which in turn excite the membrane phospholipase *(PLC)*. Activated PLC acts on membrane phosphoinositol *(PI)* to generate the intermediates inositol trisphosphate *(IP$_3$)* and diacyl glycerol *(DAG)*. IP$_3$ acts to increase intracellular calcium for activation of Ca^{2+}-dependent protein kinases, while DAG directly activates protein kinase C *(PK-C)*. Both kinases phosphorylate different substrates and altered functional activity results.

leukocytes in the peripheral blood are spherical and nonmotile, and other leukocyte functions such as oxidative burst activity, pinocytosis, exocytosis, and phagocytosis are absent or occur at a low rate. In short, these functions of leukocytes are all induced responses and require leukocyte **activation.** Considerable progress has been made in recent years in our understanding of the intracellular machinery responsible for activating the various important functional responses that occur following leukocyte stimulation (Fig. 4.36). This progress has occurred on several related fronts; better definition of the receptor systems in-

volved, the role of membrane lipid remodeling in cell activation, pathways of transmembrane surface signal transduction, the importance of "second messenger systems" in cell function, and the biology of the responses themselves. All of this program is basically targeted at addressing a single important question: **how do leukocytes do what they do?**

The answer to this question is clearly not a simple one, but our ability to control inflammation in a clinical setting as "practitioners of the healing arts" remains ultimately limited by our relative lack of detailed knowledge concerning how leukocytes function. Much of the currently employed therapy for inflammatory diseases is aimed at rather nonspecific depression of leukocyte function. Useful functions as well as damaging ones are altered. This situation will certainly change within the professional lifetimes of most of the readers of this book. We will reach into our little black bags and fill our syringes with fluids containing molecules aimed at specific mediators, selected secretory products, and precise cell functions. It will be very exciting.

Receptor Definition and Function

The biochemical definition of various systems important to the inflammatory response has reached a point of respectable sophistication. Although obviously of considerable importance, the level of available detail is beyond our scope, and we will highlight only a few examples. The reading list at the end of the chapter provides entry to the specialty literature. Activation of the **complement system** gives rise to a number of molecular species that can interact with host cells and regulate their function. This interaction, as for many other molecules, is mediated through distinct cell surface complement receptors. Receptor engagement produces biological responses that can modulate host defense reactions or enhance inflammation. Because of its importance to the inflammatory response, we will use the complement system as an example of the recent progress in the art of receptor definition.

The multiplicity and specificity of all leukocyte receptor systems is exemplified by the fact that many different complement receptors have been identified. Some recognize different regions on C3, while the other receptors display specificity for C1q, C5a, or the alternate pathway molecule, Factor H. Activation of the complement system results, among other things, in sequential limited proteolytic activation and regulation of the C3 molecule. This process gives rise to multiple C3 fragments, several of which have biological activity.

C3 receptors. Three receptors for various C3 fragments have been identified and termed **CR-1, CR-2,** and **CR-3.** CR-1 represents one of the most versatile of the CR-3 activity; defective expression of CR- executes the largest number of functions. **CR-1** regulates complement activation at the cell surface, functions in the processing of complexes of antigen and antibody, and participates in a variety of important host cell–mediated defense reactions such as neutrophil secretion and phagocytosis. CR-1 is expressed on neutrophils and macrophages as well as other cells. It is the major C3b receptor, and C3b is an important opsonin. **CR-2** is a distinct receptor predominantly expressed on B lymphocytes and apparently recognizes several C3 fragments distinct from C3b, CR-2 regulates both effector cell function (especially antibody-dependent cellular cytotoxicity, ADCC) and the proliferative responses of lymphocytes. **CR-3** is expressed on neutrophils, macrophages, and certain types of lymphocytes. The major biological responses mediated by CR-3 appear to be similar to those mediated by CR-1; however, CR-3 does not recognize C3b but a different C3 fragment called C3bi. Since C3bi is a more stable fragment than C3b, CR-3 may be a more effective receptor than CR-1 in regulating *in vivo* responses. This suggestion has been supported by recent data obtained from patients exhibiting defective CR-3 activity but normal CR-1 function. These patients have severe, recurrent bacterial infections and defective phagocyte function. Some of the functional abnormality associated with defective CR-3 activity undoubtedly relates to the fact that the **leukocyte adhesion molecule Mo1** has CR-3 activity; defective expression of CR-3 would be expected to lead to defective leukocyte adhesion responses. Thus, the molecular definition of these specific C3 receptor systems has already been shown to have clinical significance.

Anaphylatoxin receptors. Complement activation also results in the generation of two fragments, C3a (77 amino acids) and C5a (74 amino acids), which are referred to as the **anaphylatoxins,** and which have a broad range of functions in the inflammatory response (*see* Mediators section). The ability of the anaphylatoxins to elicit biological responses from a variety of cell types long suggested the presence of specific receptors. These receptors have now been identified. Current data indicate that **C3a receptors** are present on smooth muscle cells, mast cells, neutrophils, macrophages, and certain subsets of T lymphocytes. This is in keeping with the role of C3a in smooth muscle contraction, vascular permeability, histamine release from mast cells, and other functions. The number of such receptors on individual cells is impressive; estimates of millions of C3a receptors per mast cell have been given. C3a molecules from various species show remarkable sequence homology, and the "active site" carboxy terminus is always leucyl-glycyl-leucyl-alanyl-arginine. This sequence has proved to be important to receptor binding and function, since cleavage of the single carboxy-terminal arginine results in a molecule called **C3a des Arg,** which is virtually devoid of receptor binding and biological activity. It is also apparent that the two leucine residues in the carboxy-terminal pentapeptide (positions 73 and 75) of C3a are binding subsites. The functional significance of these various binding domains is still not clear; future structure/function studies with C3a and its receptor will no doubt clarify the situation.

C5a receptors are expressed on neutrophils, eosinophils, basophils and mast cells, and macrophages and mediate the broad range of functional activities of this molecule including chemotaxis, cell adhesion and aggregation, and cellular release

phenomena. Current data indicate that there are probably fewer, but still many, C5a receptors on target cells than C3a receptors (thousands instead of millions). The carboxy-terminal pentapeptide of C5a differs from that of C3a in being methionyl - glutamyl - leaucyl - glycyl - arginine. Unlike the situation with C3a des Arg, C5a from which the carboxy-terminal arginine has been cleaved **(C5a des Arg)** retains C5a receptor interaction and functional activity which varies among different species. Cleavage of the carboxy-terminal pentapeptide leaves a molecule called **C5a 1-69** (74–amino acid native C5a minus 5 residues) which is devoid of functional activity but still binds to the C5a receptor. Recent studies using such C5a derivatives and analogues have shown that the C5a receptor contains at least two binding sites for different domains of the ligand; one reacts with a recognition domain contained in the amino-terminal 69 residues of the molecule (C5a 1-69), and the other in a domain of C5a composed of the carboxy-terminal 5 residues of the peptide, within which binding subsites for methionine (position 70) and leucine (position 72) as well as the carboxy-terminal arginine (position 74) have been identified. Preliminary structure/function studies indicate that all of the binding subunits must be involved for full expression of C5a functional activity, but that partial function may be retained even with the exclusion of certain binding subunits. Such molecular studies on the C5a receptor help to explain the retention of functional activity by C5a des Arg and the fact that C5a 1-69 still exhibits receptor binding. Further clarification will be forthcoming.

Role of Membrane Lipid Remodeling in Leukocyte Activation

The receptors involved in the interaction with specified ligands important to the inflammatory response are all embedded in the lipid bilayer of the plasma membrane. It is now clear that the membrane phospholipids are not merely structural components of the membrane, but are dynamic participants in lipid-protein interactions essential to cell activation. The breakdown and resynthesis of membrane phospholipids occurs in response to stimulation, and it now seems clear that these receptor-mediated events are important in transmembrane signaling. Thus, the concept of a **phosphoinositol cycle** has emerged, in which receptor-ligand binding initiates a series of changes leading to phospholipid breakdown and the generation of biologically important intermediates followed by eventual resynthesis of the original membrane phospholipids.

The turnover of membrane phospholipids is the major transducing event in this important messenger system. Receptor-ligand interaction stimulates the activation of **phospholipase C (PLC)**, which catalyzes the hydrolysis of a specific class of membrane phospholipids, the **phosphoinositols** (PI). Precisely how specific receptor occupancy is linked to the activation of PLC is not clear, but it appears to be dependent on coupling *via* guanine nucleotide regulatory proteins **(G-proteins)** similar to those involved in the coupling of the adenyl cyclase membrane receptor system. The G-proteins are a family of proteins that functionally couple a wide array of membrane receptors to intracellular biochemical effector systems that regulate various second messengers. Both stimulatory (G_s) and inhibitory (G_i) molecules have been identified, and the system is envisioned to play an important regulatory role in cell activation. Such a system only partially explains the measurable brevity of most phosphoinositol turnover-related responses. Stimulation of cells *via* surface receptors that activate PI turnover usually elicits responses that last for only about 5 minutes or less, even with a continuing supply of the stimulant. This suggests the existence of sensitive internal receptor regulatory systems, which may be under G-protein control.

Phospholipase C hydrolyses membrane phosphoinositols to generate two different intracellular messengers, **inositol trisphosphate (IP$_3$)** and **diacylglycerol (DAG)**. These two important intermediates subsequently cause activation of two independent but synergistic pathways that lead to cell activation events. **IP$_3$** is a hydrophilic molecule that is released into the cytoplasm, where it triggers a rise in cytosol Ca^{2+} by the release of calcium from the endoplasmic reticulum and possibly other organelles. This rise in cytosolic calcium is in turn necessary for the triggering of several processes including activation of the **Ca^{2+}-calmodulin-dependent protein kinase,** and the phospholipase A$_2$-dependent release of arachidonic acid from its esterified position in membrane phospholipids to initiate the arachidonic acid metabolic pathways for prostaglandin, thromboxane, and leukotriene synthesis. **DAG,** the other product released by PLC-mediated hydrolysis of phosphoinositol, is highly hydrophobic and remains membrane bound, where it directly activates the Ca^{2+}/phosphatidylserine-dependent **protein kinase C (PK-C).** PK-C is a membrane-bound kinase, where it presumably interacts with its cofactor, phosphatidylserine, as well as the membrane-bound DAG released by PLC-induced membrane phosphoinositol hydrolysis. Once activated, PK-C catalyzes the activation by phosphorylation of a number of important endogenous proteins including the membrane NADPH-oxidase associated with the "respiratory burst of phagocytosis" leading to the generation of superoxide anion and other important oxygen metabolites.

The protein phosphorylation catalyzed by PK-C profoundly modulates a long list of Ca^{2+}-mediated processes including secretory phenomena and exocytosis, cell proliferation and differentiation, smooth muscle contraction, membrane conductance and transport, and many other metabolic processes. With respect to the cells of inflammation, PK-C activation has been implicated in serotonin release and arachidonic acid metabolism in platelets, superoxide anion generation and lysosomal enzyme release from neutrophils, and histamine release from mast cells and basophils. Since PK-C is ubiquitous and widely distributed in virtually all cells and tissues, this list will no doubt grow as additional cell functions are examined.

Transmembrane Signaling and Second Messengers

The binding of a ligand to its receptor is a critical event that initiates leukocyte activation. Such binding, however, is a surface phenomenon, which only begins the sequence of events leading to functional alteration. In order for such an initiation event to result in altered leukocyte activity (chemotaxis, secretion, phagocytosis, *etc.*), **transmembrane signaling** of the receptor-ligand binding must occur in order to connect this plasma membrane event with the intracellular mechanisms mediating cellular activity. The communication events occurring between the cell surface and the interior are still not well understood, but a better definition is emerging. Transmembrane signaling involves carrier molecules, such as the **G-proteins,** to relay the excitation signal from stimulated cell surface receptors to reactive enzymes such as **phospholipase C,** which is subsequently involved in the hydrolytic remodeling of the phospholipids in the cell membrane *via* the **phosphoinositol cycle.** In the process of signal transduction, several different intracellular "second messengers" necessary for translation of the stimulation signal into augmented cell function are produced.

Because of their ability to carry signals from activated membrane receptors to effector enzymes and channels, the **G-pro-**

teins have been intensely studied in recent years. They have a common molecular design consisting of 3 polypeptide chains, one of which contains a guanyl-nucleotide binding site. Because of their widespread distribution in cells and tissues and considerable sequence homology among various G-proteins, it is believed that they evolved by duplication and divergence from a common ancestral gene. G-proteins serve a wide variety of cellular functions. In addition to transmembrane signaling in inflammatory cells, they are apparently involved in the hormonal control of adenylate cyclase, visual excitation in retinal rod cells, translocation of macromolecules in protein synthesis, and the regulation of cell proliferation (*see* Chapter 6). All G-proteins are activated by receptors that are integral membrane glycoproteins. Receptor occupancy by specific ligand induces a conformational change in the receptor itself, which both alters receptor affinity for the ligand and triggers G-protein activation on the cytosolic face of the plasma membrane. G-proteins normally cycle between an inactive guanine diphosphate (GDP) state and an active guanine trisphosphate (GTP) state. The GDP-GTP conversion is slow in the absence of an activated receptor, but is markedly accelerated by receptor-ligand binding. One target for the activated G-protein in leukocytes seems to be **phospholipase C** which, after activation, can initiate the phosphoinositol cycle. Activated G-proteins no doubt interface with other important enzyme systems.

Why have cells evolved such complicated, multistep mechanisms for transmembrane signaling? Why transpose a G-protein between the receptor and the enzyme it is to activate? The answer to these questions is not clear, but it may be because of the remarkable **amplification** of the initial signal that such a system provides; one receptor-ligand binding event can activate many molecules of G-protein, which in turn can activate several molecules of PLC, and so forth, thereby greatly expanding the effect of the initial extracellular signal. In addition, G-protein activation allows a single type of receptor to be functionally coupled to a number of different effector systems. This may explain, for example, why C5a binding to its receptor on a neutrophil can induce several different functional alterations; chemotaxis, secretion, *etc.* Further research will be required to fully understand these reactions.

When specific ligand-receptor interaction occurs, a message is generated which initiates the process of cell activation. This "first message" is therefore a specific one that relates to the binding of the ligand to its membrane receptor, and the ligand thus becomes the "first messenger" in the communication pathway. Simple binding of a ligand to its receptor, however, does not produce functional alteration. That is, the first message is by itself insufficient to result in cell activation. Translation of the first message into cellular activity requires a "second message," which bridges the gap between the receptor-ligand event at the cell surface and the intracellular effector mechanisms necessary for specific functional alteration. As such, the **"second messengers"** are molecules of great importance, since without them the "first message" would fail to result in the stimulated change in cellular activity.

There are a large number of these "second messenger" molecules which fulfill different functions in different situations. Some of these messengers are specific to certain cell types and activation pathways. Thus, **diacylglycerol** and **inositol trisphosphate** function as second messengers following their release from membrane phosphoinositides by phospholipase C as we have explained. Some second messengers such as **cyclic AMP (cAMP)** and **divalent calcium (Ca^{2+})** are much more ubiquitous and merit our attention.

Cyclic AMP (cAMP, cyclic adenosine

monophosphate) regulates intracellular reactions in virtually all animal cells that have been studied to date. For cAMP to function as an intracellular messenger, its intracellular concentration must be closely regulated so that it can change rapidly in response to extracellular signals; cAMP levels are known to change 5-fold within seconds of stimulation. Cyclic AMP is synthesized from ATP by the plasma membrane–bound enzyme **adenylate cyclase,** and its intracellular levels are controlled through a balance of synthesis and degradation by **phosphodiesterases** that convert active cAMP to inactive 5'-AMP (adenosine 5'-monophosphate). Most stimuli for which cAMP is the intracellular messenger act by stimulating the activity of adenylate cyclase to effect a rise in cytosolic cAMP. As in other activation systems, receptor stimulation itself does not activate adenylate cyclase, but introduces conformational changes in the receptor, which stimulate the signal-coupling **G-protein** so that it binds GTP instead of GDP and can then activate adenylate cyclase for ATP conversion to cAMP. Cyclic AMP is a second messenger in a wide variety of physiologic processes ranging from hormone-induced effects like thyroxine and progesterone secretion, hepatic glycogen breakdown, and bone resorption to secretory phenomena like histamine release from mast cells.

Most, if not all, of these effects are mediated through activation of **cAMP-dependent protein kinases,** which are found in all animal cells and which catalyze the transfer of a phosphate group from ATP to protein in the cell; the resultant covalent phosphorylation regulates the activity of these proteins. Phosphorylation can both activate and inactivate enzymes; those activated by phosphorylation are usually degradative while those inactivated by phosphorylation are usually synthetic. One of the unifying themes of biochemical regulation is that **phosphorylation** of proteins by **protein kinases** and their **dephosphorylation** by **phosphoprotein phosphatases** are major means for altering cell function. Precisely how this all works, however, remains somewhat unclear. There are many different protein kinases in cells and only a few appear to be cAMP-regulated. The mechanism of regulation for most protein kinases is not known. Thus, the cAMP-dependent protein kinases join **protein kinase C** and a large number of other less-understood protein kinases in the regulation of cellular activity.

Divalent calcium (Ca^{2+}) is also an important intracellular regulator that functions as a second messenger in a large number of biologically important reactions. Indeed, it is difficult to identify biological responses in which Ca^{2+} is not involved at some stage. Muscle contraction, endocrine and exocrine secretion, fluid and electrolyte transport, numerous metabolic activities, and a long list of leukocyte functions are dependent on Ca^{2+}. Like cAMP, there is very little free Ca^{2+} in the cytosol, most of it being membrane bound particularly to organelles like the endoplasmic reticulum. A gross imbalance thus exists between cytosol Ca^{2+} and extracellular Ca^{2+}, creating an enormous gradient that tends to drive Ca^{2+} into the cell. In order to maintain this imbalance, a plasma membrane–bound enzyme system **(Ca^{2+}-ATPase)** uses the energy of ATP hydrolysis to pump Ca^{2+} out of the cell. This remarkable system in part enables the endoplasmic reticulum to take up Ca^{2+} from the cytosol against a steep 5000-fold to 10,000-fold concentration gradient across its membrane. The Ca^{2+} second messenger system is an almost universal means by which extracellular signals (receptor-ligand interactions) regulate diverse cell functions.

It now appears that the initiation of the **phosphoinositol cycle** following cell stimulation is the major transducing event in the Ca^{2+} second messenger system because of the key intermediates generated. Thus, a now familiar sequence is envisioned in which **receptor-ligand binding** induces **conformational changes** in the receptor, which activate the **G-proteins** to catalyze activation of **phospholipase C** for hydrolysis and turnover of **membrane phosphoinositides,** leading to the generation of the reactive intermediates **diacylglycerol** (DAG) and **inositol trisphosphate** (IP3). It is these reactive intermediates that initiate the flow of biochemical information in the two main branches of the Ca^{2+} second messenger system, the **calmodulin** branch, which is stimulated by IP3, and the **protein kinase C** branch, which is stimulated by DAG. IP3 appears to induce the release of Ca^{2+} from the endoplasmic reticulum and subsequent activation of the Ca^{2+}-calmodulin-dependent protein kinase, while DAG stimulates protein kinase C directly as a Ca^{2+}-dependent fashion.

It has long been observed that some of the responses mediated by Ca^{2+} as a second messenger are brief while others are quite prolonged. It now appears that these phenomena may be explained by the two branches of the Ca^{2+} messenger system. The rapid IP3-induced rises in cytosol Ca^{2+} are transient because the pool of calcium in the endoplasmic reticulum is rapidly depleted, whereas DAG induces a slower but more sustained rise because of Ca^{2+} influx across the plasma membrane. Since both systems often work simultaneously, it thus appears that the Ca^{2+}-dependent flow of information from cell surface to cell interior proceeds by the calmodulin pathway responsible for initiating responses and the protein kinase C pathway jointly in the regulation of many cell functions, as changes in the intracellular cAMP levels can influence both the calmodulin and protein kinase C branches of the Ca^{2+} messenger system.

How do leukocytes do what they

do? We stated at the outset that there were no simple answers to this question. As our collective knowledge about receptor-ligand interaction, membrane phospholipid turnover, transmembrane signaling mechanisms, and second messenger systems has grown to intelligible levels of biochemical sophistication, the answers seem to be just beyond our reach. It is likely only to be a matter of time before the new biology of leukocyte activation begins to have a substantial impact on our understanding of inflammatory diseases, and the application of this increased level of understanding to clinical problems will no doubt suggest new and exciting therapeutic approaches to those problems.

CHEMICAL MEDIATORS OF INFLAMMATION

General Features of Mediators

A simple definition of a chemical mediator might be any chemical messenger that acts on blood vessels and/or inflammatory cells to contribute to an inflammatory response. A large number of agents fulfill this definition. Since the **vascular** and **cellular** aspects of inflammation remain its central features, it stands to reason that the most important mediator molecules are those that enhance blood flow, increase vascular permeability, or induce the emigration of leukocytes from the bloodstream to the site of injury. Because of the importance of these functions in host defense, a large number of chemical mediators can induce these changes. This reiterates the theme of redundancy and inflammatory responsiveness.

Where do the mediators of inflammation come from and what are they like? Chemical mediators can be **exogenous** (coming from outside the body) such as endotoxin (LPS), or they can be **endogenous** (coming from within the body) such as histamine. In keeping with the view that inflammation is a host defense system, most of the useful chemical mediators are endogenous. The endogenous mediators can be derived from plasma sources (such as bradykinin), leukocytic sources (such as LTB_4 and IL-1), of from the tissues themselves (endothelial and fibroblast products). Although not all of the mediator receptor systems have been defined, it appears that virtually all of these chemicals interact with their targets *via* specific receptor-ligand interactions at the cell surface.

Some mediators are **preformed** and only require release from their cellular stores (such as histamine and serotonin), while others are newly **synthesized** by stimulated cells (such as platelet-activating factor) or are generated as a consequence of multiple enzymatic steps involving sequential activation of different molecules by limited proteolysis (such as the complement and coagulation systems). Some mediators are small (such as histamine, M_r 200, or bradykinin, 9 amino acids), some are intermediate in size (such as tumor necrosis factor, M_r 17,000), and some are large (such as fibronectin, M_r 500,000). Some are amines like histamine and serotonin, some are lipids like the leukotrienes and platelet-activating factor, some are glycoproteins like interferon, and many are polypeptides like C5a.

The chemical mediators of inflammation have generated intense interest among biochemists, physiologists, cell biologists, pathologists, pharmacologists, and clinicians. Research efforts have been aimed at elucidating molecular details of synthesis and secretion that might provide clues to means of specific pharmacologic intervention in inflammatory diseases. Since our focus here is on understanding the biology of the inflammatory response, we will emphasize the function of the various mediators in terms of their relationship to the phenomenology of inflammation (vascular and cellular events), their unique biochemical features, and the means by which they are generated.

Injury precipitates the inflammatory response largely by stimulating the release of chemical mediators. Their existence was long suspected because whatever the nature of the injury, the ensuing inflammatory changes comprise a fairly uniform, almost stereotyped reaction. The relative significance of different mediators to a developing inflammatory reaction varies somewhat depending upon the animal species, the location in the body, and the nature of the injurious agent. A well-developed inflammatory reaction involves many mediators acting simultaneously. Most of the mediators that we will consider have been shown to be active only in the earlier stages of inflammation; much less is known about the mediation and pathogenesis of chronicity. Although differing widely in chemical structure and in mechanisms of release or activation, the mediators have one general characteristic in common: they tend to be distributed widely throughout the body, so that release and/or activation can occur locally at any inflammatory focus.

Mediators are usually highly available, either by immediate release of a preformed substance or by rapid enzymatic formation. They usually have rather short tissue half-lives and can be quickly inactivated, also locally, and as a rule do not circulate systematically except in unusual circumstances; the presence in the systemic circulation of significant concentrations of these potent pharmacologic agents would pose a difficult problem in regulating and limiting the response, and might well prove disastrous in many instances. Lastly, natural inhibitors of most mediators are found in normal plasma. This is presumably to limit the extent of inflammatory responses.

The mediation of inflammation involves an extensive network of interacting chemicals which provide the system with a high degree of redundancy. This guarantees that both amplification and preservation of the response can be maintained even if one component or another of the system is deficient. There are virtually no parts of the inflammatory response that are dependent on a single mediator; indeed, most functions can be elicited by multiple mediators and most mediators serve multiple functions. The potent and extremely important complement fragment of C5a, for example, can stimulate neutrophil adhesiveness and aggregation, chemotaxis, and lysosomal enzyme release as well as several other functions and appears to be an important initiator of acute inflammation, yet genetic deficiency of C5 is not a major impairment to inflammatory responsiveness. This strongly argues for the value of compensatory collateral mediation systems. If there is a weak link in the system, it is the leukocytes, not the mediators. Unlike C5 deficiency, genetic defects in neutrophil function generally result in defective inflammatory responses and poor protective host defenses which, without vigorous antibiotic intervention, often prove to be incompatible with life.

Vasoactive Amines: Histamine and Serotonin

Histamine (β-imidazolylethylamine) is a **preformed** mediator immediately available largely from the granules of tissue mast cells and peripheral blood basophils and, in some species, the platelets. It is formed by the decarboxylation of the amino acid 1-histidine. Histamine has long been considered to play an important part in the initiation of the vascular aspects of a wide variety of inflammatory states. It is undoubtedly important in mediating the immediate active phase of increased vascular permeability. Histamine produces not only increased vascular permeability but has profound effects on vascular and bronchial smooth muscle as well. Histamine is unquestionably of major importance in the pathogenesis of systemic anaphylaxis (*see* Chapter 5).

In mast cells and basophils, histamine is stored within granules in the cytoplasm, and is bound to heparin within the granules. When these granules are extruded from the cell, histamine is released. By direct action, histamine promotes the contraction of extravascular smooth muscle, for example in the bronchus, and dilates arterioles. It also elicits an increase in vascular permeability by causing the endothelial cells of venules to contract and round up, so that gaps appear between the margins of adjacent cells. Soon after release it is inactivated by histaminase or by oxidative deamination.

Serotonin (5-hydrozytryptamine, 5-HT) is an important mediator of inflammation in some animal species. It is found in certain cells of the gastrointestinal tract, the brain, the lung, and the blood platelets. In many animals it is also found in mast cells and basophils. It is formed from dietary tryptophan. Serotonin has a variety of effects on smooth muscle, blood vessels, and nerves in different regions of the body and can produce pain. It is inactivated by amineoxidase.

Vasoactive amine release from mast cells occurs in response to a wide variety of stimuli such as physical injury, mechanical trauma, irradiation, heat, various chemical agents, snake venoms, mellitin from bee venom, toxins, trypsin, surfactants (such as bile salts), dextran, polyvinylpyrrolidone, alkylamines, histamine liberators (such as Compound 48/80), ATP, a neutrophil lysosomal cationic protein, immunologic processes, antigenic challenge of IgE antibody–sensitized cells, and exposure to anaphylatoxins (C3a and C5a). Release from platelets occurs during the platelet-release reaction triggered by stimuli such as thrombin, trypsin, collagen, polystyrene particles, emulsions of long-chain fatty acids, antigen-antibody complexes, globulin-coated surfaces, snake venoms, epinephrine, and ADP. In addition, vasoactive amines can be secreted from platelets following interaction with platelet-activating factor.

The mechanisms involved in the release of amines and other mediators from mast cells, basophils, and platelets have been intensively studied. Of particular interest is the role of IgE antibody in mediator release in various systems and how this can explain the pathogenesis and manifestations of anaphylactic reactions (*see also* Chapter 5). It has become clear that release depends upon a secretory (rather than cytotoxic) mechanism. Antigen bridging of cell-bound IgE is followed by a sequence of biochemical events which leads to the release of mediators (*see* Chapter 5). Both histamine and 5-HT induce contraction of smooth muscle and increased vascular permeability. Neither appears to be chemotactic for neutrophils. Recently, however, it has been reported that histamine is specifically chemotactic for eosinophils. Thus, histamine and eosinophil chemotactic factor of anaphylaxis (ECF-A), both released from mast cells, probably cause the influx and localization of eosinophils in immediate hypersensitivity reactions.

Kinins

The kinins are a group of related polypeptides that are split from protein precursors (kininogens) by enzymes termed kallikreins. The prototype kinin is **bradykinin** (to indicate that it is slow to produce a full contraction of smooth muscle in comparison to histamine). Bradykinin is a polypeptide consisting of nine amino acids and is derived from a circulating high molecular weight kininogen (HMW kininogen). The related peptides lysyl-bradykinin and methionyl-lysyl-bradykinin are also produced but are not as important as bradykinin. Other kinins are derived from tissue kininogens by the action of tissue kallikreins that may be similar to plasma kallikreins. **Leukokinins** are kinins derived from leukocytes. An additional kinin **(C-kinin)** is derived from one of the early acting complement components. After generation, kinins are quickly inactivated by kininases (carboxypeptidases), enzymes that split amino acids from the carboxy-terminal end of these polypeptides.

Bradykinin results from activation of the "contact system" of plasma when the enzyme **kallikrein** acts to cleave it from the substrate high molecular weight kininogen **(HMW kininogen)** in a contact reaction also involving coagulation factors XII (Hageman factor) and XI (plasma thromboplastin antecedent, PTA), prekallikrein, and plasminogen. This is the same plasma "contact system" responsible for intrinsic coagulation and fibrinolysis (*see* Chapter 3). This complicated "contact" system of plasma proteins constitutes one of the major groups of plasma proteins, along with the complement system, involved in inflammation. We will discuss this "tangled web" of interlacing reactions in more detail later (*see* section on the Hageman factor–dependent Pathways).

Once set into motion, the "contact system" generates kallikrein, which cleaves bradykinin and other kinins from HMW kininogen. Bradykinin is a potent mediator that has a variety of effects on blood vessels and various cell types. The kinins act on peripheral vessels to cause vasodilation and reduce arterial smooth muscle tone, they increase capillary permeability, raise intracapillary pressure by contracting the veins, and modulate the function of other cells and tissue components. Kinins can also stimulate the release of histamine from mast cells and activate the arachidonic acid cascade for prostaglandin and leukotriene production. Along with the prostaglandins, bradykinin is thought to be a major mediator of the pain of acute inflammation by virtue of its effects on afferent nerve fibers.

All the kinins promote extravascular smooth muscle contraction and vasodilation, and they are the most potent known inducers of increased vascular permeability *via* the same mechanism as histamine, namely contraction and separation of endothelial cells in venules. It remains unclear whether bradykinin promotes increased vascular permeability directly or *via* an indirect mechanism involving some intermediate. By virtue of its varied effects, bradykinin is still regarded by some as an excellent candidate for a general mediator of actual inflammation. That is, through either direct or indirect mechanisms, kinins are able to increase peripheral blood flow, affect vascular permeability, and produce pain. They can thus induce *rubor, calor, tumor,* and *dolor,* the four cardinal signs of inflammation.

Complement Fragments as Mediators

It has become increasingly clear in recent years that the complement system is the principal humoral effector and/or amplification system in inflammation. During activation of the complement system, cleavage fragments are produced from various complement proteins, which serve as ligands for receptors on many inflammatory cells. In general, there are two types of ligands produced, those which bind to microorganisms (such as C3b) and serve as opsonins, and those which are freely diffusible in plasma (such as C5a) where they may encounter and activate inflammatory cells. As we have already discussed opsonins and the process of opsonization (*see* Phagocytosis), we will focus our attention here on the **anaphylatoxins.**

Biologic characterization and structural analysis of the anaphylatoxins have advanced markedly over the last decade. Detailed features of these important polypeptides have been elucidated at the molecular level. The molecules in question are C3a, C4a, and C5a. Because they are of greater importance than C4a, we will focus our attention here on the **C3a** and **C5a** anaphylatoxins. These important complement fragments serve as local hormones to cause alterations in the secretory, locomotor, and metabolic activities of the leukocytes with which they interact. Specific receptors for each of the anaphylatoxins have been characterized. As one tabulates the various functions attributed to C3a and C5a (Table 4.17), it becomes apparent that their diversity of action is in part a biological consequence of the large number of cell types that respond to these humoral factors. **Virtually every circulating cell type except the erythrocyte responds directly to anaphylatoxin exposure.** There are also numerous examples of tissue cell types that respond to the anaphylatoxins including mast cells, tissue macrophages, endothelial cells, and perhaps fibroblasts.

Like the products of arachidonic acid metabolism, these polypeptide fragments mediate a wide variety of cellular functions. In terms of the influence of C3a and C5a on inflammatory cells, it is useful to divide the cellular responses into 4 broad categories; chemotactic behavior, metabolic activation, secretory phenomena, and

Table 4.17
Biological Activities of the Anaphylatoxins

Function	C3a	C5a
Leukocyte chemotaxis	no	yes
Smooth muscle contraction	yes	yes
Increased vascular permeability	yes	yes
Neutrophil membrane-ruffling	no	yes
Increased leukocyte stickiness	no	yes
Neutrophil aggregation	no	yes
Superoxide anion generation	no	yes
Neutrophil secretion	no	yes
Mast cell degranulation	yes	yes
Stimulate respiratory burst	no	yes

morphologic changes with increased adhesiveness and aggregation. It appears that the initial ligand-receptor interaction activates the leukocytes and thereby encourages all of these diverse activities, although C5a promotes a broader range of functional alteration than does C3a (Table 4.17). It is now clear that C5a is the major complement-derived chemotaxin and perhaps the most important chemotaxin from any source. C5a stimulates chemotaxis in neutrophils, eosinophils, basophils, and monocytes. Neutrophil activation by C5a also leads to numerous biochemical alterations including stimulation of the respiratory burst with increased oxidative metabolism and superoxide anion generation, and initiates arachidonic acid metabolism. C5a also causes increased lamellipodia formation (*see* Fig. 4.30), promotes increased adhesiveness and aggregation, and induces neutrophil secretory responses and lysosomal enzyme release.

Both C3a and C5a cause increased vascular permeability and smooth muscle contraction. The mechanisms whereby these anaphylatoxins promote increased vascular permeability and edema formation are multifactorial. They relate to the release of histamine from mast cells, which in turn mediates the vascular changes, but may also relate to prostaglandin and leukotriene release from leukocytes following activation of the arachidonic acid cascade. It was formerly thought that the anaphylatoxins could directly influence vascular permeability, but it is now generally considered that they exert their effects on vascular permeability through mast cell and leukocyte intermediaries. It appears, however, that at least part of the effects of the anaphylatoxins on smooth muscle may be direct and leukocyte-independent. This has been established by exposing strips of smooth muscle to these stimuli in culture systems in which no leukocytes are present.

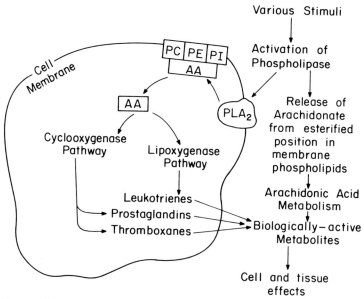

Figure 4.37. Generation of Biologically Active Arachidonic Acid Metabolites. The various potent prostaglandins, thromboxanes, and leukotrienes so important to the inflammatory process have their origin in arachidonic acid *(AA)* esterified into membrane phospholipids such as phosphatidylcholine *(PC)*, phosphatidylethanolamine *(PE)*, and phosphatidylinositol *(PI)*. Arachidonic acid is freed from these cell membrane phospholipids *via* phospholipases such as phospholipase A_2 *(PLA$_2$)* and metabolized *via* one of two major pathways.

Arachidonic Acid Metabolites

Unlike histamine, which has been known to be a mediator of inflammation for some time, our understanding of the importance of arachidonic acid and its metabolites in inflammation dates only from the early 1970s when Dr. John Vane, who was later awarded a Nobel prize for his work, discovered that drugs like aspirin work by interfering with arachidonic acid metabolism. The metabolites of arachidonic acid function in a variety of biological processes, of which inflammation is among the more important. These metabolites are sometimes referred to as **autacoids,** rapidly formed short-range hormones that decay spontaneously or are rapidly destroyed enzymatically. In addition to inflammation, arachidonic acid metabolites are important to coagulation and thrombosis and in cardioplumonary, renal, and endocrine pathophysiology.

Arachidonic acid is a 20-carbon polyunsaturated fatty acid (5,8,11,14-eicosatetraenoic acid) derived directly from dietary sources or by conversion from essential fatty acids like linoleic acid. It is never free within the cell but esterified into membrane phospholipids such as phosphatidyl-choline in many types of inflammatory cells including platelets. In order for arachidonic acid metabolism to proceed, it must first be freed from its esterified position in these membrane phospholipids. This is accomplished through the activity of various cellular phospholipases (principally phospholipase A_2) that become activated during the early phases of cell stimulation. The freed arachidonic acid is metabolized via one of two major pathways (Fig. 4.37).

The **cyclooxygenase** pathway is named for the enzyme responsible for the conversion of arachidonic acid into the unstable prostaglandin endoperoxide **PGG$_2$**, which is subsequently reduced to a second unstable endoperoxide, **PGH$_2$**, which breaks down nonenzymatically to produce prostaglandin E$_2$ (**PGE$_2$**), prostaglandin D$_2$ (**PGD$_2$**), and prostaglandin F$_{2\alpha}$ (**PGF$_{2\alpha}$**). These prostaglandins have been implicated in the production of pain associated with inflammation, and can cause vasodilation and assist other mediators in producing increased vascular permeability. PGH$_2$ may also be converted either by prostaglandin I$_2$ synthetase to **prostacyclin (PGI$_2$)**, primarily in endothelial cells, or by thromboxane A$_2$ synthetase to **thromboxane TXA$_2$)**, primarily in platelets. PGI$_2$ and TXA$_2$ are rather unstable intermediates with important biological properties in inflammation and blood coagulation (*see also* Chapter 3). PGI$_2$ is a potent vasodilator and inhibitor of platelet aggregation and TXA$_2$ is an important vasoconstrictor and potent platelet aggregator. Thus, the cyclooxygenase pathway of arachidonic acid metabolism is responsible for the production of the various prostaglandins, prostacyclins, and thromboxanes and interfaces in several ways with the mediation of inflammation.

Arachidonic acid may also be metabolized via the **lipoxygenase** pathway to produce **hydroperoxyeicosatetraenoic acid (HPETE)** compounds, which are the precursors of the potent **leukotrienes.** Some of the HPETE compounds are directly chemotactic for leukocytes, but most of the HPETEs are converted first to the unstable intermediate leukotriene A$_4$ **(LTA$_4$)**, which is subsequently metabolized to give rise to the leukotrienes, so designated because of their typical triene chain structure and the fact that they were first isolated from leukocytes. LTA$_4$ is either converted into leukotriene B$_4$ **(LTB$_4$)** or conjugated with glutathione to produce leukotriene C$_4$ **(LTC$_4$)**, which is subsequently metabolized to produce, sequentially, leukotriene D$_4$ and leukotriene E$_4$ **(LTD$_4$ and LTE$_4$)**. The combination of LTC$_4$, LTD$_4$, and LTE$_4$ accounts for the biological activity formerly known as the **slow-reacting substance of anaphylaxis.** LTB$_4$ is one of the most potent inflammatory mediators known and causes leukocyte chemotaxis, aggregation, increased adhesivenes, lysosomal enzyme release, and superoxide anion generation. The cysteinyl-containing leukotrienes C$_4$, D$_4$, and E$_4$ can produce intense vasoconstriction and, on a molar basis, are probably 1000 times as potent as histamine in producing increased vascular permeability. Thus, the leukotrienes are the major products of lipoxygenase metabolism of arachidonate and are potent mediators of inflammation. Much recent drug research has been aimed at the identification of therapeutic agents that might act specifically on either the lipoxygenase or cyclooxygenase pathways of arachidonic acid metabolism. This field is moving very rapidly.

Lymphokines

The term **lymphokine** is well entrenched in the literature, but as the size and biological activities of this extended family of molecules continues to grow, the definition becomes less and less explicit. The simplest definition of a **lymphokine** is any non-antibody, hormone-like protein or glycoprotein produced by a lymphocyte. Some lymphokines are **afferent** molecules involved, for example, in various helper and suppressor functions in antibody formation within the afferent limb of the immune response. Others are **effector** molecules that attract, mobilize, and activate leukocytes. These effector or "inflammatory lymphokines" are of greater interest to our discussion of inflammation. The related terms **cytokine** and **monokine** evolved to include lymphokine-like substances produced by nonlymphoid cells. This extended meaning of the term "lymphokine" was necessary to encompass recent progress in defining the molecular nature of lymphokines, since many lymphokines can be produced as, or have analogs in, products of nonlymphoid cells. It may be best to think of all of the members of this growing family of biologically active mediators as cytokines, with the lymphokines themselves representing only an important subset.

Much of what we know of the lymphokines comes from carefully controlled *in vitro* experiments, and most of these "factors" were first identified by assaying some functional alteration in a target cell population following addition of supernatant fluids from stimulated lymphocyte cultures. With respect to their role in disease processes, evidence for lymphokine participation comes from 3 major lines of evidence: first, that injections of lymphokines into animals can mimic disease processes; second, that lymphokines can be isolated from diseased tissues and fluids; and third, that lymphocytes from diseased patients can produce lymphokines *in vitro* when exposed to disease-related antigens.

The lymphokines are a large family of proteins and/or glycoproteins that are generally smaller than M_r 30,000. Not all of the many described lymphokines will be discussed here. With a few notable exceptions, the precise chemical structure of many of the lymphokines is not known. They are primarily products of activated T cells, but some can also be produced by B cells, macrophages, and other cell types. Lymphokines usually do not circulate, but are rather produced locally and have a relatively short chemical half-life necessitating sustained production for sustained biological activity. They are active in a wide variety of conditions; reported *in vitro* lymphokine activities include over 100 assayable functions. The targets for lymphokine action include all types of leukocytes as well as endothelium and fibroblasts, a spectrum of cellular re-

sponders that incorporates all of the cells essential to inflammatory and reparative responses. The activities stimulated by lymphokines include such vital processes as cell motility, growth and proliferation, regulation, activation, injury, and repair. With respect to inflammation, lymphokines can **attract, accumulate, activate,** and **localize** several types of leukocytes to sites of inflammatory injury. With improved molecular definition of the lymphokines, it is probable that various functional activities currently assigned to different "factors" may all be due to the same molecule.

Inflammatory Lymphokines

Much progress has been made in this field since the first report of a lymphokine appeared in 1966, but the molecular mechanisms whereby lymphokines exert their effects and the biochemical characterization of most of these "factors" is still preliminary. The best characterized of the lymphokines involved in the inflammatory process are those that affect macrophages. **Macrophage migration inhibitor factor (MIF)** was the first lymphokine described and has been extensively investigated. It is an acidic glycoprotein, heterogeneous in terms of molecular weight (M_r 12,000 to 82,000), that inhibits the migration of macrophages, presumably thereby retaining emigrated monocytes in the area. MIF is primarily a product of activated T cells, but apparently it can also be produced by B cells. MIF activity is also associated with increased clumping of macrophages (aggregation), increased stickiness (adherence), alterations in macrophage transmembrane electrical potential and electrophoretic mobility, phagocytosis, and pinocytosis. Ultrastructurally, MIF-treated macrophages exhibit retracted cell processes and extensive cytoplasmic vacuolation, accompanied by enhanced microvillus formation and a loss of cell surface glyoprotein in areas of cell contact. MIF appears to act by binding to receptors on the cell surface, but the receptor itself has yet to be defined, and the mechanisms by which MIF inhibits cell migration are not yet clear.

Some of the activities of MIF involve biochemical activation of the target macrophages (increased glucose oxidation *via* the hexose monophosphate shunt, increased glucosamine uptake, increased bactericidal activity) in a series of activities originally ascribed to **macrophage activation factor (MAF)**. Although some cloned T cell lines appear to produce distinct factors, MIF and MAF tend to co-purify, and as a result their existence as distinct molecules remains open to further investigation. Because of their similar functional activities and apparent structural homology, it has become apparent in recent years that many of the activities ascribed initially to MAF are likely due to **interferon-γ.** That is, MAF and interferon-γ may well be the same molecule.

Another lymphokine important to cell migration is referred to as **macrophage chemotactic factor (MCF)**. Produced by both B and T cells, MCF activity is distinct from MIF and apparently is due to a heterogeneous, heat-stable M_r 12,500 to 55,000 molecule. MCF induces specific directed migration (chemotaxis) in monocytes and macrophages and is presumably important in the attraction of such cells to inflammatory foci.

The lymphokines that affect the behavior of granulocytes are less well characterized and less numerous than those that affect macrophages. A lymphocyte-derived **leukocyte inhibitory factor (LIF)** has been described, which is apparently distinct from MIF and inhibits the migration of neutrophils. Lymphocyte-derived **chemotactic factors** for each of the granulocytes (neutrophils, NCF; eosinophils, ECF; basophils, BCF) have been described. These factors are distinguishable from one another and from MCF.

Similar studies have revealed lymphocyte-derived chemotactic factors for lymphocytes and even fibroblasts. Thus, apparently distinct lymphokines can induce the directed migration of virtually all of the cells important to inflammation.

A number of lymphokines have also been identified that can affect vascular permeability, such as **lymph node permeability factor (LNPF), skin reactive factor (SRF),** and **thymic permeability factor (TPF).** These "factors" remain poorly characterized, and it is not clear whether the vascular effects observed when they are injected into the skin can be directly related to these factors or are due to the secondary release of other vasoactive substances. Unlike these rather poorly characterized permeability factors, **lymphotoxin (LT)** is a well-defined, M_r 18,000 molecule produced by stimulated T and B cells, which is nonspecifically cytostatic or cytotoxic against a wide variety of tumor cells *in vitro.* The cloning of the gene for LT demonstrated about 30% amino acid homology with the cytokine **tumor necrosis factor (TNF),** *see below*). Additional lymphokines have been described which can influence the clotting system both directly and indirectly.

Taken collectively, the lymphokines provide a means of explaining some of the phenomena involved in certain kinds of immune reactions, hypersensitivities, and inflammatory reactions. Their common denominator is that they can **mobilize, attract,** and **activate** a wide variety of circulating cells that are well-known participants in local inflammation. On the basis of *in vitro* effects, the list of potential lymphokine activities is extremely large. Not all of these activities, however, appear to have *in vivo* correlates, and thus they remain open to questions of biological relevance. It is also clear that greater biochemical definition of these various "factors" will be required before their various effects can be viewed as truly distinct. Despite these shortcomings, the evidence favoring the importance of lymphokines to inflammatory reactions is overwhelming.

Interferons

Interferons are a group of somewhat different glycoprotein molecules initially discovered because of their antiviral effects. Interferon inducers include viruses, bacteria, and bacterial products like endotoxin. It is now apparent that the interferons have a wide range of effects on cells, particularly on those of the immune system, but also on inflammatory cells. It has also become clear that the interferons represent a rather large group of molecules.

There are at the present time three major groups of molecules classified as interferons, one derived initially from leukocyte cultures as **"leukocyte interferon"** (now **interferon-α, INF-α**), one of fibroblast origin called **"fibroblast interferon"** (now **interferon-β, INF-β**), and one produced by lectin-stimulated lymphocyte cultures called **"immune interferon"** (now called **interferon-γ, INF-γ**). Because of their potential clinical use, much recent attention has been directed toward applying the techniques of modern molecular biology to the interferons, some of which are probably products of a multigene family, and some of which are products of separate genes. Several of these genes have now been cloned. Interferons of the INF-α group are products of a multigene family, whereas INF-β is probably the product of a single gene. The INF-γ gene shows no homology with the INF-α and INF-β genes and is principally different in that it contains 3 introns. Also, INF-γ uses a different receptor on the cell membrane, distinct from the common receptor for INF-α and INF-β. As a product of stimulated T lymphocytes, interferon-γ is truly a lymphokine while the others are probably best termed cytokines; interferon-γ is also apparently more multi-functional and potentially more potent. All mechanisms known to result in T lymphocyte activation cause the production of INF-γ.

In addition to their well-known antiviral effects, interferons mediate a variety of other cellular activities including antiproliferative effects on tumor cells and enhancement of the expression of immunologically relevant cell surface structures such as histocompatibility antigens, as well as other immunoregulatory functions. The interferons have a wide range of reported functions of importance to the inflammatory response, most of which relate to its effects on macrophages and, to a lesser extent, neutrophils. Interferons may induce up-regulation of Fc receptors and increase phagocytosis, cause macrophage activation and increased metabolic activity, and enhance phagocyte microbicidal and cytotoxic activity. The interferon system is thus emerging as a broadly based host defense system involved both in the primary nonspecific resistance to a variety of microorganisms and in specific immune responses. Since recombinant interferon molecules are now available, a much greater amount of information will be forthcoming during the next decade.

Interleukins

Interleukins are polypeptides that act on leukocytes and other targets. The term **interleukin** reflects the fact that these mediators are both produced by and act on leukocytes. They are "messenger molecules," which allow communication between cells in order to effect certain cell functions. Some interleukins are produced by monocytes and are therefore termed "monokines," while others are lymphocyte products and appropriately termed "lymphokines." All are part of the larger "cytokine" family. Several interleukins have been described, but the best characterized (and seemingly the most important) of these to inflammation is **interleukin-1 (IL-1),** and we will direct

Table 4.18
Some of the Multiple Biological Activities
Ascribed to Interleukin-1

Induces fever (endogenous pyrogen)
Increased acute phase reactant production
T-cell activation, "inflammatory lymphokines"
Induces IL-2 production by T-helper cells
Neutrophil activation
Induces endothelial procoagulant activity
Increases endothelial stickiness for PMN[a]
Induced PMN emigration
Augments B-lymphocyte growth and
  differentiation
Fibroblast mitogenic activity
Osteoclast activation

[a] Abbreviation used is PMN, neutrophil.

most of our attention here to IL-1 (Table 4.18). Several other interleukins (termed IL-2, IL-3, IL-4, *etc.*) have been identified and serve a variety of different functions interfaced closely with the immune system (*see* Chapter 5).

Interleukin-1 (IL-1). The list of postulated functions for IL-1 has grown considerably in recent years (Table 4.18). It is now clear that it is really much more than simply an interleukin since it affects several non-leukocytic targets such as liver, pancreas, bone, cartilage, muscle, fibroblasts, and brain. IL-1 is also not a single molecule, but a family of monocyte- and macrophage-derived polypeptide "monokines" that had been described for several years under various names such as **endogenous pyrogen,** the mediator of fever, and **leukocyte endogenous mediator,** the inducer of acute phase protein synthesis. Biochemical studies have now shown all of these "factors" to be IL-1. Clarification of the present dilemma of how many of the multiple biological activities of IL-1 are due to a single substance has begun with the cloning of cDNAs coding for IL-1. At least two dissimilar gene products (IL-1$_\alpha$ and IL-1$_\beta$) have been cloned; there are probably more. The two forms cloned so far have only

26% amino acid homology, and it is likely that they represent two distinct gene products.

The host responses to challenges such as microbial invasion, injury, and inflammation are often called **acute phase responses.** They are characterized by alterations in metabolic, endocrinologic, neurologic, and immunologic functions and include such phenomena as increased hepatic synthesis of the so-called **acute phase proteins,** leukocytosis of primarily circulating immature leukocytes, decreased plasma iron and zinc levels, variable polyclonal B lymphocyte activation, transient negative nitrogen balance, and other clinical changes such as increased erythrocyte sedimentation rate, fever, and decreased appetite. A fundamental event in the acute phase response appears to be the production of and release to the circulation of IL-1, which acts somewhat like a hormone in mediating these host responses to infection and inflammation. IL-1 can directly or indirectly induce virtually all of the laboratory and clinical aspects of the acute phase response.

In response to infection, blood monocytes and tissue macrophages synthesize and release IL-1. This produces local effects by contributing to cellular infiltration and local hyperemia, stimulates the hypothalamus to result in the production of fever, and acts directly on the bone marrow to affect the release of neutrophils to the circulation. There is also increased hepatic amino acid uptake and synthesis of acute proteins such as **C-reactive protein,** although albumin synthesis is actually reduced. Local effects of IL-1 include stimulation of PGE$_2$ and latent proteinase production, fibroblast proliferation, and the attraction of inflammatory cells such as neutrophils and monocytes as well as T and B lymphocytes. Thus, while the biochemical specifics of many IL-1 activities remain to be fully elucidated, it is clear that IL-1 is an important mediator of host responses to infection and inflammation. One additional important function of IL-1 is to stimulate certain subpopulations of lymphocytes to produce "lymphokines," the most notable being interleukin-2 (IL-2). IL-2 plays an important immunologic role by providing the growth signal for clonal expansion of various helper, suppressor, and cytotoxic lymphocyte populations (*see* Chapter 5). Studies on the structure and function of different molecular forms of IL-1 will probably have enormous clinical application. Strategies for the development of IL-1 antagonists will be developed, and recombinant DNA methods may yield molecules potentially useful in selected types of therapy.

Tumor Necrosis Factor

The current knowledge about this fascinating molecule comes from two rather divergent avenues of investigation. It was originally isolated from macrophages, in a series of studies on the pathogenesis of cachexia in chronic disease, as a M_r 17,000 polypeptide hormone called **cachectin.** It was produced in considerable amounts by endotoxin-stimulated macrophages and was responsible for the lipemia and lipoprotein lipase suppression characteristic of certain chronic infections. **Tumor necrosis factor (TNF)** was first described as a protein in the serum of Bacillus-Calmette-Guerin BCG)–primed and endotoxin-treated animals that produced hemorrhagic necrosis of tumors *in vivo* and tumor cell necrosis *in vitro*. TNF was also shown to be a macrophage product of about M_r 17,000. Although initially described *via* quite different lines of investigation, one aimed at cachexia and the other at tumor necrosis, cachectin and TNF have in the last two years been shown to be the same molecule, by both amino acid homology and genetic sequence analysis. This is, of course, not the first example of how two fishing lines can end at the same fish; we have already discussed how "endogenous pyrogen" and

"leukocyte endogenous mediator" became IL-1.

What does this molecule do? Is it important? The mechanism by which TNF elicits shock and hemorrhagic tumor necrosis remains unclear, but it probably serves as a proximal mediator for the effects of bacterial lipopolysaccharide (endotoxin) by initiating a large number of secondary events including alterations in vascular endothelium and the generation of various local inflammatory mediators. As such, TNF is currently envisioned as one of the principal mediators in the pathogenesis of Gram-negative (endotoxin-induced) shock. It has also been considered as an endogenous antineoplastic agent, that is, as a potential explanation of the phenomenon of tumor surveillance (*see* Chapter 6). Irrespective of the roles in which it was originally cast, TNF has emerged in recent years as an active general mediator of inflammation. In this setting, it seems to play an important part in diverse disease processes.

TNF is an endogenous pyrogen, inducing fever both directly and by peripheral induction of IL-1. It is also capable of stimulating PGE_2 and collagenase production, activating neutrophils and endothelial cells to make them more adhesive, and enhancing phagocytosis. TNF is primarily a macrophage product, and the major stimulus for its production is bacterial lipopolysaccharide (endotoxin). TNF exhibits a remarkable number of biological activities similar to those of IL-1. Induction of IL-1 by TNF and of TNF by IL-1 is known to occur, which may account for some of their overlapping biological activities, but the functional similarity of the two molecules is still striking. Both can induce C-reactive protein synthesis, increase prostaglandin and collagenase synthesis, induce fever, activate neutrophils, enhance expression of procoagulant activity on endothelial cells, and produce filbroblast proliferation, among other things. This is all the more remarkable since IL-1 and TNF are biochemically and immunologically distinct molecules which share no structural homology and do not recognize the same cellular receptor. It may be that the importance of these various inflammatory and host defense functions has merely necessitated a redundancy in the means by which the required functions can be achieved. This would be in keeping with the concept of the inflammatory response as a fundamental survival mechanism.

Platelet-Activating Factor

This important low molecular weight phospholipid was first described as a fluid-phase mediator of acute allergic reactions, released from antigen-stimulated leukocytes (basophils), which activated platelets to aggregate and release their stores of bioactive chemicals. Platelet-activating factor (**PAF**) is now recognized to be a potent stimulus of the acute inflammatory process and to function in a much broader sense than was originally conceived. PAF is produced by a wide variety of activated inflammatory cells including neutrophils, basophils, monocytes and macrophages, eosinophils, platelets, and vascular endothelium. A long list of mediators can stimulate such cells to produce PAF, including products of complement activation (C5a) and blood coagulation (thrombin) as well as phagocytic stimuli. In these cells, PAF is not preformed but requires cell activation for its biosynthesis.

All PAFs were originally thought to be biochemically identical, but refinements in isolation procedures (especially high-performance liquid chromatography, **HPLC**) have made it clear that there are several closely related species of PAF; at least 16 different forms can be released from stimulated neutrophils. The relationship of biochemical structure to biological activity has been extensively studied, since it may provide a basis for molecular modulation of the inflammatory effects of PAF and open potential therapeutic avenues. It is not our purpose to present these biochemical details beyond noting that PAF is a unique glycerophospholipid in which a single structural feature, the acetyl group esterified at the sn-2 position, seems essential for bioactivity. Because of its importance, many pharmaceutical companies are actively working on the biochemistry and biosynthesis of PAF with an eye toward the development of specific antagonists.

PAF-induced effects on various inflammatory cell populations as well as induced intravascular, pulmonary, and cardiovascular alterations have been implicated in the development of a growing list of disease conditions. PAF causes aggregation and secretion in platelets as well as chemotaxis, enhanced adhesiveness, aggregation, lysosomal enzyme release, and superoxide anion production in neutrophils. Similar effects have been described for monocytes and macrophages. The pulmonary effects of PAF include increased airway resistance, edema formation, and decreased compliance, while a range of cardiovascular effects including conduction arrhythmias and systemic hypotension have been described. Thus, this single small mediator has a wide range of potent proinflammatory effects involving a wide variety of cells and tissue types. The precise role of PAF in the initiation and maintenance of tissue injury and in the myriad of interactions among the involved cells will require additional research, but it is clear that PAF is one of the most potent and widely distributed of the inflammatory mediators.

Products of Blood Coagulation

The interface between the clotting and fibrinolytic systems and inflammation is very clear to anyone who has spent much time in the microscopic examination of inflamed tissues. Fibrin deposits are extremely common in many types of acute inflammatory responses, and they sometimes are so predominant as to form the basis for descriptive naming of the lesions; *e.g.,* fibrinous bronchopneumonia (*see* Figs. 4.7 and 4.8). In the process of conversion of fibrinogen to fibrin, **fibrinopeptides** are formed, some of which have biological activity as mediators of vascular permeability and the chemotaxis of leukocytes. In addition, fibrinolytic activity generated to resolve tissue fibrin deposits also contributes to inflammation. The details of the proteolytic attack of plasmin on fibrin clots are important since the breakdown products of fibrinogen/fibrin (called **fibrin degradation products, FDPs**) can have considerable relevance to ongoing inflammatory reactions.

The major biological activity of the FDPs is their anticoagulant activities mediated by competitive inhibition of the clotting action of thrombin on fibrinogen substrates. In addition, the smaller FDPs impair platelet adhesiveness, aggregation, and release reactions, while the larger ones may have an opposite effect. Some of the FDPs can also cause smooth muscle contraction, increase capillary permeability, and induce the chemotaxis of granulocytes. Because of their biological importance, it is common in clinical medicine to measure the circulating levels of FDPs. Elevated levels of FDPs in the circulation are used as an indication of clinically important states of elevated fibrinolysis such as disseminated intravascular coagulation (DIC) which may follow Gram-negative sepsis, surgical trauma, shock, and different infectious and neoplastic disease states.

Lysosomal Enzymes as Mediators

We have already discussed the various means by which leukocytes, principally neutrophils and macrophages, can release lysosomal enzymes as a secretory response, as part of the phagocytic process or after death of the cells. Lysosomal enzymes may be mediators of inflammation in their own right, or they may act extracellularly on appropriate nonlysosomal substrates to produce biologically active substance. For example, certain of these enzymes can produce active cleavage products from complement proteins. In addition, the generation of factors that will attract leukocytes, through the action of lysosomal enzymes, is a potential mechanism for self-perpetuation of leukotaxis; chemotactic factors attract white blood cells, which participate in the inflammatory reaction and in so doing generate chemotactic factors and so on. Other lysosomal constituents, for example collagenase and elastase, can directly damage tissue.

The lysosomal enzymes of phagocytic cells are recognized as potential mediators of vascular injury. Because of the time sequence of appearance of these cells in evolving inflammatory reactions, lysosomal enzymes may be involved in the mediation of the delayed or prolonged phase of increased vascular permeability. They also explain why hemorrhage and thrombosis are sometimes seen in severe forms of acute inflammation. Neutrophils have a rather short life span, and they may merely disintegrate at sites of inflammation where they have accumulated, and thereby release materials that either directly promote damage or interact with other systems or cells capable of generating damage. It is becoming increasingly clear that such cells also release mediators when they phagocytose microorganisms, antigen-antibody complexes, or perhaps even fragments of necrotic tissue as part of their "clean up" function. Further, there is now good evidence that this release of enzymes can be an active secretory process not necessitating cell death.

Lysosomes represent a group of cytoplasmic organelles first described in 1955. Their existence was initially postulated solely on the basis of biochemical data, but it later was confirmed with the aid of morphologic techniques. Lysosomes are bounded by a unit membrane and have a more or less homogeneous inner core. They usually measure 0.25–0.5 microns but may become as large as 3 microns in diameter. Lysosomes that have not participated in cellular digestion are referred to as "primary lysosomes." Some of these have been called "storage granules," such as those of the neutrophil leukocytes. When a cell has ingested material by phagocytosis or pinocytosis (endocytosis), the vacuole is referred to as a "phagosome." When the phagoctic vacuole or phagosome has fused with a lysosome, the structure is called a "phagolysosome" or "digestive vacuole."

Our knowledge of the role of leukocytes in defense against bacterial invasion dates back to Metchnikoff, who showed around the turn of the century that these cells accumulate at the site of bacterial infection. He also postulated that they release their "cytases," bringing about death of the microorganisms. These "cytases" have since been identified as lysosomal hydrolases.

While the defensive role of leukocytes has been accepted generally, it was not until recently that these cells were implicated in tissue injury and inflammation. Many types of severe inflammatory lesions have been shown to be dependent on neutrophils. Such lesions cannot be elicited in leukopenic animals. Several *in vivo* studies have implicated neutrophil leukocytes and their lysosomes in inflammatory reactions. The vasculitis of serum-sickness and nephrotoxic nephritis is diminished considerably in leukopenic animals. Passive cutaneous anaphylaxis (PCA) reactions induced with homologous or heterologous antibody can be inhibited with an antileukocyte serum that causes leukopenia. Here too, phagocytosis of antigen-antibody aggregates and degranulation can be demonstrated ultrastructurally. The mode of action of leukocytes and their granules on the terminal vascular bed and on cells appears to be complex, with several substances participating. The lysosomal enzymes of leukocytes must therefore be considered as important contributors to evolving inflammatory responses. As such, they must be considered legitimate mediators of inflammation.

HUMORAL AMPLIFICATION SYSTEMS IN INFLAMMATION

As we have noted previously, the inflammatory response is essentially one of drawing blood-borne defenses into tissue sites where injury is taking place. It is now clear that in addition to the important contributions made by hemodynamic and permeability adjustments and leukocytic events, complicated and closely interdigitated humoral amplification systems exist to expand the blood-borne contribution to the inflammatory response. Of these humoral amplifiers, the **Hageman factor–dependent pathways** (contact system) for kinin generation, coagulation, and fibrinolysis, and the **complement system** have been best characterized.

Hageman Factor–Dependent Pathways

The complicated interactions of the components of the Hageman factor (HF)–dependent systems for kinin generation, fibrinolysis, and coagulation in the pathogenesis of inflammation is not completely understood, although the involved plasma proteins have been fairly well characterized. The components of this system (clotting Factors XI and XII, prekallikrein, HMW kininogen, and plasminogen) consist of a series of zymogens that, upon activation by limited proteolytic cleavage on a negatively charged surface, act sequentially to mediate three distinct processes: the generation of kinins, the generation of fibrin, and the generation of fibrinolytic agents (Fig. 4.38). A fourth function, activation of the complement cascade, can occur secondarily.

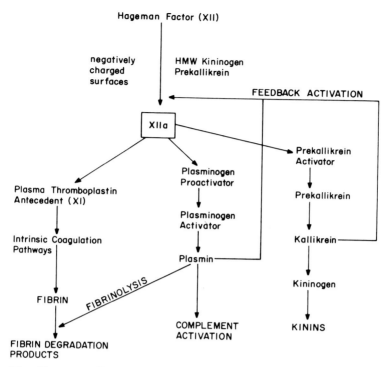

Figure 4.38. The Hageman Factor-Dependent Pathways. Activation of Hageman factor (XII) provides a means of access to four systems of importance to inflammation: intrinsic coagulation, fibrinolysis, kinin generation, and complement activation. Cyclical activation can occur *via* plasmin and kallikrein. (HMW, high molecular weight.)

We have already discussed many of the activation mechanisms and the biological activities associated with activation of the contact system related to intrinsic coagulation and fibrinolysis (*see* Chapter 3), as well as kinin generation. In brief, the component proteins are activated by limited proteolytic cleavage, which exposes the active site in each except for HMW kininogen, which acts as a sort of cofactor in bringing prekallikrein and factor XI (plasma thromboplastin antecedent, PTA) to the negative charged surface so that these molecules can interact with Hageman factor (XII). It is suspected that several biologically relevant negatively charged surfaces such as insoluble collagen, cartilage, basement membrane, sodium urate crystals, and perhaps even antigen-antibody complexes can subserve

this function. During activation, the molecules are split into light and heavy chains that are linked by disulfide bridges. Hageman factor (XII) and the complex of prekallikrein (PK) and HMW kininogen circulate in the plasma, and factor XI (PTA) and HMW kininogen may also exist in plasma as a complex. When assembled on a negatively charged surface, Hageman factor (XII) and the PK-HMW kininogen complex become bound to the surface because of the positively charged residues in the heavy chain of Hageman factor (XII) and a histidine-rich portion of the light chain of HMW kininogen. In this fashion, Hageman factor (XII) are brought into apposition on the surface and are activated. Hageman factor (XII) and PK are sometimes referred to as "active zymogens" because they can induce a triggering event leading to cleavage and activation when they are brought into contact with each other.

Initiation of this system produces activated Hageman factor (XIIa) to initiate intrinsic coagulation through factor XI (PTA) and fibrinolysis through the effects of kallikrein on phasminogen. The coagulation process itself, we must recall, is an almost constant feature of inflammation and at times the most detrimental aspect of an evolving inflammatory reaction when fibrin deposition is extensive. As we have discussed, kinin generation in the fluid phase in plasma is also intimately tied to this contact activation system. The cleavage of PK produces kallikrein, which cleaves bradykinin from HMW kininogen both on the negatively charged surface and in the nearby fluid phase. Thus, activation of the contact system initates the biochemical reactions leading to kinin generation, intrinsic coagulation, and fibrinolysis. In addition, both plasmin and kallikrein can feed back into the system to cleave additional native Hageman factor (XII), thus providing a mechanism for cyclic activation.

The link between the contact system and the complement system completes this "tangled web" of carefully balanced biochemical reactions. Activation of the complement system in this setting is secondary, and dependent on the generation of the enzymes plasmin and kallikrein during contact activation of plasma. Plasmin and kallikrein are apparently capable of cleavage activation of the complement proteins C1, C3, and C5, although the physiological significance of some of these *in vitro* cleavage reactions is questionable. In addition, thrombin generated through Hageman factor (XII)–mediated intrinsic coagulation can also cleave C3 and C5. Thus, the complement proteins may be drawn into this contact system network by the broad substrate spectrum of some of the potent enzymes generated

during contact activation. In addition, the plasmin generated liberates, from both fibrin and fibrinogen, fragments that are capable of increasing vascular permeability and eliciting a chemotactic response for neutrophils.

Lastly, there is growing evidence that activated Hageman factor (XIIa) is itself a mediator. The activated β-fragment of Hageman factor (XII) appears to be a potent permeability factor, which may be identical to a fragment identified years ago in dilute plasma and called permeability factor-dilute (**PF-dil).** More recent studies with the purified β-fragment document that it is a potent permeability-inducing agent some 10 to 100 times more potent than bradykinin. Furthermore, this β-fragment seems to work at physiological concentrations (less than a ng/ml) representing less than 1/10,000th of the amount of β-fragment present in 1 ml of plasma. As more biochemically pure components of this unique contact activation system become available, the multiplicity of function ascribed to its activation products will no doubt be further clarified.

Although the precise mechanism by which the contact system participates in the development of the inflammation are not well understood, ample evidence indicates that many of the features of the inflammatory process can be traced to activated products of the system (Table 4.19). The potentially injurious functions of the component proteins and their cleavage fragments may be of particular clinical importance. In addition to playing a broad role in inflammation, coagulation, and fibrinolysis, activation of the contact system has been linked to such diverse clinical conditions as disseminated intravascular coagulation (DIC), arthritis, shock, the nephrotic syndrome, allergic airway disease, the carcinoid syndrome, and typhoid fever.

It is clear that the contact system involves a number of biologically important

Table 4.19
Amplified Inflammatory Activities Following Contact Activation

Function	Basis
Fibrin deposition	Intrinsic coagulation
Vasodilation	Kinin generation
Vascular permeability	Kinins, activated Hageman factor, fibrinopeptides
Pain induction	Kinins
Histamine release	Kinins
Smooth muscle contraction	Kinins, FDPs[a]
Chemotaxis	Fibrinopeptides, FDPs, kallikrein
Fibrinolysis	*via* plasminogen activation
Complement activation	Plasmin, kallikrein

[a] Abbreviation used is FDPs, fibrin degradation products.

pathways. Activated Hageman factor (XIIa) can set these pathways in motion, but activation of the system is not completely tied to contact activation, since other enzymes, derived from cells, are capable of activating individual components of the system. In particular, recent studies have defined a role for leukocyte enzymes in this regard. Neutrophil elastase, for example, can activate HMW kininogen, kallikrein, and Hageman factor (XII). We can expect a far better understanding of the interactions between cellular factors and components of the contact system in plasma in the future. The contact system thus represents a major system in plasma for enhancing inflammation, and its activation can serve as a critical relating four different and important systems; blood coagulation, fibrinolysis, kinin generation, and complement activation. The contact system of plasma, summarized in Figure 4.38, thus clearly qualifies as an important humoral amplification system.

Complement System and Inflammation

The complement system really **is** a system, even though it is often referred to as a single entity, "complement." It was discovered in the late 1800s as the heat-labile principle in fresh guinea pig serum which was required for bactericidal activity in serum from immune guinea pigs. Complement thus *complements* the action of antibody in the killing of bacteria. It is the main means by which antibodies function in host defense against most bacterial infections, and many complement components participate in other functions important to host defense and the inflammatory reaction. Complement is a complex series of interacting protein components designated as C1, C2, C3, C4, C5, C6, C7, C8, and C9 for the **classical pathway,** as factor B, factor D, factor H, factor I, and properdin for the **alternate pathway** of activation, and a variety of regulatory protein molecules (Table 4.20).

Like the coagulation system, the complement proteins circulate as precursor soluble proteins (zymogens), which are generally inactive unless triggered. The activated complement components, however, are **enzymes,** and they interact sequentially in an ordered and well-understood fashion in the **classical pathway** of antibody-directed cell lysis. It is now also well established that complement components can be activated *via* pathways not requiring antibody, as in the alternate pathway that is induced by bacterial cell wall components. A variety of enzymes from sources not intrinsic to the classic complement sequence, such as plasmin, kallikrein, and the lysosomal enzymes of leukocytes, can activate some of the complement components. Consequently it is likely that complement has the potential to be activated in any situation in which leukocytes have accumulated, since lysosomal enzymes can be released from leukocytes during the course of phagocytosis or following their degeneration or death.

Upon activation, the various components of the complement sequence (Table 4.20) interact sequentially in a self-assembling cascade fashion reminiscent of the coagulation cascades. The primary target of most complement-mediated reactions is biological membranes. Complement may cause impairment of biological membranes and thus lead to cytolysis, or it can affect cell membranes *via* specific complement receptors. In this way it can cause activation of specific cellular functions such as enhanced vascular permeability, smooth muscle contraction, chemotactic attraction of leukocytes, release of mediators from mast cells, immune adherence, degranulation and release of lysosomal enzymes from neutrophils and enhanced phagocytosis. It is through these diverse biological activities of the cells affected by complement that the system participates in inflammatory reactions.

Complement Activation

Two major pathways for activating the complement sequence are now recognized. They are the **classical** pathway and the **alternate** pathway. The sequence

Table 4.20
Principal Components of the Classical and Alternate Complement Pathways

Component	Function
Classical	
C1q	Binds to antibody; reveals active site on C1r
C1r	Cleaves C1s to reveal active subunit
C1s	Cleaves C4 and C2 to form the C3 convertase
C2	Converted by C1s to C2a and C2b
C4	Converted by C1s to C4a and C4b
C4b2a	Classical C3 convertase
C3	Most abundant component; cleaved by classical C3 convertase
C3a	Cleavage product of C3; anaphylatoxin
C3b	Cleavage product of C3; opsonin; part of C5 convertase
C4b2a3b	Classical C5 convertase
C5	Substrate for C5 convertase
C5a	Cleavage product of C5; anaphylatoxin
C5b	Binds C3b on membrane; initiates membrane attack sequence
C6	Binds to C5b as bimolecular complex
C7	Binds to C5bC3b; inserts into lipid bilayer
C8	Binds to C5b-7 and inserts in membrane; initiates leakage
C9	Bound to and polymerized by C5b-8; insertion of poly C9 into membrane produces lesion leading to lysis
C1-INH	Control molecule; inhibits C1 activation as well other enzymes
Alternate	
C3	Source of C3b for alternate pathway C3 convertase activity
Factor B	Cleaved by Factor D to form Bb for C3 convertase
Factor D	Active serine protease; cleaves factor B bound to C3b
C3bBb	Alternate C3 convertase; can bind additional C3b
C3bBbC3b	Alternate pathway C5 convertase
Factor H	Control molecule; restricts alternate C3 convertase formation
Factor I	Control molecule; cleaves C3b to inactive form C3bi
Properdin	Positive regulator; binds to and stabilizes C3bBb convertase

of biochemical events involved in the classical activation of complement is a well-documented, although somewhat complicated, story. In the presence of two or more molecules of IgG or at least one molecule of IgM bound to a cell wall (bacterium), the three subunits of C1, named **C1q, C1r,** and **C1s,** become associated in equimolar amounts as a precursor macromolecular complex (Fig. 4.39). C1q is a unique globular protein with 6 protruding collagen-like appendages which is capable of interacting with a site on the Fc portion of certain complexed or aggregated immunoglobulins. This interaction leads to a conformational change in C1q which is transmitted to C1r, and the C1r subunit becomes a proteolytic enzyme (a serine protease), which activates C1s by cleavage to yield activated C1s. The natural substrates of activated C1s are C4 and C2 (Fig. 4.40). C4 is cleaved by activated C1s, and the major fragment, C4b, is bound to the complex, markedly enhancing the subsequent cleavage of C2 by activated C1s. The major fragment of C2, C2a, binds to C4b to form a new enzymatically active bimolecular complex, C4b2a, or **C3 convertase.** This complex is unstable and rapidly decays, releasing C2d into the fluid phase; but the active C42 site may be regenerated with native C2. In the course of activation of C2, a kinin-like activity, **C-kinin,** which is distinct from bradykinin, is generated.

In the next stage of the complement sequence, the newly formed enzyme, C3 convertase, splits C3 into two fragments (Fig. 4.41). The smaller fragment, **C3a,** is an anaphylatoxin and potent inflammatory mediator, as we have discussed. The larger fragment is bound to the complex as the important opsonin **C3b,** or is released into the fluid phase as the inactive decay fragment C3i. When bound to the complex, C3b confers the property of **immune adherence,** the ability of the complex to bind to erythrocytes, neutrophils, platelets, and bone marrow–derived lymphocytes. In fact, C3b can bind

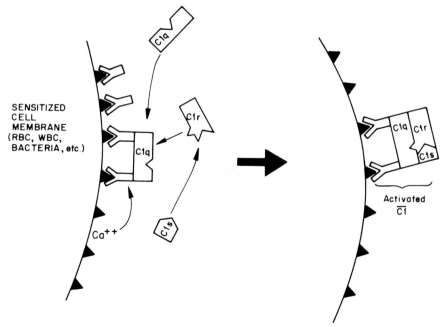

Figure 4.39.   Activation of C1. Antibody binds to antigen on the cell surface. Serum *C1q* binds to the Fc portion of immunoglobulin and then *C1r* and *C1s* attach to bound *C1q* in the presence of calcium ions. The binding and activation of *C1s* completes the activation of *C1*.

Figure 4.40. Activation of C4 and C2. The natural substrates for activated C1 are *C4* and *C2*. The cleavage fragments *C4b* and *C2a* become bound in a molecular complex in the presence of magnesium ions, and the activated *C4b2a* enzyme is known as *C3 convertase,* which can act upon native *C3* to produce cleavage.

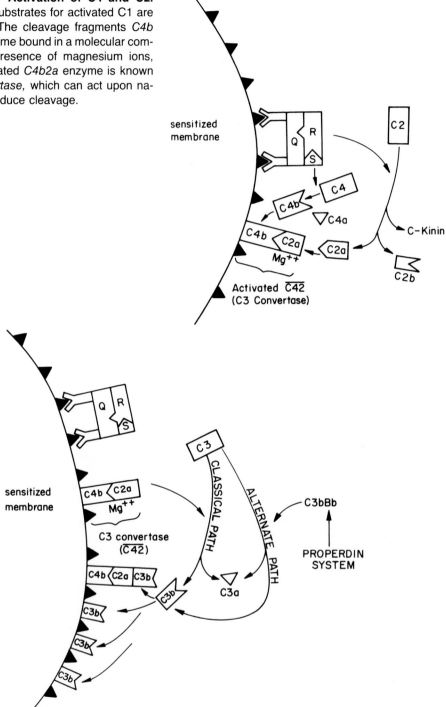

Figure 4.41. Activation of C3. Both the *C3 convertase (C4b2a)* generated *via* the classical pathway and the C3 convertase *(C3bBb)* generated *via* the alternate pathway can cleave native *C3* into two major fragments. The *C3a* fragment is an anaphylatoxin, while the *C3b* fragment becomes bound to the complex, where it modifies the activated *C4b2a* enzyme so that C5 convertase activity *(C4b2a3b)* is generated.

independent of C4 and C2. Fixation of C3b to the complex modifies the activated C4b2a enzyme so that it develops new enzymatic specifity, termed **C5 convertase** (activated C4b2a3b), able to split C5 into two fragments (Fig. 4.42). The smaller fragment, **C5a,** is released into the fluid phase and is both an anaphylatoxin and a chemotactic factor for polymorphonuclear leukocytes and monocytes. The larger fragment, **C5b,** becomes complex-bound but is unstable and rapidly decays. This nascent C5b fragment becomes the focal point for the nonenzymatic allosteric adsorption and eventual assembly of C6, C7, C8, and C9 into the **C5b-C9** cytolytic complex capable of behaving as the **"membrane attack complex" (MAC)** in complement-mediated cell lysis.

The mechanism by which the membrane attack complex functions has been detailed only fairly recently. When C5 is cleaved by C5 convertase and C5b is produced, self-assembly of the MAC is initiated. C5b and C6 form a stable bimolecular complex that binds to C7, causing C7 to express a site through which the C5b-7 complex can bind to the cell membrane. This C5b-7 complex bound to the cell membrane becomes the receptor for C8 binding, and the subsequent C5b-8 complex can bind and polymerize C9. In this regard, it should be noted that C8 has no detectable affinity for membranes by itself and is therefore entirely dependent on the mediating function of C5b-7, which not only determines the site of membrane attack but also serves as the C8 receptor. The fully assembled complex is a unique molecular creature containing a single molecule each of C5b, C6, C7, and C8 and multiple molecules of C9; it is basically an enormous complex made up of the tetramolecular C5b-8 complex (M_r

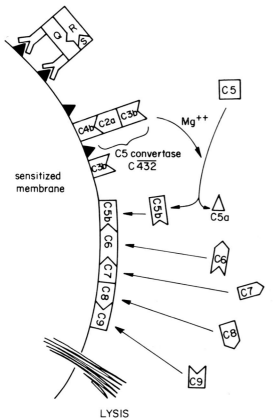

Figure 4.42. Activation of C5 and the Terminal Complement Sequence. The *C5 convertase (C4b2a3b)* generated cleaves native *C5* into two major fragments. The *C5a* fragment is a potent anaphylatoxin and chemotactic agent, while *C5b* becomes membrane bound. The binding of *C6* stabilizes the bound *C5b*, and the subsequent binding of *C7, C8,* and *C9* produces lysis by forming transmembrane channels in the lipid bilayer of the membrane.

about 500,000) and tubular poly C9 (M_r approximately 1,100,000). The MAC becomes inserted in the cell membrane, and is so large that it is actually visible in electron micrographs as "holes" in the membrane which have a 100 angstrom–wide central pore surrounded by a 50 angstrom–wide rim. These characteristic and well-known images of the MAC and the membrane lesions produced by complement are by and large due to the tubular poly C9 contained in the MAC. Current evidence strongly suggests that the tubular poly C9 inserted in the cell membrane represents the major complement transmembrane channel and that the tetramolecular C5b-8 complex is the unit that catalyzes the polymerization of C9.

Actual membrane leakiness can be detected prior to complete assembly of the MAC. In the absence of C9, the C5b-8 complex tends to aggregate in the cell membrane, and these large protein aggregates produce structural and functional membrane damage evidenced by leakiness. It appears that tubular poly C9 may not be entirely necessary for the lysis of anucleate cells such as bacteria and erythrocytes, but may be essential for the killing of nucleated cells. There are two distinct ways in which the large C5b-8 complex, with a combined M_r of close to 600,000, acts on C9: binding, and polymerization. Both the binding and the polymerization reactions can proceed irrespective of whether C5b-8 is membrane-bound or free in plasma, although the consequences in terms of cell lysis are obviously different. Binding of C9 occurs *via* the C8 part of the C5b-8 complex, but it is not known precisely how C5b-8 causes C9 polymerization. What *is* known is that polymerization of C9 occurs, and that the tubular poly C9 that results and is inserted into the cell membrane corresponds almost exactly with the electron microscopic images of complement-damaged cells; there is little doubt that the "holes" seen in such membranes are evoked by poly C9.

With the binding of C9, an accelerated influx of water and sodium ions into the cell occurs, and intracellular potassium is lost to the extracellular fluid. These water and electrolyte fluxes across the transmembrane channel create severe ionic disequilibrium, which eventually leads to osmotic rupture of the cell. The cell becomes an empty sac and is removed by the phagocytic systems.

In 1954, a new activity (termed **properdin**) was described, which participated in the activation of C3 through C9 but appeared not to be dependent on antibody. Since this **"alternate pathway"** was activated by bacterial cell wall components and did not require antibodies, it was seen to be a more natural or nonspecific mechanism of host defense and probably the major pathway for complement activation in the early stages of infection, prior to the synthesis of complement-fixing antibodies in response to the invader. It is now clear that the cofactors for properdin are distinct from the classic complement components. The properdin system is now understood to be an alternate pathway for the activation of the terminal complement components, independent of C1, C4, and C2.

The reactions of the alternate pathway system are now as well studied as those of the classical complement sequence. The properdin system consists of at least 3 activities, factor B, factor D, and C3, as well as the regulatory molecules factor H, factor I, and properdin itself. Activation of the alternate pathway may be initiated by microorganisms or by aggregated immunoglobulins of certain classes. The site on rabbit and guinea pig immunoglobulins responsible for the activation of the alternative pathway is distinct from the C1q-fixing site and resides in a part of the heavy chain near the hinge region on both the Fc fragment and the F(ab)$_2$ fragment. The alternate pathway can also be activated by certain insoluble polysaccharides independent of immunoglobulins.

The initial reactions of the alternate pathway occur when certain microbial polysaccharides interact with factors B, D, and C3 to produce cleavage of C3. The major cleavage product of C3 is C3b (as in classical cleavage), which then interacts with alternate pathway components B and D to form a C3 convertase (activated C3bBb), which can activate more C3 thus forming the so-called "C3 amplification loop." The means by which this comes to be have only recently been elucidated. C3b serves as a receptor for factor B in a magnesium-dependent binding reaction that ultimately reveals the active site in factor B for C3 cleavage. The bound factor B is then cleaved by factor E, with a smaller fragment (Ba) being removed from the major fragment (Bb). This larger fragment (Bb) remains bound to the activated complex of C3bBb, which can cleave native C3, thus gaining access to the terminal classical complement sequence beyond C3. Properdin binds to the alternate pathway C3 convertase, C3bBb, and increases the stability of the complex. Factor H also binds to C3b and modulates its functions; it is thought to restrict the formation of the C3bBb convertase by competing with factor B for its binding site on C3b. Factor I is also a regulatory molecule that cleaves and inactivates C3b as well as other components.

It should be stressed that amidst all these hieroglyphics, two major facts must emerge. **First,** the key complement component around which both the classical and alternate pathways revolve is C3. **Second,** after C3 cleavage either by C3 convertase (activated C4a2b) in the classical pathway or by C3 convertase (activated C3bBb) in the alternate pathway, activation of the terminal complement components proceeds in a similar fashion and the biological activities that result are identical. Thus, while two activation schemes provide flexibility in host defense, the ultimate functional consequences of complement activation are the same.

Complement Functions in Inflammation and Host Defense

In discussing the complement activation sequence above, we have talked largely in terms of membrane events leading to lysis of a target cell or bacterium. Equally or possibly more important to inflammation is the elaboration of soluble fluid-phase products and cell-bound fragments that act as important mediators of the inflammatory and other biological responses (Table 4.21). Some of these biological functions merit our special attention.

Virus neutralization by antibody can be enhanced in the presence of C1 and C4, and, in the case where antibody concentrations are low, by fixation of C3b. It seems likely, then, that complement may be extremely helpful in the early stages of some viral infections, when antibody titers are low.

Hereditary angioedema (HAE) is a disease of man mediated by a low molecular weight fragment derived from C2 cleavage, which has kinin-like activity (C-kinin). The action of C1 is normally regulated by a plasma glycoprotein called C1-inhibitor (C-INH). This inhibitor binds stoichiometrically with C1r and C1s in the C1qrs complex to inhibit their activities, thus preventing C1 activation and the further assembly of the C3 convertase (activated C4b2a). A deficiency of this control protein has been defined in human HAE patients. In the absence of C1-INH, uncontrolled production of the C2 kinin occurs, which is apparently responsible for producing the episodic attacks of cutaneous, respiratory, and gastrointestinal edema characteristic of HAE. There are no well defined HAE-like syndromes in animals.

Immune adherence is the phenomenon by which cells or particles bind to specific receptor sites on neutrophils, monocytes, macrophages, and platelets, thus enhancing phagocytosis (opsonization). This important biological phenom-

Table 4.21
Selected Biologic Activities of Complement-derived Mediators

Component or Fragment	Biologic Function
C1q	Binds to IgG and IgM
C14, C1423	Viral neutralization
C4a	Weak anaphylatoxin
C4b	Immune adherence and enhancement of phagocytosis; Antibody-formation
C2 fragment	C2 kinin; (increase vascular permeability, edema)
C3a	Histamine release, smooth muscle contraction, increased capillary permeability, lysosomal enzyme release
C3e	Induction of leukopenia and leukocytosis
C3b	Activation of the alternative complement pathway, immune adherence, enhanced opsonization, enhanced induction of antibody formation, enhancement of antibody-dependent cellular cytotoxicity, stimulation of B cell lymphokine production, *etc.*
C3d	Immune adherence *via* receptors on lymphocytes and macrophages
C5a	Histamine release, smooth muscle contraction, increased capillary permeability, chemotaxis of leukocytes, leukocyte secretion, increased adhesiveness and aggregation, *etc.*
C5b	Opsonization of fungi; initiates membrane damage
C6	Promotion of blood coagulation
C5b-9	Membrane attack sequence

enon is due to C3b binding to the surface of the cells or particles. C3b also has other apparent functions, as it can stimulate lymphocytes to produce a chemotactic factor for macrophages. The binding of C3b to lymphocytes also may facilitate antibody production by B cells and enhance antibody-dependent cellular cytotoxicity.

Anaphylatoxin generation refers to the biological activities of the complement cleavage peptides C3a and C5a. The C3 convertase generated from either classical or alternate pathway complement activation, along with other noncomplement proteolytic enzymes like plasmin, trypsin, lysosomal enzymes from leukocytes, and certain bacterial proteinases, can release C3a by cleavage of native C3. This fragment obeys the definition of an anaphylatoxin in that it can cause increased vascular permeability when in-

jected intradermally, causes smooth muscle contraction, and releases mediators such as histamine from mast cells. Similar activity can be generated by C5a, which is cleaved from native C5 by C5 convertase, as well as a similar group of noncomplement proteolytic enzymes that can function to cleave C5.

C5a is believed to be the classical or principal anaphylatoxin. Its biological functions are similar to those described above for C3a and include interaction with mast cell and basophil receptors to cause degranulation and histamine release, smooth muscle contraction, and increased vascular permeability. It is of further interest that C5a can promote chemotaxis and mediate the release of lysosomal enzymes from neutrophil leukocytes. This gives the system a self-amplification loop in that initial complement activation will generate C3a and C5a, which, *via* their effects on neutrophils, cause release of enzymes capable of cleaving additional native C3 and C5 to generate more C3a and C5a. Thus, certain key features of the inflammatory response are at least partially contingent on the activities of C3a and C5a. Although these peptides have similar biological activities, they differ in potency and receptor specificity. C3a is less potent than C5a, and each peptide seems to react with different membrane receptors.

Chemotaxis refers to the directed migration of leukocytes in response to specific chemical signals. The complement system is an important source of chemotactic factors that mediate the local accumulation of leukocytes at sites of acute inflammation. The most important complement-derived chemotaxin is C5a. **Other biological functions** of the complement system have been less well detailed than virus neutralization, immune adherence, anaphylatoxin generation, and chemotaxis. Recently, **C3e,** a low molecular weight fragment of C3 distinct from C3a, has been characterized and shown to either induce the release of leukocytes from bone marrow or mediate sequestration of leukocytes in the marginal pool. This fragment is probably what was once called **leukocyte immobilization factor,** and it may play a role in neutrophilia or neutropenia seen in inflammation. The complement protein **C6** has been reported to be required for normal blood coagulation, at least in rabbits. Rabbits deficient in C6 have prolonged clotting times, and this defect can be corrected by the addition of purified C6. **Neutralization of endotoxin** and protection from its lethal effects in animals may require the complement proteins, at least through C6. Target cells bearing complement components C1–C7 are more readily damaged by lymphocytes, thus providing a means for amplified cellular cytotoxicity. The complement system interacts with **plate-** lets in several ways, thus bringing into play their additive functions of coagulation and mediator release.

Our understanding of the complement system has been advanced considerably since the days of Wassermann, when it was known to medical personnel largely as something one needed in syphilis serology. It is now recognized as the most important humoral amplification system and plays a broad role in such vital reactions as the inflammatory response and other host defenses against infection.

In our discussion above, we have stressed the phlogistic properties of the complement system with little attention to control mechanisms. It should be obvious that in order to avoid total complement consumption by any single complement-fixing reaction, numerous inhibitors and built-in control mechanisms must be operational. It also should be recalled that many of the active components (cleavage products) are unstable and decay rapidly. The extrinsic factors (inhibitors or inactivators of complement peptides) combine with or destroy the activated components and thus prevent the progression of the reaction sequence or destroy the pathobiologic activity of the activated product. The importance of these regulatory molecules is well illustrated in the series of diseases that are associated with absence of one or more of the inhibitors and hence uncontrolled or poorly controlled spontaneous activation of the complement system.

PERSPECTIVES ON THE INFLAMMATORY RESPONSE

The inflammatory response is both complex and varied. The basic hemodynamic and permeability changes and the infiltration of leukocytes represent its common themes, but different mixes of these common elements, different time courses, different initiating stimuli and tissue sites, and dissimilar outcomes complicate predictions of their clinical manifestations. The underlying cellular and biochemical processes themselves encompass complicated and interlacing networks of chemical signals and responses to stimulation. It may be well at this point to reiterate or summarize the key features of this complicated host defense mechanism to ensure that the intricacies of the response do not wind up masking an appreciation for the overall nature of the reaction.

You should note that two major aspects of the response are paramount: the vascular phenomena of hemodynamic and permeability changes, and the cellular events that permit plasma proteins and leukocytes to enter inflamed tissues. Throughout the response, we continually encounter two important arms of the defense reaction, humoral and cellular, which dominate discussions of inflammation much as they do immunology. Only the uninitiated would attempt to place value judgements on which arm of the response is the most important. Clearly, they are both vital and closely interactive parts of the whole, so carefully interdigitated and interdependent as to be inseparable. Nonetheless arguments still flare, centered historically on the views of Cohnheim, who attributed the bulk of inflammation to vascular phenomenology, and those of Metchnikoff, who believed inflammation to be fundamentally dependent on the activities of the leukocytes.

Recent progress in our understanding of the biochemistry of the generation and function of the various chemical mediators and humoral amplification systems has produced a new wave of excitement regarding their fundamental importance to inflammation. The application of recombinant DNA technology to these potent chemicals will only further increase our appreciation for the intricacies and specificities of their multiple interactions. By the same token, the "new biology" of leukocytes and improved understanding of the mechanisms by which their consid-

erable functional repertoire becomes activated has greatly clarified our long-standing questions regarding how these amazing cells can perform all of their unique operations.

The relatively uncomplicated past is gone. We must continue to probe disease mechanisms with new ideas and new tools. As pathologists and clinicians, we are used to dealing with lesions in our patients, but not with their molecules. We are visually oriented scientists, trained to recognize the abnormal and to interpret its significance. It is difficult for us to think of injury to molecules when viewing a swollen joint or a focus of coagulation necrosis. We are well geared for the pathology of the liver, or the pancreas, or the lung, but less oriented in the direction of injuries to the stimulus-response coupling apparatus or the pathology of ligand-receptor interaction. We all must learn to speak the language of the cell and of the molecule, while not losing sight of what it all means to the tissues, the organs, and the entire organism. We must remember that while the underlying basis may be molecular, only the entire animal can develop clinical signs and present them for our questioning. Our ability to answer those questions at the highest possible level of resolution will continue to be the challenge of modern medicine.

"Our own wronged flesh
May work undisturbed, restoring
The order we try to destroy, the rhythm
We spoil out of spite: valves close
And open exactly, glands secrete,
Vessels contract and expand
At the right moment, essential fluids
Flow to renew exhausted cells,
Not knowing quite what has happened."
W. H. Auden

HEALING AND REPAIR

If the entire inflammatory process is the most important of the host defense mechanisms, then the healing and repair of injured tissue is undoubtedly its most requisite component. It is important to perceive from the outset that **inflammation** and **repair** are intimately linked; events aimed at healing actually begin almost as soon as injury has taken place, and features central to inflammation may persist throughout the repair phases. As such, it is highly appropriate to view healing and repair as part of a continuum of loosely timed events stretched between the moment of initial injury and the final result of healing.

The repair of injury is a phylogenetically important process that occurs virtually throughout the animal kingdom and, indeed, even occurs in vegetables. It seems that the lower one goes in the animal kingdom phylogenetic tree, the more complete is **tissue regeneration** as a type of healing response. If an earthworm is decapitated, it simply forms a new head, and this process can be repeated several times. An additional example comes from the starfish, in which species repair is a sort of extension of asexual reproduction. In lower vertebrates such as amphibians, whole limbs and tails can be regenerated. Such efficiency is not, however, the province of the higher animals with which we must deal, and the acquisition of sophisticated higher mammalian functional advantages has been accompanied by certain evolutionary exchanges. We have lost the capacity for wholesale organ regeneration, and some tissues do not regenerate at all. Instead, higher mammals have developed a phenomenal capacity for the repair and/or replacement of damaged cells and tissues with less specialized connective tissue. Because of this, even mild injuries usually result in some scar tissue formation.

Healing and repair are among the more remarkable of biological phenomena. The process of repair is so customary that it is easy to overlook. It has happened to all of us at some level. If even the most sedate and quiescent of tissues are incised or otherwise damaged, within 24 hours intense cellular activity is underway to heal the defect created by the wounding process. This commonplace activity, familiar at least superficially to all of us, is deceptively simple, but under its seemingly quiet surface the waters of cell biology run deep.

The healing and repair processes in any tissue are dependent not only on the cellular composition of that tissue, but also on the nature of the injury process itself and its impact on the integrity of tissue architecture. Using the kidney as an example, a toxic injury that destroys renal tubular epithelium without injuring the more resistant connective tissues may be repaired by **regeneration,** whereas a kidney abscess that destroys the connective tissue framework as well as the epithelium will be repaired by **scarring.** The healing responses to many types of injury may involve combinations of repair by regeneration as well as scarring, but it will enhance our understanding of the underlying biology to categorize the major healing processes. We will therefore divide the repair process into two subcategories that have clinical and biological significance: (1) healing by **parenchymal regeneration,** and (2) healing by **connective tissue replacement.**

HEALING BY PARENCHYMAL REGENERATION

At a simplistic level, repair consists of the replacement of dead or damaged cells by new healthy cells derived from either the parenchymal or connective tissue elements in the damaged tissue. If the repair is accomplished largely by the regeneration of parenchymal cells, almost perfect reconstitution of the original tissue can result. A good example can be drawn from clinical medicine. In the temperate zones of North America as well as other parts of the world where cold weather highlights the winter season, people use antifreeze in their vehicles to keep the engine cooling system from freezing. The sweet taste of the ethylene glycol in anti-freeze has brought many animals to veterinarians in acute renal failure. This is due to necrosis of the renal tubular epithelial cells caused by the toxicity of ethylene glycol and its metabolites (*see* Fig. 2.20). If these patients can be kept alive by dialysis, both functional and structural recovery is usually good. The reasons for this recovery lie in the **repair by parenchymal regeneration** that takes place in the patients' kidneys. While the **function** of those kidneys is being replaced by dialysis, the **structure** of the damaged tubular epithelial cells is being restored by the regeneration of tubular epithelial cells (Fig. 4.43).

This type of clinical example can be used to illuminate two important points about parenchymal regeneration (Table 4.22). **First,** it can only eventuate in tis-

Table 4.22
Basic Important Features of Parenchymal Regeneration

Requires an intact connective tissue framework.
Can only occur in tissues composed of labile or stable parenchymal cellular elements.

sues that have the cellular capability for parenchymal regeneration. We will discuss this in more detail later on. **Second,** it can only occur if the connective tissue framework of the tissue is maintained so that the regenerating cells have an architectural framework upon which to build. In the example above, the antifreeze kills the tubular epithelial cells, but does not destroy the underlying tubular basement membranes or the connective tissue supporting network for the tubules. Hence, the framework is maintained. To better

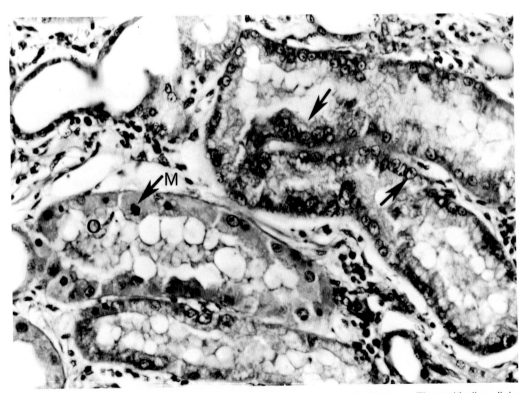

Figure 4.43.   Renal Tubular Regeneration. Ethylene glycol toxicity in a cat. The epithelium lining the tubules has proliferated *(arrows)* along the intact basement membrane, and a mitotic figure is seen *(M)*. There are oxalate crystals *(O)* in the tubules.

understand parenchymal regeneration we must understand something about the regenerative capabilities of various tissues and cells.

Cellular Regenerative Capability

The various cells of the body can be divided arbitrarily into three major groups based on their regenerative capability: **labile, stable,** and **permanent** cells. As we will see, such a classification scheme is only a generalization, but it is nonetheless a useful one for our purposes. Labile and stable cells either are in constant turnover anyhow, or retain the ability for regeneration throughout their life span. On the other hand, permanent cells cannot reproduce themselves, are terminally differentiated end-stage cells, and hence have little or no regenerative capability. From this background, it should immediately be clear that any serious attempts at regeneration as a means of tissue reconstitution after injury can occur only in tissues composed of labile or stable cell populations (Table 4.22). If cells of the permanent type become injured and die as a result of that injury, then repair will occur *via* proliferation and replacement by less specialized connective tissue cells. An additional point is worthy of emphasis: even when regeneration occurs (as in labile and stable cell populations) and the cellular mass of the injured tissue is replaced, the original architecture of the tissue may not be perfectly imitated. In this regard art and science are similar: numerous copies of the works of Van Gogh and Rembrandt have been made, but they always seem to lack something of the original masterpiece.

Labile Cells

Those cells of the various tissues and organs which under normal physiologic conditions continually multiply at a fairly rapid rate throughout life are referred to as labile cells. Their continual replication is a means of replacing cells that are continually being destroyed. Such cells usually are limited to the lymphoid and hematopoietic elements and to the surface-oriented epithelia. **Bone marrow** cells are in a constant state of proliferation throughout life in order to maintain the normal cellular composition of the circulating blood. In short, the rapid turnover of blood cells is continually being compensated for by the formation of new, mature cellular elements in the labile cell populations of the bone marrow. Only when the precursor stem cells in the marrow itself are destroyed is the proliferative capability of this system altered. Then, proliferation of fibroblasts and connective tissue replacement follows, as it might in any other tissue, and scarring (in this case called myelofibrosis) results. With respect to the **lymphoid tissues,** including the spleen, renewal of cell populations can occur from the germinal lymphoblastic cells in those tissues or from the primitive mesenchymal stem cells of the splenic and lymphoid sinuses. In a sense, what happens in the lymphoid tissues and spleen is somewhat analogous to what happens in the bone marrow.

The situation with respect to the **epithelia** is somewhat different and of considerable interest to our study of repair by regeneration. It should be stressed that the labile epithelia do not include all forms of epithelium in the body, but are limited to the epithelia that make up the cellular lining of surfaces throughout the body. This includes the stratified squamous epithelia of the skin and of mucosal surfaces such as the oral cavity, vagina, and cervix; the columnar epithelia of the respiratory and gastrointestinal mucosae; the lining cells of most excretory ducts found within glands such as the biliary tract, salivary glands, and pancreas; the columnar epithelium of the fallopian tubes and uterus; and the transitional epithelium of the urinary tract. At these various anatomical locations, a continuum of maturation and sloughing takes place, which is normally compensated for by the proliferative capability of more primitive and less well differentiated reserve or stem cells usually located deep to the surface, such as the basal cells in the epidermis. The continual turnover of the gastrointestinal epithelium forms an additional good example. Here, superficial cellular elements are continually being sloughed into the intestinal contents to be replaced by proliferative activity within the deeper crypts. Maturation proceeds as the cells move from the crypts to the surface of the villi. Indeed, it is common to see mitotic figures in the intestinal crypts of normal animals.

Following injury, almost perfect reconstitution of tissues composed of labile cell populations can occur by proliferation of remaining cells at the margins of the wound or area of injury. It must be stressed again, however, that this can only occur in the face of an intact connective tissue framework or scaffolding upon which the regenerating epithelium can grow. Epithelium on surfaces also regenerates over large, excavating defects in tissue, but here the process is delayed until the expansive tissue defect becomes filled with less-specialized fibrovascular granulation tissue. In such injuries, a combination of repair by connective tissue replacement and repair by regeneration occurs; the bulk of the defect is filled by connective tissue replacement, while the surface is healed by regeneration of the epithelium.

Stable Cells

Cells that are generally classified as stable differ from the labile cell populations discussed previously in that they normally have a rather low rate of turnover during adult life. Instead, they retain the **capacity** for rapid division and proliferation in response to a variety of kinds of stimuli. These cells also are capable of reconstitution of the injured tissue to almost perfectly normal architecture. Cells that fit into these categories are the parenchymal cells of most of the glandular tissues of the body including the pancreatic acinar cells, renal tubular epithelium, hepatic epithelium, salivary gland epithelium, vascular endothelial cells, and a wide spectrum of mesenchymal cells such as fibroblasts, osteoblasts, chondroblasts, and skeletal smooth muscle cells. A good illustration of the regenerative capability of stable cells already has been given in the example of ethylene glycol (antifreeze) toxicity and renal tubular epithelial regeneration. An additional example can be found in the regenerative capacity of the liver. The liver is a common target for toxic injury, and it is indeed fortunate in this regard that it has such an enormous functional reserve. It has been shown that up to 70–80% of the hepatic epithelium can be removed *via* surgical excision and that regeneration of the original mass of hepatic epithelium occurs quite rapidly. Such regenerative capability allows the liver to repair injuries caused by toxic, viral, or chemical injury.

It must be stressed again that although stable cells are entirely capable of regeneration, such repair does not necessarily occur. The additional necessary ingredient is again that the underlying framework or supporting connective tissue stroma be preserved (Table 4.22). With respect to most parenchymal tissues, the critical structural component in this regard appears to be the integrity of the basement membrane or, more properly, the retention of an appropriate arrangement of the basement membranes such that **tissue architecture** is maintained. Many types of epithelial as well as endothelial cells appear capable of synthesizing basement membrane components upon which to grow, but in the absence of proper architectural arrangement, an uncoordinated growth results. Thus, the stimuli for cell proliferation may be operative even in the absence of an appropriate connective tissue framework, but the result is a haphazard proliferation of cells into disorganized clusters and masses, which have little structural or functional resemblance to the original tissue. Cell proliferation by itself is inadequate to ensure regeneration, and the end result must include restoration of structure-function relationships that are dependent on the architectural arrangement of the connective tissue framework (basement membranes) if regeneration is to be successful.

An additional hindrance to proper regeneration is excessive exudation at the sites of tissue injury. Where there has been sufficient exudation that the exudate cannot be resolved by reabsorption as well as by enzymatic and phagocytic degradation, the exudate will of and by itself provoke a connective tissue response as part of the process of **organization** and lead to scarring. For example, excessive fibrin deposition on alveolar surfaces and bronchiolar walls during the acute phases of pneumonia is known to stimulate the development of fibrosis.

The proliferative capability of mesenchymal cells is well known. The intense proliferation of fibroblasts which accompanies or precedes scarring, is a good example of a stable mesenchymal cell population being called into action. In the repair of a long bone fracture, osteoblast proliferation is essential to the ultimate formation of a solid bony union. Vascular endothelium normally has a rather slow rate of turnover. If, however, a segment of a vessel becomes denuded of endothelium, cells from the margin of the wound quickly migrate into the injured area and proliferate to fill the defect. Endothelial proliferation also is a prominent component of granulation tissue formation, in which the proliferation of endothelium in small venules, arterioles, and capillaries results in the formation of a new vascular bed for the injured tissue, a process referred to as **neovascularization.** These newly formed capillary beds become the sites of egress for phagocytic cells, which invade the wound to perform their defensive functions and provide a nutrient supply for the proliferating fibroblasts in the healing wound. We will have more to say about the endothelium later on.

Somewhat analogous to endothelial cells, the smooth muscle cells making up the walls of hollow viscera and blood vessels also have a very low turnover rate in the normal adult. The smooth muscle cells do, however, have considerable proliferative capability. Possibly the best example of this can be drawn from the intense smooth muscle proliferation that occurs under hormonal influence in the pregnant uterus. Similar, if somewhat less dramatic, changes can be documented during the normal estrus cycle. Smooth muscle proliferates in the walls of blood vessels in response to various kinds of injury. It is particularly responsive to lowered oxygen tension (hypoxia) and to increases in blood pressure (hypertension). In both of these settings, smooth muscle proliferation occurs in the walls of medium and larger muscular arteries. When a vessel is severed or otherwise injured, local smooth muscle proliferation occurs. Smooth muscle proliferation in response to injury also is thought to be involved in the pathogenesis of such degenerative vascular diseases as atherosclerosis.

Permanent Cells

Cells that are classified as permanent are those in which regenerative attempts are generally abortive. To this group belong cells such as neurons and cardiac muscle cells, for which tissue repair by regeneration is, at best, of no practical importance. When neurons in the central nervous system (CNS) are lost, they are gone forever. They can be "replaced," in a sense, by the proliferation of the supportive cellular elements of the CNS, the glial cells. However, restoration of structure-function relationships does not occur, and, for all practical purposes, a neuron lost is indeed a neuron gone for good.

The situation in the peripheral nervous system (PNS) is a little different and more complicated. here, the sequellae to injury depend upon where within the peripheral neuron injury takes place. If the injury spares the cell body, damaging only the peripheral axon, then regeneration can occur from the intact proximal axonal segment or from the cell body itself. On the other hand, if the cell body is damaged and lost, the entire neuron dies, including the peripheral axon, and regeneration does not occur. Therefore, regeneration within the PNS depends largely on the anatomic location of the damage. If an axon is injured, the portion of the axon distal to the injury usually degenerates completely while the axonal segment proximal to the injury degenerates only to the level of the nearest node of Ranvier. Regeneration of the damaged distal axon can proceed from the node of Ranvier, and such regeneration can be quite rapid. Regenerating proximal segments actually have been clocked at the biologically blazing speed of 5 mm/day.

In a fashion analogous to the need for connective tissue stroma if parenchymal regeneration is to succeed, the regrowth of the damaged axon also has an important caveat. The regenerating proximal segment must contact and gain continuity with the old channel (sheath) of the original nerve fiber if successful regeneration of the distal axon is to succeed. If, for whatever cause, the regenerating proximal segment becomes separated from the distal segment, then a disorganized growth of axonal fibers results which fails to restore the continuity of the original fiber. This is basically what takes place in the formation of the **amputation or traumatic neuroma,** which is basically a mass of regenerating axonal fibers lacking orientation and a reason to be. Such growths do nothing for the patient but cause pain.

Skeletal and cardiac muscle provide an interesting biological contrast. Skeletal muscle is able to regenerate well if injured. Again, restoration of structural and functional integrity depends on the preservation of the arrangement of basement membrane and other connective tissue elements. When the basement membrane is intact, regeneration of skeletal muscle is excellent. When the basement membrane is disrupted, regeneration of muscle fibers is less effective. If the edges of a wound in skeletal muscle are separated, for example by a blood clot, muscle cells will proliferate but cannot effectively bridge the gap, which becomes filled by scar tissue. Unfortunately, cardiac muscle has little if any ability to regenerate. For this reason, injuries to the myocardium, such as infarcts, are healed by replacement with scar tissue.

The reason for the differences between cardiac and skeletal muscle, in their ability to heal, is that skeletal muscle contains a population of cells called **satellite cells.** These are essentially resting myoblasts and are found between the sarcolemma of mature muscle fibers and the basement membrane. When skeletal muscle is injured, they proliferate, fuse to form myotubes, and eventually form mature fibers in a fashion analogous to the embryological growth of skeletal muscle. Cardiac muscle lacks the satellite cells and, as a result, lacks the capacity for regeneration.

Thus, the situation with respect to permanent cells and their regenerative capability is not a happy one. Even in the face of an intact connective tissue framework, regeneration is basically not an option. Figure 4.48 should help to place the relative value of cellular regenerative capability into perspective with other features of the healing and repair process.

HEALING BY CONNECTIVE TISSUE REPLACEMENT

In many situations in which injury to tissue occurs, the amount of tissue destruction is such that not only are host tissue cells destroyed and lost, but the framework of supporting connective tissue elements is also destroyed. Healing by regeneration of the tissue then cannot occur. In these situations, the defect becomes filled with less-specialized fibroblastic cells, which ultimately effect a repair of the damaged tissue by replacing the injured portion with scar tissue. For obvious reasons, this is a less-desirable end result than is parenchymal regeneration, but it occurs so often that it is worthy of our detailed attention. Despite the fact that nearly perfect reconstitution of the tissue does not occur when repair takes place by connective tissue replacement, the biology of this form of healing is perhaps even more interesting than that of parenchymal regeneration.

These sorts of defects and injuries are characterized by the formation of **granulation tissue.** This term is derived from the appearance of the soft, developing, fibrovascular scar. Grossly, it has a granular appearance, which reflects its characteristic histologic features: the proliferation of fibroblasts and newly formed small blood vessels. Thus, granulation tissue is best defined as **fibrovascular connective tissue.** Its formation and morphology are of interest to our understanding of the biology of wound repair and healing. It also is important not to become confused by the somewhat similar-sounding terms **granuloma** and **granulomatous.** "Granuloma" is a term used to describe a particular unitized form of inflammation in which macrophages predominate, and "granulomatous" is a term used to define a similar morphologic type of inflammation in which the unitized character of the lesion is missing.

Thus, it is important to make a clear distinction between "granuloma" and "granulomatous" as types of inflammation, and "granulation tissue" as a form of healing response.

Morphology of Granulation Tissue Formation

The development of granulation tissue in a large ulcerated lesion proceeds very much as does the healing of a simple surgical incision. There are substantial quantitative differences, of course, as we will outline later, which make the appearance of a large granulating wound considerably different. In a mature granulating wound, it often is possible to recognize several different zones as one proceeds from the margins (or deep edge) to the surface (Fig. 4.44).

At the deep edge of a mature granulating wound, it often is possible to recognize a **zone of mature connective tissue,** which represents the oldest portion of the healing process. Here, the entire healing process has virtually run its course, and mature collagenous scar tissue has resulted. Because of the nature of the overlying defect, however, this mature connective tissue is still well vascularized. It is these vessels in the zone of mature connective tissue which are the source for the growth of neocapillaries seen in the **zone of capillary proliferation,** which lies superficial to the zone of vascularized mature connective tissue. Here, budding young vessels grow from the more mature vessels in the deeper zone up into the granulating wound. These vessels often have a somewhat parallel arrangement as they grow perpendicular to the surface of the defect (Fig. 4.45). There are often anastomotic branches of these neovascular structures, which ensure a substantial collateral circulatory supply. This can give the appearance of a fine gridwork of plump young vessels in the area.

Between the growing young vessels

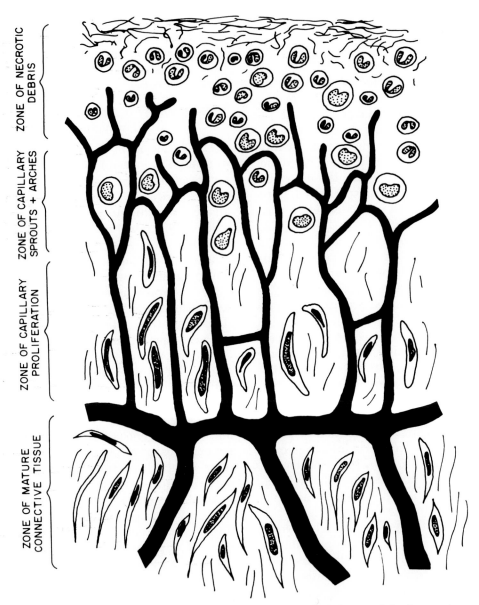

ZONE OF NECROTIC DEBRIS

ZONE OF CAPILLARY SPROUTS + ARCHES

ZONE OF CAPILLARY PROLIFERATION

ZONE OF MATURE CONNECTIVE TISSUE

Figure 4.44. Zones in Granulation Tissue. Schematic representation of the four major zones in a granulating wound. The lesion is oldest at the base where the mature connective tissue is found.

there are proliferating fibroblasts laying down extracellular matrix components, and scattered inflammatory cells. Superficial to this morphologic regions a **zone of capillary sprouts and arches** where migration and mitosis of the endothelial cells occur at the leading edge. These newly formed capillaries form by budding from existing neocapillaries in the zone of capillary proliferation. At first the buds and sprouts are not perfused with blood, as they are solid buds of endothelium. Differentiation soon proceeds, however, and the buds develop lumens to allow blood to move through them. As these sprouts advance into the inflamed area toward

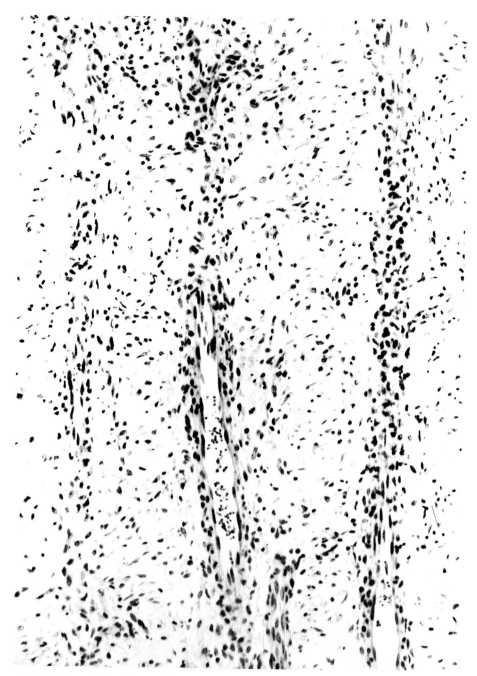

Figure 4.45. **Granulation Tissue.** The vessels are typically parallel to each other and perpendicular to the surface. Between the vessels is active fibroplasia along with a few scattered macrophages.

the surface of the wound they form delicate anastomotic arches with each other. The walls of these delicate young vessels exhibit enhanced vascular permeability, and easily permit the movement of fluids, plasma proteins, and red and white cells from the blood stream into the healing lesion. For this reason, newly forming granulation tissue is often edematous. These developing capillary sprouts and anastomotic arches are basically growing into an inflamed area which is filled with clotted blood, fibrin, and necrotic debris.

Scattered between these neocapillaries are numerous phagocytic cells performing their clean-up functions. Large numbers of **macrophages** usually are present, but closer to the ulcerated surface there may be many **neutrophils** as well. On the surface and extending down to the level of neovascular sprouts and arches is a **zone of necrotic debris,** which may or may not be covered with a scab of dried blood. Here are many dead cells, coagulation products and, usually, a fair number of neutrophils. If there is substantial contamination of the surface, the numbers of leukocytes and the percentage of them that are neutrophils will be increased.

At the epithelial edges of the wound is abundant evidence of attempts at epithelial restitution (Fig. 4.46). Much proliferation of the basal layer is seen, and there is usually a markedly thickened epithelium, which sends pegs and fronds of proliferating cells down along the margins. Such epithelium is attempting to restore surface continuity by growing down under the coverlet provided by the dessicated surface scab. As the edges in a large wound may be far apart, successful re-epithelialization usually cannot take place until wound contraction and the granulation process have proceeded to a point where closer apposition is possible. These proliferating edges of epithelium often seem to invade the edges of the granulating defect and, because of a slight morphologic resemblance to neoplastic change, have been referred to as **psuedoepitheliomatous hyperplasia.** Such changes, however, are reversible and can be seen at the margins of most granulating wounds on epithelial surfaces.

These typical morphologic characteristics of granulation tissue provide a useful temporal map for what is happening. The healing process is most advanced at the base, and proceeds from there toward the surface, laying down connective tissue components as it goes. Because the surface remains exposed, an active reaction continues, which basically can be resolved only by restitution of the epithelial surface. Clinically, this may necessitate surgical excision of the granulation tissue in an attempt to achieve better edge apposition.

There are several important cellular features of granulation tissue that warrant our attention. There are basically three cell types that always are found in a healing or granulating wound: the **macrophage,** the **fibroblast,** and the **endothelial cell.** Their activities are central to the healing process.

Macrophages

We have already discussed the arrival of macrophages at sites of inflammation, and have noted their importance and prominence in the later, more chronic stages of an evolving inflammatory reaction. It is during these more chronic phases in the evolution of a successful inflammatory response that the distinction between "inflammation" as a host defense mechanism and "healing" as a reparative effort becomes remarkably blurred. The highly important macrophages play a pivotal role in the transition between inflammation and wound healing, and are essential cells for the phagocytic removal of necrotic debris and exudate that have accumulated within the damaged tissue.

The inflammatory response resulting from tissue injury is characterized by a relatively rapid accumulation of numerous neutrophils and macrophages at the site of injury. While both of these cell types may begin to emigrate from blood vessels adjacent to the injured tissue at about the same time, the neutrophils quickly reach a maximum level in the

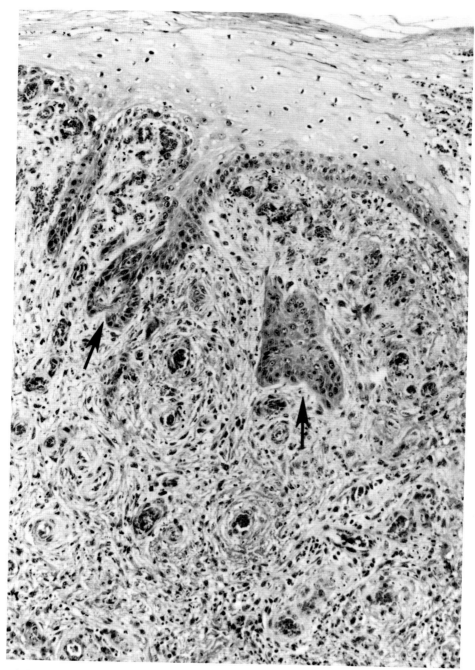

Figure 4.46.   Pseudoepitheliomatous Hyperplasia. Active proliferation of squamous epithelium at the edge of a granulating wound. There are pegs and islands of proliferating epithelium *(arrows),* which appear to "invade" the underlying fibrovascular connective tissue.

wound and then decline in number, while macrophages reach maximal levels somewhat later, usually become the principle phagocytic cell in chronic injuries, and are of prominent importance in granulation tissue.

The role of the macrophage in wound repair has perhaps best been exemplified in experiments in which attempts were made to eliminate macrophages from healing wounds and to inhibit phagocytosis by those remaining cells. Such experiments have been attempted using antimacrophage serum (AMS), but AMS alone seems to have variable effects on the macrophages in healing wounds, even though declines in circulating monocyte levels might occur. As the effects of AMS alone seem to be capricious, attempts have been made to eliminate the circulating sources of replacement cells. Since tissue macrophages are largely derived from blood monocytes, hydrocortisone has been used to produce monocytopenia. Using this system, the number of macrophages in wounds can be reduced to approximately one-third. This reduction in macrophage levels is accompanied by inhibition of wound debridement, as evidenced by increased levels of fibrin deposition and a decreased rate of disappearance of both fibrin and neutrophils. When AMS is used together with hydrocortisone in such studies, the effects are dramatic, and the result is virtually complete disappearance of macrophages from the wounds.

Two separate aspects of these studies are worthy of our attention: **first,** the continual recruitment of tissue macrophages from circulating monocytes is important if useful numbers of macrophages are to be maintained in the healing wound, and **second,** if the source of macrophages is diminished (as in monocytopenia), then a variety of agents (including AMS) can react with and destroy much of the residual population of macrophages in the healing wound. Interestingly enough, depletion of neutrophils has no apparent effect on the subsequent healing of experimental wounds in the absence of gross contamination. The main function of the neutrophil is to destroy bacteria introduced into the wound at the time of injury and to assist in the sterilization of contaminated surfaces.

What do these studies of healing wounds tell us about the functions of macrophages in normally healing wounds? The lack of wound debridement clearly implicates the macrophage as the principal phagocytic cell in healing wounds. Since severe inhibition of wound debridement results from the absence of these cells, the macrophage seems essential for this function. A marked delay in fibroplasia is also noted, both in terms of onset and rate of proliferation of fibroblasts. This suggests that macrophages may be important cells in setting the stage for fibrosis to occur, possibly because an essential prerequisite for fibroblast proliferation is adequate wound debridement. It also is possible that the macrophage is necessary for inactivation of local **inhibitors** of fibroblast proliferation known to be present in inflamed wounds. Macrophages also have been shown to produce **growth factors** that promote the proliferation of fibroblasts and other cells. It is evident that more work needs to be done in this area of research, but the essential role of the macrophage in cleaning up cellular debris and inflammatory exudates and in setting the stage for fibroblast proliferation seems clear. As such, these important cells are involved in the orchestration as well as the execution of both the degradative and reparative phases of wound repair.

Fibroblasts

For many kinds of open wounds and tissue defects, as we have discussed previously, the morphologic expression of those reparative phenomena is the formation of **granulation tissue.** Granulation tissue can be regarded as a sort of "temporary organ," present as long as it is useful and then disappearing, to ultimately be replaced by a collagenous scar. It is an interim solution to a specialized problem; the filling of large defects in tissue. Granulation tissue is not the only such "temporary organ" known to man;

an additional, more complex example of this type would be formation of the placenta during pregnancy. Along with the macrophages (and, as we shall see, endothelial cells), the fibroblasts are of critical importance to wound healing; without them, healing of most types of wounds would never proceed.

The fibroblasts are ubiquitous connective tissue cells and the most widespread of the mesenchymal cells, present in substantial numbers in virtually every organ and tissue. They are classified as "stable cells retaining proliferative capability", and certainly they maintain the capacity for rapid growth to a far greater degree than other similarly classified cells. Indeed, as anyone who has worked with tissue culture can testify, "fibroblast overgrowth" is such a common result of many attempts to isolate and grow non-fibroblasts (parenchymal cells), that it becomes a disturbing annoyance. These same growth characteristics, which often make fibroblasts the bane of the tissue culturist, are, however, of critical importance to the healing and wound repair processes.

Fibroblasts are essential to wound repair by virtue of their ability to proliferate locally and to synthesize and lay down extracellular matrix components such as collagen in order to restore functional and structural integrity to the damaged tissue and to provide the wound with tensile strength. In short, when an effective cellular defense has been mounted within the damaged tissue, the reparative phenomena that follow almost always involve at least some fibroblast proliferation; some scarring almost inevitably accompanies virtually all injuries.

ELABORATION OF EXTRACELLULAR MATRIX COMPONENTS. We have already briefly introduced some of the important components of the extracellular matrix in a general way (see Chapter 3), and it is beyond our scope to detail here the biochemical intricacies involved in the synthesis and elaboration of these important structural components of connective tissues. Interested readers seeking further details should consult the reading list given at the end of the chapter.

The importance of extracellular matrix components like collagen in wound healing has been appreciated for a very long time, for the simple reason that the ultimate result of many repair processes is the formation of collagenous scars. However, since the complex processes of cell proliferation, cell migration, cell differentiation, and cellular interaction are involved in wound healing and repair, we must take a broader look at the extracellular matrix as more than merely the source of the end stage product, collagen.

If we arbitrarily divide wound repair into inflammatory, proliferative, and reorganization or remodeling stages, evidence can be used to support the importance of the fibroblast during all three stages. **Healing begins at the moment of injury.** It is the fibroblast product collagen that is critical in the early hemostatic events that occur in the damaged tissue. Escaping blood from damaged vessels coagulates to form the blood clot. A primary step here is the adhesion of platelets to exposed collagen. Collagen also provides the negatively charged surface necessary for the activation of Hageman factor to begin the intrinsic coagulation cascade. Thus, by virtue of its initial interaction with platelets and Hageman factor, collagen occupies a key position in wound healing from the very beginning of the process.

During the inflammatory phase, the leukocytes that invade the tissue also play a role. Recent evidence suggests that in uninfected wounds, neutrophils may not be essential participants. Their removal with antineutrophil serum does not significantly impair the progress of sterile wound repair, and they apparently do not contribute significantly to wound clearance by phagocytosis. This is in contrast to the situation with macrophages, as we have discussed previously. The neutrophils appear to be largely antibacterial cells in this setting, as well as adding potent hydrolytic enzymes to the local environment. Of the long list of enzymes contained in neutrophils, **collagenase** is of particular interest to us here. Granulocyte collagenase differs from other animal collagenases in that it apparently is not inhibited by serum. Thus, its collagenolytic activity proceeds in the face of serum exudation into the wound. While the role of collagenase in wound repair is not completely understood, it seems reasonable to assume that it may serve the purpose of liberating cells (both mesenchymal and epithelial) for migration at the wound edges and facilitating the movement of connective tissue cells by enzymatic degradation of the collagenous matrix in which they are seated. Collagenolysis can, in fact, be shown to occur around the epithelium at the wound edges in experimental wounds. Thus, the collagenolytic activity assists in allowing wound healing to enter the proliferative phase by freeing cells for migration and proliferation. This in turn can be shown to be associated with a burst in collagen synthetic activity by the proliferating fibroblasts.

The final stages of healing involve the production, maturation, and removal by remodeling of collagen synthesized during the proliferation phase. The newly synthesized collagen fibrils bridge the gap between the edges of the damaged tissue to form a collagenous scar of appreciable tensile strength. It has thus become apparent that the fibroblast product, collagen, and its manufacturer, the fibroblast, are invariably involved in virtually all phases of the healing process (Fig. 4.47).

EXTRACELLULAR MATRIX REMODELING. One of the more interesting phases of wound repair and healing is the **remodeling of the extracellular matrix.** It is now clear that alterations in the nature of the extracellular matrix begin quite early in the healing process, and are not just the terminal event we recognize as "collagenous scarring." Like many of the other sequential events in healing, production and remodeling of the extracellular matrix overlaps with other active processes and is difficult to compartmentalize into a strict time frame.

Although alterations in the connective tissues are apparent even at fairly early stages of wound repair and healing, most of the matrix remodeling occurs over a more prolonged period. During granulation tissue formation and the time that follows its formation and dissolution, the extracellular matrix is constantly changing its composition. Therefore, the biochemical composition of the matrix depends, in part, on the **time** elapsed since the injury occurred; **fibronectin** is a conspicuous component of young healing wounds but is less prominent than **collagen** in older wounds.

It is also apparent that the composition of the extracellular matrix differs depending on the **location** within the wound. It makes sense that the initial deposits of extracellular matrix material occur at the **margins** of the wound, and more centrally only as the developing granulation tissue fills the more interior portions of the wound space. This means, in essence, that the margins of a healing wound will be "older" in terms of their development than the central portions, which helps to explain the differences in composition of the extracellular matrix at various distances from the center of the defect.

It is becoming more and more clear that the sequential appearance of various extracellular matrix components in wound repair has considerable functional significance. **Hyaluronic acid (HA),** a member of the general class of polysaccharides called **glycosaminoglycans (GAGs),** occurs early in granulation tissue. Evidence suggests that HA promotes cell movement by facilitating reversible adhesion of cell membranes with the matrix sub-

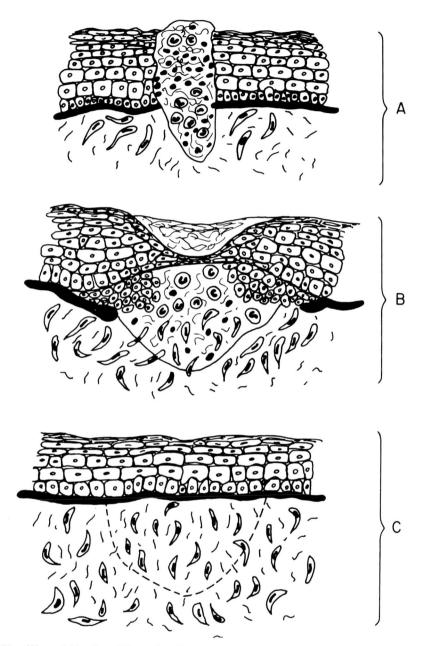

Figure 4.47.   Wound Healing. Tissue healing involves collagen and the fibroblast at all stages. *A,* The initial lesion exposes collagen to bring about coagulation and platelet aggregation for hemostasis. *B,* The infiltrating leukocytes remodel the wound using granulocyte collagenase while fibroblasts begin to proliferate and synthesize collagen at the base. *C,* The wound has been repaired and the defect filled by mature collagenous connective tissue synthesized and elaborated by the fibroblasts.

stratum, and it may promote cell division. As granulation tissue matures, there is less HA present, since it is removed enzymatically by tissue and leukocyte hy-

aluronidase. As HA content wanes, increases in **proteoglycans** such as chondroitin- and dermatan-sulfate occur. Proteoglycans contribute considerable resilience to the healing wound and may influence collagen fibrillogenesis in fibroblasts and thus facilitate collagen deposition.

Of all the extracellular matrix components, the important adhesive glycoprotein molecule **fibronectin** is certainly one of the most important because of the diversity of its interaction with various cellular and extracellular components central to wound healing (Table 4.23). Fibronectin promotes the adhesiveness and spreading of platelets at the site of injury, augments the adhesion and migration of leukocytes, and enhances macrophage phagocytosis as a nonimmune opsonin. It also promotes fibroblast and endothelial cell adhesion and migration, as well as the migration of epidermal cells over granulation tissue, thus promoting re-epithelialization. Substantial amounts of fibronectin are found in early granulating wounds, where it also serves as a sort of primitive matrix that can influence the pattern of collagen deposition. It appears that the deposition of extracellular fibronectin is important to the organization of types I and III collagen, with fibronectin serving as a temporary template for the subsequent deposition of collagen. In addition, fibronectin serves as a sort of extracellular "glue" that helps to anchor fibroblasts as well as macrophages *via* specific fibronectin receptors.

As time passes, the nature of the extracellular matrix in a healing wound changes. There is a marked decrease in the amounts of hyaluronic acid and fibronectin, and an increase in the amount of **collagen** present. Collagen is really a generic term that encompasses a growing family of at least 11 types of molecules, all of which consist largely of the unique collagen triple helical structure. The primary types of collagen deposited during fibroplasia and granulation tissue formation are **type I** and **type III** collagen; the percentage of other types of collagen participating in wound repair are low. Both type I and type III collagen are fibrillar types of collagen that have **uninterrupted** triple helices. It is the deposition of these rigid helical collagen macromolecules that gradually provides the healing tissue with increased tensile strength. This process takes time, and scar tissue never really does fully regain the tensile strength of intact tissue. It has been estimated that most skin wounds have regained only about 20% of their final strength after 3 weeks, and at maximum strength a scar is only about 70% as strong as intact skin. The increase in tensile strength that wounds develop after collagen deposition is not only related to the amount of collagen being deposited, but also to the **remodeling** of the collagen with formation of larger collagen bundles.

Depending on the nature of the wounding process and the involved tissue, formation of new **basement membrane** can also occur. This has been best documented in the process of re-epithelialization in skin wounds. It appears that epithelial cells migrate initially over a provisional matrix and that true basement membrane formation does not occur until migration has ceased and epithelial continuity has been restored. Basement membrane reformation appears to occur in sequential stages, with the deposition of **laminin** and **type IV collagen** (interrupted triple helical collagen) proceeding

Table 4.23
Roles of Fibronectin in Wound Healing

Promotes platelet spreading
Stimulates leukocyte adhesion and migration
Nonimmune opsonin for phagocytosis
Augments fibroblast adhesion and migration
Augments endothelial cell adhesion and migration
Promotes epidermal growth and re-epithelialization
Provides primitive scaffolding for collagen deposition

from the original margin of the wound toward the center in a sort of "zipper" mechanism.

The extracellular matrix components thus accumulate in wound healing and granulation tissue formation in a fairly predictable fashion, with the initial hyaluronic acid and fibronectin deposits being replaced in older wounds by types I and III collagen for greater tensile strength. This sequence of events allows each of the extracellular matrix components to exert its own special influences on the evolving cellular and biochemical activity central to wound repair.

WOUND CONTRACTION AND THE MYO-FIBROBLAST. During the evolution of granulation tissue, fibroblasts acquire ultrastructural, chemical, immunological, and functional characteristics that clearly distinguish them from fibroblasts of normal tissues. A fibrillar system develops within the cytoplasm, with the appearance of bundles of parallel fibrils resembling those of smooth muscle cells. Strips of active granulation tissue tested *in vitro* behave like smooth muscle in that they are contracted and relaxed by agents that contract or relax smooth muscle, including serotonin, angiotensin, bradykinin, epinephrine, and some of the prostaglandins.

The yield of actomyosin that can be extracted from granulation tissue is comparable to that which can be obtained from an equal mass of uterine smooth muscle, and the calcium-activated ATPase activity of the extracts is similar. Granulation tissue fibroblasts gradually develop intracellular neoantigens similar to those present in smooth muscle. Antibodies against actomyosin also fix to these cells, indicating immunologic identity. When granulation tissue regresses after the healing of a wound, these various phenomena can no longer be demonstrated. Thus, it has become widely accepted that the forces producing wound contraction reside in the modified fibro-

blasts typical of granulation tissue. Because of their functional and morphologic similarity to smooth muscle cells, these modified fibroblasts are known as **myofibroblasts.** These cells seem to progressively develop intracytoplasmic "muscles" as well as cell-to-cell and cell-to-stroma connections. They are functionally active cells that can contract either spontaneously or in response to endogenous mediators, and apparently can do so at the same time that collagen is being laid down. This provides a unique sort of "lock-step" arrangement so that the shrinkage of the scar tissue occurs simultaneously with its acquisition of additional tensile strength. This of course is a useful phenomenon in the healing of open wounds, but it also can occur where it is neither needed nor wanted. It can result in serious disfigurement and can cause postinflammatory lumenal strictures in organs such as the intestine. In short, the healing of an open wound is highlighted by the appearance of specialized granulation tissue fibroblasts or myofibroblasts that acquire morphologic and functional characteristics of typical contractile smooth muscle cells. These cells provide a contemporary explanation of the age-old observations regarding wound contraction.

Many questions remain unanswered about the biology of myofibroblasts. What factors promote their development and differentiation? What mediating agents actually are responsible for their contraction *in vivo?* What influences their ultimate disappearance from the healed wound? Only further research will answer the remaining questions, but progress to date in identifying and understanding these cells and their functions has given a new level of interest and sophistication to the formerly mundane subject of wound contraction.

Endothelial Cells

The role of the endothelium in wound repair and healing relates basically to its functional capabilities as the cell type lining the blood vessels. As we have mentioned previously, vascular endothelium normally has a fairly low turnover rate. In several different models it has been documented that endothelial cells in the microvasculature start proliferating relatively early in the course of an inflammatory injury. Precisely what the stimulus is for this proliferative activity is not clear, but at least part of the story seems to involve leukocytes.

Leukocytic infiltrates often seem to precede the ingrowth of the microvasculature into damaged areas. If the leukocytic infiltration is delayed, so will be the vascular ingrowth. Granulation tissue, it should be recalled, is basically fibrovascular connective tissue. Buds of endothelial cells grow out from existing blood vessels at the wound margins, undergo canalization, and form a series of vascular arcades by joining with their neighbors. These newly formed vessels are extremely permeable and leak protein readily so that the fluid bathing the injured area consists virtually of dilute plasma. It forms an excellent nutrient medium for the various proliferative activities of the fibroblasts and the phagocytic activities of the leukocytes. This highlights one of the major functions of endothelium in the healing process in granulation tissue (and elsewhere): to proliferate and provide a highly permeable nutrient microvasculature to support the activities of the various cellular members of the healing drama. The same newly formed vessels that are so permeable to protein also readily exude leukocytes and thus form a conduit for the movement of phagocytic cells from the vascular compartment to the injured area.

Thus, within the granulating wound, the **macrophage** is essential for the removal of necrotic debris and exudate (wound debridement) and can provide growth factors to promote fibroblast proliferation; the **fibroblast** is the synthetic source of collagen required to partially restore the structural integrity of the tissue and to provide tensile strength to the wound; and the **endothelium** provides a nutrient conduit whereby the damaged tissue is bathed in plasma and phagocytic cells. It is clear that other cell types also are important to the healing process, but without the macrophage, the fibroblast, and the endothelial cell, wound healing would be essentially impossible.

ROLE OF GROWTH FACTORS IN HEALING AND REPAIR

The entire preceding discussion has an underlying theme; in order for healing and repair to take place, much **cell proliferation** must occur. Not only must parenchymal cells proliferate if repair by regeneration is to take place, but the critical processes of re-epithelialization, neovascularization, and fibroblast proliferation central to granulation tissue formation all depend on enhanced mitotic activity within the involved cell populations. What causes these cells to proliferate?

It is becoming increasingly clear that much of the cellular activity central to healing and wound repair is under the guidance of **growth factors** derived from a variety of sources. This is a rapidly growing field in which additional biochemical details become available on a regular basis (*see also* chapter 7). Although more molecular and functional definition will certainly be forthcoming, of the several different growth factors that have been identified in recent years, 5 seem to be of sufficient importance to the healing process to warrant our brief attention here. These are: **macrophage-derived growth factor, platelet-derived growth factor, epidermal growth factor, fibroblast growth factor,** and **transforming growth factor.**

Macrophage-derived growth factor. Following up on the studies we have previously mentioned, in which depletion of circulating monocytes and tissue macrophages resulted in delayed wound healing, it was subsequently discovered that part of the biological basis for these earlier observations was related to growth factors secreted by macrophages, which could support both fibroblast proliferation and connective tissue formation. Initially referred to as **macrophage-derived growth factor (MDGF),** it now seems clear that these secretory products of stimulated macrophages probably represent a family of generic molecules that are somewhat similar to the related growth factors described below. Macrophages seem to secrete a low level of MDGF at all times, but stimulated macrophages produce much more. In addition to a proliferative influence on fibroblasts, MDGF stimulates the proliferation of smooth muscle cells and endothelium. Three important phenomena associated with healing wounds, fibroblast proliferation, neovascularization, and wound contraction, may thus be regulated, at least in part, by the secretion of growth factors from macrophages.

Platelet-derived growth factor. It seems reasonable that any growth factor that is likely to play an important role in wound healing ought to have at least two properties; it should be able to direct the migration of cells into the area being repaired, and it should be able to cause those cells to proliferate. In other words, it should be both chemotactic and mitogenic. **Platelet-derived growth factor (PDGF)** has these functional capabilities and is believed to represent one of the important influences on wound repair. Platelets are almost always at the scene where injury takes place because of hemorrhage. Released to extravascular sites by the injury process, platelets aggregate and degranulate in response to soluble stimuli or to collagen in the extracellular matrix. Degranulation releases platelet α-granule constituents, including PDGF. Several other cell types, including endothelial cells, smooth muscle cells, and ac-

tivated blood monocytes also appear capable of producing PDGF-like molecules. In addition, low levels of PDGF (of platelet origin) are normally present in plasma.

PDGF is the most potent mitogen found in plasma for mesenchymal cells such as fibroblasts and smooth muscle cells and appears to work through specific membrane receptors on such cells. PDGF is a potent attractant for mesenchymal cells like fibroblasts and smooth muscle cells. It has also been shown to be chemotactic for a variety of inflammatory cell types, including end-stage differentiated cells like neutrophils that do not respond to its mitogenic properties. It is presently envisioned that PDGF may join with other chemoattractants to favor inflammatory cell influx into acute wounds, and PDGF also contributes to the later attraction of mesenchymal cells, which may subsequently respond to the mitogenic properties of PDGF. Thus, following resolution of the acute inflammatory response, PDGF may assist in mediating local mesenchymal cell proliferation as part of the early repair process. PDGF also seems to play a role in tissue remodeling, as it can stimulate fibroblast collagenase production allowing removal of excess or damaged collagen and thus limit scar tissue formation and assist in the remodeling of repaired tissues and organs. These various functions make PDGF one of the leading candidates on a growing list of growth factors that may have potential therapeutic uses.

Epidermal growth factor. Some 25 years ago, a "factor" was isolated from the salivary glands of mice that was subsequently shown to cause premature tooth eruption and eyelid opening in newborn mice. When it was demonstrated that this "factor" could cause maturation and growth of the epidermis, it was called **epidermal growth factor (EGF).** Much more is known about EGF now, and, like PDGF, it has a number of effects that are related to the healing process. EGF is a relatively small (53 amino acid residues), single-chain polypeptide that is very stable; even boiling or acid treatment do not destroy its functional capabilities. While male mouse salivary gland tissue remains a major experimental source of EGF, it is probably much more ubiquitous, since it can be secreted by Brunner's glands in the intestine and is also found in urine and milk. Like PDGF, EGF also seems to exert its effects through specific receptor binding, and its wide spectrum of activity is suggested by the fact that EGF receptors are found on virtually all mammalian cell types. They are most abundant on epithelia. EGF has a wide range of effects, but for wound healing and tissue repair, its major attribute is the ability to stimulate the growth of a large variety of cell types. Although the mechanisms of action of EGF are not completely understood, it apparently acts as a sort of "progression factor" in the cell cycle by encouraging dividing cells to proceed through subsequent cell cycles. With its potent effects on epithelial cells as well as mesenchymal cells like fibroblasts, the facility of EGF to impact on clinical wound repair is obvious and has stimulated the commercial production of recombinant EGF for potential therapeutic applications. Indeed, initial trials with recombinant EGF have produced a 50–75% acceleration in the healing of experimental skin wounds. As such, this molecule, as well as others, have already shown the enormous potential that contemporary recombinant DNA technology has for clinical medicine.

Fibroblast growth factor. Initially isolated from bovine brain and pituitary gland extracts, **fibroblast growth factor (FGF)** now seems to be a family of related 145–155 amino acid polypeptide molecules with a wide tissue distribution, all of which share the unique property of binding tightly to **heparin,** and all of which are mitogenic for fibroblasts as well as other cell types. Although heparin is a mast cell product, the heparin-binding ca-

pacity of FGF has no proven biological function, but it may be related to extracellular matrix binding. It also aided in the purification of the molecule. Both acidic and basic forms of FGF have been identified, which have similar biological activities but different isoelectric points; they appear genetically related, with the same intron/exon structure, and share about 55% amino acid homology.

Fibroblast growth factor has the potential for involvement in wound healing and tissue repair *via* three different mechanisms; *(a)* FGF is a potent **mitogen** for fibroblasts and other cell types including endothelial cells, *(b)* FGF has been shown to be **angiogenic,** that is, it induces the growth of new capillaries into previously avascular spaces, and *(c)* FGF may be involved in regulating the synthesis of **extracellular matrix** components such as **fibronectin.** As we have discussed, wound healing, particularly the formation of **granulation tissue,** involves fibrovascular proliferation and the synthesis and laying down of new extracellular matrix components. It may well be that FGF is one of the important regulatory molecules that govern these well-known events. Recently, FGF has been shown to promote the healing of several different types of experimental wounds, and the availability of recombinant FGF molecules will certainly accelerate research into the intriguing properties of this potentially important factor.

Transforming growth factor. Like several of the other more recently identified "growth factors," **transforming growth factor (TGF)** is apparently at least two resolvable molecules called **TGF-α** and **TGF-β,** of which the latter, **TGF-β** , is apparently the more important. TGF owes its identity to a series of studies in tumor cell biology about 10 years ago related to the so-called **"autocrine theory of transformation."** This theory suggests that transformed cells (tumor cells) grew in an uncontrolled fashion because they were capable of producing growth factors for their own use; that is, tumor fibroblasts produced growth factor activity that normal fibroblasts did not. Interestingly, although normal cells did not produce the factors, they could respond and become "transformed" under the influence of the growth factors produced by their already transformed counterparts. This singular feature was responsible for the name **transforming growth factor.**

With improved methods of biochemical identification, it is now known that TGF can be produced by a wide variety of normal cell types. **TGF-β** from most sources is a two-chain dimer consisting of about 112 amino acid residues, which functions *via* a receptor distinct from the EGF receptor. **Platelets** are a particularly rich source of TGF-β, although the factor is quite distinct from PDGF. Like most of the other growth factors, interest in TGF-β with respect to wound healing and tissue repair is related to its profound effects including enhanced fibroblast proliferation, particularly in concert with EGF, and the stimulation of fibroblast collagen and fibronectin formation.

More research will be required before the complete biological potential of TGF-β, as well as the other growth factors discussed, can be fully understood. It is certain that we will all be hearing more about the clinical application of growth factors for promoting wound repair in the future, for the impact of recombinant DNA biotechnology and our increasing competence in "instructing" bacteria to make generous quantities of certain molecules hold enormous promise for clinical medicine.

WOUND HEALING

Wounds can occur in many ways. They can be deliberately inflicted as in surgery, or they can result from a wide variety of other backgrounds ranging from trauma to inflammation. All require a solution if "restitution of tissue continuity" is to result. Lesions are in fact wounds to tissue, and the manner of healing for various kinds of wounds is remarkably similar.

There is often confusion in the use of the terms healing, repair, and regeneration, but distinctions are useful. As we have discussed previously, **regeneration** refers to the replacement of lost tissue by tissue of the same type. **Repair** is a somewhat more general term that encompasses both regeneration and connective tissue replacement. There is really no precise definition of **healing,** but it generally includes all means (including connective tissue replacement and regeneration) by which restoration of tissue continuity is achieved. It is difficult to define an end point for healing. For example, a skin wound may appear "healed" when epithelial regrowth over the surface has occurred, but below the surface, remodeling and modulation of the connective tissue may continue for weeks or even months depending on the magnitude of the initial defect.

Healing is an amazing phenomenon, the ultimate value of which often is regarded as being determined by its effectiveness in restoring the tissue to complete normalcy of structure and function. Therefore healing by connective tissue replacement must be considered less effective than healing by parenchymal regeneration.

A number of important concepts in cell biology are central to the healing process. First, the **movement** of cells is essential. Second, the ability of cells to **proliferate** is vital, for without cell proliferation, neither parenchymal regeneration nor scarring could take place. Third, the phenomenology behind cell **differentiation** and **maturation** is ultimately responsible for the restitution of normalcy. It is also pertinent to mention that **cell death** and the removal of dead cells play a large part in the inflammatory and maturational phases of healing. Exudates must be resolved, and dead cells removed, before tissue continuity can be restored. The entire healing process is thus exemplary of the various kinds of closely integrated cellular activity that comprise many of the mammalian defense reactions against injury and invasion.

There are considerable gaps in our knowledge of how all of this comes to be. Much is known, for example, about fibroblasts and the means by which they synthesize and lay down collagen but, despite recent progress, we remain relatively ignorant about the importance of the extracellular matrix environment in which these activities occur. This complicated bath of molecules in which the connective tissue develops may be exerting greater influences over the whole healing process than was previously realized.

The cell proliferation so central to wound healing is basically tied to controls over mitosis. We usually think of the increased mitotic activity in, for example, regenerating epithelium as being a result of the stimulus produced by the injury process itself. However, the epithelial proliferation may in fact not be due to stimulation, but to the release from inhibitory influences that normally act to keep mitosis in check. The various growth factors also promote cell proliferation, but less is known about what turns the system off. Why, for example, do proliferating fibroblasts in a healing wound eventually stop proliferating? What are the signals?

The regulatory processes responsible for determining the end points of the re-epithelization are similarly complicated and poorly understood. The cessation of cell proliferation, which occurs when epithelia from opposite sides of a wound meet, implies the existence of a mechanism that recognizes that coverage is complete, otherwise there would be a piling up of epithelium. The cellular events involved in this **contact inhibition** are not well understood, but they may involve cell-to-cell communication *via* changes in membrane permeability or surface electrical charge. Such events in cellular biology are clearly important and illustrate for us the vital contributions that basic approaches can have to real-life problems in clinical medicine.

HEALING AND REPAIR IN PERSPECTIVE

In retrospect, several well-defined stages can be reconstructed in the progression of a simple healing skin wound. First, there is formation of the **blood clot** within the incised tissue and the subsequent development of a scab. Second, **epithelial continuity** is restored, often as quickly as the first 24–48 hours if edge apposition is good. Third, an **inflammatory reaction** develops in the incised dermis with neutrophil infiltration followed by macrophage infiltration. Fourth, **neovascularization** occurs with the ingrowth of tender new capillary buds to bridge the wound. Fifth, **fibroblast proliferation** occurs to provide a sufficient cellular base for the manufacture and laying down of **collagen.** Thereafter, the process is one of progressive accumulation of collagen within the wound, which eventually produces the sixth event, gradual **devascularization** of the incision site. In the absence of a nutrient vasculature, the seventh stage of **egress of inflammatory cells** occurs, and, as the wound becomes progressively avascular, **fibroblast regression** takes place as an eighth step. The ninth stage leaves us with the relatively acellular and avascular, pale, collagenous **scar** as an end product of wound healing.

It must be emphasized that while it is possible to arbitrarily divide the process into these sorts of staged events, there is considerable overlap between the stages of this dynamic process, which forms a continuum from initiation of the wound to the terminal scar. Thus, several different stages are going on simultaneously.

The clinical relevance of an increased

understanding of the biology of healing should be readily apparent. Through an enlightened approach to understanding the healing process at the cellular and molecular levels we are best able to know how to proceed as clinicians to create the appropriate local environments to favor the various phases of the healing process. Similar processes keyed to the nature of the injury and the tissue itself characterize the healing and repair mechanism no matter where it occurs. It is thus clear that advances in the treatment of wounds and the healing of tissue damage are less

likely to come from new surgical techniques than they are to come from improved understanding and the application of new basic knowledge.

We also must reiterate that healing and repair can take place by either tissue regeneration or by connective tissue replacement. In an inflammatory injury, the ultimate outcome depends on a wide variety of factors, some host dependent and some agent dependent. If the host destroys the invader and little tissue is lost, then a return to normal is possible so long as the organization of exudate does not

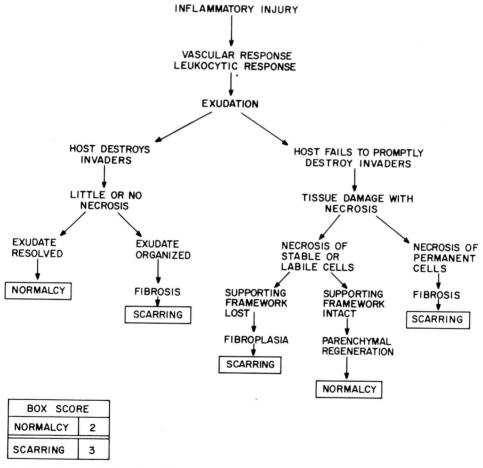

Figure 4.48. Routes to Healing: Restitution of Normalcy *versus* Scarring. The achievement of normalcy at the end of a repair process depends upon how well the host handles the invaders, how much necrosis occurs, how much exudate is present and how it is resolved, the nature of the injured tissue cells, and the condition of the supporting connective tissue framework. Scarring is more common than complete restitution of normalcy.

promote scarring. If the invader is not promptly destroyed, the outcome depends most often on whether or not the tissue-supporting structures necessary for regeneration are intact or destroyed. Regeneration cannot occur satisfactorily in the absence of an intact connective tissue framework, and scarring is the inevitable end result. We also must recall that the nature of the host cells damaged is of considerable importance, as permanent-type cells cannot regenerate even if the connective tissue framework remains intact. The various options with respect to healing and repair are graphically summarized in Figure 4.48. The unfortunate truth is that for most kinds of injury, some scarring almost inevitably results. The combination of ingredients and factors necessary for the restitution of complete normalcy are much less likely to occur in a real-life setting than are the combination of ingredients and factors that lead to scarring. The end result of tissue damage is, therefore, more often scarring than complete restitution of normalcy. To appease our annoyance at the inherent unfairness of this biological game, we need only remind ourselves once again that the entire inflammation and repair process is **survival oriented,** and that the other alternative, death, is even less acceptable than is scarring.

Reference Material

Inflammation

Adams, D.O., and Hamilton, T.A.: The cell biology of macrophage activation. *Ann. Rev. Immunol.* 2:283–318, 1984.

Anderson, D.C., and Springer, T.A.: Leukocyte adhesion deficiency: an inherited defect in the Mac-1, LFA-1, and p150,95 glycoproteins. *Ann. Rev. Med. 38*:175–194, 1987.

Babior, B.M.: Protein phosphorylation and the respiratory burst. *Arch. Biochem. Biophys. 264*:361–367, 1988.

Baggiolini, M.: Proteinases and acid hydrolases of neutrophils and macrophages and the mechanisms of their release. *Adv. Inflamm. Res. 3*:313–327, 1982.

Baggiolini, M., and Dewald, B.: The neutrophil. *Int. Arch. Allergy Appl. Immunol.* 76(2):13–20, 1985.

Beilke, M.A.: Vascular endothelium in immunology and infectious disease. *Rev. Infect. Dis.* 11:273–283, 1989.

Benveniste, J., and Pretolani, M.: Paf-Acether (platelet-activating factor): its role in inflammation. *Adv. Inflamm. Res. 10*:7–21, 1986.

Berridge, M.J.: Inositol trisphosphate and diacylglycerol: two interacting second messengers. *Ann. Rev. Biochem. 56*:159–194, 1987.

Bertram, T.A.: Neutrophilic leukocyte structure and function in domestic animals. *Adv. Vet. Sci. Comp. Med. 30*:91–130, 1985.

Bevilacqua, M.P., and Gimbrone, M.A., Jr.: Inducible endothelial functions in inflammation and coagulation. *Sem. Thromb. Hemostas. 13*:425–433, 1987.

Bielefeldt Ohmann, H., Lawman, M.J.P., and Babiuk, L.A.: Bovine interferon: its biology and application in veterinary medicine. *Antiviral Res. 7*:187–210, 1987.

Black, H.S.: Role of reactive oxygen species in inflammatory processes. In: *Nonsteroidal Antiinflammatory Drugs,* (C. Hensby and N.J. Lowe, eds). Karger, Basel, 1989, pp. 1–20.

Bray, M.A.: Leukotrienes in inflammation. *Agents and Actions 19*:87–99, 1986.

Brown, E.J.: The role of extracellular matrix proteins in the control of phagocytosis. *J. Leukocyte Biol. 39*:579–591, 1986.

Bruijn, J.A., Hogendoorn, P.C.W., Hoedemaeker, P.J., and Fleuren, G.J.: The extracellular matrix in pathology. *J. Lab. Clin. Med. 111*:140–149, 1988.

Buck, C.A., and Horwitz, A.F.: Cell surface receptors for extracellular matrix proteins. *Ann. Rev. Cell Biology 3*:179–206, 1987.

Butcher, E.C., Lewinsohn, D., Duijvestijn, A., Bargatze, R., Wu, N., and Jalkanen, S.: Interactions between endothelial cells and leukocytes. *J. Cellular Biochem. 30*:121–131, 1986.

Cohen, S.: Physiologic and pathologic manifestations of lymphokine action. *Human Pathol. 17*:112–121, 1986.

Colditz, I.G.: Margination and emigration of leukocytes. *Surv. Synth. Path. Res. 4*:44–68, 1985.

Curtis, A.: Cell activation and adhesion. *J. Cell Sci. 87*:609–611, 1987.

Cybulsky, M.I., Chan, M.K.W., and Movat, H.Z.: Biology of disease: acute inflammation and microthrombosis induced by endotoxin, interleukin-1, and tumor necrosis factor and their implication in gram-negative infection. *Lab. Invest. 58*:365–378, 1988.

Dana, N., Todd, R.F., III, and Arnaout, M.A.: Mo1 surface glycoprotein: structure, function and clinical importance. *Pathol. Immunopathol. Res. 5*:371–383, 1986.

Davies, P., Bailey, P.J., and Goldenberg, M.M.: The

role of arachidonic acid oxygenation products in pain and inflammation. *Ann. Rev. Immunol.* 2:335–357, 1984.

Dinarello, C.A.: An update on human interleukin-1: from molecular biology to clinical relevance. *J. Clin. Immunol.* 5:287–297, 1985.

Dinarello, C.A., and Mier, J.W.: Interleukins. *Ann. Rev. Med.* 37:173–178, 1986.

Fantone, J.C., and Ward, P.A.: Polymorphonuclear leukocyte-mediated cell and tissue injury. *Human Pathol.* 16:973–978, 1985.

Fearon, D.T.: Cellular receptors for fragments of the third component of complement. *Immunol. Today* 5:105–112, 1984.

Fearon, D.T., and Wong, W.W.: Complement ligand-receptor interations that mediate biological responses. *Ann. Rev. Immunol.* 1:243–271, 1983.

Ferrante, A., Nandoskar, M., Walz, A., Goh, D.H.B., and Kowanko, I.C.: Effects of tumor necrosis factor alpha and interleukin-1 alpha and beta on human neutrophil migration, respiratory burst and degranulation. *Int. Arch. Allergy Appl. Immunol.* 86:82–91, 1988.

Feuerstein, G., and Hallenbeck, J.M.: Leukotrienes in health and disease. *FASEB J.,* 1:186–192, 1987.

von Figura, K., and Hasilik, A.: Lysosomal enzymes and their receptors. *Ann. Rev. Biochem.* 55:167–193, 1986.

Ford-Hutchinson, A.W.: Leukotrienes as potential mediators of inflammation. *Adv. Inflamm. Res.* 7:29–37, 1984.

Forman, H.J., and Thomas, M.J.: Oxidant production and bactericidal activity of phagocytes. *Ann. Rev. Physiol.* 48:669–680, 1986.

Freissmuth, M., Casey, P.J., and Gilman, A.G.: G proteins control diverse pathways of transmembrane signalling. *FASEB J.* 3:2125–2131, 1989.

Gallin, J.I., Goldstein, I.M., and Snyderman, R.: *Inflammation: Basic Principles and Clinical Correlates.* Raven Press, New York, 1988.

Gallin, J.I.: Neutrophil specific granules: a fuse that ignites the inflammatory response. *Clin. Res.* 32:320–328.

Giger, U., Boxer, L.A., Simpson, P.J., Lucchesi, B.R., and Todd, R.F. III.: Deficiency of leukocyte surface glycoproteins Mo1, LFA-1, and Leu M5 in a dog with recurrent infections: an animal model. *Blood* 69:1622–1630, 1987.

Gilman, A.G.: G proteins: transducers of receptor-generated signals. *Ann. Rev. Biochem.* 56:615–650, 1987.

Gleich, G.J., and Adolphson, C.R.: The eosinophil leukocyte: structure and function. *Adv. Immunol* 39:177–253, 1986.

Gordon, D.L., and Hostetter, M.K.: Complement and host defence against microorganisms. *Pathology* 18:365–375, 1986.

Gordon, S.: Biology of the macrophage. *J. Cell Sci.* 4:267–286, 1986.

Hallet, M.B. (ed): *The Neutrophil: Cellular Biochemistry and Physiology.* CRC Press, Boca Raton, Fla., 1989.

Halliwell, B., Hoult, J.R., and Blake, D.R.: Oxidants, inflammation, and anti-inflammatory drugs. *FASEB J.* 2:2867–2873, 1988.

Harlan, J.M.: Consequences of leukocyte-vessel wall interactions in inflammatory and immune reactions. *Semin. Thromb. Hemostas.* 13:434–444, 1987.

Henson, P.M., and Johnston, R.B., Jr.: Tissue injury in inflammation: oxidants, proteinases and cationic proteins. *J. Clin. Invest.* 79:669–674, 1987.

Hokin, L.E.: Receptors and phosphoinositide-generated second messengers. *Ann. Rev. Biochem.* 54:205–235, 1985.

Horwitz, M.A.: Phagocytosis of microorganisms. *Rev. Infect. Dis.* 4:104–123, 1982.

Hugli, T.E.: Structure and function of the anaphylatoxins. *Springer Sem. Immunopath* 7:193–220, 1984.

Hurst, N.P.: Molecular basis of activation and regulation of the phagocyte respiratory burst. *Annals Rheum. Dis.* 46:265–272, 1987.

Hynes, R.O.: Fibroectins. *Sci. Amer.* 254:42–51, 1986.

Hynes, R.O.: Integrins: A family of cell surface receptors. *Cell* 48:549–554, 1987.

Janoff, A.: Elastase in tissue injury. *Ann. Rev. Med.* 36:207–216, 1985.

Kampschmidt, R.F.: The numerous postulated biological manifestations of interleukin-1. *J. Leukocyte Biol.* 36:341–355, 1984.

Kaplan, A.P., and Silverberg, M.: The coagulation-kinin pathway of human plasma. *Blood* 70:1–15, 1987.

Kay, A.B.: Eosinophils as effector cells in immunity and hypersensitivity disorders. *Clin. Exp. Immunol.* 62:1–12, 1985.

Kikkawa, U., and Nishizuka, Y.: The role of protein kinase C in transmembrane signalling. *Ann. Rev. Cell Biol.* 2:149–178, 1986.

Kirchner, H.: Interferons: a group of multiple lymphokines. *Springer Sem. Immunopath.* 7:347–374, 1984.

Kluger, M.J., Oppenheim, J.J., and Powanda, M.C. (eds): *The Physiologic, Metabolic and Immunologic Actions of Interleukin-1.* Alan R. Liss, New York, 1985.

Lachmann, P.J., and Hughes-Jones, N.C.: Initiation of complement activation. *Springer Sem. Immunopath.* 7:143–162, 1984.

Lagente, V., and Fortes, Z.B.: Role of PAF-Acether in the vascular events of inflammation. *Progr. Biochem. Pharmacol.* 22:149–155, 1988.

Larrick, J.W., and Kunkel, S.L.: The role of tumor necrosis factor and interleukin-1 in the immunoinflammatory response. *Pharmaceut. Res.* 5:129–139, 1988.

Larsen, G.L., and Henson, P.M.: Mediators of inflammation. *Ann. Rev. Immunol.* 1:335–360, 1983.

Le, J., and Vilcek, J.: Tumor necrosis factor and interleukin-1: cytokines with multiple overlapping biological activities. *Lab. Invest. 56:*234–248, 1987.

Lehrer, R.I.: Neutrophils and host defense. *Ann. Int. Med. 109:*127–142, 1988.

Lewis, R.E., and Granger, H.J.: Neutrophil-dependent mediation of microvascular permeability. *Fed. Proc. 45:*109–113, 1986.

Linscott, W.D.: Biochemistry and biology of the complement system in domestic animals. *Progr. Vet. Microbiol. Immunol. 2:*54–77, 1986.

Lundberg, C., Bjork, J., Lundberg, K., and Arfors, K.-E.: Polymorphonuclear leukocyte (PMNL) dependent and independent microcirculatory plasma leakage. *Progr. Appl. Microcirc. 1:*86–99, 1983.

Maddox, D.E.: Eosinophils: Assays and interpretation. *Clin. Rev. Allergy 6:*163–190, 1988.

Majno, G.: *The Healing Hand: Man and Wound in the Ancient World.* Harvard University Press, Cambridge, Mass., 1975.

Marchalonis, J.J.: *The Lymphocyte: Structure and Function.* Marcel Dekker, New York, 1987.

Metchnikoff, E.: *Lectures on the Comparative Pathology of Inflammation (1893).* Reprint by Dover Publications, New York, 1968.

Morrison, D.C., and Ryan, J.L.: Endotoxins and disease mechanisms. *Ann. Rev. Med. 38:*417–432, 1987.

Movat, H.Z.: *The Inflammatory Reaction.* Elsevier, Amsterdam, 1985.

Movat, H.Z., Cybulsky, M.I., Colditz, I.G., Chan, M.K.W., and Dinarello, C.A.: Acute inflammation in Gram-negative infection: endotoxin, interleukin 1, tumor necrosis factor, and neutrophils. *Fed. Proc. 46:*97–104, 1987.

Muller-Eberhard, H.J.: The membrane attack complex of complement. *Ann. Rev. Immunol. 4:*503–528, 1986.

Nathan, C.F.: Secretory products of macrophages. *J. Clin. Invest. 79:*319–326, 1987.

Needleman, P., Turk, J., Jakschik, B.A., Morrison, A.R., and Lefkowith, J.B.: Arachidonic acid metabolism. *Ann. Rev. Biochem. 55:*69–102, 1986.

Neer, E.J., and Clapham, D.E.: Roles of G protein subunits in transmembrane signalling. *Nature 333:*129–134, 1988.

Nomura, H., Nakanishi, H., Ase, K., Kikkawa, U., and Nishizuka, Y.: Inositol phospholipid turnover in stimulus-response coupling. *Progr. Hemostas. Thromb. 8:*159–184, 1986.

Omann, G.M., Allen, R.A., Bokoch, G.M., Painter, R.G., Traynor, A.E., and Sklar, L.A.: Signal transduction and cytoskeletal activation in the neutrophil. *Physiol. Rev. 67:*285–322, 1987.

Oppenheim, J.J., and Jacobs, D.M. (eds): *Leukocytes and Host Defense.* Alan R. Liss, New York, 1986.

Pangburn, M.K., Muller-Eberhard, H.J.: The alternative pathway of complement. *Springer Sem. Immunopath 7:*163–192, 1984.

Parker, C.W.: Lipid mediators produced through the lipoxygenase pathway. *Ann. Rev. Immunol. 5:*65–84, 1987.

Parrott, D.M.V.: Lymphocyte locomotion: the role of chemokinesis and chemotaxis. *Monogr. Allergy 16:*173–186, 1980.

Pestka, S., Langer, J.A., Zoon, K.C., and Samuel, C.E.: Interferons and their actions. *Ann. Rev. Biochem. 56:*727–778, 1987.

Petreccia, D.C., Nauseef, W.M., and Clark, R.A.: Respiratory burst of normal human eosinophils. *J. Leukocyte Biol. 41:*283–288, 1987.

Pober, J.S.: Cytokine-mediated activation of vascular endothelium: physiology and pathology. *Amer. J. Pathol. 133:*425–433, 1988.

Pollard, T.D., and Cooper, J.A.: Actin and actin-binding proteins. A critical evaluation of mechanisms and functions. *Ann. Rev. Biochem. 55:*987–1035, 1986.

Powanda, M.C., Oppenheim, J.J., Kluger, M.J., and Dinarello, C.A. (eds): *Monokines and Other Non-Lymphocytic Cytokines.* Alan R. Liss, New York, 1988.

Proud, D., and Kaplan, A.P.: Kinin formation: mechanisms and role in inflammatory disorders. *Ann. Rev. Immunol. 6:*49–84, 1988.

Rasmussen, H.: The calcium messenger system. *New Engl. J. Med. 314:*1094–1101, 1164–1170, 1986.

Reichard, S., and Kojima, M. (eds): *Macrophage Biology.* Alan R. Liss, New York, 1985.

Reynolds, H.Y.: Lung inflammation: normal host defense or a complication of some diseases? *Ann. Rev. Med. 38:*295–323, 1987.

Riches, D.W.H., Channon, J.Y., Leslie, C.C., and Henson, P.M.: Receptor-mediated signal transduction in mononuclear phagocytes. *Progr. Allergy 42:*65–122, 1988.

Roch-Arveiller, M., Giroud, J.P., and Regoli, D.: Kinins and inflammation: emphasis on interactions of kinins with various cell types. *Progr. Appl. Microcirc. 7:*81–95, 1985.

Ross, G.D.: *Immunobiology of The Complement System: An Introduction For Research and Clinical Medicine.* Academic Press, New York, 1986.

Rossi, F., Berton, G., Bellavite, P., and Della Bianca, V.: The inflammatory cells and their respiratory burst. *Adv. Inflamm. Res. 3:*329–340, 1982.

Rotrosen, D., and Gallin, J.I.: Disorders of phagocyte function. *Ann. Rev. Immunol. 5:*127–150, 1987.

Ruoslahti, E., and Pierschbacher, M.D.: New perspectives in cell adhesion: RGD and integrins. *Science 238:*491–497, 1987.

Russell, S.W., and Pace, J.L.: The effects of interferons on macrophages and their precursors. *Vet. Immunol. Immunopath. 15:*129–165, 1987.

Ryan, U.: The endothelial surface and responses to injury. *Fed. Proc.* 45:101–108, 1985.

Saito, H., Hayakawa, T., Yui, Y., and Shida, T.: Effect of human interferon on different functions of human neutrophils and eosinophils. *Int. Archs. Allergy Appl. Immunol.* 82:133–140, 1987.

Sandborg, R.R., and Smolen, J.E.: Biology of disease: early biochemical events in leukocyte activation. *Lab. Invest.* 59:300–320, 1988.

Sbarra, A.J., and Strauss, R.R. (eds): *The Respiratory Burst Oxidase and Its Physiological Significance.* Plenum Press, New York, 1988.

Schiffman, E.: Leukocyte chemotaxis. *Ann. Rev. Physiol.* 44:553–568, 1982.

Schreiber, R.D.: The chemistry and biology of complement receptors. *Springer Sem. Immunopath.* 7:221–250, 1984.

Schumaker, V.N., Zavodszky, P., and Poon, P.H.: Activation of the first component of complement. *Ann. Rev. Immunol.* 5:21–42, 1987.

Sha'afi, R.I., and Molski, T.F.P.: Activation of the neutrophil. *Progr. Allergy* 42:1–64, 1988.

Sibley, D.R., Benovic, J.L., Caron, M.G., and Leftkowitz, R.J.: Regulation of transmembrane signaling by receptor phosphorylation. *Cell* 48:913–922, 1987.

Sklar, L.A.: Ligand-receptor dynamics and signal amplification in the neutrophil. *Adv. Immunol.* 39:95–143, 1986.

Slocombe, R.F., Malark, J., Derksen, F.J., and Robinson, N.E.: Importance of neutrophils in the pathogenesis of acute pneumonic pasteurellosis in calves. *Amer. J. Vet. Res.* 46:2253–2258, 1986.

Smedegard, G.: Mediators of vascular permeability in inflammation. *Progr. Appl. Microcirc.* 7:96–112, 1985.

Stossel, T.P., Hartwig, J.H., Yin, H.L., Southwick, F.S., and Zaner, K.S.: The motor of leukocytes. *Fed. Proc.* 43:2760–2763, 1984.

Stryer, L., and Bourne, H.R.: G proteins: A family of signal transducers. *Ann. Rev. Cell Biol.* 2:391–419, 1986.

Styrt, B.: Species variation in neutrophil biochemistry and function. *J. Leukocyte Biol.* 46:63–74, 1989.

Sundsmo, J.S., and Fair, D.S.: Relationships among the complement, kinin, coagulation, and fibrinolytic systems. *Springer Semin. Immunopathol.* 6:231–258, 1983.

Takemura, R., and Werb, Z.: Secretory products of macrophages and their physiological functions. *Amer. J. Physiol.* 246 *(Cell Physiol. 15)*:C1–C9, 1984.

Tauber, A.I.: Protein kinase C and the activation of the human neutrophil NADPH-Oxidase. *Blood* 69:711–720, 1987.

Tracy, K.J., Lowry, S.F., and Cerami, A.: Cachectin: a hormone that triggers acute shock and chronic cachexia. *J. Infect. Dis.* 157:413–420, 1988.

Vadas, P., and Pruzanski, W.: Role of secretory phospholipases A_2 in the pathobiology of disease. *Lab. Invest.* 55:391–404, 1986.

Vane, J.R., and Botting, R.: Inflammation and the mechanism of action of anti-inflammatory drugs. *FASEB J.* 1:89–96, 1987.

Wallis, W.J., and Harlan, J.M.: Effector functions of endothelium in inflammatory and immunologic reactions. *Pathol. Immunopathol. Res.* 5: 73–103, 1986.

Ward, P.A.: Host defense mechanisms responsible for lung injury. *J. Allergy Clin. Immunol.* 78:373–378, 1986.

Wardle, E.N.: *Cell Surface Science in Biology and Medicine.* Elsevier, New York, 1985.

Warner, A.E., Molina, R.M., and Brain, J.D.: Uptake of blood-borne bacteria by pulmonary intravascular macrophages and consequent inflammatory responses in sheep. *Amer. Rev. Resp. Dis.* 136:683–690, 1987.

Wedmore, C.V., and Williams, T.J.: Control of vascular permeability by polymorphonuclear leukocytes in inflammation. *Nature* 289:646–650, 1981.

Weiss, E.R., Kelleher, D.J., Woon, C.W., Soparkar, S., Osawa, S., Heasley, L.E., and Johnson, G.L.: Receptor activation of G proteins. *FASEB J.* 2:2841–2848, 1988.

Weissmann, G.: *The Woods Hole Cantata: Essays on Science and Society.* Raven Press, New York, 1985.

Winkler, G.C.: Pulmonary intravascular macrophages in domestic animal species: Review of structural and functional properties. *Amer. J. Anat.* 181:217–234, 1988.

Worthen, G.S.: Lipid mediators, neutrophils, and endothelial injury. *Amer. Rev. Resp. Dis.* 136:455–458, 1987.

Wright, S.D., and Griffin, F.M., Jr.: Activation of phagocytic cells' C3 receptors for phagocytosis. *J. Leukocyte Biol.* 38:327–339, 1985.

Zigmond, S.H., and Lauffenburger, D.A.: Assays of leukocyte chemotaxis. *Ann. Rev. Med.* 37:149–156, 1986.

Healing and Repair

Barbul, A., Pines, E., Caldwell, M., and Hunt, T.K. (eds): *Growth Factors And Other Aspects of Wound Healing: Biological and Clinical Implications.* Alan R. Liss, New York, 1988.

Baserga, R.: Multiplication and division of mammalian cells. In: *Biochemistry of Disease,* Vol. 6. Marcel Dekker, New York, 1976.

Brown, E.J.: The role of extracellular matrix proteins in the control of phagocytosis. *J. Leukocyte Biol.* 39:579–591, 1986.

Bruijn, J.A., Hogendoorn, P.C.W., Hoedemaeker, P.J.,

and Fleuren, G.J.: The extracellular matrix in pathology. *J. Lab. Clin. Med. 111:*140–149, 1988.

Buntrock, P., Jentzsch, K.D., and Heder, G.: Stimulation of wound healing using brain extract with fibroblast growth factor (FGF) activity. I. Quantitative and biochemical studies of formation of granulation tissue. *Exper. Pathol. 21:*46–53, 1982.

Buntrock, P., Jentzsch, K.D., and Heder, G.: Stimulation of wound healing using brain extract with fibroblast growth factor (FGF) activity. II. Histologic and morphometric examination of cells and capillaries. *Exper. Pathol. 21:*62–67, 1982.

Buck, C.A., and Horwitz, A.F.: Cell surface receptors for extracellular matrix proteins. *Ann. Rev. Cell Biol. 3:*179–206, 1987.

Carpenter, G.: Epidermal growth factor: biology and receptor mechanisms. *J. Cell Sci. 3*(suppl.):1–9, 1985.

Carrico, T.J., Mehrhof, A.I., Jr., Cohen, I.K.: Biology of wound healing. *Surg. Clin. N. Amer. 64:*721–733, 1984.

Clark, R.A.F., and Henson, P.M. (eds): *The Molecular and Cellular Biology of Wound Repair.* Plenum Press, New York, 1988.

Cohen, I.K.: An update on wound healing. *Ann. Plast. Surg. 3:*264–272, 1979.

Cvapil, M.: Pharmacology of fibrosis; definitions, limits and perspectives. *Life Sci. 16:*1345–1362, 1976.

Dvorak, H.F.: Tumors: wounds that do not heal. Similarities between tumor stroma generation and wound healing. *New Engl. J. Med. 315:*1650–1659, 1986.

Eckersley, J.R.T., and Dudley, H.A.F.: Wounds and wound healing. *Br. Med. Bull. 44:*423–436, 1988.

Eisinger, M., Sadan, S., Silver, I.A., and Flick, R.B.: Growth regulation of skin cells by epidermal cell-derived factors: implications for wound healing. *Proc. Natl. Acad. Sci. USA 85:*1937–1041, 1988.

Gabbiani, G.: The role of contractile proteins in wound healing and fibro-contractive diseases. *Methods Achiev. Exp. Pathol. 9:*187–206, 1979.

Gabbiani, G., Hirschel, B.J., Ryan, G.B., Statkov, P.R., and Majno, G.: Granulation tissue as a contractile organ; a study of structure and function. *J. Exp. Med. 35:*719–734, 1972.

Gabbiani, G., and Montandon, D.: Reparative processes in mammalian wound healing: the role of contractile phenomena. *Int. Rev. Cytol. 48:*187–219, 1977.

Gabbiani, G., and Runggerbrandle, E.: The fibroblast. In: *Tissue Repair and Regeneration*, pp. 1–50, edited by L.E. Glynn. Elsevier-North Holland, Amsterdam, 1981.

Glynn, L.E.: The pathology of scar tissue formation. In: *Tissue Repair and Regeneration*, Handbook of Inflammation, Vol. 3, (L.E. Glynn, ed.), pp. 285–308, Elsevier–North Holland, Amsterdam, 1981.

Glynn, L.E. (ed): *Tissue Repair and Regeneration*, Handbook of Inflammation, Vol. 3, Elsevier–North Hollands, Amsterdam, 1981.

Grinnell, F.: Fibronectin and wound healing. *J. Cellular Biochem. 26:*107–116, 1984.

Hunt, T.K., Knighton, D.R., Thakral, K.K., Goodson, W.H., and Andrews, W.S.: Studies on inflammation and wound healing: angiogenesis and collagen synthesis stimulated *in vivo* by resident and activated macrophages. *Surgery 96:*48–54, 1984.

Igishi, K.: The role of fibronectin in the process of wound healing. *Thromb. Res. 44:*455–465, 1986.

King, L.E., Jr.: What does epidermal growth factor do and how does it do it? *J. Invest. Derm. 84:*165–167, 1985.

Knapp, T.R., Daniels, J.R., and Kaplan, E.N.: Pathologic scar formation: morphologic and biochemical correlates. *Am. J. Pathol. 86:*47–70, 1977.

Koch, A.E., Polverini, P.J., and Leibovitch, S.J.: Induction of neovascularization by activated human monocytes. *J. Leukocyte Biol. 39:*233–238, 1986.

Kurkinen, M., Vaheri, A., Roberts, D.J., and Stenman, S.: Sequential appearance of fibronectin and collagen in experimental granulation tissue. *Lab. Invest. 43:*47–51, 1980.

Leitzel, K., Cano, C., Marks, J.G., and Lipton, A.: Growth factors and wound healing in the hamster. *J. Derm. Surg. Oncol. 11:*617–622, 1985.

Liebovich, S.J., and Ross, R.: The role of the macrophage in wound repair: a study with hydrocortisone and anti-macrophage serum. *Am. J. Pathol. 78:*1–100, 1975.

Majno, G.: *The Healing Hand: Man and Wound in the Ancient World.* Harvard University Press, Boston, 1977.

Makarski, J.S., Jr.: Mechanisms in neovascularization: sprouting. *Surv. Synth. Path. Res. 1:*79–86, 1983.

McMinn, R.M.H.: The cellular morphology of tissue repair. *Int. Rev. Cytol. 22:*63–92, 1967.

Minor, R.R.: Collagen metabolism: a comparison of diseases of collagen and diseases affecting collagen. *Am. J. Pathol. 98:*227–280, 1980.

Mosher, D.F.: Physiology of fibronectin. *Ann. Rev. Med. 35:*564–575, 1984.

Oda, D., Gown, A.M., Vande Berg, J.S., and Stern, R.: The fibroblast-like nature of myofibroblasts. *Exp. Mol. Pathol. 49:*316–329, 1988.

Peacock, E.E., Jr.,: *Wound Repair*, ed. 3. W.B. Saunders, Philadelphia, 1984.

Roberts, A.B., Anzano, M.A., Lamb, L.C., Smith, J.M., and Sporn, M.B.: Type beta transforming growth factor: a bifunctional regulator of cellular growth. *Proc. Natl. Acad. Sci. USA 82:*119–123, 1985.

Roberts, A.B., Sporn, M.B., Assoian, R.K., Smith, J.M., Roche, N.S., Wakefield, L.M., Heine, U.I., Liotta, L.A., Falanga, V., Kehrl, J.H., and Fauci, A.S.: Transforming growth factor type beta: rapid induction of fibrosis and angiogenesis *in vivo* and stimulation of collagen formation *in vitro*. *Proc. Natl. Acad. Sci. USA 83:*4167–4171, 1986.

Ross, R.: The fibroblast and wound repair. *Biol. Rev. 43:*51–96, 1968.

Ross, R.: Platelet-derived growth factor. *Ann. Rev. Med. 38:*71–80, 1987.

Rudolph, R., Guber, S., Suzuki, J., and Woodward, M.: The life cycle of the myofibroblast. *Surg. Gynecol. Obstet. 145:*389–394, 1977.

Rungger-Brandle, E., and Gabbiani, G.: The role of cytoskeletal and cytocontractile elements in pathologic processes. *Am. J. Pathol. 110:*359–392, 1983.

Ryan, G.B., Cliff, W.J., Gabbiani, G., Irle, C., Montandon, D., Statkov, P.R., and Majno, G.: Myofibroblasts in human granulation tissue. *Human Path. 5:*55–67, 1974.

Sholley, M.M., Ferguson, G.P., Seibel, H.R., Montour, J.L., and Wilson, J.D.: Mechanisms of neovascularization: vascular sprouting can occur without proliferation of endothelial cells. *Lab. Invest. 51:*624–634, 1984.

Simpson, D.M., and Ross, R.: The neutrophilic leukocyte in wound repair. *J. Clin. Invest. 51:*2009–2023, 1972.

Sporn, M.B., and Roberts, A.B.: Peptide growth factors and inflammation, tissue repair, and cancer. *J. Clin. Invest. 78:*329–332, 1986.

Sporn, M.B., Roberts, A.B., Wakefield, L.M., and Assoian, R.K.: Transforming growth factor-beta: biological function and chemical structure. *Science 233:*532–534, 1986.

Van Brunt, J., and Klausner, A.: Growth factors speed wound healing. *Bio/Technology 6:*25–31, 1988.

Walton, G.S., and Neal, P.A.: Observations on wound healing in the horse: the role of wound contraction. *Equine Vet. J. 4:*1–5, 1971.

Woodley, D.T., O'Keefe, E.J., and Prunieras, M.: Cutaneous wound healing: a model for cell-matrix interactions. *J. Am. Acad. Derm. 12:*420–433, 1985.

Yamada, K.M.: Cell surface interaction with extracellular matrix materials. *Ann. Rev. Biochem. 52:*761–799, 1983.

5

Immunopathology

Maja M. Suter

Cellular Components of the Immune Response
  Lymphocytes
    T Cells: Helper, Suppressor and Cytotoxic cells
    B cells
    Null Cells
  Mononuclear Phagocyte System
  Mast Cells, Basophils, and Eosinophils
  Lymphoid System
Interaction of Cells of the Immune Response
  Antigen Presentation and Recognition
    Antigen Presentation to T Helper (T_h) Cells
    Antigen Recognition by Cytotoxic T (T_c) Cells
    Antigen Recognition by B Cells
  Role of Immunoglobulins in the Immune Response
  Lymphokines and Monokines
    Interleukins
    Interferons
    Tumor Necrosis Factor
    Lymphotoxins
    Platelet-Activating Factor (PAF)
Target Cell Killing
  Cytolytic Attack Mechanism of Complement
    One-Hit Kinetics
    Lipid-Bilayer Target
    Transmembrane Channel
    Mechanisms of Transmembrane Channel Formation
    Colloid-Osmotic Nature of Lysis
    Control of Membrane Attack by Complement
  Target Cell Killing by Cytotoxic Cells
    Recognition of the Target Cell by Cytotoxic Cells
    Triggering or Activation of Cytotoxic Cells
    Release of Cytotoxic Activity
    Lysis of the Target Cell
Immune-Mediated Tissue Injury
  Types of Hypersensitivity: Introduction and Classification
    Immediate-Type Hypersensitivity (Type I)
    Cytotoxic, or Tissue-Specific Antibody Hypersensitivity (Type II)
    Immune-Complex Disease (Type III)
    Cell-Mediated or Delayed-Type Hypersensitivity (Type IV)
  Mechanisms of Hypersensitivity
    Mechanisms of Immediate-Type Hypersensitivity (Type I)
      Initiation of Immediate-Type Hypersensitivity and the IgE Response

Activation of Mast Cells and Mechanisms of Mediator Release
Mediators: Histamine, Leukotrienes and Prostaglandins, Platelet-Activating Factor, Eosinophil Chemotactic Factor of Anaphylaxis and the Eosinophil
Lesions of Immediate-Type Hypersensitivity
Mechanisms of Cytotoxic Hypersensitivity (Type II)
  Reactions Against Specific Cell Types
  Immunohematologic Diseases
Mechanisms of Immune-Complex Disease (Type III)
  Formation and Deposition of Immune Complexes
  Experimental Basis for Understanding Immune-Complex Disease
  Deposition Process for Immune Complexes
  Mediation of Immune-Complex Lesions
  Case 5.1: Immune-Complex Disease
Mechanisms of Delayed-Type Hypersensitivity (Type IV)
  Initiation of Type IV Hypersensitivity
  Nature of the Cellular Infiltrate in Delayed-Type Hypersensitivity and Lesions
  Mediators of Cellular Hypersensitivity (Lymphokines)
  Delayed-Type Hypersensitivity in Perspective
Diseases of the Immune System
  Immunodeficiency Diseases
    Defects of the Mononuclear Phagocyte System
    Antibody (B Cell) Deficiencies
    Cellular (T Cell) Deficiencies
    Combined Immunodeficiencies (CID)
  Acquired Immunodeficiency Diseases
Autoimmune Diseases
  Mechanisms of Injury Associated with Autoimmunity
  Important Mechanisms of Induction of Autoimmunity
  Classification of Autoimmune Diseases
    Case 5.2: Pemphigus, an Autoimmune Skin Disease
Assessment of Immune System Function
  Assessment of Antibody Production
  Lymphocyte Function Tests
  Histopathology
  Immunohistochemistry
  Flow Cytometry
  Reference Material

Immunology and immunopathology are rapidly expanding fields which makes it both important and difficult to assemble the various new pieces of information to meet the needs and demands of contemporary veterinary medical science. Enormous advances have been made in immunologic concepts and methods. Both pathologists and clinicians find it necessary to be familiar with and to coordinate the concepts and methods of immunology.

A number of areas of emphasis have emerged from the study of immunology which help to focus attention on the breadth of the field. **Immunobiology** deals with the origin, induction, and mechanisms of the immune response. **Immunochemistry** is concerned with the physicochemical structure and molecular actions of antigen and antibody either *in vivo* or *in vitro*. In recent years, immunochemical principles and methods have also been applied to the cell surface receptors with which antigens and antibodies interact. **Serology** classically has dealt with antibodies and their reactions with antigens foreign to the host. **Immunohematology** encompasses the immunology and immunochemistry of certain constituents of the blood, as well as the immunology of blood groups. **Immunogenetics** deals with the genetic control of immune responses and its application to events such as organ transplantation. **Clinical Immunology** is devoted to the diagnosis and evaluation of immune status in the various immune-mediated disorders, immune deficiency diseases, allergic disorders, transplantation, and problems of immune function in neoplastic diseases. **Immunopathology** may be defined broadly as the study of lesions induced by or resulting from immune mechanisms. It is primarily concerned with the untoward consequences of immunologic responses, and will be our primary emphasis in this chapter. Obviously, these various subdivisions of immunology do not define distinct borderlines, and there is frequent overlap.

When most of us consider immunology, we think of it as the study of a vital part of those host defenses which serve to protect against threatening microorganisms. While the immune system obviously is important in protection, it is now clear that many kinds of immune responses may prove deleterious to the host. We must, therefore, make a distinction between **immunity** as a phenomenon associated with beneficial effects and **hypersensitivity** as a phenomenon associated with deleterious effects. The curious thing is that the development of immunity or hypersensitivity subsequent to antigen exposure occurs through basically the same mechanisms. It is not well understood why hypersensitivity reactions occur in certain individuals whereas immunity is conferred on most individuals under similar conditions of antigen exposure. The field of **immunopathology** is really a subset of the larger fields of pathology, immunology, and biochemistry, and thus encompasses a variety of phenomena. It deals with various kinds of derangements of biologic processes that arise as a consequence of immunologic reactions.

When abnormal, aberrant, excessive, or otherwise inappropriate immunologic responses lead to pathologic changes, these reactions are termed **immunopathologic.** The common denominator is that the **immune response causes tissue damage.** Allergies, autoimmunity, anaphylaxis, and the various kinds of immune complex–induced injuries are good examples. Even immunologic responses initiated as part of normal defense reactions can lead to pathologic insult to the host. When a pig suffering from hog cholera mounts an immune response against the causative virus, part of the chronic damage that results is due to the immune response and the ensuing immunopathologic reaction, rather than the virus itself. In the battle between host defenses (the immune system) and the invader (hog cholera virus), the battlefield itself (the pig) may become badly damaged, even if the host ultimately wins the war.

An additional important general point must be made. Almost without exception, the tissue injury resulting from immunopathologic reactions involves no new mediators, pathways, or molecules that are not already built into the scheme of inflammation. While the initiation of the reactions involves immunologic phenomena rather than the usual sorts of causes of inflammation such as microorganisms, the final common pathway leading to tissue injury involves the same cells and mediators that characterize *all* inflammatory reactions. The effector arm leading to tissue injury in most immunopathologic reactions is *inflammation,* and it obeys most of the same rules that are true for inflammatory reactions of a more classical background. This fact allows us to focus our attention on immunopathologic mechanisms rather than on end points. There are exceptions to this general rule, most notably immunopathologic injuries resulting from direct cell-to-cell contact between specifically sensitized lymphocytes and their target cells in tissue. Even here, however, inflammation ensues. In essence, the immunopathologic reactions trigger the release of a highly focused constellation of chemical mediators which leads to the accumulation of inflammatory cells and plasma constituents. As in "ordinary" inflammation, it is the presence of blood-derived elements which ultimately leads to tissue injury. Antibody or cell-mediated immune responses may initiate the reaction, but it is the leukocytes, the plasma proteins and their cleavage products, and the various other mediators of inflammation that actually effect most of the damage.

CELLULAR COMPONENTS OF THE IMMUNE RESPONSE

Before we discuss the various mechanisms by which immune-mediated diseases develop, we will briefly review the participants in this drama, the different components of the immune system. It will soon become clear that the same cells and soluble factors active in normal immune or inflammatory defense reactions also play a major role in immune-mediated tissue destruction and disease, but we will look at them in a different light than when we examined them as participants in inflammation (Table 5.1).

Lymphocytes

The various subcategories can be divided into three major groups, based on the ability of the different types of cells to express certain cell surface markers as well as functional differences; **T cells, B cells,** and **Null cells.** Depending on the animal species, lymphocytes constitute between 20% (dog), 40% (cat, horse), and 60% (cow) of peripheral blood leukocytes. All lymphocytes either differentiate to exert their function or expand to form a pool of memory cells that respond when the immune system again experiences contact with the same antigen.

T CELLS. This group of lymphocytes proliferates and differentiates in the thymus before seeding secondary peripheral lymphatic organs. They carry the **T cell receptor,** which is a cell surface molecule called TCR2 associated with the CD3 complex. The TCR2 molecule is a disulfide-linked heterodimer comprised of an α and a β chain that form the antigen binding site. The **CD3 complex** is a group of 3 transmembrane molecules thought to transduce the activation signal across the cell membrane. This T cell receptor is distinct from, but related to immunoglobulin, and is present on all mature T cells. The T cell receptor/CD3 complex is associated with a CD4 molecule in helper T cells or a CD8 molecule in suppressor/cytotoxic T cells, both of which are thought to stabilize the antigen-receptor complex. Essentially all leukocytes, including T cells, express a member of the **leukocyte cell adhesion molecule (Leu-CAM)** family of adhesion molecules called **lym-**

Table 5.1
Cellular Components of the Immune System

Cell	Morphology	Markers	Receptors	Products	Function
T_h	Small lymphocyte, lymphoblast	CD4(man)	IL-2,[a] IL-1, TCR, LFA-1, CD2	IL-2, IL-4, IL-5, γIFN	Help $\uparrow$ B/T cells (class II restricted) Memory cells
T_s	As above	CD8(man)	As above	SF	Suppress B/T cells Memory cells
T_c	As above	CD8(man)	As above	Perforin, TNF	Kill tumor and virus-infected cells (class I restricted) Memory cells
B	As T cells, mature: plasma cells	Surface Ig	Fc, IL-2, IL-4, IL-5, iC3b	Ig's	Antibody production Memory cells
NK	LGL	None	Fc, LFA-1, IL-1, IL-2	Perforin, γIFN, IL-1, IL-2	Kill virus-infected and tumor cells (not MHC-restricted)
Mϕ	Variable	Class II Ag	Fc, C3b, iC3b	Cytokines (IL-1, etc)	Phagocytosis, APC
Mast cells	Granules (metachromatic)		Fcϵ	Vasoactive amines, LT's PAF, PG's	Chemotaxis for eos, vasodilation, $\uparrow$ vascular permeability, smooth muscle contraction
Eos	Granules		Fc, C3b	Enzymes	Proinflammatory, antiparasitic

[a]Only when stimulated; Abbreviations used are: IL, interleukin; TCR, T-cell receptor; IFN, interferon; SF, suppressor factor; LFA, lymphopcyte function-associated; TNF, tumor necrosis factor; Ig, immunoglobulin; LGL, large granular lymphocyte; Mϕ, macrophage; APC, antigen presenting cell; eos, eosinophils; LT, leukotrienes; PAF, platelet-activating factor; PG, prostaglandins.

phocyte function-associated antigen (**LFA-1**). LFA-1 is expressed in greater quantity (up to 40,000 per cell) on T cells than on B cells, and is generally not found on nonhematopoietic cells. Through the use of specific anti-LFA-1 monoclonal antibodies, it has been shown that this molecule is involved in a variety of adhesion-dependent leukocyte functions such as cell-mediated cytotoxicity and induction of T helper cell proliferation. LFA-1 may also be involved in the homing of lymphocytes to certain anatomic sites *via* specific recognition within **high endothelial ven-**ules (**HEV**). T cells also express a **CD2 receptor,** a molecule that is important in lymphocyte adhesion to other, nonhematopoietic cells.

T cells are divided into three major subgroups depending on their function (Table 5.1). **Helper T cells (T_h)** are activated by the interaction of their T cell receptor with a specific antigen presented in context with the class II major histocompatibility (MHC) antigen on the surface of antigen-presenting cells such as macrophages. Activated T cells also express receptors for interleukin 1 (IL-1) and interleukin 2 (IL-2), and respond to these molecular stimuli. Upon activation, T_h cells stimulate B cells to differentiate to plasma cells and produce immunoglobulins, and activate cytotoxic T cells to kill their targets. To exert these various functions, T_h cells secrete a large number of regulatory molecules called **lymphokines,** which also act on other cell types including macrophages. **Suppressor T cells (T_s)** are regulatory lymphocytes that specifically suppress the immune response to a specific antigen by releasing suppressor factors that inhibit T helper or B cells. **Cytotoxic T cells (T_c)** are activated by T_h cells upon antigen stimulation. They are able to kill virus-infected cells or tumor cells. They recognize the antigen on the cell surface of the target cell in conjunction with the MHC class I antigen.

B CELLS.   The effector cells of the humoral immune response responsible for antibody production are the B cells and their terminally differentiated counterpart, the plasma cells. B cells recognize antigen with their surface membrane–bound immunoglobulin. They also express receptors for components of the complement system, including C3b, and several B cell growth factors such as IL-4 (Table 5.1). In their activated state they also express the IL-2 receptor. To be able to respond to a specific antigen, B cells usually require stimulation by antigen-specific T_h cells. That is, they respond best to what are usually referred to as **T-dependent antigens.** Certain unusual antigens that have multiple identical binding sites are able to stimulate B cells independent of T_h cells and thus function as **T-independent antigens.** The most commonly cited T-independent antigens are the polysaccharide **lectins** which can cross-link the antigenic determinants of the surface immunoglobulins.

NULL CELLS.   The null cells form an interesting population of lymphocytes that cannot be defined by markers for either B or T cells. They constitute between 5 and 20% of peripheral blood lymphocytes depending on the animal species. Mature null cells have the morphology of **large granular lymphocytes (LGL).** Null cells are nonadherent, nonphagocytic cells most of which possess IgG Fc receptors, but lack complement receptors, T cell receptors, or surface immunoglobulins. This cell population includes cells with various functions such as killer (K) cell activity and natural killer (NK) cell activity. **K cells** are leukocytes that recognize their target cell *via* an antibody bound to their Fc receptor and kill their target through an antibody-dependent cellular cytotoxicity reaction (ADCC). **NK cells** recognize determinants on tumor cells or virus-infected cells and kill the target cells directly. The precise definition of K cells and NK cells is, however, still emerging, as some lymphocyte populations appear to exert cytotoxicity *via* both NK-like and ADCC mechanisms, and both these killing activities may actually be performed by the same cells.

Mononuclear Phagocyte System

We have already become acquainted with macrophages in the context of inflammation and wound healing in the previous chapter, but this group of phagocytes is also very important in the development of both the immune response and immune-mediated tissue injury. The various bone marrow-derived members of the mononuclear phagocyte system are found in virtually all organs and connective tissues. They include the monocyte-derived macrophages central to inflammation as well as the "fixed" mononuclear phagocytes such as the Kupffer cells of the liver, Langerhans cells of the skin, dendritic cells and interdigitating cells of the lymph nodes, mesangial cells of the kidney, microglia of the central nervous system, and osteoclasts of bone. They adhere to glass or plastic, carry receptors for the Fc fragment of immunoglobulins and for activated complement components (C3b, C3bi) on their surface, and may be stimulated to express MHC class II antigens. These various receptors are important for both of the most important mononuclear phagocyte functions: phagocytosis and antigen presentation.

The Fc receptor and the complement receptors are involved in the phagocytosis of opsonized antigens, and the MHC class II antigen is needed for interaction with T cells. After phagocytosis, macrophages usually "process," or partially degrade and digest, the antigen and present critical components on their surface in combination with the MHC class II antigen to activate T cells. Upon activation, they secrete a large number of monokines, the most important being **interleukin 1 (IL-1)**. Cells that present antigens to T cells are called **antigen-presenting cells.** However, not only the members of the mononuclear phagocyte system can present antigens; other cell types, such as B cells, or under certain circumstances epithelial cells that may aberrantly express MHC class II antigens, have this capability too.

Mast Cells, Basophils, and Eosinophils

We have previously discussed mast cells and basophils as important sources of vasoactive agents in acute inflammatory reactions (*see* Chapter 4). They are also the predominant cells involved in the rapid mediator-release reaction characteristic of **anaphylaxis** and other forms of **type I (immediate-type) hypersensitivity.** As we have discussed, mast cells are found largely in perivascular sites in tissues, while basophils are rare circulating granulocytes. The cytoplasm of both types of cells is packed with granules that contain various potent chemical mediators. Both cell types also have abundant membrane receptors (Fcε receptors) that bind the Fc portion of IgE antibody with high affinity. With appropriate bridging of IgE molecules bound to these cell surface receptors, an explosive degranulation with mediator release occurs. At least two populations of mast cells exist, the **mucosal** mast cells, found principally in the gastrointestinal and respiratory tracts, and the **connective tissue** mast cells, found in the skin. The circulating basophils are functionally related to mast cells in that their cytoplasmic granules have similar mediator profiles, and they respond similarly to antigenic challenge. Like all granulocytes, basophils are of bone marrow origin, but they are never abundant members of the peripheral leukocyte pool. Among mammals, the rabbit is unique in having up to 4% circulating basophils; in all other species they are rare members of the circulating leukocyte pool. The role of these cells in type I (immediate-type) hypersensitivity will be discussed later in this chapter.

The role of eosinophils as "killer cells" in parasitic disease and as "regulatory cells" in acute inflammation and immediate-type hypersensitivity has already been introduced (*see* Chapter 4). Eosinophils respond to many of the same influences as the neutrophil, including soluble bacterial factors and activated components of complement, and a number of eosinophil-specific chemotaxins have been defined. They are also responsive to antigen-antibody complexes and have membrane receptors for both IgG and C3 fragments. IgE-dependent activation of mast cells leads to the elaboration of a wide array of chemical mediators including **histamine** and the **eosinophil chemotactic factor of anaphylaxis (ECF-A),** both of which exhibit considerable specific chemotactic activity for eosinophils. Although the importance of eosinophils as "regulator cells" in type I hypersensitivity has recently been challenged, these fascinating cells can secrete several chemicals of potential importance in dampening the local effects of a hypersensitivity reaction involving mast cell degranulation. The eosinophil major basic protein neutralizes heparin, histaminase inactivates histamine, a type B arylsulfatase inactivates leukotrienes LTC_4, LTD_4 and LTE_4 (SRS-A), and eosinophil phospholipase D can apparently inactivate platelet-activating factor (PAF). The generation of prostaglandins by eosinophils exposed to IgE-containing immune complexes and their phagocytosis of extruded mast cell granules may also constitute mechanisms by which the eosinophil can limit the effect of certain kinds of allergic reactions, but it is clear that the proinflammatory contributions of eosinophils are more important than their antiinflammatory properties.

Lymphoid System

Lymphocytes originate in the bone marrow and mature in primary lymphoid organs. B cells mature in the bone marrow in mammals and the bursa of Fabricius in birds, and T cells mature in the thymus. From these organs they migrate to specific locations in secondary lymphoid organs. B cells localize in the lymphoid follicles of the lymph nodes, the spleen, and the **gut-associated lymphoid tissue** (GALT, Peyer's patches) of the intestine. T cells localize in the paracortex of the lymph nodes, the periarterial sheaths of the spleen, and in parafollicular areas of the GALT. The localization of these cells in various tissues can be assessed by immunohistochemistry. Resident lymphocyte populations are also found in the lung and the skin. In the lung they form lymph follicles associated with bronchi and bronchioles (the **bronchial-associated lymphoid tissue**, BALT). The skin-resident lymphocytes (mostly T cells) together with epidermal antigen-presenting cells (Langerhans cells), the keratinocytes (which are known to secret soluble factors and under certain influences to express MHC class II antigens), and the regional lymph nodes form the **skin-associated lymphoid tissue** (SALT).

Lymphocytes reside temporarily in these secondary lymphoid tissues, but many return to the blood where they circulate briefly prior to returning to the secondary lymphoid organ from which they came. This process is called lymphocyte **homing,** and it plays a major role in immunological surveillance. It is antigen-independent and occurs in hours. The main components of homing lymphocytes are memory T and B cells, some virgin T cells, and perhaps also some NK cells. In secondary lymphoid organs such as peripheral lymph nodes, tonsils, GALT, and BALT, **high endothelial venules (HEV)** are present and are involved in the recognition of the "home" organ (*see also* Chapter 4). Lymphocytes enter lymph nodes only by crossing HEV and not by migrating through other endothelia. Two different **homing receptors (high endothelial binding factors, HEBF)** have been found on HEV of Peyer's patches and lymph nodes, and the receptors are recognized preferentially by the cells that home back to the respective organ. No HEV are present in thymus, bone marrow, and nonlymphoid organs such as the skin or mucous membranes. In these organs the **CD2 adhesion receptor** is thought to be important because it binds to the cell adhesion molecule **lymphocyte function-associated molecule 3 (LFA-3),** which has a broad tissue distribution including endothelial, epithelial, and connective tissue cells.

INTERACTION OF CELLS OF THE IMMUNE RESPONSE

The various members of the cellular family making up the immune system communicate with each other in a variety of ways. Antigens are recognized, processed, and presented by one group of cells to other members of the immune cell family. It is important to understand how these cells communicate with each other and what factors are involved in this interaction. Only a thorough understanding of these interactions will enable us to understand the pathogenesis of immune-mediated tissue injury. This is a finely tuned system with many complex interactions. When the system works, immunity can result. Conversely, if it does not function properly, immune deficiency or immune-mediated disease may be the result.

Antigen Presentation and Recognition

In the last 10 years or so, it has become clear that antigen recognition by T or B cells follows distinctly different mechanisms. Antigens in their native conformation bind to immunoglobulin receptors on B cells while T cell receptors bind denatured antigens presented on the cell membrane.

ANTIGEN PRESENTATION TO T HELPER (T_h) CELLS   The presentation of antigens to T_h cells is a crucial first step in the induction of an immune response and involves **antigen-presenting cells (APC)** of which the prototype is the macrophage. Other cells that are able to present antigens include dendritic cells of the spleen, Langerhans cells of the skin, and interdigitating cells of the lymph nodes. More recently, B cells have also been shown to present antigen to T cells. For effective antigen presentation, the APC must be able to take up the antigen, internalize it by phagocytosis, and process it (Fig. 5.1). Processing of antigen by APC involves denaturation in endosomes by lysosomal enzymes, leading to the unfolding of the protein and the exposure of hydrophobic sites. These sites are then capable of interacting with the lipid bilayer of the cytoplasmic membrane and are subsequently expressed on the cell surface in combination with MHC class II antigens. It has been shown that macrophages, in which antigen processing is diminished through inhibition of lysosomal enzymes, are unable to activate T_h cells.

The expression of the MHC class II molecules is also critical to antigen presentation. After antigen/class II molecule presentation to the T_h cell receptor, helper cells are activated by this receptor-mediated interaction with the macrophage. T cells express cell surface molecules that seem to stabilize the T cell receptor–antigen/class II interaction (CD4 on helper T cells, CD8 on suppressor/cytotoxic T cells). Additionally, soluble factors secreted by the macrophage are important for T cell activation, especially **interleukin-1** (IL-1). The influence of IL-1 on T cells is twofold: IL-1 stimulates IL-2 production and also induces the expression of receptors for IL-2, which then allows the T cells to respond to this growth factor. Activated T cells then proliferate and differentiate to exert their effector function as helper cells. The production of γIFN by these cells increases the MHC class II antigen expression on APC and thus potentiates antigen presentation. Induction of MHC class II antigen expression as a response to γIFN is not limited to the cells of the mononuclear phagocyte system but extends, with prolonged antigenic stimulation, to many cell types including epithelial, endothelial, and connective tissue cells. Such mechanisms may be involved in the activation of autoreactive T cells, and may thus be involved in the initiation of autoimmune disease.

ANTIGEN RECOGNITION BY CYTOTOXIC T (T_c) CELLS.   Recognition of antigenic determinants on target cells by T_c cells depends on the combined expression of a denatured antigenic determinant and an MHC class I antigen on the surface of target cells. In target cells, antigens such as viral glycoproteins or nucleoproteins are synthesized in the endoplasmic reticulum, transported to the Golgi apparatus, and then to the cell surface where they are presented in combination with the MHC class I antigens. This combination of antigen/class I molecule is then recognized by antigen-specific activated T_c cells.

ANTIGEN RECOGNITION BY B CELLS.   In contrast to T cells, B cells do not require

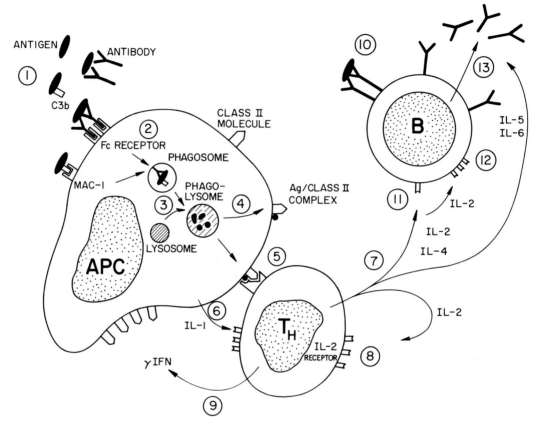

Figure 5.1. Antigen Presentation: Induction of the Humoral Immune Response. Several features of the interactions of antigen presenting cells *(APC)*, T helper cells *(T$_h$)*, and B cells are shown. *Antigen Presenting Cell (APC): (1)* opsonization of the *antigen, (2) antigen-APC* contact *via Fc receptor* or *MAC1* (iC3b receptor) and phagocytosis (opsonization is not essential but probably occurs frequently *in vivo*), *(3)* fusion of *phagosome* and *lysosome* leading to processing of the *antigen, (4)* presentation of antigenic epitopes on cell surface in context with MHC *class II molecule,* *(5)* interaction of the *antigen/class II complex* with the T cell receptor on the *T$_h$* cell, *(6)* secretion of *IL-1. T helper Cell (T$_h$):* activation of the T cell receptor and influence of *IL-1* lead to activation of *T$_h$;* there is *(7)* secretion of *IL-2, IL-4, IL-5,* and *IL-6* (all influence *B* cell maturation and differentiation), *(8) IL-1* and *IL-2* (autocrine) induced expression of *IL-2 receptors* on *T$_h$,* and *(9)* secretion of γ*IFN* and subsequent increased expression of MHC *class II molecule* on *APC. B cell:* activation of *B* cell by *(10)* binding of the native antigen to the surface immunoglobulin antigen receptor, *(11)* stimulation by *IL-2, IL-4, IL-5,* and *IL-6* from *T$_h$,* and *(12)* increased expression of IL-2 receptors leading to maturation and differentiation of *B* cells to plasma cells with *(13)* antibody production.

the expression of MHC molecules for their activation. They carry surface membrane–bound immunoglobulins that serve as the antigen receptors (Fig. 5.1). These immunoglobulin receptors bind the antigen in its native state. B cells may also function as APC by unfolding antigens in order to express them in conjunction with MHC class II molecules for T$_h$ cells.

Role of Immunoglobulins (Ig) in the Immune Response

Antibodies are produced by B cells in two forms: membrane-bound or secreted.

As mentioned above, the membrane-bound Ig serves as the B cell antigen receptor and is an integral membrane protein. The secreted Ig is the effector molecule of the B cell. Antibodies are divided into five classes or **isotypes** according to their structure and function; IgM, IgG, IgA, IgD, and IgE. IgG is subdivided further into subclasses, which vary from species to species. Table 5.2 summarizes the properties of the different immunoglobulin classes.

Antibodies are composed of heavy and light chains, which differ among the various isotypes; the heavy chain determines the isotype. During their differentiation, B cells can change the type of heavy chain that they produce, a process called **iso-type switching.** The first antibody expressed on the cell surface is IgD, followed by IgM, and then IgG or one of the others. Any individual B cell, however, appears capable of expressing specificity for a single antigenic epitope. Immunoglobulin light and heavy chains each have a constant and a variable region, and the variable regions of the two chains combine to form the antigen binding site. The constant region interacts with Fc receptors on cell surfaces and binds complement components. Most of the effector functions of antibodies are mediated by the constant region and are important in our

discussion of immune-mediated tissue injury.

IgG Fc receptors are present on many phagocytic cells, such as the cells of the mononuclear phagocyte system or neutrophils, and enable these cells to engulf antigenic particles (e.g., bacteria) that are coated with antibody (opsonized). Other types of Fc receptors (such as for IgE or IgM) are present on killer cells and are mediators of **antibody-dependent cellular cytotoxicity (ADCC).** This mechanism is involved in cytotoxic reactions (type II hypersensitivity) and will be discussed later. Fc receptors for IgA are present on certain epithelial cells and are needed for the mucosal transfer and excretion of IgA. IgE receptors are present on mast cells and basophils. Binding of IgE to this receptor sensitizes these cells to a specific antigen and, with subsequent antigenic challenge, these surface-bound IgE molecules are cross-linked by the antigen which triggers stimulation of the cells and release of a number of inflammatory mediators. This response is called **immediate-type hypersensitivity** and will be discussed in greater detail later.

Lymphokines and Monokines

This heterogenous group of water-soluble, nonhormone, nonantibody factors

Table 5.2
Properties of Immunoglobin Classes

	IgM	IgG	IgA	IgE	IgD
Serum half-life (days)	5.1	23	5.8	2.8	2.3
Complement fixation	+ +	+[a]	—	—	—
Opsonization	—	+	—	—	—
Mast cell sensitization	—	—	—	+ +	—
Transplacental	—	±[b]	—	—	—
Transepithelial	±[e]	±[c]	+ +	—	—
ADCC	—	+	—	—	—

[a] Only some subclasses.
[b] Depends on type of placentation (hemochorial and endothelial).
[c] Minor importance.
ADCC, antibody-dependent cellular cytotoxicity.

that are produced by lymphocytes (lymphokines), macrophages (monokines), or other cells (cytokines) form an important part of the "messenger" system for intercellular communication. Some of the lymphokines (*e.g.*, IL-1) are important mediators of inflammation (*see* Table 4.18), but, as a family, they are probably more important to the regulation and interaction of the cells involved in the immune response.

Lymphokines are ideal molecules for the regulation and modulation of the immune response because their short half-life (usually a few hours or less) confines their physiologic effect to a local environment over a short time frame. This aids in the fine tuning of complex interactive processes among many different cell types. It is now abundantly clear that lymphokines are important for normal immune responses, and they are intimately involved in the pathogenesis of certain kinds of immune-mediated tissue injury.

Interleukins

Interleukin-1 (IL-1) was originally described as a factor synthesized by macrophages, but it is now known that it can be produced by virtually all nucleated cells. We will concentrate here on the effects of macrophage IL-1 on the immune response. IL-1 binds to cells that express the IL-1 receptor. Two distinct forms of IL-1 have been identified, IL-1$_\alpha$ and IL-1$_\beta$, which have similar if not identical functional activities and bind to the same receptor, but are not completely homologous at the functional site. IL-1 has many different functions, affects a variety of target cells, and enhances the immune response by activating all cellular components of the immune system (Fig. 5.2). In some of its actions, such as increasing the activity of cytotoxic cells, IL-1 has a synergetic effect with γIFN and IL-2. Its effects on cells outside of the immune system include the induction of acute phase proteins by hepatocytes; increased proliferation and mediator release by endothelial cells; enhanced procoagulant activity of endothelial cells; increased proliferation and prostaglandin synthesis by fibroblasts, muscle cells, and synovial cells; induction of collagenase and other enzymes by chondrocytes and osteoblasts; and the induction of fever (*see also* Table 4.18). Some of the effects of IL-1 on lymphocytes can be inhibited by immunosuppressive agents such as cyclosporine, corticosteroids, and certain of the prostaglandins. This effect is often desired in the treatment of autoimmune diseases such as rheumatoid arthritis. However, these agents also interfere with the action of IL-2 and may act primarily on the IL-1 target cell. Cyclooxygenase inhibitors seem to interfere with those effects of IL-1 that are prostaglandin-mediated, such as fever and muscle proteolysis.

Interleukin 2 (IL-2) is a true "interleukin" with a specific effect on T cells. IL-2 is one of the most thoroughly studied and characterized lymphokines. The gene that codes for IL-2 has been cloned, and recombinant molecules are available. IL-2 plays an important immunologic role by providing the growth signal for clonal expansion of various helper, suppressor, and cytotoxic lymphocyte populations. IL-2 interacts with T lymphocytes by binding to specific membrane receptors not present on resting cells, but which appear rapidly after T lymphocyte activation (Fig. 5.1). Sustained T cell proliferation depends on the presence of both specific IL-2 receptors and IL-2; if either is absent, the cells will stop proliferating and die. This process is antigen-dependent; if antigen is removed, IL-2 receptors disappear from the cell surface, and T cell proliferation stops.

Two receptor molecules have been shown to bind IL-2, a p55 molecule (also called the Tac antigen) and a p75 molecule; however, only p75 binding results in internalization of the receptor-ligand com-

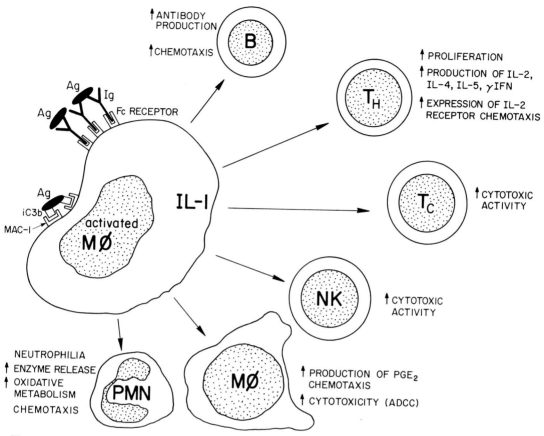

Figure 5.2.   Effects of IL-1 on the Immune System. Macrophages secrete *IL-1* after stimulation by opsonized antigen *via* the *Fc receptor* or *via* the *MAC-1* receptor *(iC3b)*. Macrophage *IL-1* is an important initiator of the immune response and stimulates practically all of the necessary cells. (*Mφ*, macrophage; *Ag*, antigen).

plex and the transmembrane signaling of the activation event. Certain antiinflammatory drugs (dexamethasone), chemical mediators of inflammation (PGE₂, serotonin), and immunosuppressive drugs (cyclosporine) stop lymphocyte proliferation by interfering with IL-2 production or receptor expression.

An important link between IL-1 and IL-2 arises from the fact that a critrical signal for lymphocyte production of IL-2 is their stimulation by IL-1. IL-2 is not just a growth factor, it also stimulates T lymphocytes to release a variety of other lymphokines including γIFN and IL-4. IL-2 also has a direct effect on B cell prolif-

eration. Hence, IL-2 seems to play an important role in initiating and modulating B cell proliferation and differentiation (Fig. 5.3). Additionally, IL-2 enhances the cytotoxic activity of T_c cells and NK cells (in synergy with γIFN and IL-1). Direct evidence for the importance of IL-2 has been obtained by injection of anti–IL-2 antibodies into laboratory animals, creating a severely immuno-suppressed state.

Interleukin 3 (IL-3) also evolved through a series of name changes (such as panspecific hemopoietin, PSH) while its true molecular identity was being established. It is a heavily glycosylated, 166

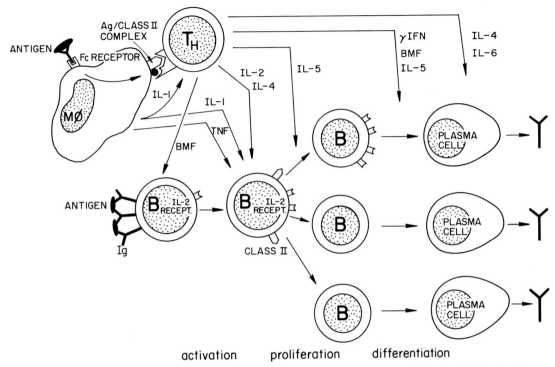

Figure 5.3. Role of "B Cell Growth Factors" in B Cell Activation and Antibody Production.
Various factors are secreted by activated T_h cells and macrophages which stimulate *activation,*
proliferation, and *differentiation* of resting *B* cells at different stages of their development. (*IL,*
interleukin; *γIFN, γ*interferon; *TNFα,* tumor necrosis factor; *BMF,* B cell maturation factor).

amino acid protein of M_r around 25,000
and is a product of activated T-lympho-
cytes. IL-3 appears to be the only hemopoietin able to directly stimulate the production of pluripotential hemopoietic stem
cells *in vitro;* it stimulates the growth of
colonies of mast cells, neutrophils, macrophages, and megakaryocytes. It is also
important to note that the action of IL-3
is not limited to immature hematopoietic
cells, as it can also stimulate the division
of well-differentiated mast cells and enhance cell division and phagocytosis in
mature macrophages. The interaction of
IL-3 with various target cells occurs *via*
a recently identified specific IL-3 surface
receptor. Because of the variety of cells
which respond to IL-3, it has been suggested that it functions as a sort of mo-

lecular link between the hematopoietic
system and the immune system.

  **Interleukin-4 (IL-4, BSF-1, BCGF I,
IgE switch factor)** also has evolved
through a variety of name changes, most
of which relate to its function as a B cell
stimulatory factor. IL-4 is a 20,000 M_r
protein produced by activated T cells which
acts on resting B cells to increase their
expression of class II MHC molecules and
to markedly increase the production of
immunoglobulins by endotoxin-stimulated B cells. As a growth factor, IL-4 acts
in concert with anti-idiotypic antibodies
to stimulate the proliferation of **resting**
B cells, a step important in the clonal
expansion of antigen-specific B cells (Fig.
5.3). It also increases viability and stimulates growth of normal T-cells, and serves

as a co-stimulant (along with, for example, IL-1) for the growth of mast cells as well as several hematopoietic lineage cells such as granulocytes, megakaryocytes, erythroid precursors, and macrophages. Thus, IL-4 is an interleukin with a broad range of effects.

Interleukin-5 (IL-5, BCGF II) is produced by T cells and is another pleiotropic lymphokine that acts on B cells and other cells. IL-5 modulates **activated** B cells by stimulating their proliferation, increasing production of immunoglobulins (IgG, IgM, and IgA), and inducing expression of IL-2 receptors (Fig. 5.3). In addition, IL-5 stimulates differentiation of bone marrow stem cells and induces differentiation of eosinophils and T_c cells (the latter co-stimulated with IL-2).

Interleukin-6 (IL-6, BSF 2, interferon β_2 is another cytokine produced not only by T cells, but also by macrophages and fibroblasts. It induces antibody secretion from activated normal B cells (Fig. 5.3).

Interferons

The three major types of IFN (α, β, and γ), originally described as factors produced following viral infections and exerting antiviral effects, were introduced in Chapter 4. In this chapter we will limit our discussion to **γ Interferon (γIFN)**, the lymphokine produced by mitogen- or antigen-activated lymphocytes, which plays a major role in immune regulation. Due to the availability of recombinant bovine interferons, we probably know more about bovine γIFN than about this lymphokine in other domestic animal species. Bovine γIFN is a protein of 145 amino acids, and is the product of a single gene. γIFN has several distinct effects on cells of the immune system (Fig. 5.4). It increases the expression of high-affinity Fc and C3b receptors on the cell surface of macrophages and other cells bearing these receptors. This effect may be of primary importance in the clearance of immune complexes through phagocytosis and in antibody-dependent cellular cytotoxicity (ADCC). γIFN increases the expression of class II MHC molecules on cells bearing these molecules, such as macrophages, and increases the activity of these cells in antigen presentation. Additionally, it induces class II MHC antigens on cells that normally do not express these molecules, such as keratinocytes and glandular epithelial cells. This action may promote the induction of autoimmune phenomena, as aberrantly expressed class II MHC molecules have been demonstrated in autoimmune thyroiditis and diabetes. γIFN also functions as a growth factor late in B cell differentiation, acting synergistically with other B cell growth factors. γIFN has certain synergistic effects with IL-1 and tumor necrosis factor (TNFα), such as enhanced cytotoxicity against tumor cells; however, some of these effects may relate to the fact that both IL-1 and TNFα can induce γIFN production, and that γIFN induces TNFα production by macrophages and TNFα receptor expression on target cells.

Tumor Necrosis Factor

Tumor Necrosis Factor (TNFα) is an important cytokine not only in inflammation and shock but in immune mechanisms. It is produced by activated macrophages and to a much lesser extent secreted by activated T lymphocytes. The various influences of TNFα on the immune system are shown in Figure 5.5. TNFα increases both T and B lymphocyte proliferation in synergy with IL-1. It also works with IL-6 to enhance the development of hematopoietic precursor cells. TNFα augments expression of IL-2 receptors, increases expression of MHC class II molecules, and enhances the IL-2 response of T cells. Furthermore, TNFα is secreted by cytotoxic cells and is involved

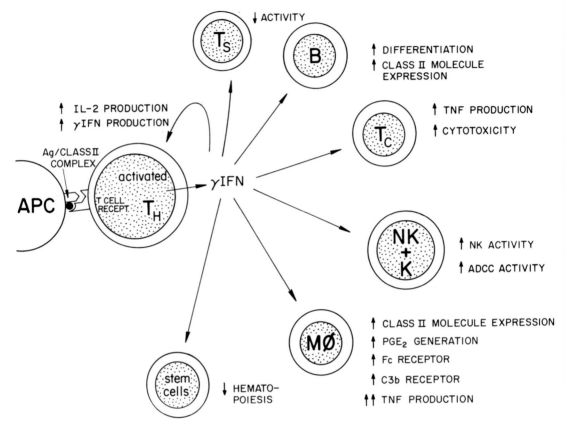

Figure 5.4.   Effects of γInterferon (γIFN) on the Immune System. *γIFN is secreted by T*h *cells that have been activated by the interaction of their T cell receptor with the antigen/MHC class II complex on an antigen presenting cell (APC). γIFN often increases the activity of immune cells, sometimes synergistically with IL-1.*

in target cell lysis by promoting **apoptosis** (*see also* Chapter 2). It remains possible that some of the effects ascribed to TNFα could be because TNFα induces production of other lymphokines such as IL-1 or **granulocyte-macrophage colony stimulating factor (GM-CSF)**. Glucocorticosteroids strongly suppress TNFα synthesis.

Lymphotoxins

   Lymphotoxins (LTS) are a heterogeneous population of cytolytic factors released by lectin- or antigen-stimulated lymphocytes which have cytotoxic effects.

In contrast to perforins and the complement fragment C9, lymphotoxins appear to function *via* mechanisms other than formation of pores. The best-characterized lymphotoxin is usually referred to as **TNFβ** (often just called **lymphotoxin**) and is produced by T$_c$ cells and NK cells. TNFα and TNFβ are distinct but related molecules, bind to the same receptor, and have similar functions such as a strong cytotoxic activity against tumor cells. There are several other less well defined cytotoxic factors produced by activated lymphocytes, such as **NK cytotoxic factor (NKCF)**, which is distinctly different

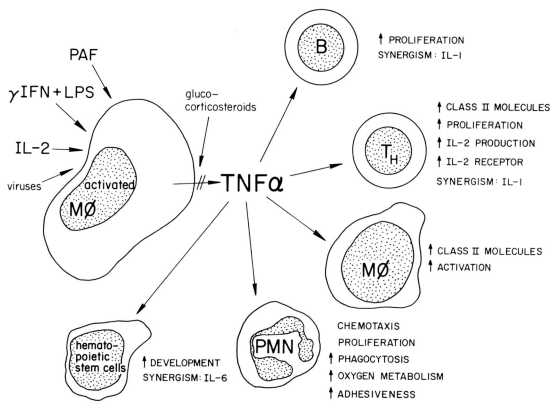

Figure 5.5. Effects of Tumor Necrosis Factor (TNFα) on the Cells of the Immune System. The major source of *TNFα* is the activated macrophage. *TNFα* enhances the immune response, often in synergism with IL-1. *TNFα* production is increased by various stimuli such as *PAF, γIFN, LPS, IL-2,* and many infectious agents. *Glucocorticosteroids* inhibit *TNFα* production. (*PAF,* platelet-activating factor; *γINF, γ*interferon; *LPS,* lipopolysaccharide [endotoxin]; *IL,* interleukin).

from TNFβ and not inhibited by anti-TNF antibodies.

Platelet-Activating Factor (PAF)

The cytokine PAF is a low molecular weight phospholipid that has been characterized as a glyceryl ether containing phosphoglyceride, with the basic structure of 1-O-alkyl-2-acetyl-sn-glyceryl-3-phosphorylcholine, abbreviated simply AGEPC. PAF was originally found to be released from sensitized basophils and mast cells in response to antigen-IgE interaction. In this situation it was found to be a potent mediator of anaphylaxis

and hyperreactivity involved in type I and type III hypersensitivities. Extensive studies in recent years have shown that PAF is produced by a variety of other cells including macrophages, neutrophils, platelets, endothelial cells, and even lymphocytes (Fig. 5.6). PAF has a variety of effects on many different cells. Besides its strong *proinflammatory activities* (*see* Chapter 4), PAF is considered a potent modulator of cellular immune responses. Its influence as an immunoregulator relates to the ability of PAF to inhibit lymphocyte proliferation, stimulate suppressor cells and NK cells, and increase IL-2 responses. PAF is thought to be an im-

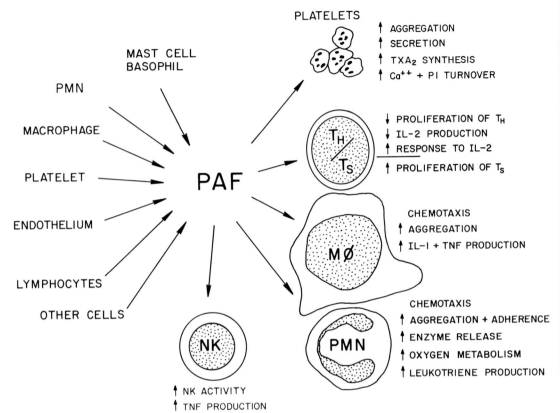

Figure 5.6. Effects of Platelet-Activating Factor (PAF) on the Cells of the Immune System.
PAF is produced by a variety of activated cells; mast cells and basophils release PAF after antigen-IgE interaction, PMN after phagocytic stimuli, endothelial cells and platelets after thrombin activation, etc. In addition to its strong proinflammatory influences, PAF also has a modulating effect on lymphocyte activity.

portant mediator of immune-mediated tissue injury.

TARGET CELL KILLING

The killing of target cells occurs either through the action of cytotoxic cells of the immune system or by the action of complement components. It is one of the important functional expressions of normal immune surveillance against both tumor cells and virus-infected cells, but it can also be an important part of the pathogenesis of immune-mediated tissue injury. In order to understand target cell killing, we must first understand the cytotoxic cells and the cytolytic components

of the complement system in order to compare the mechanisms that are involved in the killing of target cells.

Cytolytic Attack Mechanism of Complement

Cytolysis by complement (C) exhibits certain characteristic features that are central to an understanding of the process (Table 5.3). **First,** it has one-hit kinetics, as established by studies of dose-response curves and of reaction kinetics. This means that once initiated, the reaction goes to completion. **Second,** the lipid bilayer of the cell membrane is the target of C attack; **third,** the membrane lesion produced by C is a transmembrane channel;

Table 5.3
Cytolysis by Complement:
Five Characteristics

One-hit kinetics
Lipid bilayer is the target
Lesion is a transmembrane channel
Insertion of hydrophobic C peptides into lipid bilayer
Colloid-osmotic nature of actual cell lysis

fourth, the cytolytic mechanism is colloid-osmotic cell lysis.

ONE-HIT KINETICS. The cytolytic attack by C demonstrates one-hit kinetics. Once the activation of C components is initiated and C5 binds to the cytoplasmic membrane, the reaction always proceeds to cell lysis. The distinction between a one-hit and a multihit, or cooperative, process is based on the shape of the dose-response curve. A one-hit reaction will yield a curve that is entirely concave to the abscissa, whereas a multihit process will produce a sigmoidal dose-response curve (Fig. 5.7).

LIPID-BILAYER TARGET. This central issue of C-mediated cytolysis has been investigated with experimental lipid bi-

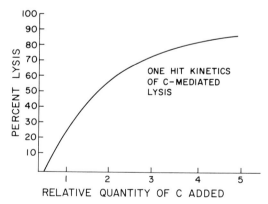

Figure 5.7. One-hit Kinetics of C-Mediated Lysis. Summarized data from several studies were used to form this transposed data curve, which shows that lysis is related to the number of complement (C) fixation sites per cell and that lysis occurs *via* discrete channels. This conforms to theoretical expectations of one-hit kinetics.

layers which are excellent models for the cytoplasmic membrane of cells *in vivo*. Two types of lipid bilayers have been used. One of these is the **liposome,** a structure consisting of concentric lipid bilayers with alternating compartments that contain water. The other type is a **planar lipid bilayer,** which is basically an artificial membrane interfaced with an aqueous surface. When lipsomes are damaged by C, the low molecular weight solutes in the aqueous compartment leak out, and appropriate markers are used to measure the leakage. In such studies, it has been shown that the C attack is initiated by the C5b67 complex, followed by assembly of C8 and C9.

TRANSMEMBRANE CHANNEL. Since membrane damage is due to channel formation, it is expected that the rate of marker release from the inside to the outside of the membrane depends on the molecular weight of the marker. This is in contrast to a mechanism involving overall destruction of the membrane (such as that induced by detergents), in which case markers of different size are released simultaneously. Differential release of markers of different size has demonstrated that the transmembrane channel has an internal diameter of approximately 10 nm. Therefore, molecules smaller than this diameter are released immediately following complement attack, while larger ones are released only after the membrane has been ruptured as a consequence of subsequent osmotic swelling.

MECHANISMS OF TRANSMEMBRANE CHANNEL PRODUCTION. The mechanism by which the membrane attack complex functions has been detailed only fairly recently. When C5 is cleaved by C5 convertase of either classical or alternate pathway origin, C5b is produced, and self-assembly of the **membrane attack complex (MAC)** is initiated. C5b and C6 form a stable bimolecular complex that binds to C7, causing C7 to express a site through which the C5b-7 complex can bind to the cell membrane. This C5b-7 complex bound to the cell membrane becomes the receptor for C8 binding, and the subsequent C5b-8 complex can bind and polymerize C9. It is this C5b-C9 complex, in association with a bilayer membrane, which produces the transmembrane channel.

In the first step, C5b interacts with C6 and C7 to expose hydrophobic sites in the phospholipid moiety of the membrane in which actual insertion of the molecule occurs (Fig. 5.8). This reaction proceeds without obvious damage to the membrane, and no membrane leakage can be detected. C8 has no detectable affinity for membranes by itself and is therefore entirely dependent on the mediating function of C5b-7, which determines not only the site of membrane attack, but serves

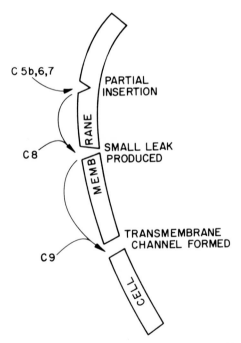

Figure 5.8. Transmembrane Channel Formation. The reactions of the terminal complement components with the cell membrane lead to lysis. Some leakage is apparent after fixation of *C8* but the transmembrane channel is not fully formed until *C9* is inserted into the membrane.

as the C8 receptor. The fully assembled complex is a unique molecular species containing a single molecule each of C5b, C6, C7, and C8 and multiple molecules of C9; it is basically a enormous complex made up of the tetramolecular C5b-8 complex (M_r about 600,000) and tubular poly-C9 (M_r approximately 1,100,000). The MAC becomes sequentially inserted in the cell membrane, and it is so large that it is actually visible in electron micrographs as "holes" in the membrane which have a 10 nm–wide central circular pore surrounded by a somewhat wider rim (Fig. 5.9). These characteristic and well-known images of the MAC and the membrane lesions produced by complement are largely due to the tubular poly-C9 contained in the MAC. Current evidence strongly suggests that the tubular poly-C9 inserted in the cell membrane represents the major complement transmembrane channel, and that the tetramolecular C5b-8 complex is the unit that catalyzes the polymerization of C9.

Actual membrane leakiness can be detected prior to complete assembly of the MAC. In the absence of C9, the C5b-8 complex tends to aggregate in the cell membrane, and these large protein aggregates produce structural and functional membrane damage evidenced by leakiness. It appears that tubular poly-C9 may not be entirely necessary for the lysis of anucleate cells such as bacteria and erythrocytes, but may be essential for the killing of nucleated cells. There are two distinct ways in which the large C5b-8 complex acts on C9: binding and polymerization. Both the binding and polymerization reactions can proceed irrespective of whether C5b-8 is membrane-bound or free in plasma, although the consequences in terms of cell lysis are obviously different. Binding of C9 occurs *via* the C8 part of the C5b-8 complex, but it is not known precisely how C5b-8 causes C9 polymerization. It is clear, however,

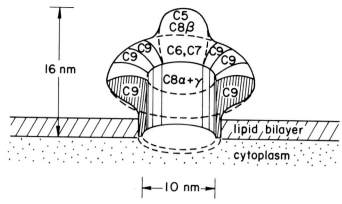

Figure 5.9. Arrangement of Complement Components in the Membrane Attack Complex.
After the binding of C5b67 to the cytoplasmic membrane of the target cell, the α and β chains of the C8 component insert into the lipid bilayer, initiating the binding of *C9* and the subsequent polymerization of C9 to form a transmembrane channel. (Modified from: Pollack, E.R.: Molecular mechanism of cytolysis by complement and by cytolytic lymphocytes. *J. Cell Biochem. 30:*133–170, 1986.)

that polymerization of C9 occurs, and that the tubular poly-C9 that results and is inserted into the cell membrane corresponds almost exactly with the electron microscopic images of complement-damaged cells; there is little doubt that the "holes" seen in such membranes are evoked by poly-C9.

With the binding of C9, an accelerated influx of water, sodium, and calcium ions into the cell occurs and intracellular potassium is lost to the extracellular fluid. These water and electrolyte fluxes across the transmembrane channel create severe ionic disequilibrium which eventually leads to osmotic rupture of the cell.

COLLOID-OSMOTIC NATURE OF LYSIS. Important evidence for the development of transmembrane channels is derived from the two-stage character of cytolysis by C. When a cell is attacked by C, it first swells. In a second step the membrane is explosively ruptured and the cell contents spill out. The damage caused by the MAC permits salt, water, and other small molecules to flow across the cytoplasmic membrane, but the membrane damage is too small to allow macromolecules, such as proteins and nucleic acids, to leave the

cell. The formation of the membrane channels leads to loss of the ionic gradient across the membrane and disappearance of the membrane potential. This leads to disturbance of the important intracellular-extracellular, colloid-osmotic equilibrium. Loss of this equilibrium causes swelling of the cell, calcium influx, and subsequent rupture. Additionally, other factors (such as lysozyme) may be able to enter the cell and cause further damage. A simple scheme of the major steps of complement-mediated lysis is given in Figure 5.10.

CONTROL OF MEMBRANE ATTACK BY COMPLEMENT. The assembly of the MAC is controlled at two stages, the insertion step and the polymerization of C9. **S-protein** or other plasma **lipoproteins** inhibit the insertion of C5b-7 into the lipid bilayer by physical association with the complex. S-protein binds to the hydrophobic membrane binding site of the C5b-7 complex and renders it water soluble. When S-protein and lipoproteins such as high-density lipoprotein (HDL) associate with the C5b-8 complex, they inhibit polymerization of poly-C9 *via* a mechanism which remains unclear.

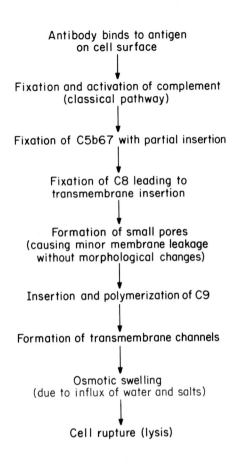

Antibody binds to antigen
on cell surface

↓

Fixation and activation of complement
(classical pathway)

↓

Fixation of C5b67 with partial insertion

↓

Fixation of C8 leading to
transmembrane insertion

↓

Formation of small pores
(causing minor membrane leakage
without morphological changes)

↓

Insertion and polymerization of C9

↓

Formation of transmembrane channels

↓

Osmotic swelling
(due to influx of water and salts)

↓

Cell rupture (lysis)

Figure 5.10. Complement-Mediated Lysis.
The sequence of events in the lysis of cells by
complement begins with antigen-antibody reactions and ends with swelling of the cell and
eventual cell rupture.

Target Killing by Cytotoxic Cells

Four different cell types act as the effector cells in cytotoxicity: **cytotoxic T
(T_c) cells, killer (K) cells, natural killer
(NK) cells,** and **"NK-like" T cells** (also
known as **lymphokine-activated killer
cells, LAK**). T_c cells are a distinct and
readily defined cell population, while NK
and K activity is associated in part with

cells characterized as **large granular
lymphocytes (LGL).** It has been suggested that the term "NK cell" should be
applied only in a functional sense, that
is, to a non-MHC-restricted, nonimmune
cytotoxicity, and not to a particular cell
population. Cells with NK activity often
have different phenotypes and lineages.

The process of killing a target cell by
cytotoxic cells can be divided into four
different phases: **first,** recognition of the
target cell by the cytotoxic cell leading to
cell-cell contact; **second,** triggering or activation of the effector cell; **third,** release
of the cytotoxic activity by the effector
cell, and **fourth,** killer cell–independent
lysis of the target cell. Table 5.4 summarizes the mechanisms of recognition
and action of the different cytotoxic
cells.

RECOGNITION OF THE TARGET CELL BY
CYTOTOXIC CELLS. T_c cells use largely
the α and β chains of their T cell receptor
(TCR) to recognize a specific antigenic
determinant in association with class I
MHC molecules on the target cell. As
mentioned above, the CD8 cell surface
molecule seems to stabilize the T cell receptor–target cell interaction. The presentation of the antigen on the target cell
surface occurs after intracellular antigen
processing. Rarely it may happen as direct integration of an unprocessed antigen into the cell membrane. Antigen recognition requires prior exposure to antigen
by the T_c cell and is therefore a true
immune response. While much is known
about how T_c cells recognize their target
cells, the receptor structure of **NK cells**
has not yet been determined. It is clear
that the putative NK cell receptor is a
glycoprotein, distinct from both the Fc
receptor and the T cell receptor. A leukocyte adhesion molecule, LFA-1, present
on the NK cell surface, stabilizes the receptor–target cell complex. NK activity
is directed against a wide variety of target cells; however, there is heterogeneity

Table 5.4
Mechanisms of Cell-Mediated Cytotoxicity

	T_c	NK	K^a	"NK-like" T cell[b]
MHC restriction	+[c]	—	—	—
Receptor involved	TCR	NKR?	FcR?	—
Prior sensitization required	+	—	+	—
IL-2 stimulates function	+	+	+	+
Cytolysis *via* perforin	+	+	+	+

[a] Not a uniform cell population, NK cells and some "NK-like" killer cells exhibit this function.
[b] Formerly LAK (lymphokine-activated killer cells.
[c] Rarely MHC class II antigens are involved; Tc, cytotoxic T cell; TCR, T cell receptor; NKR, NK cell receptor; FcR, Fc receptor; ?, putative.

in target cell recognition, because some cells kill a wide variety of target cells while others have a more restricted target spectrum. In contrast to T cells, target cell recognition by NK cells is not dependent on prior exposure to antigen and is therefore **not** a true immune response. The killing activity of NK cells appears to be part of the natural resistance of an individual to virus-infected cells and tumor cells, and it has been suggested that the major role of NK cells may be to assist in antibody-dependent cellular cytotoxicity *in vivo*.

A third mechanism of antigen recognition comes about by **K cells** *via* their Fc receptor. This cytotoxicity is called **antibody-dependent cellular cytotoxicity (ADCC)** because antibody mediates the cytotoxic cell–target cell contact by forming a bridge between antigen on the target cell membrane and the Fc receptor on the K cell. **"NK-like" T cells** (lymphokine-activated killer cells, LAK) kill their targets in a NK-like way, that is, the killing is non-MHC restricted and does not require prior sensitization. Less is known about the cytotoxic mechanism of LAK cells.

TRIGGERING OR ACTIVATION OF THE CYTOTOXIC CELL. While target cell recognition in the different forms of cytotoxic-

ity may be accomplished by distinctly different mechanisms, the events following recognition seem to be similar in all forms of cell-mediated cytotoxicity. Immediately following binding to the target cell, the cytotoxic cell begins to reorient its granules and other cytoplasmic organelles toward the region of target cell contact. Additionally, cytoskeletal reorganization (microtubules and actin) leads to an increased surface area of membrane contact with the target cell, and may actually involve membrane interdigitation. These are events that take place quickly; internal reorganization requires only several minutes and prepares the cells for the lethal hit. Recognition of the target thus leads to activation of the cytotoxic cell, and the events of cytotoxicity are initiated.

RELEASE OF CYTOTOXIC ACTIVITY. Following activation of the cytotoxic cell and reorientation of its organelles, granule membranes fuse with the cytoplasmic membrane, leading to **exocytosis** of granule contents. The importance of these events is emphasized in clinical patients with functional deficiencies; patients with the Chédiak-Higashi syndrome exhibit decreased cytotoxic activity related to abnormal granule formation and impaired exocytosis.

In addition to other enzymes, cytolytic granules from NK cells and T_c cells contain monomeric **perforins** (also called pore-forming protein [PFP] or cytolysin) as the major source of cytolytic activity. Perforins are acidic proteins of M_r 66–77,000 which, upon activation, polymerize to form **polyperforins** (Fig. 5.11). Polymerization of perforins is thought to be one of the essential mechanisms for target cell lysis. Cytotoxic cells can recycle cytolytic perforins and sequentially kill several target cells, yet are not themselves injured. Perforins are thought to bind to chondroitin sulfate A within the granules which inhibits spontaneous polymerization. After exocytosis, perforins dissociate from chondroitin sulfate A because of the higher pH in the extracellular milieu. Furthermore, detectable levels of perforins can only be demonstrated in cytotoxic cells that have been activated by IL-2; this may explain some of the

protection provided to the resting cytotoxic cell against autodigestion.

LYSIS OF THE TARGET CELL. While target cell recognition may be highly antigen-specific, the lethal hit delivered by the cytotoxic cell is nonspecific; any cell can be killed once the cytotoxic cell is activated. This situation is analogous to complement-mediated cytolysis in which the cytolytic process follows without cellular specificity. Like the MAC of complement lysis, cellular cytotoxicity also obeys the laws of one-hit kinetics; once it is initiated, it goes to completion.

Upon activation of the cytotoxic cell, granule contents are released by **calcium**-dependent exocytosis (Fig. 5.11). After secretion, perforins bind to the membrane of the target cell and, in the presence of **calcium,** polymerize to form tubular structures that insert as poreforming units into the target cell membrane. This process is amazingly similar

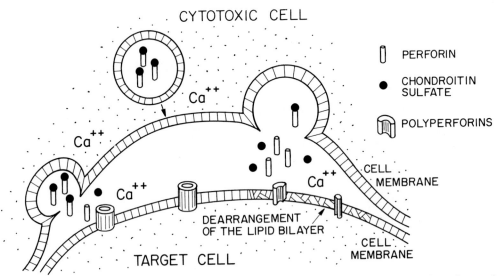

Figure 5.11. Cell-Mediated Killing of the Target Cell. After activation, the *cytotoxic cell* secretes *perforins* by exocytosis in a calcium-dependent manner. The secreted *perforins* bind to and insert into the plasma *membrane* of the *target cell* and in the presence of calcium polymerize to form *polyperforins* and a transmembrane channel. Within the lysosomal granule perforins are bound to *chondroitin sulfate* proteoglycan, which inhibits polymerization and damage to the lysosomal membrane. After exocytosis perforins dissociate from the proteoglycan. (Modified from: Ding, J., Young, E., and Chau-Ching, L.: Multiple mechanisms of lymphocyte-mediated killing. *Immunol. Today* 9:140–144, 1988.)

to complement-mediated cytolysis; 10–20 aggregated perforins form transmembrane channels analogous to those formed by the MAC, and monoclonal antibodies raised against perforins cross-react remarkably with all the members of the membrane attack complex (C5b-6, C7, C8, and C9). Indeed, a substantial degree of amino acid sequence homology has been demonstrated between the functional sites of C9 and perforins. The transmembrane channel formed by polyperforins is a highly functional one, which permits a flux of 10^9 ions per second, leading to membrane depolarization and severe electrolyte and macromolecule leakage. The primary damage to the target cell is a **colloid osmotic lysis** similar to what occurs following complement attack. It is interesting that these two processes, one based on cell-to-cell contact and exocytosis and the other on molecular assembly of complement proteins, should be so analogous. The similarities and differences between complement-mediated cytolysis and cellular cytotoxicity are summarized in Figure 5.12.

It is also clear that calcium- and perforin-independent pathways of killing must exist, since some cytotoxic cells (especially T_c) retain their cytolytic activity without calcium and perforin. Additionally, it has been shown that perforin-mediated membrane damage alone does not kill all the target cells, and that nuclear disintegration is necessary for cell death by **apoptosis** (*see also* Chapter 2). Shortly after membrane damage and release of small molecules, DNA breakdown products can be demonstrated in cells attacked by cytotoxic cells. This aspect of cellular cytotoxicity is most likely due to rather poorly characterized soluble nucleolytic factors that are antigenically related to TNF and lymphotoxin. These nucleolytic factors work much more slowly than do the perforins, and require several hours to lyse their target. It is thus currently envisioned that perforins open up the cytoplasmic membrane rather quickly, while nucleolytic factors enter the cell through the pore to reach the nucleus somewhat more slowly.

IMMUNE-MEDIATED TISSUE INJURY

The initiating mechanisms involved in immunopathologic events are principally the same as those underlying normal immune responses. It is therefore appropriate to remind ourselves of the distinction between **immunity** as a phenomenon associated with beneficial effects and **hypersensitivity** as a phenomenon associated with deleterious effects. It is still not well understood why hypersensitivity reactions occur in certain individuals, while immunity is conferred on most individuals by similar exposure.

During the past two decades, enormous advances have been made in the elucidation of the fundamental mechanisms of immunologic reactions in both host defense and disease. The knowledge and techniques of modern immunology have lead to a better understanding of the pathogenesis of immunologically mediated disease as well as more rational therapy. All hypersensitivity reactions involve immune responses and are therefore dependent on prior sensitization of the host with a specific antigen. The traditional classification of hypersensitivity into four major types by Coombs and Gell has stood the test of time (Table 5.5). The first three types are **antibody-mediated** and develop rather quickly, while the fourth type is mediated by T cells and macrophages and is a **delayed reaction.** Such a classification scheme is based on the kinds of antibodies and cells involved. In most forms of naturally occurring immunological disease, however, multiple types of hypersensitivity responses may participate simultaneously in the pathogenesis of tissue injury. We will briefly introduce the four types of hypersensitivity and then discuss each type in greater detail.

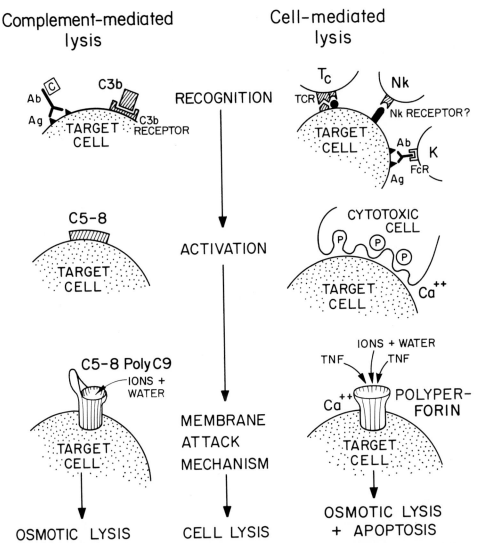

Figure 5.12 Similarities and Differences in Cytolysis Mediated by Complement and Cytotoxic Cells. In *complement-mediated lysis,* antibody or *C3b* interact with antigen or Mac-1 (iC3b) as a *recognition* event, and the attack sequence involves formation of a transmembrane channel by C components with insertion of *poly-C9* into the membrane. In *cell-mediated lysis,* antigen with or without MHC molecules form the *recognition* event, and *activation* of the cytotoxic effector cell initiates receptor-antigen interaction with release of cytotoxic granules. The secreted perforins insert into the lipid bilayer of the *target cell* in a fashion analogous to complement-mediated lysis. Transmembrane channel formation leads to *osmotic lysis* of the *target cell.* In cell-mediated lysis, the additional secretion of TNFα causes nuclear damage and *apoptosis.*

Types of Hypersensitivity: Introduction and Classification

IMMEDIATE-TYPE HYPERSENSITIVITY (TYPE I). This includes **anaphylaxis** and the allergic reactions to extrinsic aller- gens which occur in sensitized individu- als. These reactions are mediated by an- tibody of the **IgE** class triggering the release of **chemical mediators** from mast cells and basophils. Bronchial asthma, hay fever, milk allergy, allergic rhinitis, ur-

Table 5.5
Classification of Hypersensitivity Reactions

Reaction Type	Immunologic Mediator	Mechanism	Disease Example
Type I	IgE	Mediator release	Anaphylaxis
Type II	IgG, IgM	Cytotoxic	Autoimmune hemolytic anemia
Type III	IgG, IgM	Immune complexes	Glomerulonephritis
Type IV	Sensitized cells	Delayed-type hypersensitivity	Tuberculosis

ticaria, and atopy are good examples. The reaction begins within seconds or minutes after the binding of inhaled or circulating antigens with IgE bound to the Fcε receptor on the surface of tissue mast cells, located primarily near surfaces exposed to the external environment (skin, respiratory, and gastrointestinal tracts), or circulating basophils. This binding initiates reactions that lead to the release of histamine and other mediators from granules within the sensitized mast cells or basophils (Fig. 5.13). It is the **mediators** that are responsible for clinical disease. The major lesion is derangement of the intra- and extravascular fluid circulation; there is usually little cell destruction, and the complement system is not involved.

CYTOTOXIC, OR TISSUE-SPECIFIC ANTI-BODY HYPERSENSITIVITY (TYPE II.   Reactions of this type often lead to cellular or tissue damage. An antibody (usually of the IgG or IgM class) reacts with an antigenic determinant on a cell or tissue element. There are two principle mechanisms involved in this hypersensitivity:

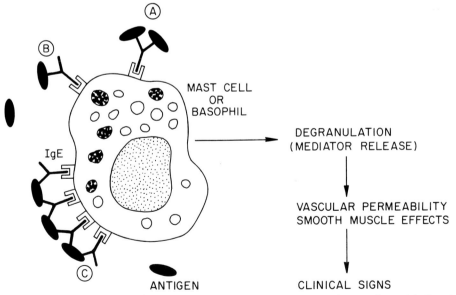

Figure 5.13.   Immediate-Type (Type I) Hypersensitivity. Bridging of two adjacent *IgE* molecules on the cell surface by specific antigen *(C)* and subsequent aggregation of the Fcε receptors lead to mediator release by the *mast cell*. Forms of antigen binding *(A, B)* which do not bridge adjacent *IgE* molecules fail to initiate the membrane events which lead to mediator release.

complement-mediated cytotoxicity and **antibody-dependent cellular cytotoxicity (ADCC),** both resulting in cellular death and other pathologic change in tissues, such as swelling or fragmentation of basement membrane (Fig. 5.14). Many of the **autoimmune diseases** (reactivity against self antigens) are representative of this type of cytotoxic immune reaction. Examples are autoimmune hemolytic anemia, some forms of immune-mediated leukopenia, and thrombocytopenic purpura. In these diseases, antibodies are formed against red blood cells, white blood cells, or platelets. The antigenic determinants are located on the cell surfaces. It also is believed that certain forms of renal disease are caused by the action of anti-kidney antibodies. A variation of type II hypersensitivity involves reactions in which antibodies bind to specific cell surface receptors. In such cases, the binding of antibodies to the receptor does not lead to cell lysis but stimulates or inhibits cellular responses normally induced by the binding of a specific ligand, such as a hormone. Neither complement nor killer cells are involved. Examples of this type of reaction are anti-TSH receptor antibodies in hyperthyroidism (Grave's disease), anti–gastric mucosal antibodies in pernicious anemia, and anti–acetylcholine receptor antibodies in myasthenia gravis. The autoimmune dermatosis pemphigus is a disease in which autoantibody binding to cell surface antigens of keratinocytes causes loss of cell-cell adhesion and subsequent blister formation, thus representing a unique, direct, antibody-mediated tissue derangement.

IMMUNE-COMPLEX DISEASE (TYPE III). Immune complexes are large molecular aggregates formed by the binding of antigen and antibody and sometimes complement (Fig. 5.15). They are constantly being formed and removed in the course of a normal immune response. Under appropriate conditions, immune complexes

may initiate pathologic processes. Experimental observations have indicated that the conditions under which the complexes are formed determine their pathogenetic activity. That is, when antigens are present in slight or moderate excess over specific antibody, the immune complexes that are formed remain small and soluble and may become trapped beneath endothelial cells along capillary basement membranes, or the internal elastic laminas of arteries, where complement is subsequently activated. The deposition of immune complexes in vessels and the activation of complement subsequently causes neutrophil leukocytes to migrate toward the lesions (chemotaxis) which, in turn, induce inflammation or necrosis in blood vessels or adjacent structures. Immune complexes initiating complement activation can liberate histamine from mast cells and cause increased vascular permeability. To some extent this may determine where vasculitis occurs. We will consider the deposition process in more detail later. One of the best examples of this form of immunologically mediated tissue injury is **immune-complex glomerulonephritis.**

CELL-MEDIATED OR DELAYED-TYPE HYPERSENSITIVITY (TYPE IV). This type of immunologic reaction is mediated by sensitized cells (lymphocytes) and activated macrophages. Neither circulating antibody nor complement are involved. The antigens responsible for its development are often, but not always, derived from infectious agents. When these antigens interact with the sensitized cells, macrophages are immobilized in the area and are induced to release enzymes that cause local edema, granulomatous inflammation, vascular thrombosis, and necrosis. This is probably the least understood of the four main types of hypersensitivity reactions. Delayed hypersensitivity probably occurs during the course of many infections, and is an important

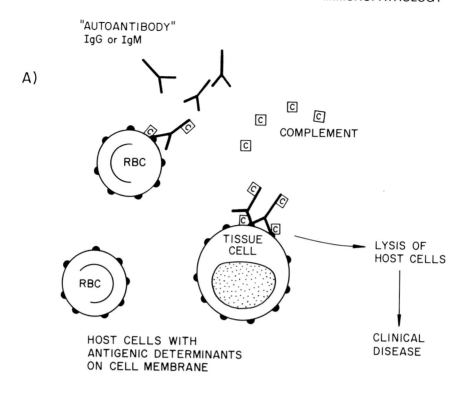

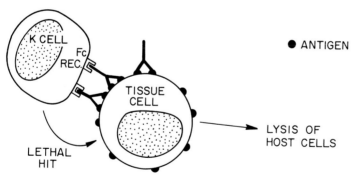

Figure 5.14.   Cytotoxic (Type II) Hypersensitivity. Antibody *(IgG or IgM)* directed at cell membrane components (often autoantigens) binds to the specific antigen on the cell surface. Two different mechanisms may be involved in the pathogenesis of cell injury: *A,* complement-mediated cytotoxicity. *Complement* fixation and activation follows antibody binding and cell lysis results; *B,* antibody-mediated cellular cytotoxicity. *K cells* bind the *Fc* fragment of antibodies (IgG) directed against cell surface antigens. After antibody binds to the cell, the *lethal hit* is executed *via* perforins and other cytotoxins. (*RBC,* red blood cell; *C,* complement.)

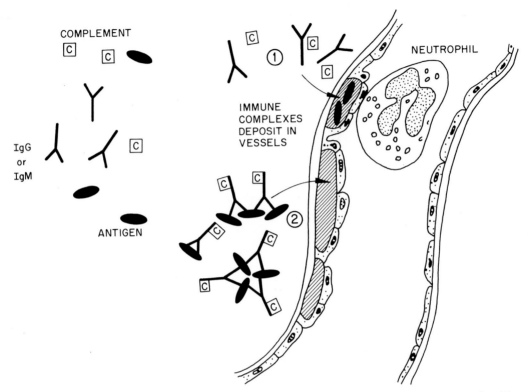

Figure 5.15. Immune-Complex Disease (Type III). *Immune complexes* may form *in situ (1),* or may form in the circulation and be deposited *(2). Antigen* combines with *IgG* or *IgM* antibody, fixes *complement,* and the resulting activation generates C5a for chemotactic attraction of *neutrophils,* which are responsible for much of the tissue damage.

factor in the development of some diseases caused by viruses, bacteria, and most fungi and parasites. Cell-mediated hypersensitivity is responsible for graft rejection and for immunity against some tumors. Thus, we must once again attempt to understand that the same orderly processes that can be protective (cell-mediated immunity) may, under appropriate conditions, become harmful (delayed-type hypersensitivity). The characteristic lesion of delayed hypersensitivity is a reaction composed of mononuclear cells often located near venules. These infiltrating cells are lymphocytes and cells of the mononuclear phagocyte system, and the lymphocytes have a dominant role in the production of the reaction by secretion of a number of lymphokines which attract macrophages, influence other lymphocytes, and kill target cells (Fig. 5.16).

MECHANISMS OF HYPERSENSITIVITY

Understanding the pathogenesis of immunologically mediated tissue injury requires an integration of information derived from studies in pathology, immunology, and biochemistry which are collectively useful to both pathologists and clinicians. In this section, we will continue to refer to hypersensitivity reactions in terms of the Coombs and Gell types I-IV scheme, but we must be constantly aware that in many types of clin-

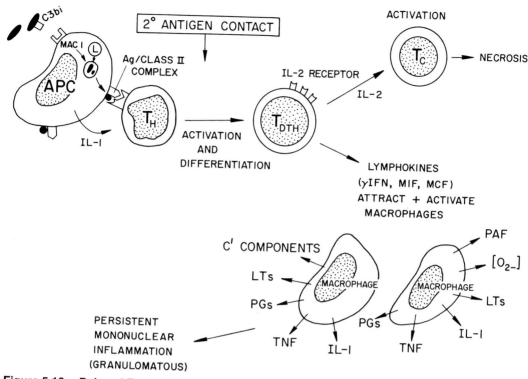

Figure 5.16.   Delayed-Type Hypersensitivity (Type IV). T_h become sensitized by the antigen/MHC complex presented by the antigen-presenting cell *(APC)*. Upon secondary antigenic challenge they will be activated and differentiate into delayed-type hypersensitivity cells *(T_{DTH})*. Following activation the T_{DTH} cells release lymphokines *(IL-2, γIFN, migration inhibition factor (MIF)*, macrophage chemotactic factor (MCF))*, which attract and activate other inflammatory cells *(macrophages)* and activate cytotoxic T cells *(T_c)*. This leads to tissue damage and a typical mononuclear cell infiltrate.

ical disease combinations of various immunopathologic networks and pathways are involved.

Mechanisms of Immediate-Type Hypersensitivity (Type I)

The type I hypersensitivity reactions are sometimes referred to as **mediator diseases** because the effects produced by such reactions result from pharmacologically active substances released by the reaction of antigen with effector cells sensitized by IgE antibody. IgE is locally produced by cutaneous and mucosal plasma cells after the primary contact of

the body with antigen. The mast cells (tissue) or basophils (peripheral blood) are the primary effector cells. They are sensitized by the binding of the locally produced IgE to their cell surface Fcϵ receptor. During a secondary challenge with the antigen, cell-bound antibody is cross-linked by antigen which subsequently clusters the occupied Fcϵ receptors in the membrane. Mast cells (or basophils) are activated to secrete a variety of mediator substances including histamine, serotonin, heparin, eosinophil chemotactic factor, platelet activating factor, prostaglandins, leukotrienes, and others (Table 5.6).

The diseases considered to have a type

Table 5.6
Mast Cell-Derived Mediators of Type I Hypersensitivity

Mediator	Chemical Structure	Functions
Preformed mediators		
Histamine	β-Imidazolylethylamine	Vasodilation and increased vascular permeability, smooth muscle contraction.
Serotonin	5-Hydroxytryptamine	Vasoconstriction and smooth muscle contraction.
ECF-A[a]	Acidic peptide (M_r 500–600)	Chemotaxis of eosinophils.
NCF	MW > 10,000	Chemotaxis of neutrophils.
Kininogenases		Generation of kinins.
Newly synthesized mediators		
LT's	A mixture of LTC_4, LTD_4, LTE_4 (SRS-A)	Contraction of bronchial and vascular smooth muscle, ↑ vascular permeability.
PAF	AGEPC (MW 300-500)	Aggregation and degranulation of platelets, chemotaxis and activation of PMN and Mϕ.
PGD_2	Eicosanoid	Contraction of bronchial smooth muscles, vasodilation and increased vascular permeability.
LTB_4	Eicosanoid	Chemotaxis of neutrophils.

[a] Abbreviations used are: ECF-A, eosinophil chemotactic factor of anaphylaxis; NCF, Neutrophil chemotactic factor; LT, leukotrienes; SRS-A, slow reacting substance of anaphylaxis; PAF, platelet activating factor; AGEPC, 1-0-alkyl-2-acetyl-sn-glyceryl-3-phosphorylcholine; Mϕ, macrophage; PG, prostaglandins.

I pathogenesis range from the relatively benign, such as ragweed, tree, or grass pollinosis, affecting 10–15% of the entire human population, through the less common and serious disorders, such as urticaria and asthma, to rare and life-threatening episodes of systemic anaphylaxis. **Anaphylaxis** is the prototype of immediate hypersensitivity and its most devastating manifestation. Anaphylaxis is caused by the massive release of mediators from mast cells and basophils, which then induce the dramatic, immediate, and life-threatening pathophysiologic effects. The pathophysiology of anaphylaxis is understood in some detail, and therapeutic maneuvers, such as the administration of drugs like epinephrine, can be understood in terms of mechanism. In the other disease processes, such as allergic rhinitis or asthma, similar immediate hypersensitivity reactions initiate the episode, but it appears that more prolonged inflammatory responses also contribute. This is illustrated, in clinical terms, by the fact that the antiinflammatory effects of corticosteroids, which have little or no effect on anaphylaxis or mediator release, have profound effects on the symptomatology of rhinitis and asthma.

To some extent, the diseases and location of primary tissue damage associated with type I hypersensitivity reflect the tissue distribution of the effector mast cells. Since the skin and the respiratory and gastrointestinal tracts have the most mast cells, they are common sites for type I reactions.

INITIATION OF IMMEDIATE-TYPE HYPER-SENSITIVITY AND THE IgE RESPONSE. Like every immune response, immediate-type hypersensitivity depends on an initial contact of the host with an antigen that induces the primary response, which in this case is the production of IgE by local plasma cells. Antigens that induce type I hypersensitivity contact the body largely at surfaces exposed to the external environment, such as the skin and the respiratory and intestinal mucosa. IgE secretion is a local phenomenon that follows local antigen processing and presentation, activation of T_h cells, and final immunoglobulin production by plasma cells. The production of IgE is also regulated by T_s cells. IgE first binds by its Fc fragment to the Fcϵ receptor of local tissue mast cells, and later spills over into the circulation to sensitize basophils and mast cells throughout the body. IgE is detectable only in minute quantities in the circulation (0.05 μg/ml) and has a very short circulating half life (2.3 days), but it may remain "fixed" to the mast cells in tissue for long periods of time (up to 12 weeks). Due to such long-lived "fixed" antigen-specific IgE, the host remains in prolonged sensitization.

There are a few other compounds that can activate mast cells directly, without utilizing the Fcϵ receptor. The most important of these are the **anaphylatoxins** C5a and C3a, which react through a separate receptor and may have an enhancing effect on the reaction *in vivo*. Additionally, T cells seem to modulate immediate-type hypersensitivity *via* two T cell–derived factors, **histamine releasing factor** (HRF) and an **antigen-specific T cell factor** (TCF) which are able to activate mast cells.

ACTIVATION OF MAST CELLS AND MECHANISMS OF MEDIATOR RELEASE. The release of mediators by effector cells is an active, energy-requiring secretory process (Fig. 5.17). In recent years, great progress has been made in the under-standing of this process. Many of the mechanisms involved in mediator release from mast cells are similar to the **stimulus-response coupling** and **signal-transduction** processes central to the activation of leukocytes in inflammation (*see* Chapter 4). Some details pertinent to hypersensitivity reactions are reiterated here.

Activation of mast cells and basophils in immediate-type hypersensitivity begins with the binding of multivalent antigens to the membrane-bound IgE (Fig. 5.17). This leads to cross-linking of IgE and the subsequent **aggregation of Fcϵ receptors.** It has been shown that the number of aggregated receptors and the size of receptor clusters is related to the intensity of the stimulatory signal. This receptor clustering most likely initiates the activation of **G-proteins** which are located within the lipid bilayer of the plasma membrane. Two signal pathways resulting from the hydrolysis of membrane phospholipids are thought to provide synergistic signals for granule secretion: the stimulation of G-proteins activates **phospholipase C,** a membrane-bound enzyme that hydrolyzes membrane phosphoinositols to produce two different intracellular second messengers, **inositol trisphosphate (IP$_3$)** and **diacylglycerol (DAG).** IP$_3$ is released into the cytoplasm and acts on intracellular membrane receptors to release calcium from intracellular stores, mainly from the endoplasmic reticulum. Seconds after addition of a stimulant to mast cells an increase of intracellular free calcium ($[Ca^{2+}]_i$) can be demonstrated *in vitro.* Additionally, there is evidence for an increased **calcium influx from outside the cell** after activation of mast cells and basophils, probably due to the formation of a membrane channel. It is not clear, however, if the calcium influx from the extracellular space is mainly used to replenish the intracellular stores or if it is directly responsible for the measurable increase in $[Ca^{2+}]_i$. **DAG,** the other sec-

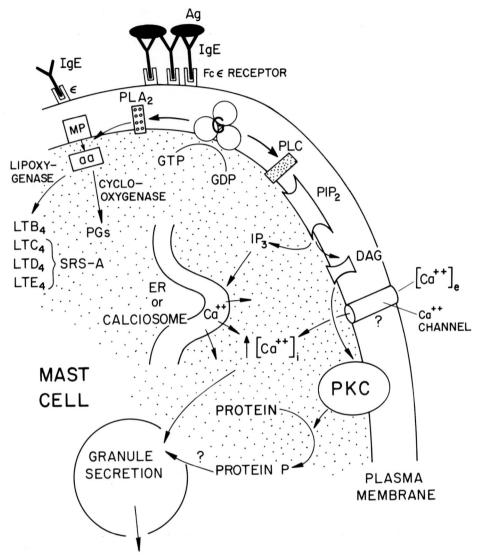

Figure 5.17. Mast Cell Activation and Transmembrane Signaling. *Mast cells* are activated by the interaction and cross-linking of *IgE* with the antigen *(Ag)* and the subsequent aggregation of *Fcε* receptors on their cell surface. This leads to activation of G proteins *(G)* that bind *GTP* and activate phospholipase C *(PLC)*. *PLC* is a phosphodiesterase that degrades membrane phosphoinositols *(PIP$_2$)* to two intracellular second messengers: inositoltrisphosphate *(IP$_3$)* and diacylglycerol *(DAG)*. *IP$_3$* causes the release of calcium *(Ca^{2+})* from intracellular stores, especially the endoplasmic reticulum and *calciosomes.* Extracellular calcium enters through a putative membrane channel. *DAG* activates a membrane-bound protein kinase C *(PKC)*, which in turn initiates the phosphorylation of various cytoplasmic proteins. The increase in intracellular free calcium *[Ca^{2+}]i* and the phosphorylation of cytoplasmic proteins results in *granule secretion.* The clustering of *Fcε* receptors and G protein activation also activates phospholipase A$_2$ *(PLA$_2$)* which cleaves arachidonic acid *(aa)* from membrane phospholipids *(MP)* and produces leukotrienes *(LTB$_4$, LTC$_4$, LTD$_4$, LTE$_4$)* and prostaglandins *(PG)* via the *lipoxygenase* and *cyclooxygenase* pathways. *(SRS-A,* slow reacting substance of anaphylaxis).

ond messenger resulting from the action of phospholipase C, activates **protein kinase C (PK-C)**. PK-C is a membrane-bound enzyme that, upon activation by DAG and in the presence of increased $[Ca^{2+}]_i$, binds cofactors (phosphatidylserine and calcium) and phosphorylates many intracellular proteins. Presently this step is poorly understood, and the relationship of intracellular protein phosphorylation to the final secretion of granules is unclear. A third pathway has been shown to be of primary importance in the activation of mast cells: the formation of **arachidonic acid metabolites.** The activation of G-proteins may also stimulate a **phospholipase A$_2$**, which in turn hydrolyzes membrane lipids to form arachidonic acid. This leads to the activation of the cyclooxygenase and lipoxygenase pathways and results in the formation of **prostaglandins, thromboxanes, and leukotrienes.**

Other intracellular second messengers such as cyclic nucleotides (cAMP and cGMP) were previously thought to be important in mast cell activation. Stimulation of β-adrenergic receptors by substances like isoproterenol were shown to increase intracellular cAMP and decrease mediator release, while stimulation of α-adrenergic receptors by agents like norepinephrine decreased intracellular cAMP and increased mediator release. However, the significance of these nucleotides in *in vivo* mast cell secretion is now thought to be minimal.

Ultrastructural examination of mast cells during IgE-induced degranulation reveals swelling and fusion of cytoplasmic granules. The fused granules form tortuous cytoplasmic canalicular channels which fuse with the plasma membrane and open to the cell surface to permit the explosive release of mediators.

Mediators

Following activation of mast cells and basophils, two important events occur; (1) the release of **preformed mediators** from cytoplasmic granules, and (2) the production of **newly synthesized mediators.** Table 5.6 summarizes the different mediators released by mast cells. The effects of these agents reflect their biological activity and include contraction of smooth muscle; increased vascular permeability leading to edema; early increase in vascular resistance which can be followed by vascular collapse (shock) if sufficient amounts of mediators are available; and increased gastric, nasal, and lacrimal secretion. In a later stage, eosinophils may be active in modulating anaphylactic reactions, and in some species platelets also appear to be important sources of pharmacologically active mediators. The type and severity of lesions observed depends upon the dose of antigen, the route of contact with antigen, the frequency of contact with antigen, the tendency for a given organ system to react, and the sensitivity of the involved individual. This final factor appears to be genetically controlled, but it may be altered by environmental conditions (such as temperature) or unrelated inflammation (such as the presence of a viral upper respiratory tract infection).

HISTAMINE.   Histamine is stored, preformed, in mast cells and basophils and, in some species, in platelets. It is formed from *l*-histidine and degraded either by oxidative deamination or by methylation and oxidative deamination. The *in vivo* pathobiologic effects of histamine include enhanced venular permeability, attributed to partial discontinuity of the endothelium, and elicitation of a profound increase in respiratory airway resistance with concomitant reduction in pulmonary compliance. Some of the actions of histamine on pulmonary mechanics, conductance, and compliance are significantly altered by pretreatment of the experimental animal with atropine, and to this extent they are attributed to vagal reflexes initiated by airway irritant receptors rather than to a direct effect on smooth muscle.

LEUKOTRIENES AND PROSTAGLANDINS. Leukotrienes and prostaglandins are synthesized and released by mast cells or basophils after IgE-induced stimulation. The activation of phospholipase A_2 in the cytoplasmic membrane leads to the release of arachidonic acid from its esterified position in membrane phospholipids such as phosphatidylcholine. A mixture of leukotrienes LTC_4, LTD_4, and LTE_4 is produced *via* the lipoxygenase pathway. This mixture used to be called **"slow-reacting substance of anaphylaxis."** PGD_2 and other prostaglandins are produced *via* the cyclooxygenase pathway. The leukotriene LTB_4, also a lipoxygenase pathway product, is a potent chemotactic factor for leukocytes, while PGD_2, LTC_4, and LTD_4 cause smooth muscle contraction, mucosal edema, and secretion. They are 100–1000 times more potent than histamine in constricting bronchial smooth muscle. Logically, the effects of these newly synthesized mediators begin after the effects of the preformed mediators, but this difference cannot always be appreciated in a clinical setting. The distinction between these timed events is, however, a useful one, since the immediate phase (due to preformed histamine) may respond to antihistamines but is not influenced by cyclooxygenase inhibitors such as indomethacin; the later phase, conversely, is due to prostaglandins and leukotrienes, and may be inhibited by various nonsteroidal antiinflammatory drugs.

PLATELET-ACTIVATING FACTOR. PAF was introduced earlier in the section lymphokines. Here we will examine its function as an important mediator of anaphylaxis. PAF is one of the mediators that are newly formed in and released from mast cells and basophils after IgE-induced stimulation. It has extremely potent effects on platelets and for this reason was termed PAF. It causes platelets to aggregate, sequester, and release vasoactive amines during IgE-induced ana-phylaxis. This leads to thrombocytopenia and marked platelet sequestration in the microvasculature of organs such as the lung which are primary sites of allergic responses. The release of vasoactive amines from platelets enhances the effect of the mediators released by mast cells and causes vasodilation and edema. PAF is chemotactic for neutrophils and macrophages which also sequester within the local microvasculature. In addition, PAF may play a role in immune-complex disease (Type III hypersensitivity) by causing release of vasoactive amines from platelets, leading to increased vascular permeability and enhanced deposition of circulating immune complexes along filtering vascular membranes.

EOSINOPHIL CHEMOTACTIC FACTOR OF ANAPHYLAXIS AND THE EOSINOPHIL. As one result of an antigen-IgE interaction on the surface of a mast cell or basophil, there is the release of a family of low molecular weight compounds that have highly specific eosinophil chemotactic activity. ECF-A is a preformed mediator that has been associated specifically with the mast cell and the basophil by its extraction from essentially pure populations of these cell types. Its association with the mast cell granules also has been demonstrated by subcellular fractionation. ECF-A extracted or released immunologically from either mast cells or basophils has an M_r of 500–600. With respect to ECF-A, there is a distinct difference between basophils and mast cells. In mast cells, ECF-A is completely preformed, so that 100% release can be obtained on sonication of appropriate tissues. In the basophil, however, numerous experiments have failed to demonstrate eosinophil chemotactic factor activity on sonication, but complete production occurs within minutes after antigenic or other appropriate stimulation. It is not known whether the ECF-A from basophils is identical in structure to the mast cell ECF-A, but its molecular size is quite similar. It also has been shown that an ECF with similar molecular size and chemotactic specificity can be generated from human neutrophils by phagocytic events or by nonspecific stimuli. Whether this generation and release is of physiologic importance has not been ascertained.

The function of eosinophils, long known to be associated with allergic reactions, has been extensively debated. It was believed that the eosinophil acted as a control cell in the anaphylactic response. It contains an arylsulfatase which degrades leukotrienes, a histaminase which can metabolize histamine, PGE_1 which is a vasoconstrictor, and a phospholipase D which inactivates PAF. It recently has been shown, however, that the **proinflammatory potential** of the eosinophils is far greater than their antiinflammatory capacity. Proinflammatory factors secreted by the eosinophil include PAF, LTC_4 (producing vasodilatation and smooth muscle contraction), reactive oxygen metabolites, and certain proteases that stimulate mast cell degranulation.

Lesions of Immediate-Type Hypersensitivity

Given the plethora of vasoactive and smooth muscle–stimulating chemicals released during anaphylaxis and other forms of immediate-type hypersensitivity, it should come as no surprise that the tissue lesions in the diseases associated with this form of hypersensitivity reflect those target tissues. Characteristic changes include vasodilatation with increased vascular permeability leading to tissue edema, sequestration of platelets in the local microvasculature and microthrombosis, leukocyte infiltrates (especially eosinophils), constriction of bronchial smooth muscle, and increased mucous secretions. To help place these lesions in perspective in a clinical setting, we will briefly consider a few of the diseases in which immediate-type hypersensitivity forms an apparent part of the pathogenesis.

BOVINE ANAPHYLAXIS. Anaphylactic reactions have been suspected as the underlying cause of various disease syndromes of cattle, including "fog fever" or "atypical interstitial pneumonia," systemic release of antigens from *Hypoderma* spp., and skin hypersensitivity to *Fasciola hepatica* antigens. The lung serves as the major shock organ in bovine anaphylaxis, resulting in dyspnea, coughing, pulmonary hypertension, systemic hypotension, increased salivation, lacrimation, and nasal discharge. Gross pathologic findings include severe pulmonary edema and congestion of the abdominal viscera. Experimentally, calves sensitized to foreign protein exhibit acute systemic anaphylaxis when challenged by aerosol exposure to the antigen during the period of maximum circulating IgE antibody production. Inhalation of the antigen at the appropriate time produces respiratory changes associated with bronchoconstriction and exudative alveolitis resembling certain features of atypical interstitial pneumonia.

MILK ALLERGY. Milk allergy may be seen in highly lactating Jersey cattle. It is an allergic reaction to the milk protein α-casein. This protein is normally synthesized in the mammary gland and secreted into the milk and does not, therefore, come in contact with the immune system for recognition as a self-antigen. Upon delayed milking, the increased intramammary pressure may force the α-casein into the circulation where it is thought to serve as an antigen and elicit sensitization. A second encounter may result in an immediate-type hypersensitivity reaction, presenting with lesions ranging from localized urticarial skin lesions and multifocal cutaneous edema to possibly severe acute systemic anaphylaxis and death.

ATOPY. Atopy has been defined as an inherited predisposition to develop IgE antibodies to certain environmental antigens such as pollens, fungal spores, animal danders, and house dusts, resulting in hypersensitivity upon repeated exposure. It occurs with increased frequency in certain breeds and families, particularly the terriers such as Cairn Terriers, West Highland Whites and Scotties. Offspring of dogs with atopic disease are also predisposed and produce more antigen-specific IgE than normal puppies. Additional studies have suggested that the basis for the abnormal IgE response may actually lie in abnormalities of the T suppressor cell network. Repeated contact of atopic individuals with the offending antigen(s) results in conditions such as allergic rhinitis, bronchitis, or dermatitis. The tissue injury that develops has been classified as immediate-type hypersensitivity, although the pathogenesis is incompletely understood, and the role of IgE antibodies in atopic dermatitis remains under considerable debate. Some dogs with atopic dermatitis may exhibit elevations of other immunoglobulin isotypes such as IgGd, while other are hypogammaglobulinemic.

Mechanisms of Cytotoxic Hypersensitivity (Type II)

Type II reactions are classically referred to as cytotoxic in character because the end result is usually lysis of a target cell against which an antibody is directed. The reaction is always mediated by an antigen-specific antibody. The lysis of target cells occurs by two major mechanisms (1) **complement-mediated lysis,** and (2) **antibody-dependent cellular cytotoxicity (ADCC).** The reaction of specific IgG or IgM antibody with the antigenic determinants on the plasma membrane of the target cell usually leads either to complement fixation or to the binding of an Fc receptor–bearing cytotoxic cell (K cell). If such reactions are directed against normal antigenic determinants of the target cell membrane, the reaction is referred to as **autoimmune** and the antibody is thus termed an **autoantibody.** If a free antigen from another source or a hapten is

adsorbed onto a cell surface, a similar lytic reaction may ensue, again leading to lysis. In the latter case, even though immunologically directed lysis of host cells occurs, the reaction is not autoimmune, as the antigen is not native to the host. Such reactions occur in some of the drug-induced hemolytic anemias. Alternatively, destruction of host cells also occurs if **exogenous antigens** cross-react with surface antigens on host cells. An immune response directed against the exogenous antigen may then lead to lysis of the cells that express the cross-reacting antigen. A typical example of such a reaction is the production of anti-myocardial antibodies in human rheumatic heart disease patients, which develop after an infection with β-hemolytic streptococci.

Since the necessary reactants (antibody, complement) for such cytotoxic reactions are found in the plasma, it is not surprising that many of the disease settings in which type II hypersensitivity reactions are implicated involve reactions against cellular elements that are in intimate contact with the plasma (Fig. 5.18). Most of the hematologic type II hypersensitivity diseases are caused by the production of antibodies against autoantigens and involve complement-mediated lysis. Examples of this form of hypersensitivity are reactions against red blood cells, white blood cells, platelets, and even endothelial cells.

The ADCC form of type II hypersensitivity is thought to be involved in the destruction of certain kinds of targets which are too large to be phagocytosed, such as parasites and tumor cells, and it may also be involved in graft rejection.

One interesting variation of type II hypersensitivity is related to those diseases mediated purely by antibodies, without involvement of complement or cytotoxic cells. The involved antibodies are not necessarily cytotoxic, and the diseases involve other mechanisms leading to functional alterations. An important group of

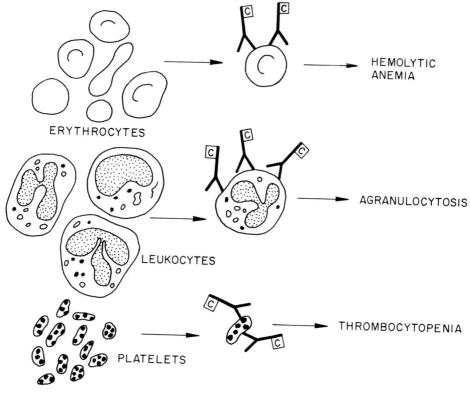

Figure 5.18. Hematologic Type II Hypersensitivity. Type II reactions are commonly directed against cellular elements in direct contact with plasma. *Hemolytic anemia* and *thrombocytopenia* are probably the most common and best documented naturally occurring examples. (*C*, complement).

skin diseases, the **bullous dermatoses,** including the pemphigus complex and bullous pemphigoid, fits into this category. In these diseases, antibodies are formed which are directed against surface antigens of dermal and mucosal keratinocytes. The reaction of the antibodies with the keratinocytes leads to loss of cell-cell adhesion (pemphigus) or loss of cell–extracellular matrix adhesion (bullous pemphigoid) without actually causing keratinocyte death. A second group of related diseases are the **anti-receptor antibody diseases** such as myasthenia gravis and Grave's disease. In these situations, antibodies are directed against specific receptors, and the binding of the antibody either increases or decreases receptor function. In myasthenia gravis, the anti-

body binds to the acetylcholine receptor, while in Grave's disease antibody binds to the TSH receptor.

Reactions Against Specific Cell Types

IMMUNOHEMATOLOGIC DISEASES. By far the best studied and characterized clinical forms of Type II hypersensitivity relate to the immunologic destruction of cellular elements in intimate contact with the blood (Table 5.7). Clinical situations in which antibodies are directed against red blood cell antigens are probably the most common and are exemplified by **transfusion reactions** and by the various forms of **acquired autoimmune hemolytic disease.**

Transfusion reactions occur when cir-

Table 5.7
Immunohematologic Disorders

Name	Mechanism
Transfusion reaction	Blood group incompatibility
Erythroblastosis fetalis	Rh incompatibility
Neonatal isoerythrolysis	Blood group incompatibility
Autoimmune hemolytic anemia	Anti-RBC antibody
Neonatal leukopenia	Anti-WBC antibody
Acquired agranulocytosis	Anti-WBC antibody
Idiopathic thrombocytopenic purpura	Antiplatelet antibody
Hemolytic reactions to drugs	Drug acts as hapten

culating antibody of host origin contacts erythrocytes from an incompatible donor. Such reactions are called **isoimmune.** These are not "autoimmune" diseases as the antigen is exogenous while the antibody is endogenous. In humans, ABO and Rh systems are the most important red cell antigenic determinants. The major blood groups of domestic animals are shown in Table 5.8.

Hemolytic disease of the newborn or **neonatal isoerythrolysis** represents a special category of transfusion-like reaction in which transfer of antigens and antibodies between the fetus and the dam can lead to destruction of the red cells of the newborn. This situation occurs fairly commonly in horses and donkeys. Since the red cell antigenic makeup of the fetus is determined by genetic contributions from both the sire and the dam, the fetal red cells are antigenically distinct from those of the dam even though they have some common antigenic determinants. If, during fetal life, these red blood cells gain access to the circulation of the dam, they elicit an immune response in the dam in the same way that any incompatible blood

transfusion would. That is, the dam makes antibodies against those fetal red cell antigens that are determined by the sire. Since the majority of maternal passive transfer of antibody in domestic animals takes place *via* the colostrum (rather than *via* placental transfer), the antibodies reactive against the fetal red cells are not present in the fetal circulation until after birth, when they are transferred in the maternal colostral antibody supply. These antibodies then attack the antigenic determinants on the newborn's red cells derived from the sire's genetic material, and red cell destruction and hemolytic disease results.

In man, where transplacental transfer of antibody occurs, a similar situation results in the disease called **erythroblastosis fetalis.** Here, the infants are born with hemolytic anemia rather than developing it after birth, because of the timing of the transfer of maternal antibody to the fetus. Neonatal isoerythrolysis is common in newborn horses and mules, but occurs rarely in dogs, cats, piglets, and calves. In piglets and calves it has occasionally been seen after vaccination of the

Table 5.8
Important Blood Groups of Domestic Animals

Species	Blood Groups
Cattle	Eleven total, B and J most important (serum lipid, passively adsorbed to erythrocytes).
Sheep	Seven total, important: B and R system (R is soluble and passively absorbed like cattle J).
Pig	Fifteen, most important the A system (has factor A and O).
Horse	Seven total, most important Aa, Qa, R, and S; commonly involved in neonatal isoerythrolysis.
Dog	Eleven total, important A system.
Cat	Only one system: AB

dam with blood-containing vaccines (*e.g.*, against hog cholera, anaplasmosis, or babesiosis). Thrombocytopenia can develop from similar mechanisms where antibody against the fetal platelets is transferred in the colostrum. Neonatal thrombocytopenia of this type of immunologic background has been described in puppies and piglets.

Autoimmune hemolytic anemia has been best characterized in dogs in which a fairly typical syndrome of anemia, spherocytosis, and a positive direct antiglobulin (Coombs) reaction develops. The Coombs test detects antibody coating the surface of the patient's red cells. The direct test is conducted by incubation of washed erythrocytes from the patient with anti-immunoglobulin antibody. The most puzzling aspect of the so-called autoimmune hemolytic diseases is that the factors responsible for initiating the production of antibody directed against self-antigens are largely unknown. Animals that die of autoimmune hemolytic anemia have massive splenomegaly with marked hemosiderosis as a direct result of the splenic removal of large numbers of damaged red cells.

Autoimmune and immunologically mediated responses similar to those described for red blood cells have also been reported to occur against leukocytes, although such reactions have generally not been described in domestic animals.

Immune reactions against platelets can occur *via* mechanisms similar to those that occur against erythrocytes and leukocytes. The result is usually purpura or other manifestations of the coagulation defect produced by severe thrombocytopenia. Such immune reactions probably form the basis for much of what has been known as **idiopathic thrombocytopenic purpura.** Immune injury to platelets following antigen-antibody reactions on the platelet surface membrane can result in lysis or in accelerated removal of the injured platelets by the mononuclear

phagocyte system of the liver and spleen. The pathogenesis of immune-mediated thrombocytopenia can include true **autoimmune thrombocytopenia,** with antibody directed against some structurally altered component of the platelet plasma membrane. Such a situation is occasionally seen together with autoimmune hemolytic anemia. The pathogenesis of other forms of immune-mediated thrombocytopenia have diverse mechanistic backgrounds. In addition to specific autoantibody directed against platelet membranes, thrombocytopenia can result from the binding of antibodies to platelets bearing adsorbed viral, bacterial, or drug antigens (haptens), or the action of immune complexes on platelets, where **innocent bystander** lysis can ensue (*see* type II hypersensitivity). In most of these situations, the presence of such immune reactions at the platelet surface can lead to either accelerated removal of the platelets from the circulation *via* the mononuclear phagocyte system, or platelet lysis, or both.

Those diseases in which antibody is directed against tissue cell surface specificities or receptors such as the **bullous dermatoses** and the **anti-receptor antibody diseases** such as myasthenia gravis are variations of type II hypersensitivity resulting from the interaction of **autoantibodies** with **self-antigens.** As such they are truly **autoimmune** diseases, and we will discuss them as examples of autoimmunity in the appropriate section of this chapter.

Mechanisms of Immune-Complex Disease (Type III)

The idea that tissue injury might occur as a result of events that follow the deposition of complexes of antigen and antibody in tissue is not a new one; such a scheme was in fact proposed almost 75 years ago. It has only been in the last 20 years or so, however, that a sufficient amount of reliable data has accumulated to firmly establish **antigen-antibody complexes** as potential pathogenic structures capable of initiating a series of events that lead to inflammatory tissue injury.

Immune complexes are formed by the reaction of antibodies with antigens that are located or deposited (in the case of circulating immune complexes) in certain vascular tissue sites. Leukocytes are attracted to the site of immune complex deposition through the generation of chemotaxins from the activation of complement, and the leukocytes become activated leading to local injury. The actual tissue-damaging mechanism in immune-complex disease involves an interdependent series of events involving antigen and antibody, components of the complement system, leukocytes and their products (especially toxic oxygen radicals and lysosomal enzymes), platelets, vascular permeability phenomena, and most of the various essential components of a localized inflammatory reaction. This fascinating pathogenetic scheme can be divided into two major phases: **first,** the formation of immune complexes and their deposition in certain tissue sites, and **second,** the initiation of tissue injury by these immune complexes and the actual mechanisms of tissue injury (Fig. 5.19).

FORMATION AND DEPOSITION OF IMMUNE COMPLEXES. Immune complexes may be formed by two different pathways, *in situ* **immune-complex formation** or **formation of circulating immune complexes.** Complexes formed *in situ* develop after the production of antibodies directed against exogenous or endogenous tissue-bound antigens. Antibodies leave the circulation to bind to the antigenic determinant in certain tissue sites, such as the glomerular capillary wall. Some clinical forms of **immune-complex glomerulonephritis** develop in this way. The second pathway involves the formation of immune-complexes that are formed in the circulation. Complexes so formed are, for the most part, taken up and catabolized to harmless end products by the cells of the mononuclear phagocyte system. However, a small fraction of appropriate size

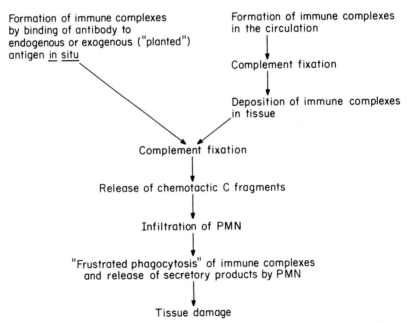

Figure 5.19. Immune Complex–Mediated Tissue Injury. Immune complexes in tissue are formed in two different ways; *in situ* formation, or formation within the circulation with subsequent deposition.

(about 19S) elude this phagocytic process and accumulate in filtering structures throughout the body such as glomeruli, blood vessels, synovial membranes, and the choroid plexus. This accumulation is governed by anatomic and physiologic determinants, not immunologic factors, so that the sites of injury have no immunologic relationship to the inducing antigen or antibody. This is an important point that requires reiteration; although tissue injury certainly occurs in immune-complex disease, in most cases the antibody is *not* directed against any host tissue component. That is, the sites of tissue injury are determined by the sites of immune complex deposition, not by the specificity of the antibody.

The pathogenicity of circulating immune complexes is largely determined by their antigen-antibody ratio. The size of the complexes and the biologic properties of the antibody thus become important in determining pathogenicity. Complexes formed in **antibody excess** tend to be large and insoluble and are rapidly phagocytosed by cells of the mononuclear phagocyte system. They do not circulate and have little opportunity to accumulate in filtering sites where immune-complex injury characteristically occurs. Complexes formed in **extreme antigen excess** are usually too small to become trapped in physiologic filters, and such complexes do not contain an arrangement of immunoglobulin molecules capable of complement activation. Complexes of about 19S size, formed in **slight antigen excess,** are usually the most pathogenic, mainly because they are the right size for deposition in tissue. The nature of the antibody involved in the immune complex is also essential to complement activation, since only some antibody isotypes are capable of complement activation.

Immune complexes can form in different locations outside the vascular lumen. This has been studied best in immune-complex disease of the kidney. Location of the complexes in the glomerular capillary wall may be either subendothelial, intramembranous (within the basement membrane), or subepithelial. In the glomerulus, certain immune complexes are also found within the mesangial matrix or within mesangial cells, which are macrophages and hence phagocytic. These anatomic localizations are determined largely by **antibody avidity** and **antigen charge.**

Subendothelial deposition usually occurs with neutral or anionic antigens, since a negative charge inhibits migration through the negatively charged basement membrane. Subendothelial localization of immune complexes also occurs with highly avid antibodies, which do not dissociate after binding. **Subepithelial** deposition, in contrast, is probably due to low avidity of the antibody and/or the cationic nature of the antigens. Antibodies with low avidity may dissociate after primary subendothelial deposition, thus antigen and antibody may migrate separately through the basement membrane and reform in a subepithelial location. Cationic antigens are thought to migrate more readily through the negatively charged basement membrane. **Intramembranous** deposition of immune complexes is rare and may represent a transitional stage of migration through the basement membrane. Immune complexes also diffuse through the mesangial matrix of the glomerulus, where they may be phagocytosed by mesangial macrophages.

The location of immune-complex deposits within the vascular structures may influence the severity and character of the inflammatory changes that occur subsequent to immune-complex deposition. Subendothelial complexes are situated close to the circulation, where they may bind more antibody and activate increased amounts of complement, thereby inducing more severe inflammatory changes. Subepithelial complexes are distinctly separated from the circulation and therefore are usually associated with thickening of the basement membrane without inflammatory infiltrates. Such a pathogenesis explains the morphologic changes seen in **membranous glomerulonephritis** where striking capillary wall thickening without leukocyte infiltrates is typically observed. In turn, mesangial deposits may activate mesangial macrophages to proliferate, attract more macrophages, and produce increased amounts of mesangial matrix leading to a **proliferative glomerulonephritis.** It is likely that these various patterns of immune-complex deposition overlap with each other in most clinical forms of immune-complex disease.

NATURE OF THE ANTIGEN. The antigen itself does not seem to be of great importance in immune-complex disease, and in many cases the exact antigen cannot be determined. However, a few types of antigens are known to be commonly involved in type III hypersensitivities, and can be divided broadly into three groups: repeatedly inhaled antigens, autoantigens, and antigens derived from persistent infectious agents.

Repeatedly inhaled allergens may encounter antibody at several levels of the respiratory tract and form immune complexes, which then deposit in bronchiolar and alveolar walls. A typical example is the extrinsic allergic alveolitis of cattle, horses, and man. Inhalation of spores of the actinomycete *Micropolyspora faeni* that grows in moldy hay leads to induction of antibody production and, after repeated exposure, can cause an interstitial pneumonia. The classical histopathological lesion is a lymphocytic interstitial pneumonia and bronchiolitis, a lesion that suggests that the pathogenesis of the disease probably involves delayed-type hypersensitivity (type IV) as well.

The **autoantigens** most often implicated in immune-mediated tissue injury are those that are **persistently** available for interaction with circulating antibody. If appropriate levels of autoantibody are formed, the requirements for immune-

complex formation and deposition may be fulfilled. An example is **systemic lupus erythematosus (SLE),** a disease in which autoantibodies are produced against several autoantigens including DNA. These diseases are, by definition, **autoimmune.**

A third group of antigens known to lead to immune-complex formation and deposition are derived from **persistent infectious agents.** Chronic staphylococcal dermatitis can lead to type III hypersensitivity with immune-complex deposition in vessel walls and dermal vasculitis. Immunization of dogs with live adenovirus type I vaccine sometimes leads to an ophthalmic syndrome known as **blue eye,** an anterior uveitis with corneal edema caused by the deposition of immune complexes of viral antigens and specific antibody. Again, we should point out that neither the antibody nor the antigen in this situation have anything to do with the eye; the injured tissue is simply a site of immune-complex deposition. Other related examples in which immune-complex disease forms an important part of the pathogenesis can be drawn from such infectious diseases of domestic animals as feline infectious peritonitis, Aleutian disease of mink, equine infectious anemia, and hog cholera (Table 5.9). In each of these situations, the repetitive or persistent presence of moderate amounts of antigen accompanied by fairly low level antibody production fulfills the requirements for immune-complex formation, deposition, and subsequent tissue injury. We should also note that not all animals with these infections develop immune-complex disease; very strong or very weak antibody producers may not develop suitable conditions for the formation of immune complexes of the proper size for deposition in tissue.

Experimental Basis for Understanding Immune-Complex Disease

While a variety of types of naturally occurring lesions are now known to be caused by the inflammatory reaction that

Table 5.9
Examples of Virally-Induced Immune Complex Diseases

Species	Virus	Organs Affected
Cat	Feline infectious peritonitis virus	Phlebitis in many organs, serositis, uveitis
Mink	Aleutian disease virus	Vasculitis, glomerulonephritis
Horse	Equine infectious anemia	Liver, spleen
Pig	Hog cholera virus	Endothelial lesions; hemorrhages, lymphoid depletion

follows immune-complex deposition in tissue, much of what we know of the mechanisms responsible for tissue injury comes from the careful dissection of three different experimental models: the Arthus reaction, acute serum sickness, and nephrotoxic nephritis. Each of these experimental models has permitted much relevant information on the pathogenesis of immune-complex disease to be gained.

ARTHUS REACTION. The simplest immune complex–induced lesion is the Arthus reaction, a localized, acute, necrotizing cutaneous vasculitis. The formation of relatively large amounts of antigen and antibody precipitating in the vessel walls is essential to the full development of an Arthus reaction. In order to localize the reaction, one of the reactants (antigen or antibody) must be in the circulation and the other injected locally. Usually, the Arthus reaction is studied by intracutaneous injection of antigen into animals having high circulating levels of precipitating antibody specific for the antigen.

Early in the reaction, antigen and antibody diffuse toward each other, meet, and precipitate in the vessel walls. This antigen-antibody precipitate binds complement to release fragments chemotactic for polymorphonuclear leukocytes (PMNs), and within a few hours these cells infiltrate the involved vessels. The PMNs phagocytose and degrade the antigen-antibody complexes and attempt to carry them away from the site of the reaction. The polymorphonuclear cells that migrate to and accumulate at the scene secrete granule enzymes and other mate-

rials that damage the vessel walls. Necrosis of vascular structures follows, permeability is increased, and red blood cells and plasma are exuded. Edema and erythema develop, and eventually, if the reaction is severe enough, hemorrhage and necrosis of the skin may occur at the site of antigen injection. The initial reaction between antigen and antibody with the fixation of complement and influx of polymorphonuclear cells occurs rapidly. If some dye such as Evans blue (which binds to albumin) is injected intravenously at the time the skin test is made, increased vascular permeability can be visualized as bluing of the test area. Maximal visible extravasation of the labeled albumin is usually apparent within 3–6 hours after injection of the antigen. The Arthus reaction has been widely studied as a prototype of immune complex–induced tissue injury.

SERUM SICKNESS. While largely an experimental model today, serum sickness first occurred as a complication of serum therapy with massive amounts of heterologous antibody. Before immunology was very well understood, patients were occasionally treated with large volumes of heterologous (mostly equine) serum in order to provide antibodies against, for example, tetanus toxin. What ensued now seems intuitively obvious: the equine serum proteins acted as antigens, and the patient's immune system responded with the production of antibody. About 8–10 days after having been given the injection of antiserum, many patients developed serious cardiovascular, joint, and

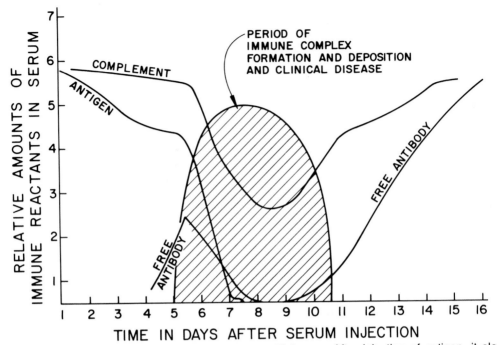

Figure 5.20. **Sequential Events in Acute Serum Sickness.** After injection of antigen, it slowly decays from the circulation until specific antibody is formed, at which time rapid antigen elimination and complement consumption occur. After deposition, the lack of antigen allows free antibody to reappear and complement levels to return to normal. It is during the period of immune-complex formation and deposition that tissue injury occurs.

renal disease, which sometimes was fatal. The basis for this "serum sickness" is now clear.

Serum sickness is induced by the intravenous infusion of a large dose of foreign serum or purified serum protein, and a series of fairly predictable events follows (Fig. 5.20). The antigen level in the serum declines in three distinct phases. The first decline results from equilibration of the injected protein between intra- and extravascular protein pools. This is followed by slower loss caused by nonimmune catabolism of circulating free antigen at a rate characteristic for the particular protein injected and the recipient species. Lastly, a phase of rapid antigen loss from the circulation occurs as a result of specific antibody production, immune-complex formation, and immune elimination of antigen from the circulation. There is initially an extreme antigen excess with the

formation of small complexes capable of remaining in the circulation. As the amount of antibody formed increases, the antigen-antibody complexes become larger and finally are removed rapidly by phagocytosis. During the immune elimination of antigen, immune complexes are formed which deposit in the characteristic tissues. Coincidental with the formation of antigen-antibody complexes in the circulation, there is a fall in the serum complement level and the appearance of acute inflammatory lesions in the kidneys, heart, arteries, and joints. In such lesions **antigen, antibody,** and host **complement components** can be detected by modern immunohistochemical techniques.

Clinical serum sickness is an extremely rare disease now that the consequences of administering large amounts of foreign protein are understood. The disease is now studied largely as an animal model in rabbits, from which much has been learned. Consistent with the timing of the spontaneous disease, animals are usually injected intravenously with a soluble foreign protein and, after about 6 to 8 days, antibodies are produced which may form immune complexes for deposition along the glomerular basement membrane causing renal injury. Affected animals develop a progressive glomerulonephritis with proteinuria and hematuria, hypoproteinemia, and elevated serum cholesterol and urea levels. The most common anatomic form of this disease is a membranous glomerulonephritis characterized by thickened glomerular capillary basement membranes, with little or no endothelial and mesangial proliferation. Lumpy, dense deposits can be seen by electron microscopy along the outer aspect of the basement membranes which correspond with the localization of antigen, antibody, and complement components as visualized using fluorescent antibody techniques. Thus, the clinical and morphologic spectrum of the experimental disease mimics the clinical situation almost exactly.

An important fact emerged from such experiments; not all of the rabbits in a given study developed the disease. Upon further dissection of this finding, it became clear that only those rabbits producing moderate amounts of antibody became sick, that is, only those which formed large amounts of immune complexes of the appropriate size for deposition developed the disease. The strongest and the weakest antibody producers did not become sick because they failed to produce sufficient **depositable** complexes of the right size. Thus, it became apparent that the individuality of the animals, not the scientists conducting the experiments, determined the outcome; *the rabbits determined their own fate by how much antibody they produced.* This is, of course, nicely analogous to the clinical situation in which not all members of any given

Table 5.10
Important Features of Immune-Complex Disease Caused by Circulating Complexes

Immune reaction is not directed at target tissues; rather they are injured by virtue of being deposition sites.

Host determines if injury will occur, depending on how much antibody is produced for a given amount of antigen.

The reaction is mediated largely by complement.

Neutrophils are responsible for much of the tissue damage.

The antigen may be totally innocuous of and by itself.

population will develop immune-complex disease under like conditions of exposure. The central features of immune-complex disease caused by circulating immune complexes are shown in Table 5.10.

NEPHROTOXIC NEPHRITIS (MASUGI) AND HEYMANN NEPHRITIS. Nephrotoxic nephritis is another experimental model of glomerulonephritis caused by the *in situ* **formation of immune complexes.** Anti–glomerular basement membrane antibodies (produced in a rabbit) are injected into rats. These antibodies subsequently leave the circulation to bind to the antigen(s) in the basement membrane. Complement activation then leads to immune-complex glomerulonephritis in these rats. Heymann nephritis represents an active model for the development of renal glomerular lesions due to *in situ* immune-complex formation. An endogenous antigen of the proximal convoluted tubule which cross-reacts with an antigen of the glomerular basement membrane is injected. Antibodies against this antigen are produced and form *in situ* immune complexes along the glomerular basement membrane, leading to membranous glomerulonephritis. Similarly, exogenous antigens could be trapped within the glomerular capillary wall and antibodies would form *in situ* immune complexes that activate complement and lead to inflammatory changes within the glomerular tufts. These various models of glomerulonephritis have collectively focused attention on the importance of the process by which immune complexes deposit in tissue, since it is now abundantly clear that if they do *not* deposit, tissue injury does not occur.

IgA nephropathy is a recently described form of glomerulonephritis in man. It is characterized by the presence of prominent IgA deposits in the mesangial regions of the glomerulus. The diagnosis is based on immunofluorescence findings. It is a common cause of glomerulonephritis in man which may progress to the nephrotic syndrome. The pathogenetic mechanism involved is thought to be the trapping of circulating IgA immune complexes within the mesangial matrix. Large mesangial IgA aggregates then activate the alternate complement pathway, leading to inflammatory changes. Circulating IgA immune complexes can be demonstrated in these patients and correlate with disease activity. IgA nephropathy is thought to be genetically determined in man, and predisposition correlates with increased production of mucosal IgA. The importance of IgA nephropathy in domestic animals is not known, although a high percentage of IgA positive glomerulonephritides have been found in mink with Aleutian disease.

Deposition Process for Immune Complexes

Circulating immune complexes encounter one of two fates: either they are phagocytosed and removed by the cells of the mononuclear phagocyte system, or they become deposited in blood vessels and tissues, setting the stage for subsequent injury. Locally **increased vascular permeability** is necessary to achieve immune-complex deposition and this permeability change is mediated by vasoactive amines. Immune complexes initiate the release of vasoactive amines in at least two different ways; **first,** they can pro-mote vasoactive amine release from basophils, which are, however, rare in the circulation, and **second,** immune complexes can interact directly with the platelet Fc receptor, stimulating platelet aggregation and the release of vasoactive mediators. Immune complexes can also fix and activate complement, which leads to formation of the C3a and C5a anaphylatoxins that can directly activate basophils to release vasoactive amines and platelet activating factor (PAF). The released PAF in turn is a potent platelet agonist that triggers the release of further vasoactive mediators. These vasoactive amines (histamine and serotonin) increase vascular permeability and lead to subsequent deposition of immune complexes in filtering vascular membranes, a process that was called the "anaphylactic trigger" for immune-complex deposition (Fig. 5.21).

Mediation of Immune-Complex Lesions

Immune complexes by themselves do not cause much tissue injury. Rather, injury results from their ability to activate humoral and cellular mediation systems. The most important step is the activation of the complement system, which promotes increased vascular permeability and the attraction and activation of polymorphonuclear leukocytes (neutrophils) that are largely responsible for the ensuing tissue damage and inflammation.

COMPLEMENT. We have previously discussed the interface between the complement proteins and inflammation in a more general way (*see* Chapter 4) and will therefore restrict our remarks here to complement as a reactant in immune-complex disease (Table 5.11). The Fc fragment of the antibodies binds C1, initiating the activation of the classical complement pathway. In immune-complex disease, the complement-derived peptides C3a and C5a deserve special attention because of their biological activities.

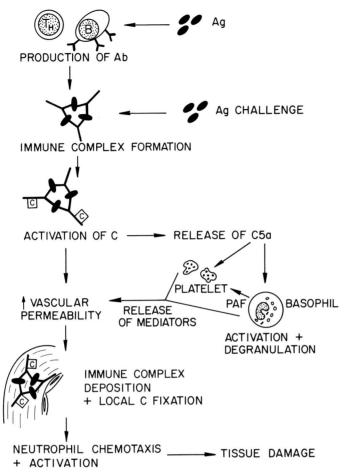

Figure 5.21.   Anaphylactic Trigger for Immune-Complex Deposition. Antigen induces synthesis of both IgG or IgM antibody, which leads to *immune complex formation* within the circulation. The local *vascular permeability* increase necessary for their deposition is mediated via *C5a-basophil-platelet activation and degranulation,* called the "anaphylactic trigger" mechanism (*Ag,* antigen; *Ab,* antibody; *PAF,* platelet-activating factor).

The peptides C3a and C5a are termed **anaphylatoxins.** They are capable of inducing several of the basic vascular phenomena characteristic of inflammation. Although structurally related, the anaphylatoxins exhibit some differences in their biologic specificity and pharmacologic potency (*see* Table 4.17). Their biologic functions include interaction with receptors on mast cells and basophils to cause degranulation and release of histamine, thereby enhancing vascular permeability. On a molar basis, the rela-

tive efficiency of C3a or C5a in releasing histamine from mast cells exceeds that of bradykinin by more than 10-fold. The anaphylatoxins are also capable of inducing smooth muscle contraction. On a molar basis, C5a is more potent than C3a. C5a possesses chemotactic activity and can stimulate PMN leukocytes, macrophages, and monocytes to undergo directional migration along the concentration gradient of the chemotactic agent. The induced influx of these phagocytic cells to the site of inflammation permits efficient

Table 5.11
Complement Function in Immune-Complex Disease

Component or Fragment	Biological Function
C1	Increases Ag-Ab association
C kinin	C2 fragment, increases permeability
C3a	Histamine release
	Smooth muscle contraction
	Increased permeability
	Lysosomal enzyme release
C3b	Immune adherence
	Alternate complement pathway activation
	Enhanced antibody formation
C5a	Histamine release
	Smooth muscle contraction
	Increased permeability
	Chemotaxis of leukocytes
C6	Promotion of coagulation
C567	Chemotaxis of leukocytes (?)

phagocytosis of microorganisms coated with C3b. It also stimulates neutrophils to produce toxic oxygen radicals that lead to tissue damage.

NEUTROPHILS. The presence of neutrophils is essential for the development of immune-complex-induced tissue injury. C5a is a strong chemotactic agent for neutrophils, leading to the accumulation of these cells at sites of immune-complex deposition. Following phagocytosis of immune complexes, activated neutrophils produce highly reactive oxygen products and release lysosomal enzymes that may cause tissue injury.

TISSUE ATTACK MECHANISM. Having explored how antigen-antibody complexes form and deposit, fix complement, and generate chemotactic activity for neutrophils, we now need to turn our attention to the means by which injury actually takes place. It has been shown that lysates of neutrophils (PMN) or of the PMN cytoplasmic granules (lysosomes) are ca-

pable of damaging glomerular basement membrane. The neutrophil-derived agents responsible for tissue damage are enzymes such as cathepsins D and E, neutral proteases such as collagenase and elastase, and other hydrolytic enzymes. Fibrinolytic activity also is present in PMN specific granules. The enzymes appear in both active and activatable form. At least four basic proteins capable of increasing vascular permeability have been isolated from the lysosomes of neutrophils. Another series of injurious PMN products are the free radicals derived from oxygen. These include superoxide anion (O_2^-), hydrogen peroxide (H_2O_2), hydroxyl radical ($\cdot OH$), and singlet oxygen. These potent oxidants have microbicidal activity and have been shown to be central to the production of tissue injury (Fig. 5.22). Ionic iron (ferric, Fe(III)) is a requirement for some reactions. H_2O_2 can cause tissue damage by its reaction with myeloperoxidase and halides, while $\cdot OH$ directly causes membrane damage. O_2^- may also enhance the inflammatory reaction by producing a chemotactic lipid from arachidonic acid.

The mechanisms by which neutrophils release their injurious constituents are not entirely known. In immune-complex disease, the complexes deposited at tissue sites form a phagocytic stimulus for the accumulating neutrophils. Since the complexes usually are fixed to a nonphagocytosable surface (glomerular basement membrane, synovial membrane), the neutrophils cannot interiorize the stimulus. Thus, as fusion of the lysosomes with the plasma membrane takes place as a result of intracellular events initiated by the membrane perturbation provided by the phagocytic stimulus (immune complex), lysosomal enzymes are discharged against the deposition site through the "frustrated phagocytosis" mechanism discussed in Chapter 4. The constituents of PMNs capable of injuring tissue in various ways were most likely designed to rid the host of invaders, but at times they

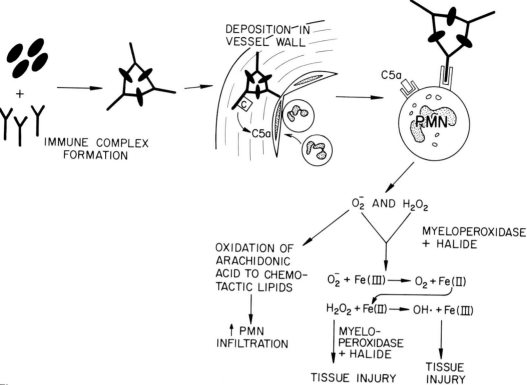

DEPOSITION IN VESSEL WALL

C5a

PMN

O_2^- AND H_2O_2

OXIDATION OF ARACHIDONIC ACID TO CHEMO- TACTIC LIPIDS

MYELOPEROXIDASE + HALIDE

$O_2^- + Fe(III) \longrightarrow O_2 + Fe(II)$

$H_2O_2 + Fe(II) \longrightarrow OH\cdot + Fe(III)$

↑ PMN INFILTRATION

MYELO- PEROXIDASE + HALIDE

TISSUE INJURY

IMMUNE COMPLEX FORMATION

C5a

TISSUE INJURY

Figure 5.22. Role of Toxic Oxygen Products in Immune Complex–Induced Tissue Injury. Circulating immune complexes are formed and deposited within the vascular wall. Activation of complement leads to formation of *C5a,* which is chemotactic for neutrophils *(PMN).* Release of toxic oxygen products by activated *PMN* causes direct tissue damage: Hydroxyl radical *(OH·)* by direct oxidation of lipid membranes, hydrogen peroxidase *(H_2O_2)* by its interaction with myeloperoxidase and halides, and superoxide anion *(O_2^-)* by the production of chemotactic lipids, which further recruits neutrophils.

Table 5.12
Injurious Constituents of Neutrophils

Constituent	Biological Activity
Proteases	Hydrolysis of base- ment membranes and proteoglycans
Plasminogen activator	Fibrinolysis
Collagenase	Destruction of colla- gen
Elastase	Destruction of elastin
Basic peptides	Mast cell activation; permeability increase
Acid cathepsins	Membrane damage
Free radicals of oxygen	Membrane damage

are, unfortunately, directed against the host's own tissues (Table 5.12).

CASE EXAMPLE

Case 5.1: Immune-Complex Disease

History. Ralph was a 7-year-old intact male cocker spaniel when first presented for evaluation of slight weight loss, anorexia, occasional emesis, polydipsia, and polyuria. Physical examination revealed a somewhat thin and listless, normothermic dog with moderate tachypnea and tachycardia. The distal limbs were slightly edematous. The packed cell volume (PCV) was 40, the hemo- globin 12.5 g/100 ml, the total white blood cell count (WBC) 18,700/cu mm, with a nor- mal differential cell count. A serum chemistry panel revealed an elevated blood urea nitrogen (BUN) of 90 mg/100 ml, a low total serum protein of 4.3 g/100 ml, with 0.6 g/100 ml albumin and 3.7 g/100 ml globulins, an elevated serum cholesterol of 319 mg/100 ml and normal serum electrolyte values. Urinalysis showed a specific gravity of 1.023 and 4+ protein. A 24-h urine collection contained 3.2 g of protein. The centrifuged urinary sediment contained 1–3 RBC, 3–5 WBC, 1–3 casts, and 1–3 epithelial cells/high-power field. A diagnosis of protein-losing renal disease (nephrotic syndrome) was made, and on the 4th hospital day a renal biopsy was performed to assist in making a definitive diagnosis.

Biopsy Results. The lesions in the kidney were largely confined to the glomeruli, which were uniformly abnormal. There were slightly increased numbers of fixed glomerular cells and an increase in mesangial matrix. Irregular, periodic acid-Schiff (PAS)-positive eosinophilic thickening of peripheral capillary basement membranes was seen in virtually all glomeruli (Fig. 5.23). Interstitial and tubular changes were mild and consisted largely of focal areas of fibrosis and infiltration by scattered lymphocytes and plasma cells. Some tubular lumina contained eosinophilic, proteinaceous debris and casts. Immunofluorescence microscopy of the biopsy specimen revealed granular, irregular deposits of host IgG and complement component C3 outlining the peripheral portions of glomerular capillary loops and scattered in the mesangium (Fig. 5.24). Ultrastructural examination revealed amorphous, electron-dense deposits within the mesangial regions as well as scattered within the thickened glomerular basement membrane (Fig. 5.25). There was widespread fusion of parietal epithelial cell foot processes.

Follow-Up. After a diagnosis of glomerulonephritis was made, the owners were advised to provide the dog with unlimited access to water and high-quality protein in the diet to help compensate for renal loss. No specific treatment is available for glomerulonephritis. The dog was seen every 6 months for 3 years thereafter. Each visit showed a further gradual decline in renal function, and the dog finally died of progressive uremia and the nephrotic syndrome at the age of 10.5 years.

Case Analysis. Ralph had the typical clinical features of protein-losing renal disease. The combination of hypoproteinemia, proteinuria, hypercholesterolemia, and edema constitutes what is known as the "nephrotic syndrome" and is typical of severe protein-losing renal disease. In dogs, this usually is due to either renal amyloidosis or glomerulonephritis. The microscopic findings in this case were typical of what occurs when the glomeruli are slowly bombarded over a period of time by immune complexes. Since Ralph's disease was a progressive, chronic one, we must assume that the antigen(s) involved were being provided constantly (or at least intermittently) to a dog that was making an appropriate level of antibody to form immune complexes of a depositable size. What was the antigen? Where did it come from? As in most cases of naturally occurring immune-complex glomerulonephritis, we do not know the answer. In that respect it is a somewhat strange disease, as we know a good deal more about the **pathogenesis** than we do about the ultimate **cause.** It remains clear, however, that the fatal disease in this dog was due to glomerular immune-complex deposition and the ensuing inflammatory injury to the glomeruli, with eventual loss of a sufficient number of nephrons to produce renal failure.

Mechanisms of Delayed-Type Hypersensitivity (Type IV)

Delayed-type hypersensitivity reactions (type IV) differ in many respects from the other forms of hypersensitivity, the major difference being the **lack of dependence on antibody.** Hypersensitivity cannot be transferred with serum but can be adoptively transferred by T lymphocytes. These are **cellular** hypersensitivity reactions, with immunologic specificity lying in the **sensitized T lymphocyte** rather than antibody. The cells and factors central to this type of hypersensitivity are those of a normal immune response and inflammation; as such, many of the mechanisms involved are already familiar to us. It is not always easy to visualize a clear distinction between **de-**

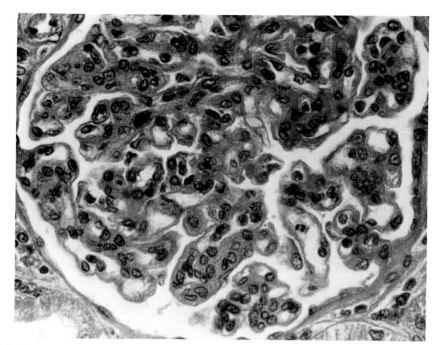

Figure 5.23.   Immune-Complex Glomerulonephritis: Histopathology. Glomerular basement membranes are thickened, and there are adhesions to Bowman's capsule.

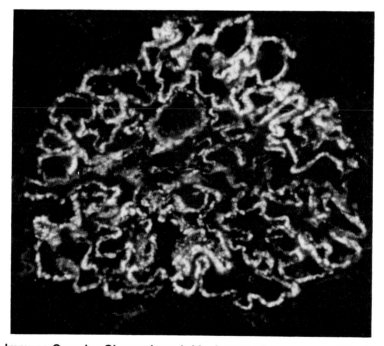

Figure 5.24.   Immune-Complex Glomerulonephritis: Immunofluorescence. This glomerulus shows irregular, lumpy deposits of host IgG. Similar results could be obtained by staining for C3. The immunofluorescence results indicate glomerular deposition of immune complexes. (Micrograph courtesy of Dr. R.M. Lewis.)

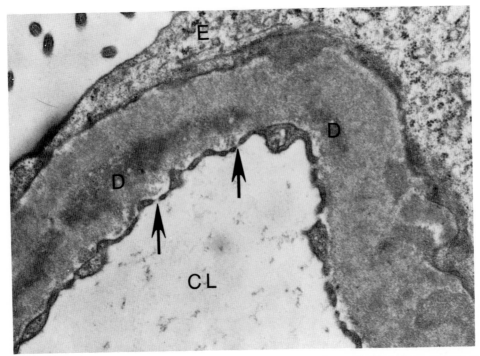

Figure 5.25. Glomerulonephritis: Electron Microscopic Findings. In this micrograph, there are irregular dense deposits *(D)* within the glomerular basement membrane. These correspond to the irregular pattern seen by immunofluorescence. The epithelial foot processes *(E)* are fused over the basement membrane, a common change in proteinuria. Typical fenestrated glomerular endothelium *(arrows)* lines the capillary lumen *(CL)*.

layed-type hypersensitivity (DTH) as an immunopathologic process, and **cell-mediated immunity** (CMI) as an expression of host defense. The mechanisms involved are almost identical. We must reiterate a point made earlier: if the reaction proves deleterious to the host it is referred to as **hypersensitivity,** but if the outcome is beneficial we call it **immunity.** It is probable that in many of these lymphocyte-mediated reactions, both CMI and DTH occur to some degree, simultaneously. That is, both beneficial and harmful results ensue.

The classic tuberculin reaction has been extensively studied as a prototypic type IV reaction, and it provides a basis for understanding the molecular and cellular events comprising DTH. Of more clinical importance, however, are the type IV hypersensitivity reactions that lead to chronic granulomatous inflammation, such as infections with mycobacteria, fungi, and protozoa. Allergic contact dermatitis is another typical type IV hypersensitivity with importance for the clinician.

The complexity of these immune-mediated mechanisms makes it increasingly difficult to provide a cohesive and workable definition of DTH, but three features are worthy of our attention: **first,** DTH reactions are antigen-specific immune reactions characterized by tissue infiltration of blood-derived mononuclear cells (lymphocytes, monocytes); **second,** DTH reactivity can be transferred between animals or individuals with viable lymphoid cells but not with immune serum; **third,** DTH reactions are dependent on T lymphocytes. As the name suggests, DTH reactions usually exhibit a maximum intensity at a delayed time (24–72 h or even more), rather than within a few minutes (type I reactions) or a few hours (type III reactions). This class of immunologic reaction is no more or less cell mediated than antibody-dependent reactions, which are ultimately due to the participation of a lymphocyte or plasma cell. With the exception of those reactions that involve direct cell killing, most reactions of cell-mediated immunity are not dependent upon the lymphocyte as an effector cell, but rather upon soluble lymphocyte products called **lymphokines** and their influence on the major effector cell population, the macrophages.

Initiation of Type IV Hypersensitivity

Type IV hypersensitivities are immune responses that depend on primary contact with an antigen leading to the development of sensitized T cells. Antigens that cause CMI and DTH are often infectious organisms that escape killing by the immune system and survive and multiply in macrophages by various mechanisms; *Toxoplasma* can inhibit phagosome-lysosome fusion, trypanosomes can escape from phagosomes and survive free within the cytoplasm, and mycobacteria and *Leishmania* are able to resist digestion by lysosomal enzymes (Table 5.13). These organisms are readily phagocytized, but because of their unique intracellular survival skills, they persist over a long period of time (*see also* Chapter 7). Some organisms that die can be digested, processed, and their antigenic parts then presented by macrophages to the cooperating cells of the immune response. Similar mechanisms appear to be involved in some viral infections. Lymphocytic choriomeningitis virus, for example, induces a severe lymphocytic inflammation in brain and meninges in immunocompetent mice, while mice with suppressed cell-mediated immunity do not demonstrate any such lesions despite viral proliferation in the brain.

Cellular Infiltrate and Lesions in Delayed-Type Hypersensitivity

The major pattern of protective CMI and injurious DTH involves collaboration between antigen-sensitized T cells and antigen-presenting cells. Delayed-type hypersensitivity reactions are composed predominantly of mononuclear cells. Only some of these cells are sensitized by the antigen, while many are recruited and activated by soluble factors (lymphokines).

The nature of the T cells involved in DTH has long been controversial and, to

Table 5.13
Examples of Escape Mechanisms of Infectious Organisms

Organism	Mechanism of Immunologic Escape
Bacteria	
Mycobacterium spp.	Resistance to lysosomal enzymes
Brucella spp.	Resistance to lysosomal enzymes
Fungi	
Systemic Mycoses	
Blastomyces dermatitidis	Capsule, difficult to degrade
Cryptococcus neoformans	Capsule, difficult to degrade
Histoplasma capsulatum	Capsule, difficult to degrade
Protozoa	
Toxoplasma gondii	Inhibition of phagosome-lysosome fusion
Leishmania spp.	Resistance to lysosmal digestion
Trypanosoma cruzi	Escape the phagosome, survive free in cytoplasm

some extent, it still is. It has been proposed that **T$_h$ cells** proliferate and differentiate into so-called **delayed-type hypersensitivity effector T cells (T$_{DTH}$),** which, upon antigenic challenge, release lymphokines that mediate local inflammation and tissue injury. Additionally, cytotoxic T cells have been demonstrated in the lesions of DTH which may indicate their direct involvement in tissue injury. Many of the infiltrating cells in DTH lesions are macrophages, including both the primary antigen-presenting macrophages and many other nonspecific macrophages attracted to the site and activated by lymphokines. In many DTH lesions, macrophages fuse to form scattered **multinucleated giant cells.** Macrophages that change from a phagocytic and antigen-presenting stage to a secreting stage are known to change their morphologic appearance. They develop an elongated shape with an eccentric nucleus and an eosinophilic cytoplasm. Their resemblance to epithelial cells gave them the name **epithelioid cells,** but it is important to recognize that they are really modified macrophages. In addition, DTH responses such as tuberculin reactions at skin test sites are usually indurated firm swellings as a result of fibrin deposition in the lesions, possibly in association with bound extravascular water.

The histologic pattern of DTH reactions is usually fairly predictably mononuclear with abundant macrophages, but DTH lesions may be accompanied by variable amounts of tissue necrosis, which can be extensive in tuberculosis, and minor accumulations of neutrophils may highlight such lesions. In certain experimental autoimmune disorders in which DTH is thought to play a pathogenetic role, such as thyroiditis or encephalomyelitis, the predominant infiltrating cell is often the lymphocyte. Despite these variations, most DTH lesions continue to be characterized by extensive macrophage infiltrations, and lesions of unknown etiology having such

a morphologic picture often suggest DTH to an experienced pathologist.

Allergic contact dermatitis is a typical example of a cutaneous type IV hypersensitivity which has been recognized in dogs, horses, and rarely cats. The initiating substances are haptens which are by themselves not immunogenic, but which may bind to carrier proteins in the epidermis and thus initiate an allergic reaction. Surface molecules on epidermal Langerhans cells (the antigen-presenting cell of the skin) are thought to act as carrier proteins. In some instances, such as under the influence of γIFN, keratinocytes may also express MHC class II antigens and be able to present antigens. Langerhans cells that present antigens migrate to the dermis and to local lymph nodes where they gain contact with T cells. These T cells become sensitized and recirculate back to the skin. Here, after secondary stimulation by the antigen, they are activated and secrete lymphokines leading to local vasodilation, dermal and epidermal edema, and infiltration of mononuclear inflammatory cells, largely macrophages.

It has become clear that the histologic picture of type IV hypersensitivity may vary somewhat, but the central feature common to all DTH reactions is that a small number of specifically sensitized lymphocytes interact locally with antigen. As a consequence of that interaction, a series of events takes place which generates an inflammatory response at the reaction site. Those events involve the production and release of lymphokines from specifically sensitized T cells, which subsequently function to recruit large numbers of other nonspecifically activated cells, especially macrophages.

Mediators of Cellular Hypersensitivity (Lymphokines)

A unique feature of DTH reactions is the production and release of soluble mediator substances, the **lymphokines,** from sensitized T cells. We have discussed lymphokines in several other contexts (*see also* Chapter 4), and these same lymphokines are the main effector molecules in DTH. There are many different lymphokines which support or modify a large number of different cell functions, and the fluid milieu of a DTH reaction is no less complicated than the mediator-rich soup that characterizes an ordinary inflammatory reaction. Unlike ordinary inflammation, in which all of the infiltrating cells are more or less equal participants, only a small percentage of the infiltrating cells in a DTH reaction are specifically sensitized cells. The inflammatory lymphokines thus provide a means of explaining this phenomenon. A few specifically sensitized T cells, responding to antigen, release a large number of different lymphokines which collectively serve to **attract, activate,** and **immobilize** large numbers of nonspecifically stimulated leukocytes.

Although several different cell types may be involved, the major influence of the secreted lymphokines is on macrophages. Upon secondary contact with an antigen, the sensitized T cells are activated and secrete a variety of lymphokines such as **IL-2, γIFN,** and **migration inhibitory factor (MIF).** Numerous other less well defined factors have been isolated from cultures of activated lymphocytes, such as **mononuclear phagocyte chemotactic factor (MCF)** or **skin reactive factor (SRF). Lymphotoxin** (now called **TNFβ**) has a strong cytotoxic activity and is largely responsible, together with the membrane attack activity of the **perforins,** for the tissue necrosis occurring in DTH reactions.

It has been known for some time that antigen preparations inhibit the migration of cells from spleen or peripheral blood taken from actively immunized animals. A soluble factor, **migration inhibition factor (MIF),** released from sensitized lymphocytes, is responsible for this inhibition of normal macrophage migration. Another important lymphokine affecting the migration properties of macrophages is the **mononuclear phagocyte chemotactic factor (MCF).** Activated lymphocyte supernatants can alter many macrophage functions in addition to migration, including increased adherence, enhanced phagocytic and pinocytotic activity, increased glucosamine uptake, increased glucose oxidation *via* the hexose monophosphate shunt, and increased bacteriostatic or bactericidal activity. These activities have been associated mainly with γIFN. γIFN acts synergistically with IL-2 on cytotoxic cells, and also stimulates macrophages to produce TNFα, to increase the expression of MHC class II antigens, Fc receptors, and Mac-1 receptors on their surface, and it induces PGE$_2$ production by these cells. This leads to increased phagocytic activity and antigen presentation by macrophages.

In addition to those factors responsible for chemotaxis, migration inhibition, and cellular activation, other less well defined factors have been described which enhance the DTH inflammatory response by promoting increased vascular permeability and by affecting the clotting system. Directly acting lymphokines, *e.g.,* **skin reactive factor (SRF),** promote vascular permeability independent of vasoactive amine release from mast cells or basophils. Fibrin accumulation in cutaneous DTH reactions begins when fibrinogen is extravasated. Procoagulant activity, principally due to tissue factor, induces extrinsic coagulation and fibrin formation. Many cells, including activated macrophages, express tissue factor. The expression of macrophage procoagulant activity in inflammatory skin disease is often a hallmark of DTH, and macrophage tissue factor can be up-regulated by a recently defined lymphokine called **macrophage procoagulant-inducing factor (MPIF)** as well as by γIFN and other cytokines. Fibrin so formed may then be cross-linked by factor XIII. These fibrin deposits contribute to the swelling and firmness of a classical cutaneous DTH reaction.

The lymphokines secreted by sensitized T cells thus collectively explain many of the well-known features of a classical DTH reaction. As an amplifying consequence of lymphokine secretion, cytokines such as **IL-1** and **tumor necrosis factor** α (TNFα) secreted by the activated macrophages also play an important role in the evolution of DTH lesions. TNFα, for example, may activate additional T cells by increasing their expression of IL-2 receptors, stimulate MHC class II antigen expression on macrophages, and attract and activate neutrophils. Thus, initial secretion of lymphokines by a relatively small number of cells provides the opportunity for considerable expansion of the reaction *via* various interlacing activation pathways. These carefully coordinated cellular events raise the interesting possibility that lymphokine production may be a much more generalized biological phenomenon than was originally suspected, of importance to both immunologically specific and nonspecific inflammatory reactions. Despite recent progress in molecular definition of the various "factors" apparently involved in DTH reactions, we still have much to learn about the coordinated nature of these unique responses as they occur in a living animal.

Delayed-Type Hypersensitivity in Perspective

It is becoming increasingly clear that tissue injury and the development of lesions in DTH reactions relate to organized interactions between T lymphocytes and macrophages, with the subsequent release of macrophage secretory products into the extracellular environment (Fig. 5.26). Through secretion of a wide variety of materials, the macrophages can damage host tissues and modulate the activity

of surrounding inflammatory cells as well. Among the secreted macrophage products are enzymes such as lysosomal hydrolases, lysozyme, plasminogen activator, collagenase, and elastase, as well as other important molecules like tumor necrosis factor, complement proteins, interferons, various other bioactive chemicals like colony-stimulating factors, lymphostimulatory factors, and a growing list of other inhibitory or cytolytic molecules. If something is worth synthesizing and secreting, macrophages seem to be able to do it.

The reactions of **cell-mediated immunity** and its immunopathologic counterpart **delayed-type hypersensitivity** fall into two broad categories: **first,** those that involve direct participation of intact lymphocytes in the effector arm of the reaction, and **second,** those that involve mediation by soluble lymphokines. The first type of reaction is essentially limited to lymphocyte-dependent cytotoxicity. The second category appears to comprise the bulk of the so-called cell-mediated or DTH-immune responses, and provides a link between this system and the inflammatory response. Various lymphokines have been shown to exert profound influences upon inflammatory cell metabolism, cell surface properties, patterns of cell migration, and the activation of cells for various biologic functions essential to host defense. In this regard, it is worth reiterating that despite the sophistication of the immune response necessary for the initiation of DTH, the effector arm largely revolves around the secretory functions of the macrophage, one of the most elemental of all inflammatory cells.

DISEASES OF THE IMMUNE SYSTEM

Not all of the diseases associated with the immune system involve **offensive** threats like the hypersensitivities. Equally important are situations that arise when the **defensive** functions of the immune system become defective, either when some infection that would normally be re-

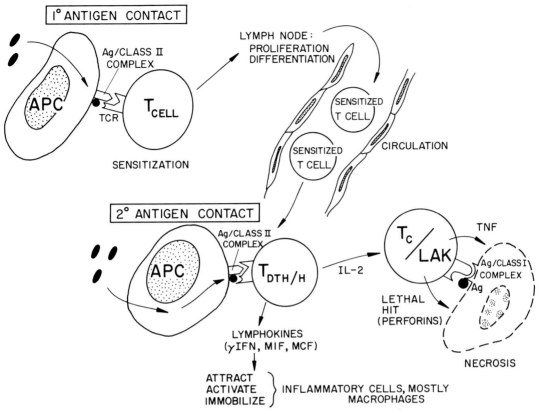

Figure 5.26.   Delayed Hypersensitivity in Infectious Diseases. Certain viral, bacterial, protozoal, or fungal antigens presented by antigen-presenting cells *(APC)* induce sensitized lymphocytes, which proliferate and recirculate so that upon subsequent interaction with the sensitizing antigen, a hypersensitivity reaction develops in which macrophages play an important effector cell role. They are attracted, activated, and localized by lymphokines *(γIFN, MIF,* and *MCF)*. Tissue destruction occurs *via* the activation of cytotoxic cells such as T_c and *LAK* cells, and their soluble factors *(perforins,* lymphotoxin *(TNFβ))*. *(IFN,* interferon; *MIF,* migration inhibition factor; *MCF,* macrophage chemotactic factor, *LAK,* lymphokine-activated killer cells.)

strained by the immune system is permitted, such as occurs in the **immunodeficiency diseases,** or when the immune system incorrectly reacts against host antigens in the **autoimmune diseases.** The immunopathologic consequences of the hypersensitivities and recurrent infections due to immune deficiencies collectively highlight the fundamental power of the immune system; when it doesn't function properly, infection results, and when it is hyperfunctional or misdirected, tissues become injured.

Immunodeficiency Diseases

The inability to mount an appropriate immune response after antigenic stimulation can result from defects of any part of the delicately balanced immune network. Defects in antigen presentation may occur if mononuclear phagocyte function is altered, disturbances of antigen recognition and stimulation of B cells or cytotoxic cells can result from defective T cells, and insufficient or inappropriate antibody production may ensue if B cell function is modified. The immunodeficiency diseases are thus classified according to the underlying functional deficit into four major groups: **first,** defects of the mononuclear phagocyte system; **second,** antibody (B cell) deficiencies; **third,** cellular (T cell) deficiencies; and **fourth,** combined immunodeficiencies (B and T cells). Many of the immunodeficiency diseases are **inherited** and occur with increased frequency in certain families and breeds. In addition, different infectious agents and toxic compounds are known to cause immune suppression and immunodeficiency, and for this reason the immunodeficiency diseases are often divided into **inherited** and **acquired** types.

DEFECTS OF THE MONONUCLEAR PHAGOCYTE SYSTEM. Defects in several different aspects of macrophage function have been described in animals, including **defects in phagocytosis** and **defects in antigen processing.** In both of these situations, antigen presentation is impaired. Defective phagocytosis has been described in Irish Setters that lack the common β subunit of the cell surface molecule Mac-1 on macrophages and neutrophils. Since Mac-1 is a receptor for C3bi, opsonized particles cannot be properly phagocytized. Animals with this defect consequently suffer severe recurrent infections because they are unable to eliminate the infectious agents. Another inherited disease, the **Chédiak-Higashi Syndrome (CHS),** involves a defect in antigen processing which may be due to an abnormality of microtubule polymerization. Animals with the defect have abnormally large, functionally altered macrophage and neutrophil lysosomes. Phagocytosis may proceed normally, but bactericidal activity and antigen processing are defective. Abnormal, extremely large granules are also found in many other CHS cells such as eosinophils and melanocytes. Associated with this abnormality are increased lymphoreticular neoplasms and heightened susceptibility to microbial infections. This recessively inherited disease has been described in man, Hereford cattle, Persian cats, Aleutian mink, beige mice, white tigers, and killer whales.

ANTIBODY (B CELL) DEFICIENCIES. Primary B cell defects have been occasionally described in several animal species. A primary **agammaglobulinemia** has been identified in foals with recurrent bacterial infections. Selective deficiencies of one immunoglobulin type have also been observed in several animal species, such as selective IgG_2 deficiency in Red Danish cattle and selective IgA deficiencies in dogs, horses, and chickens. The clinical significance of these selective deficiences is not clear.

CELLULAR (T CELL) DEFICIENCIES. The T cell deficiency occasionally seen in certain Black Pied Danish and Fresian cattle **(trait A-46)** is an example of an immunodeficiency of the cellular part of the immune system. Such animals exhibit a normal antibody response when B cells are tested in a lymphoblastogenesis assay, but cell-mediated immunity is depressed. Animals with the disease suffer from severe skin lesions, with hair loss and parakeratosis. The immune defect is believed to be a deficiency in thymic hormone, since animals that are treated with zinc oxide (an essential component of thymulin) recover fully when kept on the zinc treatment. A similar T cell defect has been reported in English Bull Terriers with acrodermatitis; however, their disease is unaltered by zinc treatment.

COMBINED IMMUNODEFICIENCIES (CID). The most devastating immunodeficiencies are usually those that involve combined immunodeficiencies, that is, defects of the humoral (B cells) as well as the cellular (T cells) part of the immune system. The most thoroughly documented CID in domestic animals is the autosomal recessive CID that occurs in up to 3% of Arabian foals. Affected foals are unable to produce functional B or T cells and exhibit marked peripheral lymphopenia as well as depleted lymphoid tissues. The deficiency in gammaglobulin production can be detected at a very young age by the lack of IgM after decline in colostral IgM, which has a half life of only a few days. During the first two months foals are protected against infection largely by passive immunity acquired from the colostrum, but as maternal antibodies decline in the blood of affected foals, they develop a remarkable incidence of recurrent infections and usually die within a few months. The lymphoid tissues of such foals lack primary and secondary lymphoid tissue in both B cell areas, such as the germinal centers of spleen and lymph nodes, and T cell areas, such as the thymus, paracortex of lymph nodes, and periarteriolar sheaths of the spleen. Death in Arabian foals with CID is often caused by opportunistic microorganisms such as equine adenovirus, *Pneumocystis carinii, Toxoplasma gondii, Cryptosporidia* spp., and others which have limited pathogenicity in animals with functional immune systems.

Acquired Immunodeficiency Diseases

Intense interest in acquired immunodeficiency diseases of animals has evolved from the recent world-wide attention directed at the fatal **acquired immunodeficiency syndrome (AIDS)** in man. Human AIDS is caused by a retrovirus (a lentivirus) called the human immunodeficiency virus (HIV) that specifically infects T helper cells and cells of the mononuclear phagocyte system (Langerhans cells of the skin and alveolar macrophages) carrying the CD4 cell surface receptor. Affected patients show a marked decrease in their helper T cell population and suffer from a severe immunodeficiency syndrome. It is the high affinity of the viral envelope glycoprotein gp120 for the CD4 molecule which enables the virus to bind to and enter the cells.

Several different **cytotoxic pathways**

are currently believed to produce the marked decline in CD4-positive cells observed in affected individuals; (1) direct killing of the HIV-infected cells by the virus; (2) lysis by cytotoxic cells or antibodies of HIV-infected cells that express viral antigens on their membrane; (3) indirect killing of uninfected cells that bind free circulating gp120 to CD4 receptors and thus resemble infected cells; or (4) formation of poorly functional and short-lived multinucleated syncytial giant cells by fusion of infected and uninfected cells with bound gp120 on the syncytial cell surface.

Infection with HIV is detectable by seroconversion within six months to a year after infection. Initial clinical signs may include chronic and persistent lymphadenopathy with skin rash and hypergammaglobulinemia. Later on, CD4 cell counts slowly and persistently drop until signs of cell-mediated immune dysfunction are detectable by intradermal skin tests. Because of the profound cellular immune deficiency, patients suffer and eventually die from various chronic opportunistic infections caused by *Pneumocystis carinii, Toxoplasma gondii,* adenoviruses, cytomegalovirus, *Cryptosporidia* spp., *Candida, Cryptococcus neoformans, Histoplasma,* and *Legionella.* An increased incidence of Kaposi's sarcoma and other forms of malignancy is also observed.

Since the description of human AIDS and the identification of the HIV virus, research has focused on animal retroviral diseases that can produce immunodeficiency and potentially serve as models for the human disease (Table 5.14). Some of the best-characterized acquired immunodeficiencies in domestic animals occur in cats. **Feline leukemia virus** (FeLV) is a C-type retrovirus responsible for the development of several different diseases in cats including lymphosarcoma of several different cytologic and phenotypic variants, granulocytic and myelomonocytic leukemia, aplastic and hemolytic anemia,

Table 5.14
Animal Models of Acquired Immunodeficiency Syndrome

Disease	Virus	Species	Similarities to H-AIDS[a]
Simian AIDS	SIV (LV)	Rhesus	Immunodeficiency, CD4 and T cell tropism, lymphadeno-pathy, hypergammaglobulinemia, opportunistic infections, encephalopathy, skin rashes.
	SRV-1	Rhesus	Immunodeficiency, lymphadenopathy, subcutaneous and abdominal fibromatosis.
	SRV-2	Rhesus, Celebes	Immunodeficiency.
Feline AIDS	FeLV	Cat, cheetah	Immunodeficiency, T cell defect, opportunistic infections, lymphoid hyperplasia, enteritis.
	FIV (LV, FTLV)	Cat	Immunodeficiency, CD4- and T cell tropism, Mg^{2+}-depen-dent reverse transcriptase, lymphadenopathy, opportun-istic infections.
Murine AIDS	MuLV	Mouse	Immunodeficiency, hypergammaglobulinemia, lymphade-nopathy.
Bovine LV	BIV (LV)	Cattle	No immunodeficiency, early infection lymphadenopathy, Mg^{2+}-dependent reverse transcriptase, cross-reactivity with HIV.

[a] Abbreviations used are: AIDS, acquired immunodeficiency syndrome; SIV, simian immunodeficiency virus; LV, lentivirus; SRV, simian retrovirus; FeLV, feline leukemia virus; FIV, feline immunodeficiency virus; FTLV, feline T-lymphotropic virus; MuLV, murine leukemia virus; BIV, bovine immunodeficiency-like virus; HIV, human immunodeficiency virus.

vimmune-complex disease with glome-rulonephritis, and acquired immuno-deficiency with multiple opportunistic infections. The precise mechanism of immunodeficiency in FeLV-infected cats is not completely understood, but the viral envelope protein pE15 has been associ-ated with immunosuppression, although there is often no consistent correlation between the extent of viremia and the extent of immunosuppression. Recently, the production of a replication-defective mutant of FeLV (called **FeLV-FAIDS mutant**) has been demonstrated in cats with severe spontaneous immunosuppres-sion.

Feline immunodeficiency virus (FIV) is a recently recognized agent that can cause an acquired immunodeficiency syn-drome in cats (feline AIDS). Unlike FeLV infection, however, FIV does not appear to induce malignancies. Like HIV, FIV is a retrovirus of the lentivirus group. Prior to the discovery of FIV, many cats thought to have clinical signs attributable to im-munodeficiency were tested and found to be FeLV negative, but it now appears that some 20% of these clinically affected but FeLV-negative cats are infected with FIV. The primary target of FIV is the T cell and, in a fashion similar to the effects of HIV, both cytotoxic effects and giant cell formation have been demonstrated in infected feline T cell cultures. FIV infec-tion eventually leads to severe leukopenia with neutropenia and generalized lymph-adenopathy.

OTHER ACQUIRED IMMUNODEFICIEN-CIES. In addition to the retroviral diseases, which cause AIDS-like immu-nodeficiency syndromes, many other in-fectious agents have been shown to be immunosuppressive. Organisms that be-long to this group are canine distemper virus in dogs, infectious bursal disease virus and Newcastle disease virus in chickens, feline panleukopenia virus, bovine viral diarrhea virus in cattle, African swine fever virus in pigs, equine herpesvirus 1, and the ectoparasite *Demodex*. Certain environmental toxins may also have a suppressive effect on the immune system. These include polychlorinated biphenyls, polybrominated biphenyls, iodine, lead, cadmium, methyl mercury, and DDT. Additionally, the T_2 toxin from the fungus *Fusarium* that grows in moldy hay depresses the immune system. Many drugs such as cyclosporine or cyclophosphamide have been used to induce immunosuppression as part of the therapy for certain diseases.

AUTOIMMUNE DISEASES

Autoimmune diseases are severe, often crippling, or even fatal diseases that occur in many different species. The cause of these diseases, however, is still largely unknown, and the pathogenesis often extremely complex. **Autoimmunity** is defined as reactivity of the immune system against **self-antigens (autoantigens),** that is, antigens expressed by normal constituent cells or proteins of the host. Normally, the immune system will distinguish between self- and nonself-antigens so that self-antigens are recognized as such and no immune response is mounted. This is referred to as **self-tolerance.** When this normal state is somehow perturbed, humoral or cell-mediated immunity can develop against autoantigens. Our understanding of the pathogenesis of autoimmunity has been complicated, however, by the discovery that reactivity against autoantigens is also part of the normal immune response and is a necessary part of immune regulation. In many different situations, autoantibodies directed against self-antigens can be detected in the serum, but the development of autoantibodies does not necessarily imply the development of tissue injury and disease. If tissue injury develops as a result of autoimmunity, the disease is called

an **autoimmune disease.** As noted earlier, the basic immune mechanisms operative in the development of immune-mediated tissue injury are similar to those that define a normal immune response, and the same holds for autoimmune reactions.

Autoimmunity that is part of the normal immune response is called **physiological autoimmunity.** One example is the mechanism of removal of senescent red blood cells (RBC). This form of physiological autoimmunity involves the expression of a new antigen on the aging RBC surface, which leads to an immune response. **Band 3 antigen** is an anionic transporter in the RBC membrane which is enzymatically cleaved when the cells age. This cleavage exposes a new epitope that is then recognized as nonself, antibodies are developed against these exposed determinants, and the opsonized red cells are removed by mononuclear phagocytes in the liver and spleen. An additional example of physiological autoimmunity is the development of **anti-idiotypic antibodies.** Idiotypes are specific sets of epitopes expressed by antigen receptor molecules on B and T cells. Anti-idiotypic antibodies are directed against these receptors and help regulate the production of antibodies or lymphocytes. This complicated idiotype-anti-idiotype regulatory network, first hypothesized by Jerne in 1974, has been shown to be of considerable importance to immune regulation.

The phenomenon of physiological autoimmunity allows us to underscore an important paradigm of modern pathobiology introduced first in Chapter 1: most diseases do not represent the acquisition of new cellular functions or biochemical pathways. Rather, functions that already exist are accentuated or diminished, and the incredible variations that we call **disease** really only mirror the fascinating complexity of **normal** biologic processes. This is certainly true for the mechanisms thought to be involved in the development of autoimmune tissue injury and autoimmune disease.

Mechanisms of Injury Associated with Autoimmunity

As we have outlined above, the development of autoantibodies does not necessarily mean that an autoimmune disease is occuring. Different mechanisms can be involved in injury associated with autoimmunity, and the clinician and pathologist often have to struggle with establishing what is real and what is artefact. For example, an unrelated disease process may, through the production of tissue damage, lead secondarily to the development of autoantibodies. Post–myocardial infarct patients often develop antimyocardial autoantibodies, but nobody has seriously suggested that "heart attacks" might be autoimmune. Similarly, patients with severe burns may develop antibodies directed against keratinocytes of the skin. This "autoimmune" reaction is due to the novel exposure of keratinocyte antigens to the immune system as a result of the burn injury. Another example of this type of "autoimmunity" is the development of anti-sperm antibodies in vasectomized males. The point to be made should be clear enough; the simple development of autoantibodies, even in association with some disease process, does not necessarily imply that the antibodies played a causal role.

In a true **autoimmune disease,** the autoimmunity is responsible for producing the lesions characteristic of the disease; that is, a cause-effect relationship can be demonstrated. Despite the difficulties associated with establishing such a cause-effect relationship, the demonstration of circulating or *in vivo* bound autoantibodies by immunohistochemical or immunofluorescence techniques remains an important diagnostic tool, especially when used in combination with appropriate clinical signs and histopathological lesions.

Important Mechanisms of Induction of Autoimmunity

The development of autoimmunity is a complex process, and several different induction mechanisms have been proposed (Table 5.15). The situation *in vivo* may be even further complicated by the fact that the tissue injury in any given disease may actually result from multiple mechanisms and multiple pathogenetic schemes.

One induction mechanism for which there is substantial evidence involves the *exposure of sequestered antigens,* that is, antigens that do not normally contact the immune system and therefore are not recognized as self antigens. Due to tissue damage by inflammation or trauma, the blood-tissue barrier may become disrupted, and the "hidden" antigens thus become exposed to the immune system. Not all examples of this mechanism, such

Table 5.15
Possible Induction Mechanisms for Autoimmunity

Exposure of sequestered antigens
 Antigens of brain, spermatozoa, lens, and milk
 α-casein
Exposure of hidden epitope
 Erythrocyte band 3, IgG molecule in rheumatoid arthritis, immunoconglutinins
Antigenic mimicry between self and foreign antigen
 Mycoplasma hyopneumoniae—normal pig lung
 Mycoplasma mycoides—normal bovine lung
 Mycobacterium tuberculosis—proteoglycan in joint cartilage
 β-hemolytic streptococci—cardiac myofibers and heart valve fibroblasts
Failure of immunological control mechanisms
 $\downarrow$ suppressor T (T_S) cells, $\uparrow$ contrasuppressor cells, or disequilibrium of the idiotype-anti-idiotype network
 Examples: Systemic lupus erythematosus ($\downarrow$ T_S), antibodies to the insulin or TSH receptor (idiotype-anti-idiotype network dysfunction)
Aberrant expression of Ia antigens
 Autoimmune thyroiditis
 Some forms of diabetes mellitus

as the anti-sperm antibodies in vasecto-mized men, actually lead to autoimmune tissue injury, but some do. The milk allergy that has been described in Jersey cattle and the demyelination of human multiple sclerosis or canine distemper may be caused, at least in part, by exposure of otherwise sequestered antigens.

Epitopes that normally are not antigenic due to the tertiary structure of a molecule may be newly exposed if the molecule is altered, which may lead to autoimmune disease through the *exposure of hidden epitopes*. Such a mechanism is proposed for the development of antibodies to IgG in human rheumatoid arthritis. An additional mechanism for the induction of autoimmunity is **antigenic mimicry** between self and foreign antigens. In porcine enzootic pneumonia, antibodies to *Mycoplasma hyopneumoniae* have been shown to cross-react with porcine lung tissue. Similar cross-reactivity has also been demonstrated in contagious bovine pleuropneumonia between *Mycoplasma mycoides* and normal bovine lung tissue. It is not clear, however, if these antibodies are involved in the development of lesions.

Dysfunction or **failure of immunological control mechanisms** may be involved in certain autoimmune reactions and may include dysfunction of regulatory T cells, or a disequilibrium of the idiotype-antiidiotype network. In certain patients with **systemic lupus erythematosus,** decreased numbers of T_s cells can be demonstrated. A disequilibrium of the idiotype-antiidiotype network is thought to be involved in the production of antibodies to insulin and to the TSH receptor. Anti-idiotypic antibodies may normally regulate the binding of insulin or TSH to their receptors on thyroid or pancreatic islet cells. Disturbance of this regulation could lead to an overproduction of anti-idiotypic antibodies and these may stimulate or inhibit the receptor.

A final mechanism for the induction of autoimmunity is **aberrant expression of MHC Class II antigens.** Class II antigens are usually expressed only on selected cells of the immune system where their expression is crucial to normal antigen presentation and immune regulation. In abnormal situations, however, other non–immune system cells are able to express Class II antigens and therefore may present new antigens to T_h cells. Aberrant expression of Class II antigens has been demonstrated in **autoimmune thyroiditis** as well as some forms of **autoimmune diabetes mellitus.** The lymphokine γIFN induces Class II molecule expression on keratinocytes and many other epithelial cells *in vitro,* and may be involved in the induction of abnormal Class II antigen expression *in vivo.*

It is clear that several complicated pathways can lead to autoimmune reactions. It is still unknown, however, what factors are truly important in initiating these aberrant responses, or why and under what circumstances they may or may not lead to tissue injury. In general, a much higher percentage of female animals suffer from autoimmune diseases than do males. A genetic component also seems to be involved since some families or breeds show an increased frequency of certain autoimmune diseases, such as lupus erythematosus in the Collie dog, or pemphigus in people with certain MHC class II antigens.

Classification of Autoimmune Diseases

Autoimmune diseases can be divided into two distinct groups based on the distribution of the autoantigen involved in the disease. In the **organ-specific** autoimmune diseases, autoantigen and lesions are essentially localized to a given organ, such as occurs in autoimmune thyroiditis, pemphigus, myasthenia gravis, and autoimmune hemolytic anemia. In the **non-organ-specific** autoimmune diseases, autoantigens are widespread throughout the body and may actually circulate in the blood stream. As might be suspected, such a situation frequently leads to systemic deposition of immune complexes in tissues and to type III hypersensitivity reactions involving characteristic target tissues including kidneys, joints, and skin. The prototypes of these non-organ-specific autoimmune diseases are **systemic lupus erythematosus (SLE)** and **rheumatoid arthritis.** In SLE, antibodies against a variety of different autoantigens are produced including anti-DNA (single- and double-stranded) antibodies, other anti-nuclear antibodies, anti-erythrocyte, anti-lymphocyte and anti-platelet antibodies.

To a large extent, then, the nature and tissue distribution of the inciting antigens determines the nature of the autoimmune disease produced. Several different types of antigenic structures may serve as **autoantigens:** cell membrane **receptors** like the TSH receptor in Grave's disease, the insulin receptor in some diseases in man, and the acetylcholine receptor of the motor end plate in myasthenia gravis; cell surface **proteins** such as the pemphigus antigen on keratinocytes and certain red blood cell antigens in autoimmune hemolytic anemia; **nuclear components** like single- and double-stranded DNA in SLE; and **immunoglobulins** like IgG in rheumatoid arthritis. It is important to reiterate, however, that the immunopathologic reactions that evolve after binding of the autoantibody usually follow the same general pathogenetic mechanisms that hold for type II and type III hypersensitivity reactions (Table 5.16).

Case 5.2: Pemphigus, an Autoimmune Skin Disease

History. A seven-year-old male Poodle exhibited progressive skin lesions for a period of four months. He had been treated by

Table 5.16
Types of Hypersensitivity and Antigens involved in Autoimmune Diseases

Hypersensitivity	Disease	Antigen
Type II	**Anti-blood cell diseases**	
	Autoimmune hemolytic anemia	RBC[a] membrane
	Autoimmune neutropenia	PMN membrane
	Autoimmune lymphopenia	Lymphocyte membrane
	Autoimmune thrombocytopenia	Platelet membrane
	Anti-receptor disease (not cytotoxic)	
	Myasthenia gravis	Acetylcholine receptor
	Grave's disease	TSH receptor
	Anti-keratinocyte diseases (not cytotoxic)	
	Pemphigus complex	Keratinocyte surface
	Bullous pemphigoid	Hemidesmosomes
	Anti-endocrine cell disease	
	Autoimmune thyroiditis	Thyroglobulin, thyroid epithelia
	Autoimmune diabetes mellitus	β cells of pancreatic islets
Type III	Systemic lupus erythematosus	Nuclear components (DNA, histone *etc.* [ANA]); cell surface components on RBC, platelets, PMN, Ly; complement, IgG(RF); cytoplasmic components.
	Rheumatoid arthritis	IgG (RF)

[a]Abbreviations used: RBC, red blood cell; PMN, neutrophil; TSH, thyroid stimulating hormone; ANA, anti-nuclear antibody; Ly, lymphocyte; RF, rheumatoid factor.

various forms of therapy including dietary restriction, topical and systemic antibiotics, and low-dose corticosteroids, but except for some occasional temporary improvements, the skin disease slowly progressed. Physical examination revealed a dog in good general condition but with severe ulceration and crusting along the mucocutaneous junctions of lips, eyes, and anus. On the palate and buccal mucosa of the oral cavity there were multiple discrete ulcers, and the dog showed increased salivation. At the time of the examination, the dog had received no corticosteroid treatment for about three weeks. The differential diagnoses included systemic lupus erythematosus, pemphigus vulgaris, erythema multiforme, and epidermotropic lymphoma.

Clinical Work-Up. The dog was kept at the clinic for three days for further observation with repeated examination every two or four hours. During that time a whitish yellow vesicle developed at the inside of one ear flap, and two vesicles appeared in the mucosa of the oral cavity. One of these vesicles was opened and the contents smeared onto a glass slide for cytological examination. The cytological evaluation revealed many neutrophils and numerous rounded, acantholytic keratinocytes. Based on the clinical signs and the cytological evaluation, a tentative diagnosis of pemphigus vulgaris was made.

Histopathology. Two of the newly formed primary lesions, a pustule in the ear skin and a vesicle from the oral cavity, were completely excised for histopathologic and immunohistochemical examination. The biopsy material was fixed in Michel's medium, a specific fixative that preserves the morphological structures and the antigenicity of possible intralesional antibody deposits. The histopathological examination revealed a suprabasilar to intraepithelial vesicular and pustular dermatitis with ulceration and abundant acantholytic cells (Figs. 5.27 and

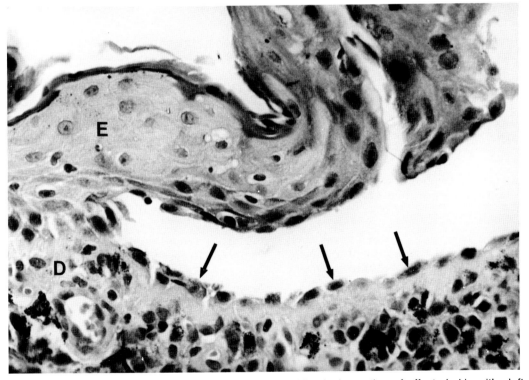

Figure 5.27.   Pemphigus vulgaris: Histopathology. Histologic section of affected skin with cleft formation above the basal cell layer and suprabasilar vesicle formation. Basal cells *(arrows)* remain on the basement membrane while all suprabasilar epithelial layers are lifted off. (*E,* epidermis; *D,* dermis.)

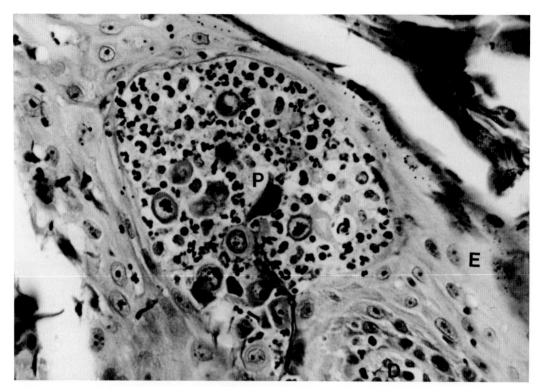

Figure 5.28.   Pemphigus vulgaris: Histopathology. Histologic section of an intraepidermal pustule *(P)* containing many acantholytic cells *(arrows)* and abundant neutrophils. (*E,* epidermis; *D,* dermis.)

5.28). The acantholytic cells appeared as single, round epidermal cells that had lost cohesion to neighboring cells. Such cells are strongly suggestive of pemphigus when found in sufficient numbers within the vesicles.

Immunofluorescence Study. Immunofluorescence staining of perilesional skin and oral mucosa for immunoglobulin and complement components showed a strong keratinocyte surface fluorescence of all suprabasilar layers of the stratified squamous epithelium (Fig. 5.29). Based on the histopathologic and immunohistochemical findings, a definitive diagnosis of **pemphigus vulgaris** was made.

Treatment. The dog was treated with high doses of corticosteroids and aurothioglucose. The lesions improved markedly within a few weeks. The owner was advised, however, that life-long treatment would be necessary to control this severe autoimmune disease.

ASSESSMENT OF IMMUNE SYSTEM FUNCTION

In order for the immune system to perform its critical functions of protecting the host from external and internal influences, carefully coordinated normal functioning of all the components of its various cellular and humoral components is required. As we have seen, both hypersensitivity and immunodeficiency can lead to disease. Therefore the clinical veterinarian must be well acquainted with the various means of assessing immune system function. It is not our purpose here to try to serve as a sourcebook for clinical immunology, since excellent texts on the subject are available, but we will briefly describe some of the more important means of assessing immune function in order to

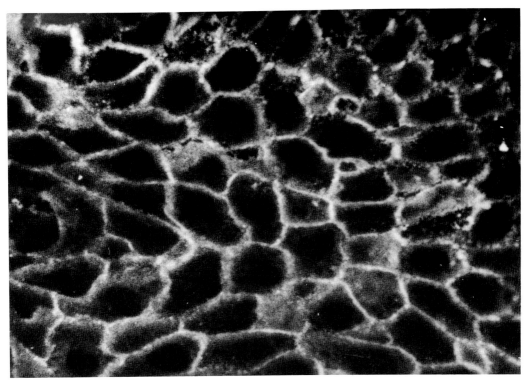

Figure 5.29. Pemphigus vulgaris: Immunofluorescence. Direct immunofluorescence method using rabbit anti-canine IgG reveals a distinct pattern of cell surface staining of keratinocytes in the perilesional epidermis representing *in vivo* deposition of the autoantibody.

place immunopathology, hypersensitivity, and immunodeficiency in a more practical and realistic setting.

Assessment of Antibody Production

Immunoglobulin (Ig) levels can be crudely measured by **serum protein electrophoresis.** Serum proteins are separated electrophoretically and quantitated by densitometry. Immunoglobulins migrate within the gammaglobulin fraction. Marked overproduction or severe deficiency of Ig can be detected by either a distinctly increased gammaglobulin peak or a lack of this fraction, respectively. Immunoglobulins can be more precisely quantitated by the determination of individual immunoglobulin classes (IgG, IgM, and IgA). This can be done by **radial**

immunodiffusion or **radioimmunoassay;** individual Ig classes are determined by the reaction of anti–specific Ig class antibodies. In the radial immunodiffusion test, the patient's serum diffuses outward from a well in an agar plate and forms a precipitation line with the anti-Ig antibody which diffuses radially from another well. In the radioimmunoassay, the specific Ig is demonstrated by its reactivity with a radiolabeled anti-Ig antibody. Quantitation allows detection of selective Ig deficiencies and measurement of immunoglobulin levels. An even more specific measurement of antibody production is the determination of **antigen-specific antibodies,** which can be measured using various immunological tests such as **indirect immunofluorescence** or **im-**

munoperoxidase assays, **enzyme-linked immunosorbant assay** (ELISA), **hemagglutination,** or **complement-fixation** assays. Most clinical immunology laboratories are equipped for several different methods of assessing Ig levels and specific Ig quantitation.

Lymphocyte Function Tests

Cell-mediated immunity can be measured *in vitro* in various lymphocyte function tests. In the **lymphocyte blastogenesis assay,** the potential of lymphocytes to proliferate in response to nonspecific (mitogens) or specific (antigen) stimuli is assessed. The lymphocytes are stimulated and the increased proliferation is measured by the increase of radiolabeled thymidine incorporation into DNA. In the **mixed lymphocyte reaction (MLR),** patient lymphocytes are stimulated by co-cultivation with irradiated lymphocytes (unable to proliferate) from another individual, and reactivity against heterologous MHC antigens is measured. Again, increased thymidine incorporation is determined. *In vivo* assessment of cell-mediated immunity is performed by **intradermal testing** for hypersensitivity to certain antigens. A specific antigen is injected intradermally, and reactivity of the immune system is demonstrated by the formation of an inflammatory focus visible as a swollen area of edema, redness, and pain. In delayed-type hypersensitivity the reaction peaks at 2–4 days, while a type I hypersensitivity may produce swelling after a few minutes. Such tests are commonly used, for example, to screen for reactivity against *Mycobacterium bovis* in cattle or *M. tuberculosis* in primates. Intradermal skin testing is also often used to determine the specific antigen responsible for allergic dermatoses. Frequent allergens are flea components and staphylococcal antigens.

Histopathology

The histologic examination of tissues obtained from affected animals is a crude and somewhat unsophisticated tool for the assessment of immune function, but an experienced pathologist can learn much from the morphologic assessment of lesions. Presented with a dead animal in the postmortem room or in the field, histopathology may be the only tool available with which to estimate immune function. The pathologist may pay special attention to the lymphoid organs in a suspected immunodeficiency case. Are all of the primary and secondary lymphoid organs present? What is their size? Arabian foals with combined immunodeficiency, for example, usually have a very small thymus that is sometimes even difficult to find. Histologically, the remnants of thymus are devoid of lymphocytes, lack a well-defined distinction between cortex and medulla, and the interlobular septa are widened. The spleens of these horses lack germinal centers and periarteriolar sheaths, and their lymph nodes may be virtually devoid of follicular and paracortical lymphocytes.

Histopathologic examination can be highly useful, but it is rarely definitive. There are certain patterns of tissue reaction, however, that are strongly suggestive of involvement of the immune system. For example, immunodeficiency diseases commonly exhibit thymic hypoplasia or atrophy, and lymphoid depletion in spleen, lymph nodes, and Peyer's patches. Hyperreactivity might be indicated by generalized hyperplasia of secondary lymphoid organs, but chronic inflammation can produce similar changes if caused by antigenic stimuli. Usually only rather marked immune malfunctions can be recognized by histopathologic examination; more subtle immune defects cannot be determined histologically, and more sophisticated approaches, such as immunohistochemistry to detect specific changes in lymphoid organs, are usually necessary to define a diagnosis.

Many of the immunopathologic and immune-mediated diseases have rather characteristic histopathologic pictures that are strongly suggestive of a certain diagnosis. The two cases presented in this chapter, immune-complex glomerulonephritis (Case 5.1) and pemphigus vulgaris (Case 5.2) illustrate this principle quite well. The histopathologic lesions can be quite characteristic for many of the immune-mediated diseases, and examination of tissue obtained by **biopsy** can often provide a great deal of information about the staging of the disease as well as suggesting a specific diagnosis.

Immunohistochemistry

The application of specific immunological methods to tissues sections has allowed an advanced level of diagnostic sophistication to be applied to many disease settings. Since the development of **fluorescein-labeled antibodies** by Coons in 1941, this technique has become a fundamental tool in many areas of pathology and has provided answers to many practical diagnostic problems. More recently, the highly sensitive **peroxidase antiperoxidase method** developed in the early 1970s has brought a markedly increased level of sensitivity to immunohistochemical techniques. Immunoperoxidase methods are based on the interaction of a specific antibody with a tissue-bound antigen and the subsequent demonstration of the antibody binding site with a label visible by normal light microscopy. The most widely used techniques are **direct** and **indirect immunofluorescence** or **immunoperoxidase,** the **peroxidase anti-peroxidase (PAP) method,** the **(strept)avidin-biotin complex (ABC and Strept-ABC),** and the **protein-A method.** The principles involved in these various techniques are illustrated in Figure 5.30.

The "multilayer" immunohistochemical techniques such as PAP, ABC, and Strept-ABC depend upon the use of additional antibody layers or the highly specific binding of avidin or streptavidin to the vitamin, biotin. All of the multilayer techniques increase the amount of label for a given amount of antigen and can increase sensitivity up to 100-fold. The labels used are either substances that fluoresce when excited by UV light of the appropriate wave length, or chromogens that change color upon reduction to become visible by normal light microscopy. The most commonly used chromogens are 3,3-diaminobenzidine (DAB) and 3-amino 9-ethylcarbazole (AEC). Various enzymes are used to reduce the chromogen such as peroxidase, alkaline phosphatase, or glucose oxidase. For electron microscopic evaluation, highly electron dense colloidal gold particles that give a clear image in electron micrographs, are commonly used.

To assess immune function, specific components of the immune system such as antibodies, complement components, or cell populations are demonstrated with specific antibodies. Using these techniques, deficiencies of selected cell populations in lymphoid organs can be demonstrated. The immune-mediated nature of tissue injuries can be assessed by the demonstration of tissue-bound immunoglobulins in autoimmune diseases, complement components in immune-complex lesions, and clonal populations of lymphocytes in B or T cell neoplasia.

Flow Cytometry

The recent development of two new techniques, the production of **monoclonal antibodies** and **flow cytometry** (Fig. 5.31), has provided researchers and diagnosticians with a powerful tool to evaluate the presence of leukocyte subpopulations and their functional state. Today, these methods are becoming widely

A) Direct peroxidase or immunofluorescence

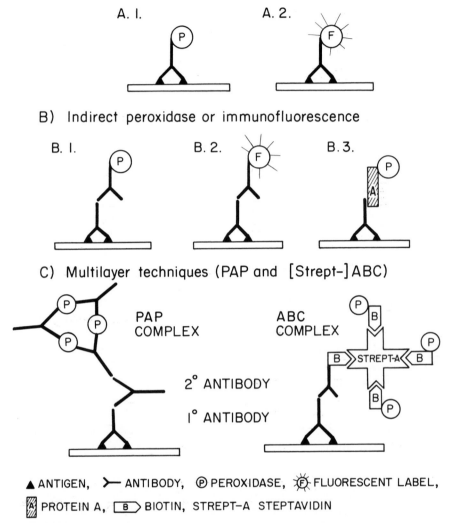

A. I.   A. 2.

B) Indirect peroxidase or immunofluorescence

B. I.   B. 2.   B. 3.

C) Multilayer techniques (PAP and [Strept-] ABC)

PAP
COMPLEX

ABC
COMPLEX

STREPT-A

2° ANTIBODY

1° ANTIBODY

▲ ANTIGEN, ⊱ ANTIBODY, Ⓟ PEROXIDASE, ⊕ FLUORESCENT LABEL,
⬚ PROTEIN A, ⬡ BIOTIN, STREPT-A STEPTAVIDIN

Figure 5.30. Principles of the Common Immunohistochemical Procedures. Various techniques are used to identify antigens or antibodies in tissues: *A,* direct immunofluorescence and immunoperoxidase assay. *B,* indirect techniques: *B1,* immunoperoxidase; *B2,* immunofluorescence; *B3,* protein A-peroxidase test. *C,* multilayer techniques: peroxidase anti-peroxidase *(PAP)* and (strept)avidin-biotin complex *(ABC)* method.

used in veterinary medicine. Flow cytometry requires single-cell suspensions, and cells of the immune system and other hematopoietic cells are particularly well suited for this type of analysis. Briefly, flow cytometry is based on the distinction and separation of labeled cell populations by a narrow beam of laser light. The cells are bound to monoclonal antibodies (labeled with a fluorochrome) that are directed against specific cell surface markers, and then individually passed through a laser beam. When a fluorochrome-labeled cell passes, it is registered by the

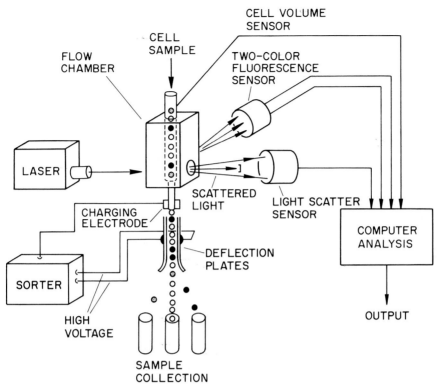

Figure 5.31.   Principles of Flow Cytometry. Cells labeled with different fluorescent markers (such as labeled monoclonal antibodies) can be analysed or sorted by the influence of the laser beam on the light scattering qualities of the various labels employed.

diffraction of the light, and the fluorochrome intensity is monitored. The information is analyzed by a computer and can be plotted in one-, two-, or three-dimensional plots. Cells can also be sorted according to their fluorochrome label. This provides the opportunity to perform function tests on specifically defined cell populations after flow cytometric sorting.

Early applications of flow cytometry simply quantitated subpopulations of cell suspensions carrying specific cell surface markers. Such quantitation, however, does not permit functional assessment of the cells being sorted and hence has limited application to the study of the immunodeficiency states. The more recent identification of function-associated surface markers has greatly enhanced the diagnostic value of flow cytometric analysis.

Good examples of such function-associated markers are the IL-2 receptor on T cells, the MAC-1 on neutrophils, the Fc receptor on macrophages, and the MHC class II molecules on antigen-presenting cells. The expression of many of these cell surface molecules is markedly increased after stimulation of the cells, and only functionally intact cells can respond with such increased expression (Fig. 5.32).

A further application of flow cytometry is the quantitation of cells in the active phase of the cell cycle (G_2/M). This is performed by staining the cellular DNA with DNA-specific fluorochromes. The degree of staining is directly proportional to the amount of DNA present in the cell, and the amount of cell proliferation can be determined by quantitating the amount of DNA.

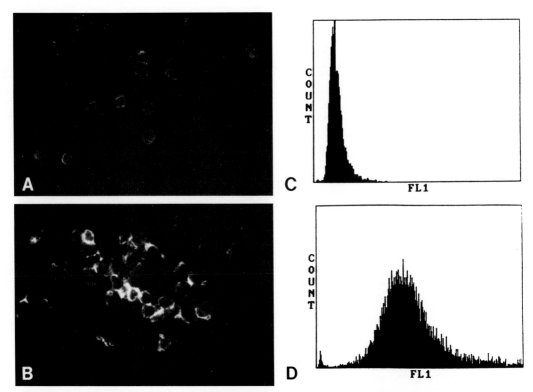

Figure 5.32.   Flow Cytometric Analysis of Equine Neutrophils. Resting equine neutrophils express very low levels of the MAC-1 leukocyte cell adhesion molecule (Leu-CAM), as shown by weak immunofluorescence when stained with a labeled monoclonal antibody directed at the common β submit *(A)*, but there is much more staining (indicating up-regulation of the receptor) when the cells are stimulated with C5a *(B)*. Flow cytometric assessment of resting *(C)* and C5a-stimulated *(D)* neutrophil populations shows a marked shift to the right in the cytometric analysis, indicating greater fluorescence intensity, which correlates with increased binding of the monoclonal antibody to the up-regulated receptor. (Courtesy of Dr. P.N. Bochsler.)

So long as researchers and diagnosticians continue to be interested in finding the answers to fundamental questions about immune-mediated diseases, additional technical means of answering those questions will be developed. In this age of high technology, it seems likely that our continuing progress will not be limited by the technical means of approaching important questions about disease, but by the ultimate complexity of the questions themselves. This is, perhaps, as it should be. The technology should be driven by the need to find appropriate answers to important questions, rather than the technology itself attempting to define for us what the questions should be.

Reference Material

Beaven, M.A., Maeyama, K., WoldeMussie, E., Lo, T.N., Ali, H., and Cunha-Melo, J.R.: Mechanism of signal transduction in mast cells and basophils: studies with RBL-2H3 cells. *Agents and Actions* 20:137–145, 1987.

Benacerraf, B.: Antigen processing and presentation. The biologic role of MHC molecules in determinant selection. *J. Immunol. 141*:S17–S20, 1988.

Beutler, B., and Cerami, A.: Tumor necrosis, cachexia, shock, and inflammation: a common mediator. *Ann. Rev. Biochem. 57*:505–518, 1988.

Bielefeldt Ohmann, H., Lawman, M.J.P., and Babiuk, L.A.: Bovine interferon: its biology and application in veterinary medicine. *Antiviral Res.* 7:187–210, 1987.

Braquet, P., and Rola-Pleszczynski, M.: Platelet-activating factor and cellular immune responses. *Immunol. Today* 8:345–352, 1987.

Breathnach, S.M., and Katz, S.I.: Cell-mediated immunity in cutaneous disease. *Human Pathol.* 17:161–167, 1986.

Cohen, I.R.: The self, the world and autoimmunity. *Sci. Amer.* 258:52–60, 1988.

Cohen, S.: Physiologic and pathologic manifestations of lymphokine action. *Human Pathol.* 17:112–121, 1986.

Dinarello, C.A.: An update on human interleukin-1: from molecular biology to clinical relevance. *J. Clin. Immunol.* 5:287–296, 1985.

Dinarello, C.A., and Mier, J.W.: Interleukins. *Ann. Rev. Med.* 37:173–178, 1986.

Dvorak, A.M., Schulman, E.S., Peters, S.P., Mac-Glashan, D.W. Jr., Newball, H.H., Schleimer, R.P., and Lichtenstein, L.M.: Immunoglobulin E-mediated degranulation of isolated human lung mast cells. *Lab. Invest.* 53:45–56, 1985.

Dvorak, H.F., Galli, S.J., and Dvorak, A.M.: Cellular and vascular manifestations of cell-mediated immunity. *Human Pathol.* 17:122–137, 1986.

Emancipator, S.N., and Lamm, M.E.: IgA nephropathy: pathogenesis of the most common form of glomerulonephritis. *Lab. Invest.* 60:168–183, 1987.

Fligiel, S.E.G., Ward, P.A., Johnson, K.J., and Till, G.O.: Evidence for a role of hydroxyl radical in immune-complex-induced vasculitis. *Am. J. Pathol.* 115:375–382, 1984.

Gallo, R.C., and Montagnier, L.: AIDS in 1988. *Sci. Amer.* 259:41–48, 1988.

Geczy, C.L.: The role of lymphokines in delayed-type hypersensitivity reactions. *Springer Semin. Immunopathol.* 7:321–346, 1984.

Germain, R.N.: The ins and outs of antigen processing and presentation. *Nature* 322:687–689, 1986.

Gonda, M.A., Braun, M.J., Carter, S.G., Kost, T.A., Bess, J.W. Jr., Arthur, L.O., and Van Der Maaten, M.J.: Characterization and molecular cloning of a bovine lentivirus related to human immunodeficiency virus. *Nature* 330:338–391, 1987.

Gordon, S., Keshav, S. and Chung, L.P.: Mononuclear phagocytes: tissue distribution and functional heterogeneity. *Current Opinion Immunol.* 1:26–35, 1988.

Halliwell, R.E.W., and Gorman, N.T.: *Veterinary Clinical Immunology.* W.B. Saunders, Philadelphia, 1989.

Hamilton, T.A., and Adams, D.O.: Molecular mechanisms of signal transduction in macrophages. *Immunol. Today* 8:151–158, 1987.

Herberman, R.B., Reynolds, C.W., and Ortaldo, J.R.: Mechanism of cytotoxicity by natural killer (NK) cells. *Ann. Rev. Immunol.* 4:651–680, 1986.

Ho, D.D., Pomerantz, R.J., and Kaplan, J.C.: Patho-genesis of infection with human immunodeficiency virus. *New Engl. J. Med.* 317:278–286, 1987.

Hoover, E.A., Mullins, J.I, Quackenbush, S.L., and Gasper, P.W.: Experimental transmission and pathogenesis of immunodeficiency syndrome in cats. *Blood* 70:1880–1892, 1987.

Horwitz, M.A.: Intracellular parasitism. *Current Opinion Immunol.* 1:41–46, 1988.

Johnson, K.J., Chensue, S.W., Kunkel, S.L., and Ward, P.A.: Immunopathology. In: *Pathology,* edited by E. Rubin and J.L. Farber. J.B. Lippincott Co., Philadelphia, 1988, pp. 96–139.

Kirchner, H.: Interferons, a group of multiple lymphokines. *Springer Semin. Immunopathol.* 7:347–374, 1984.

Koren, H.S. *et al.*: Proposed classification of leukocyte-associated cytolytic molecules. *Immunol. Today* 8:69–71, 1987.

Le, J., and Vilcek, J.: Tumor necrosis factor and interleukin 1: cytokines with multiple overlapping biological activities. *Lab. Invest.* 56:234–248, 1987.

Lewis, R.M., and Picut, C.A.: *Veterinary Clinical Immunology: From Clinics to Classroom.* Lea & Febiger, Philadelphia, 1989.

Male, D., Champion, B., and Cooke, A.: *Advanced Immunology.* J.B. Lippincott Co., Philadelphia, 1987.

Malkovsky, M., Sondel, P.M., Strober, W., and Dalgleish, A.G.: The interleukins in acquired disease. *Clin. Exp. Immunol.* 74:151–161, 1988.

Martin, T.W., and Lagunoff, D.: Mast cell secretion. In *Cell Biology of the Secretory Process.* Karger, Basel, 1984, pp. 481–516.

Matthews, J.B.: Immunocytochemical methods: a technical overview. *J. Oral Pathol.* 16:189–195, 1987.

McManus, L.M.: Pathobiology of platelet-activating factors. *Pathol. Immunopathol. Res.* 5:104–117, 1986.

Mosier, D.E.: Animal models for retrovirus-induced immunodeficiency disease. *Immunol. Invest.* 15:233–261, 1986.

Nathan, C.F.: Secretory products of macrophages. *J. Clin. Invest.* 79:319–326, 1987.

O'Garra, A., Umland, S., De France, T., and Christiansen, J.: "B-cell" factors are pleiotropic. *Immunol. Today* 9:45–54, 1988.

Old, L.J.: Tumor necrosis factor. *Sci. Amer.* 258:59–60, 69–75, 1988.

Oppenheim, J.J., Kovacs, E.J., Matsushima, K., and Durum, S.K.: There is more than one interleukin 1. *Immunol. Today* 7:45–56, 1986.

Ortaldo, J.R.: Comparison of natural killer and natural cytotoxic cells: characteristics, regulation, and mechanism of action. *Pathol. Immunopathol. Res.* 5:203–218, 1986.

Pedersen, N.C., Ho, E.W., Brown, M.L., and Yamamoto, J.K.: Isolation of a T-lymphotropic virus from domestic cats with an immunodeficiency-like syndrome. *Science 235*:790–793, 1987.

Perlmutter, R.M.: T-cell signaling. *Science 245*:344, 1989.

Podack, E.R.: Molecular mechanisms of cytolysis by complement and by cytolytic lymphocytes. *J. Cell. Biochem. 30*:133–170, 1986.

Rappolee, D.A., and Werb, Z.: Secretory products of phagocytes. *Current Opinion Immunol 1*:47–55, 1988.

Redfield, R.R., and Burke, D.S.: HIV infection: the clinical picture. *Sci. Amer. 259*:90–98, 1988.

Reynolds, C.W., and Ortaldo, J.R.: Natural killer activity: the definition of a function rather than a cell type. *Immunol. Today 8*:172–174, 1987.

Robb, R.J.: Interleukin 2: the molecule and its function. *Immunol. Today 5*:203–209, 1984.

Roitt, I., Brostoff, J., and Male, D.K.: *Immunology.* C.V. Mosby Co., St. Louis, 1985.

Shinkai, Y., Takio, K., and Okumura, K.: Homology of perforin to the ninth component of complement (C9). *Nature 334*:525–527, 1988.

Slauson, D.O., Walker, C., Kristensen, F., Wang, Y., and de Weck, A.L.: Mechanisms of serotonin-induced lymphocyte proliferation inhibition. *Cell. Immunol. 84*:240–252, 1984.

Springer, T.A., Dustin, M.L., Kishimoto, T.K., and Marlin, S.D.: The lymphocyte function associated LFA-1, CD2, and LFA-3 molecules: cell adhesion receptors of the immune system. *Ann. Rev. Immunol. 5*:223–252, 1987.

Stelzer, G.T., and Robinson, J.P.: Flow cytometric evaluation of leukocyte function. *Diag. and Clin. Immunol. 5*:223–231, 1988.

Tizzard, I.R.: *An Introduction to Veterinary Immunology,* ed. 2. W.B. Saunders, Philadelphia, 1987.

Unanue E.R., and Allen, P.M.: The basis for the immunoregulatory role of macrophages and other accessory cells. *Science 236*:551–557, 1987.

Weber, J.N., and Weiss, R.A.: HIV infection: the cellular picture. *Sci. Ameri. 259*:101–109, 1988.

Williams, T.J., Hellewell, P.G., and Jose, P.J.: Inflammatory mechanisms in the Arthus reaction. *Agents and Actions 19*:66–72, 1986.

Woodruff, J.J., Clarke, L.M., and Chin, Y.H.: Specific cell-adhesion mechanisms determining migration pathways of recirculating lymphocytes. *Ann. Rev. Immunol. 5*:201–222, 1987.

Yamamoto, J.K., Sparger, E., Ho, E.W., Andersen, P.R., O'Connor, T.P., Mandell, C.P., Lowenstine, L., Munn, R., and Pedersen, N.C.: Pathogenesis of experimentally induced feline immunodeficiency virus infection in cats. *Am. J. Vet. Res. 49*:1246–1258, 1988.

Zychlinsky, A., Joag, S., and Young, J.D.–E.: Cytolytic mechanisms of the immune system. *Current Opinion Immunol. 1*:63–69, 1988.

6
Disorders of Cell Growth

Developmental Anomalies
Acquired Lesions
  Atrophy and Hypertrophy
  Hyperplasia
  Metaplasia
  Dysplasia
Neoplasia
  Nomenclature
  Morphologic and Behavioral Features of
    Benign and Malignant Neoplasms
    Case 6.1: Histogenetic Origin
  The Stroma of Neoplasms
  Growth of Neoplasms
  Spread of Tumors—Invasion and Metastasis
Pathogenesis of Neoplasia
  Control of Cell Growth
    Growth Factors
    Overview of GF Mechanisms in the
      Regulation of Cell Growth
    Other Growth Control Mechanisms
    Role of Intracellular Messengers
  Properties of Neoplastic Cells
  The Etiology of Neoplasia
  Mechanisms of Carcinogenesis
    Initiation and Promotion
    Progression of Neoplasia and Tumor
      Latency
  Genetic Aspects of Neoplasia
    Tests for Carcinogenicity
    Chromosomal Abnormalities and Neoplasia
    Oncogenes and Cancer Suppressor Genes
    The Role of Suppressor Genes
  Viral Oncogenesis
    Mechanisms of Viral Oncogenesis
      DNA Viruses
      Retroviruses
      Examples of Virus-Induced Neoplasms in
        Animals

      Marek's Disease
      Feline Lymphosarcoma
      Bovine Leukemia
    The Clonal Nature of Neoplasms
    Vascularization of Neoplasms
  Mechanisms of Invasion and Metastasis
    Tumor Heterogeneity
    Tumor Cell Invasion
    Metastasis
      The Metastatic Process
      Vascular Invasion
      Dissemination of Embolic Tumor Cells
      Arrest of Embolic Tumor Cells
      Organ Preference of Metastasis
      Heterogeneity, Metastasis, and Cellular
        Interactions
Effect of the Tumor on the Host
  Paraneoplastic Syndromes
  Cancer Cachexia
Neoplasia and Immunity
  Tumor Antigens
  The Concept of Immunologic Surveillance
  Evidence for Immunity Against Tumors
  Effector Mechanisms in Tumor Immunity
    Cellular Cytotoxicity
    Antibody
    Natural Killer Cells
    Macrophages
    Tumor Immunity and Metastasis
  Possible Escape Mechanisms
  Enhancement of Tumor Growth by
    Suppressor Cells
Neoplasia in Perspective
    Case 6.2: Paraneoplastic Syndrome
Reference Material

A number of diseases involve abnormalities of tissue growth. These vary from congenital defects in organ development, to neoplasia (or cancer), one of the most serious diseases of both animals and man. In this chapter we consider these diseases and current knowledge of their pathogenesis. Before doing so, however, we will briefly discuss normal tissue growth and differentiation as a background against which such diseases can be considered.

Throughout the embryonic and postnatal development of an individual, tissues grow mainly by cell proliferation. Admittedly, tissue mass also can be increased by an increase in cell size, but, as a component of growth, this mechanism is relatively unimportant. Many tissues retain the capacity for cellular proliferation throughout the life of the individual, and in some there is continual mitotic division in order to replace cells that are lost. In the skin, for instance, there is continual loss of keratinized epithelial cells requiring replacement by proliferation of basal cells. Similarly, in the bone marrow there is continual cell proliferation to replace cells of the peripheral blood whose lifetime is limited. Other cells, such as those of the renal tubular epithelium or of the liver, do not continually proliferate but retain the capacity for mitotic division as a mechanism for repair.

Most of the daughter cells that result from cell proliferation undergo differentiation, adopting the structural and functional characteristics of the tissue they are destined to become. Although somatic cells are believed to retain all of the individual's genetic information, at some point differentiation involves the regulated expression of particular genes, providing the commitment to a particular course of development and specialization. Thus, cells committed to be epidermal cells only reproduce epidermal cells, liver cells produce liver cells, and so on. In most cases fully differentiated cells lose the capacity to divide, so loss of this ca-

pacity may be regarded as one feature of the process of differentiation. Although differentiation apparently involves alteration or restriction of genetic expression, the exact mechanisms by which it is accomplished are poorly understood. The most important point is that these modifications of cell behavior apparently are accomplished by regulating the expression of the genetic information in each cell and not by any process analogous to mutation.

Most tissues therefore can be regarded as containing a mixture of cells, some continually dividing, some that are not dividing but are capable of returning to the mitotic pool, and some that are terminally differentiated and no longer able to undergo mitosis. The sequence of events comprising mitosis is called the **cell cycle** and is depicted diagrammatically in Figure 6.1. G_1 is the most variable phase in terms of length, and the time taken to go through G_1 largely determines the length of the cycle and therefore the rate of cell proliferation. Critical molecular regulatory events also occur during G_1. During the S phase of the mitotic cycle, DNA and chromosomal proteins are synthesized. Of

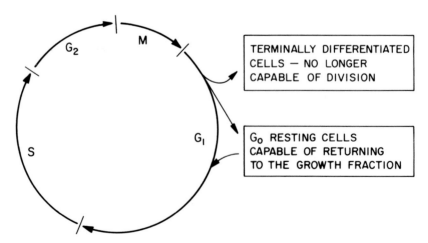

Figure 6.1.   The Cell Cycle. The cycle consists of four stages, G_1, S, G_2 and M. Cell division occurs during the M phase. In the S phase, synthesis of DNA occurs. Daughter cells may undergo differentiation and no longer be capable of division, or they may enter G_0. Cells in G_0 are mitotically inactive but may be recalled to the growth fraction under appropriate conditions.

course, proliferating cells also must synthesize all their other components in order to avoid a progressive reduction in size during mitotic division.

It also is important to realize that the rate of proliferation of cells is not the only determinant of the rate of tissue growth. The latter is a function of three factors: the rate of cell proliferation, the fraction of cells in the mitotic pool (the growth fraction), and the rate of cell loss. Under normal circumstances there are constraints placed on the proliferation of somatic cells, the mechanisms of which are incompletely understood.

In growth, as in all biological phenomena, there is variation between normal individuals. However, when outside the normal range, these variations may be regarded as pathologic and may result in functional abnormalities that we recognize as illness. Disturbances of growth may result in an excess or a deficit of tissue, or may produce an abnormal pattern of development.

DEVELOPMENTAL ANOMALIES

Malformations may occur during the growth and development of a tissue or organ and are present at birth as congenital lesions. Although they may be due to genetic defects, it is important to realize that such abnormalities also may be caused by toxins (including drugs used for therapeutic purposes), infections, and other factors. Therefore, isolated cases of developmental anomalies cannot be assumed to be inherited. The types of defects which occur are too numerous to list here, but their effect on the animal varies from negligible to lethal. Common examples are interventricular septal defects in the heart, palatoschisis, polydactyly, coloboma, renal cysts, renal hypoplasia, and ectopic location of tissue such as thyroid or pancreas.

Certain types of developmental abnormalities can be conceptualized more easily as abnormalities of growth. These include agenesis, aplasia, and hypoplasia.

Agenesis of an organ or tissue indicates a complete failure of that tissue to develop. **Aplasia** indicates a failure to grow and therefore implies the presence of a rudimentary organ. The clinical consequences of such lesions clearly depend on the organ or tissue involved. For example, aplasia of one kidney would be expected to be clinically inapparent, whereas bilateral aplasia of the kidneys would be lethal. The term aplasia also is used to refer to the failure of a tissue to renew itself, one example being the term aplastic anemia.

Hypoplasia refers to the failure of an organ to reach normal size. It is, therefore, a developmental defect occupying the spectrum between aplasia and normal development. Examples that are seen regularly are renal hypoplasia (Fig. 6.2) and testicular hypoplasia. Hypoplasia of an organ may cause clinical disease. Its severity and the life expectancy of the animal depend on the organ affected and the degree to which function is reduced.

ACQUIRED LESIONS

The lesions discussed below may be regarded as adaptive responses of cells to changes in the demands made upon them.

Atrophy and Hypertrophy

These have been discussed in Chapter 2, and are mentioned again here simply as a reminder that they are processes that can result in alterations in tissue mass or organ size.

Hyperplasia

Hyperplasia is defined as an increase in organ size or tissue mass due to an increase in the number of constituent cells. Thus, hyperplasia can occur only in those cells capable of mitotic division. It often occurs concurrently with hypertrophy and usually is classified as either physiologic or pathologic.

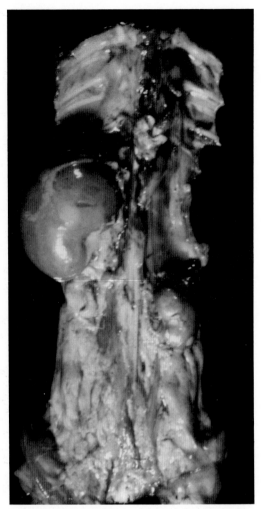

Figure 6.2. Unilateral Renal Hypoplasia. In this 2-week-old goat the left kidney was much smaller than normal. This was a congenital but not necessarily an inherited lesion. As the right kidney was normal, no signs of renal failure were present in this animal.

Physiologic hyperplasia occurs either in response to an increased level of a normal stimulus, such as a hormone, or as a regenerative or compensatory response. For example, the mammary gland undergoes hyperplasia in response to increased hormonal stimulation during pregnancy and lactation, and the adrenal cortex undergoes hyperplasia in response to increased ACTH levels. The kidney undergoing enlargement as a result of loss of the contralateral organ undergoes hyperplasia, as well as cellular hypertrophy, as a compensatory response. The liver in which there has been appreciable loss of hepatocytes undergoes regenerative hyperplasia.

Pathologic hyperplasia is said to occur when the response is excessive or abnormal in some other way, such as the arrangement of the cells. It is usually associated with excessive stimulation or chronic irritation. It should be understood that there is no well-defined cutoff between physiologic and pathologic hyperplasia. A response that at one level is regarded as physiologic may be considered pathologic when it exceeds some rather arbitrarily selected limit. Examples of pathologic hyperplasia include those due to excessive hormonal stimuli such as endometrial hyperplasia associated with prolonged progesterone secretion (Fig. 6.3) and hyperplastic goiter due to prolonged stimulation of the thyroid gland in iodine deficiency. Examples of hyperplasia due to chronic irritation usually are associated with inflammation, such as chronic otitis externa, in which there is hyperplasia of the ceruminous glands, or chronic bronchitis in which the bronchial epithelium becomes hyperplastic (Fig. 6.4A). Irritation of the biliary epithelium, in the rabbit, by *Eimeria steidiae* causes profound epithelial hyperplasia (Fig. 6.4B).

In general, hyperplasia is a relatively orderly process, but an exception is **nodular hyperplasia.** This lesion occurs commonly in the liver and pancreas of dogs and consists of variably sized nodules of well-differentiated parenchymal cells within the tissue. It is difficult to differentiate from benign neoplasia. This raises a critical point in the definition of hyperplasia and its differentiation from neoplasia. Hyperplasia, by definition, remains responsive to control, and, in the absence of the causative stimulus, will

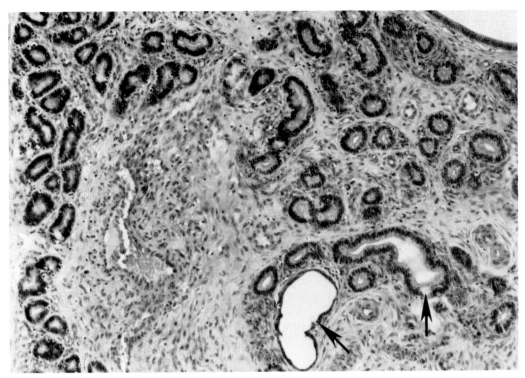

Figure 6.3.   Endometrial Hyperplasia. In the dog, hyperplasia of the endometrium occurs during the estrus cycle in response to stimulation by progesterone. Continued stimulation may lead to cystic dilatation of the endometrial glands *(arrows)* and, eventually, to infection and inflammation of the uterus.

not progress. Unfortunately, the stimuli for hyperplastic lesions, in particular nodular hyperplasia, are not always known, making it impossible sometimes to definitively distinguish benign neoplastic nodules from hyperplastic nodules.

Metaplasia

Metaplasia is an adaptive response in which one type of mature differentiated cell is replaced by a different type. Although metaplasia of epithelial to mesenchymal tissue and *vice versa* can possibly occur, in natural disease settings the two tissue types usually are related. Metaplasia can occur in either epithelial or mesenchymal tissue, and in epithelia is usually a response to chronic irritation, including inflammation. Commonly a highly specialized epithelial tissue is re-placed by less-specialized, but more resistant, stratified squamous epithelium. For example, the respiratory epithelium lining the trachea, bronchi, and bronchioles may be replaced by stratified squamous epithelium (Fig. 6.5). Clearly, such a change has some undesirable consequences; in this example these include loss of mucous secretion, loss of cilia, and consequently loss of clearance mechanisms from the airways. In metaplasia of mesenchymal tissue, fibrous tissue may be replaced by bone or cartilage (Fig. 6.6). In these cases, the change is less easily regarded as an adaptive response, and the cause is usually unknown.

In most cases metaplasia does not occur as the result of alterations in existing mature cells. Rather it depends on proliferation of germinal, or stem, cells whose

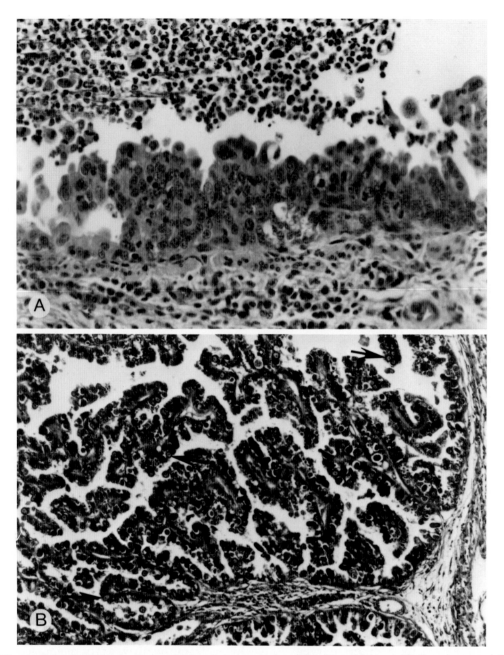

Figure 6.4. Pathologic Hyperplasia. *A,* hyperplasia of the bronchiolar epithelium is associated with bronchiolitis caused by bovine PI3 virus infection. Instead of the normal columnar epithelial cells, the bronchiole is lined by multiple layers of epithelial cells. The cells are immature and lack specialized structures such as cilia. This lesion would be expected to result in abnormal clearance of material from the airways. Inflammatory cells are present in the lumen of the bronchiole *(top). B,* hyperplasia of the biliary epithelium in hepatic coccidiosis in a rabbit. There has been remarkable proliferation of biliary epithelium, producing folded, papillary ingrowths into the lumen. The causative organism, *Eimeria stiedae,* is visible *(arrows)* in many of the cells.

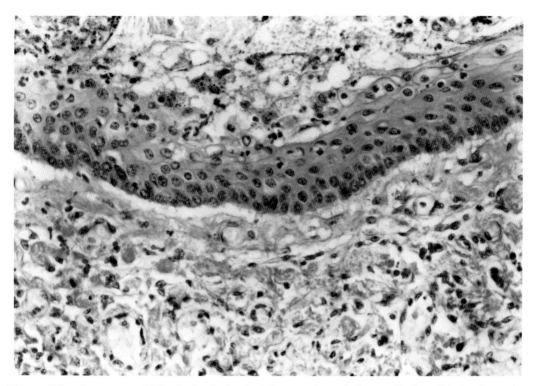

Figure 6.5. Squamous Metaplasia. Instead of the usual respiratory epithelium this trachea of a cow is lined by typical stratified squamous epithelium. This epithelium lacks specialized ciliated cells and goblet cells. As a result, there would be impairment of clearance of material from the trachea. This lesion resulted from chronic tracheitis, and the inflammatory cells and debris are present in the lumen.

progeny undergo modified differentiation. Less commonly, existing differentiated cells appear to be able to undergo direct metaplastic transformation. For example, epithelial cells lining injured renal tubules may become flattened, presumably to maintain a continuous epithelial lining. In such cases, however, it may be difficult to distinguish adaptive changes occurring in existing differentiated cells from similar changes occurring in proliferating cells.

Stable metaplastic conversion of epithelia, for example from pancreatic exocrine cells to hepatocytes, has been reported after treatment with low doses of carcinogens. However, in most naturally occurring disease settings epithelial metaplasia is reversible, the normal tissue being restored if the stimulus is removed. Metaplastic change often is associated with hyperplasia and is usually orderly. Loss of orderly arrangement leads to dysplasia.

Dysplasia

Dysplasia literally means "abnormal growth" and sometimes is used in that sense in terms such as chondrodysplasia. Commonly, however, it is used in a more restricted sense to describe a **proliferative** response accompanied by loss of regular differentiation and by cellular atypia and disorderliness. It may be thought of as disorderly or atypical hyperplasia. These changes most frequently are observed in epithelia subjected to chronic irritation or inflammation. Cellular atypia is charac-

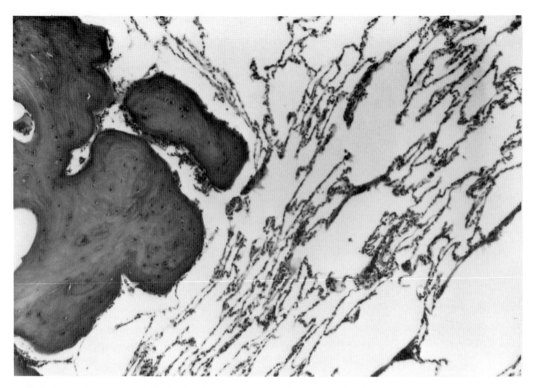

Figure 6.6. Osseous Metaplasia. A focus of bone is present in the interstitial tissue of this lung. This lesion is common in dogs and is of no functional consequence. Its cause is unknown.

terized by **pleomorphism** (variation in size and shape) and **hyperchromicity** (increased staining). There is a loss of the normal regular progression from germinal to fully differentiated cells, and mitoses are found in abnormal positions. These changes are illustrated in Fig. 6.7. By definition, dysplasia is nonneoplastic and therefore is **reversible** if the cause is removed. However, based on statistical evidence, it is known that many of these lesions, if left alone, will progress to become neoplasms. They are therefore often regarded as "preneoplastic." Morphologically there may be no way to distinguish a severely dysplastic lesion from a neoplastic one. Sometimes highly dysplastic lesions are called carcinoma *in situ* as described below.

Dysplastic lesions occur commonly in the prepuce of horses due to irritation by smegma. It also is known that there is a significant risk of squamous cell carcinoma developing at this site, illustrating the relationship between the development of dysplastic and later neoplastic lesions. To the clinician then, the importance of dysplastic lesions is the increased risk of an invasive carcinoma developing at the site of the lesion.

NEOPLASIA

Neoplasia literally means "new growth," but a more strict definition is needed to properly define the process. The proper definition of neoplasia has been traditionally controversial, but one of the better attempts is that of Willis: "A neoplasm is an abnormal mass of tissue, the growth of which exceeds and is uncoordinated with that of the normal tissues, and persists in the same excessive manner after cessation of the stimulus which evoked the change." The key features of neopla-

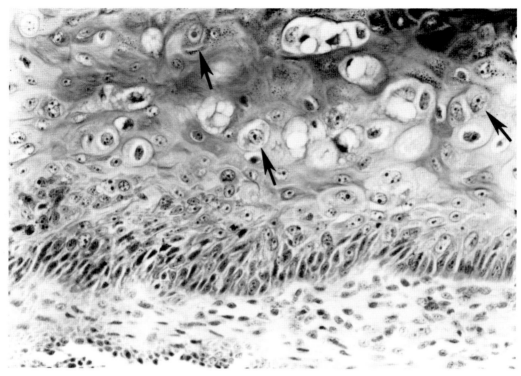

Figure 6.7.   Dysplasia of Epithelium. In this severely dysplastic lesion from the lip of a dog there are large, poorly differentiated cells in the spiny layer of the epidermis *(arrows)*.

sia which distinguish it from other forms of cell proliferation therefore are:

1. Excessive tissue growth;
2. Lack of responsiveness to control mechanisms;
3. Lack of dependence on the continued presence of the stimulus.

Nomenclature

There are several commonly used synonyms for neoplasia. The term **tumor,** strictly speaking, means a tissue swelling or mass, but by common usage it has come to mean neoplasm. **Cancer** is a term commonly used to mean malignant neoplasm.

Neoplasms are named according to the features of differentiation which can be recognized on histologic examination and which reflect the tissue of origin. Nomenclature and classification are important as they form the basis of the language by which pathologists and clinicians communicate the nature and significance of the lesion to one another. Because many forms of treatment are specific to a particular type or even subtype of neoplasm, it is imperative that the pathologist be able to convey to the clinician the nature of the neoplastic lesion involved.

As should become clear from the following discussion, the classification of neoplasms is traditionally based on their **histogenesis,** that is their putative cell or tissue of origin, and the degree to which they **differentiate** to come to resemble that origin. This tradition continues to serve us well, but as more and more tools become available to help in classifying neoplasms, it becomes apparent that there are difficulties with it. The major problem is that oncogenesis does not always mimic embryogenesis, and neoplastic cells may not closely resemble their parentage either morphologically or functionally. For example, neoplasms derived from neuroepithelial cells may come to resemble squamous or glandular epithelium, and cells that normally secrete only one hormone, or those that normally do not secrete one at all, may secrete several once they undergo neoplastic transformation. These occurrences lead to a changing world of classification, but from the clinical point of view, particularly, the most important thing is that classification be based on consistent criteria and, whenever possible, correlated with clinical behavior.

Broadly, neoplasms are classified as being of either **mesenchymal** or **epithelial** origin. Most are of one neoplastic cell type and fit into one or the other of these two groups. A few types of neoplasms contain more than one neoplastic cell type. When these are apparently derived from the one embryonic germ layer, they are called **mixed neoplasms.** A common example is the mixed mammary tumor of dogs in which proliferating epithelial tissue is intermixed with mesenchymal components, myoepithelium, bone, and cartilage (Fig. 6.8). **Teratomas** are neoplasms containing tissue derived from more than one germ cell layer. They occur most commonly in the testes or ovaries and apparently are derived from primitive pluripotential stem cells. Teratomas may contain any number of tissues of any type including bone, skin, nervous tissue, intestinal epithelium, muscle, hair, and others (Fig. 6.9).

The behavior of neoplasms is described by the terms **benign,** for those that are relatively inoffensive, and **malignant** for those that are aggressive and potentially life threatening. These terms are explained in some detail below. Benign mesenchymal neoplasms are named by add-

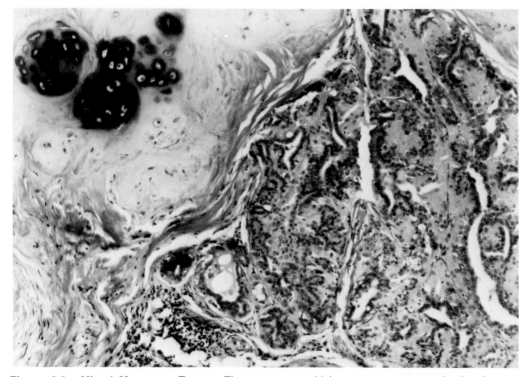

Figure 6.8. Mixed Mammary Tumor. These tumors, which are very common in the dog, are characterized by an intimate mixture of glandular epithelium and mesenchymal tissue, such as the cartilage shown here.

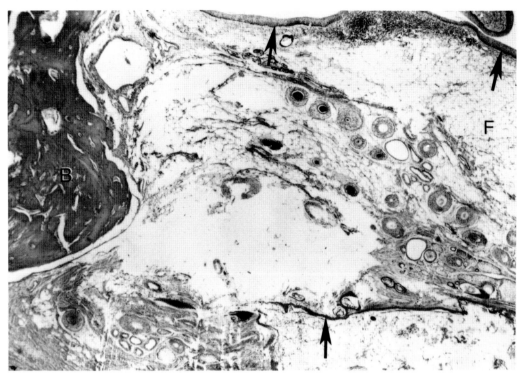

Figure 6.9.   Teratoma. This neoplasm, from the ovary of a dog, is characterized by the presence of well-differentiated tissues derived from more than one germ layer. In this case bone *(B),* fat *(F),* stratified squamous epithelium *(arrows),* hair follicles, sebaceous glands, and sweat glands are present.

ing the suffix "oma" to a prefix indicating the tissue or origin. For example, a benign neoplasm of fibroblasts is called a **fibroma** and a benign neoplasm of endothelial cells a **hemangioma.** Benign neoplasms of epithelial origin are called **adenomas.** This term refers to both those with a solid lobular pattern of growth and those with recognizable tubules, ducts, or acini. Because the term adenoma is relatively nonspecific, the tissue of origin is usually indicated, such as adenoma of sweat gland, adenoma of thyroid gland, or adenoma of adrenal cortex. Also, many modifying descriptive terms are applied to the names of neoplasms of epithelial origin. For example, **cystadenoma** describes an adenoma in which the glandular spaces are cystic, **papillary adenoma** is one in which branching, finger-like processes of neoplastic tissue extend into the lumen, **ductular** adenoma is one derived from ducts, and so on. Papillary neoplastic masses growing at a surface are known as **polyps** or **papillomas,** papillomas on the skin being known, in lay terms, as warts.

Malignant neoplasms of mesenchymal origin are called **sarcomas.** As in their benign equivalents, a prefix is used to indicate the tissue of origin. For example, a malignant neoplasm of fibroblasts is called a **fibrosarcoma,** the malignant counterpart of a fibroma. A malignant neoplasm of endothelial cells is a **hemangiosarcoma.** Malignant neoplasms of epithelial cells are called **carcinomas.** In this case, only those that form recognizable ducts, tubules, or acini are called **adenocarcinomas.** Those that form a

Table 6.1
Classification of Some Neoplasms[a]

Tissue of Origin	Benign	Malignant
Mesenchymal		
Fibrous tissue	Fibroma	Fibrosarcoma
	Myxoma	Myxosarcoma
Bone	Osteoma	Osteosarcoma
Cartilage	Chondroma	Chondrosarcoma
Adipose tissue	Lipoma	Liposarcoma
Endothelium of blood vessels	Hemangioma	Hemangiosarcoma
Endothelium of lymphatics	Lymphangioma	Lymphangiosarcoma
Skeletal muscle	Rhabdomyoma	Rhabdomyosarcoma
Smooth muscle	Leiomyoma	Leiomyosarcoma
Mast cells	Mast cell tumor	Malignant mast cell tumor
Synovium	Synovioma	Synovial sarcoma
Meninges	Meningioma	Malignant meningioma
Mesothelium	Mesothelioma	Malignant mesothelioma
Hematopoietic tissue		
Lymphocytes		Lymphosarcoma, lymphoma, lymphocytic leukemia
Plasma cells		Myeloma (multiple myeloma)
Granulocytes		Granulocytic leukemia
Monocytes		Monocytic leukemia
Erythroid cells		Erythroid leukemia
Epithelial		
Stratified squamous epithelium	Papilloma	Squamous cell carcinoma
	Basal cell tumor	
Glandular epithelium	Adenoma	Adenocarcinoma, carcinoma
Bronchial epithelium		Bronchogenic carcinoma, bronchoalveolar carcinoma
Liver	Hepatoma	Hepatoma, hepatocellular carcinoma
Urinary tract, transitional epithelium	Polyp, papilloma	Transitional cell carcinoma
Spermatogenic epithelium	Seminoma	Malignant seminoma
Endocrine epithelium	Adenoma	Carcinoma
Neuroendocrine Tissue		
Adrenal medulla	Pheochromocytoma	Malignant pheochromocytoma
Carotid body and aortic body	Paraganglioma	Malignant paraganglioma
Kulchitsky cells	Carcinoid	Malignant carcinoid
Islet cells of the pancreas	Insuloma, adenoma of β cells, etc.	Malignant insuloma, carcinoma of β cells, etc.
Neuroectoderm		
Melanocytes	Melanoma	Malignant melanoma

[a] This list is not exhaustive but indicates most of the common neoplasms as well as showing that, despite attempts to name neoplasms logically, many exceptions remain.

solid pattern are called simply carcinomas. Those forming stratified squamous epithelium are called **squamous cell carcinomas.** Again, if the tissue of origin can be recognized it is included in the name, for example, adenocarcinoma of sweat gland, adenocarcinoma of thyroid gland, or carcinoma of adrenal cortex. Some neoplasms, of course, fail to mimic their tissue of origin sufficiently for it to be recognized. In such a case, the neoplasm is said to be a **poorly differentiated** sarcoma or carcinoma, as the case may be. Table 6.1 lists commonly encountered neoplasms, their tissue of origin, and how benign and malignant lesions are named.

Despite these rules and regulations for classifying and naming neoplasms, inconsistencies persist. For example, melanoma is used to describe tumors arising from melanocytes but does not indicate the malignancy of these neoplasms. Pathologists often use the term "malignant melanoma" to overcome this problem.

The term "carcinoma *in situ*" is also something of an oddity. As explained earlier, it is sometimes very difficult to differentiate between epithelial dysplasia and frankly neoplastic lesions. When the features of disorderliness and cellular atypia become marked enough to conclude that the lesion is in fact neoplastic, but when there is no invasion of the adjacent tissue and the changes are confined to the epithelial layer, the term carcinoma *in situ*

often is applied. The term, of course, implies neoplasia and malignancy, but it should be emphasized again that there is no way to be certain that such a lesion is neoplastic. Studies of large numbers of cases do, however, support the conclusion that many such lesions are, in fact, incipient carcinomas. It is the individual case in which it is difficult to be sure.

Morphologic and Behavioral Features of Benign and Malignant Neoplasms

It is obviously important to distinguish benign from malignant neoplasms. Generally the pathologist and the clinician are attempting to predict the behavior of a particular neoplasm, and the classification as either benign or malignant is one way to express this (Table 6.2). It must be realized, however, that neoplasms do not always fall neatly into one category or the other. A spectrum exists between completely benign and highly malignant, and errors are bound to occur in trying to predict the future behavior of neoplasms. In addition, the features we use to judge malignancy, which are discussed below, do not always hold true. Some neoplasms, although having histologic features suggesting malignancy, characteristically behave in a benign fashion. It is, therefore, very important for the pathologist and the clinician to be aware not only of the usual clinical and histologic features of neoplasms, which suggest their likely behavior, but also of

Table 6.2
Characteristics of Benign and Malignant Neoplasms

Feature	Benign Tumors	Malignant Tumors
Differentiation	Well differentiated; resemble tissue of origin	Often poorly differentiated
Invasiveness	Noninvasive, circumscribed	Invade surrounding tissues and sometimes vessels
Rate of growth	Slow	Often rapid
Mitotic index	Usually low	Often high
Metastasis	Never	Sometimes

the characteristic behavior of particular types of neoplasms in each species. As an example, in the dog, basal cell tumors of the skin may show histologic features, such as a high mitotic index, which usually are suggestive of malignancy. Despite this, these neoplasms are known to be almost invariably benign. Species differences can be illustrated by contrasting mammary neoplasms in dogs and cats. In dogs, mammary tumors vary greatly in behavior, and, although malignant tumors certainly occur, most are relatively benign. In the cat, this is certainly not the case. Most feline mammary tumors are carcinomas, and they metastasize readily. This knowledge therefore suggests a very cautious prognosis to the clinician as soon as a mammary tumor is recognized in a cat. In assessing the likely behavior of a neoplasm, that is in assessing malignancy, several features are considered.

Differentiation

The differentiation of neoplastic cells refers to the degree to which they resemble, morphologically and functionally, the tissue from which they originate. Again, there is great variability in the degree of differentiation. **Benign tumors** usually are well differentiated and resemble the tissue from which they arose both cytologically and architecturally. Nuclear and cytoplasmic morphology is similar to that in the precursor tissue and usually mitotic figures are very rare (Fig. 6.10).

Malignant tumors, on the other hand, vary greatly in the degree to which they differentiate, but generally they exhibit some degree of **anaplasia.** Anaplasia means "failure to differentiate" or "loss of differentiation," and is one of the most important morphologic features of malignancy. Anaplasia should not be thought of as dedifferentiation, which would imply that cells already differentiated revert to a more primitive form. It is not generally accepted that this can occur. Anaplastic cells usually exhibit **pleomorphism.** Nuclear characteristics often are the most informative in the diagnosis of malignant neoplasms. The nuclei of such neoplasms are often large, hyperchromatic or vesicular, have an abnormal shape, and may contain one or more prominent nucleoli (Fig. 6.11). The nuclear to cytoplasmic ratio usually is abnormal. In addition to these cytologic features, the cells in malignant neoplasms often do not grow in well-differentiated architectural patterns. For example, the neoplastic cells of an adenocarcinoma of thyroid gland may form solid lobules, with only occasional acinar structures or none at all. This failure to differentiate may make it difficult or impossible to classify a neoplasm, but often a careful search will reveal the evidence of an attempt to mimic the tissue from which the neoplasm is derived, thus allowing definitive diagnosis (Fig. 6.11). Sometimes it is necessary to resort to special techniques to demonstrate the differentiation that allows classification of a neoplasm, light microscopy being only one tool by which the nature of neoplastic cells can be identified. More and more, sophisticated techniques such as electron microscopy, immunohistochemistry, biochemical analysis, and identification of specific receptors are being used to detect evidence of specific features of differentiation not discernable with the light microscope. Immunohistochemical techniques are now widely used in the study and diagnosis of neoplasms. A particular example is the use of antibodies against different types of **intermediate filaments** to identify poorly differentiated neoplasms. Carcinomas are expected to express cytokeratins, most sarcomas express vimentin, and tumors of muscle origin, whether smooth muscle or skeletal muscle, should express desmin. In the central nervous system, the expression of glial fibrillary acidic protein can be used to identify neoplastic astrocytes from other cell types. The following is illustrative of the usefulness of electron microscopy to identify the cell of origin in one case of neoplasia.

Case 6.1: Histogenetic Origin

Mickey, a 10-year-old, male, mixed-breed dog, was presented because of a steadily enlarging mass on the third digit of the right front foot. The lesion had first been noticed by the owners about 1 month previously, but, because it was not unduly worrying the dog, no immediate attention had been sought. On clinical examination the dog was normal in all respects except for the mass, which was about 1.5 cm in diameter, covered with ulcerated haired skin, and firm to palpation. No discomfort was apparently associated with its presence. The clinician advised the owners to have the mass removed and submitted for histologic examination.

The mass was submitted in neutral buffered formalin. Its cut surface was firm and white, but no clear demarcation between the mass and surrounding normal tissue could be seen. Histologically (Fig. 6.12), the cells making up the mass were very pleomorphic. They had large, or very large, vesicular nuclei that varied from round to elongate in shape and contained very prominent nucleoli. There was a high mitotic index, one to six mitoses being counted in each high-power field. The cytoplasm was faintly basophilic and moderate in amount. The cells were arranged in cords and clusters, separated by strands of fibrous tissue. In some areas elongate cells were arranged in parallel arrays. Similar cells were present in the basal layer of the epidermis and extended deep into the dermis.

No definitive evidence of differentiation was found, and, based on the arrangement of the cells, a diagnosis of **anaplastic carcinoma** was made. In an attempt to obtain a definitive diagnosis, small pieces of tissue were processed for electron microscopy.

Ultrastructurally (Fig. 6.13), the neoplastic cells were tightly packed, with closely apposed plasma membranes that sometimes displayed specialized intercellular junctions. The nuclei contained abundant eu-

chromatin, with less heterochromatin, and prominent nucleoli. The cytoplasm contained mitochondria, a moderate amount of rough endoplasmic reticulum (RER), and abundant free polysomes. In addition there were relatively rare, electron-dense organelles that, at high magnification, had an appearance consistent with that of melanosomes. Based on this evidence the diagnosis was amended to malignant melanoma.

Comments on Case 6.1. In this particular case, the neoplasm exhibited many features, at the light-microscopic level, indicative of malignancy. The cells were anaplastic, pleomorphic, had vesicular nuclei with prominent nucleoli, and there was a high mitotic index. In addition there was evidence of tissue invasion. Two types of neoplasm would be likely to occur at this site. One is squamous cell carcinoma, and the other is melanoma. Together these tumors make up most of the malignant tumors occurring on the toe of the dog. In this case it was considered to be important to determine which tumor, if either, this represented, as the prognosis would differ in each case. Squamous cell carcinomas at this site are very locally invasive but metastasize less rapidly than malignant melanomas. Melanomas, in dogs, vary in malignancy, depending, for one thing, on their site of occurrence. When on the toe, they are often extremely malignant and metastasize widely and rapidly. Following the diagnosis of malignant melanoma, therefore, a poor prognosis was offered. Two months later the dog was subjected to euthanasia because of general malaise thought to be related to the neoplasm. At postmortem examination, multiple metastases were found in the local lymph nodes and in the lung.

This case demonstrates several principles. The neoplasm had histologic features on which a diagnosis of malignancy could be based. Although no evidence of differentiation was present at the light-microscopic level, the application of a special technique was able to show definitive features of differentiation characteristic of melanocytes. In addition, the case illustrates that a knowledge of the usual behavior of specific neoplasms in particular species is valuable in formulating a prognosis, over and above

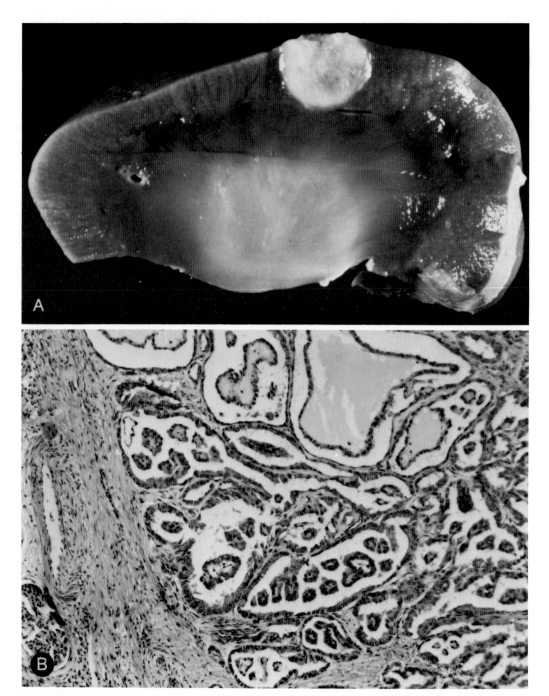

Figure 6.10 *A* and *B*.   Features of Benign Neoplasms. *A,* adenoma of renal tubular epithelium in the kidney of a horse. The neoplasm is discrete and has sharply defined borders. *B,* histologically, the neoplasm is made up of uniform, well-differentiated cells arranged in a papillary pattern.

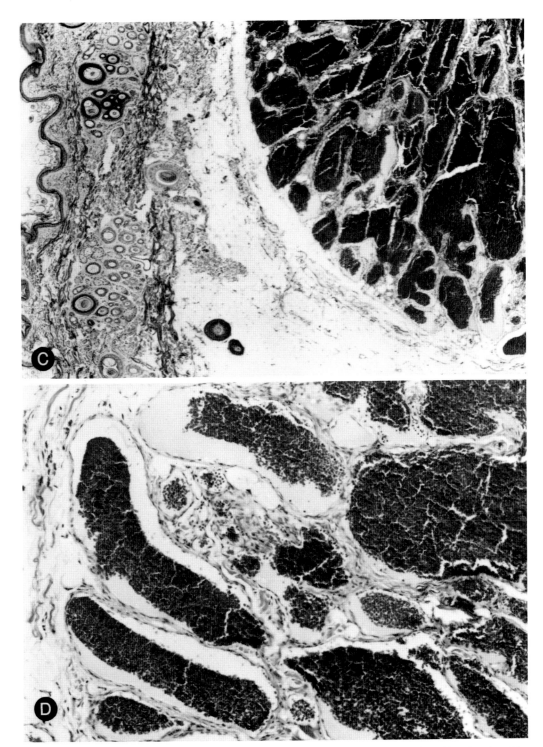

Figure 6.10 *C* and *D*.   Features of Benign Neoplasms. *C*, hemangioma in the skin of a dog. The neoplasm is discrete and has sharply demarcated borders. It forms large blood-filled spaces lined by neoplastic endothelium. *D*, the neoplastic cells are well differentiated and closely resemble normal endothelial cells. They are supported on a fibrous stroma.

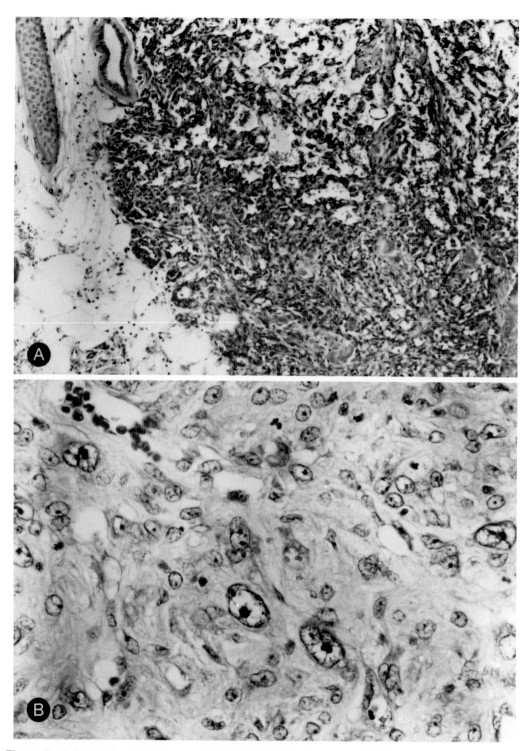

Figure 6.11 *A* and *B*. Features of Malignant Neoplasms. *A,* hemangiosarcoma in the skin of a dog. The neoplasm is relatively poorly differentiated but in some areas it forms recognizable blood-filled spaces. In others it forms solid cellular masses. It is poorly demarcated from the surrounding normal tissue. Contrast this lesion with its benign equivalent, the hemangioma shown in the preceding figure. *B,* anaplastic sarcoma. This neoplasm is very poorly differentiated, its tissue of origin not being recognizable. There is marked nuclear pleomorphism, and many of the nuclei are vesicular and contain prominent nucleoli.

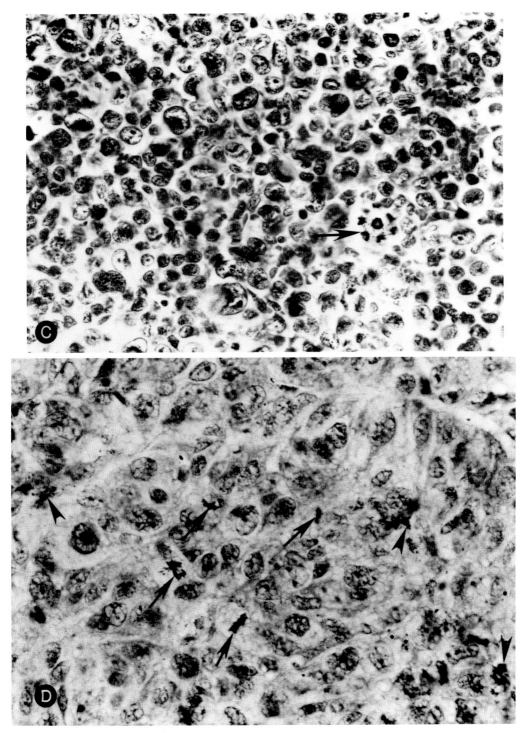

Figure 6.11 *C* and *D*.   Features of Malignant Neoplasms. *C,* anaplastic carcinoma of the lung of a dog. There is nuclear pleomorphism and the neoplastic cells are anaplastic. A bizarre, abnormal mitotic figure is present *(arrow)*. *D,* malignant melanoma from the skin of a horse. There are many mitotic figures *(arrows)*. Although this neoplasm is poorly differentiated, a number of cells contain melanin granules *(arrow heads)* allowing it to be classified as a melanoma.

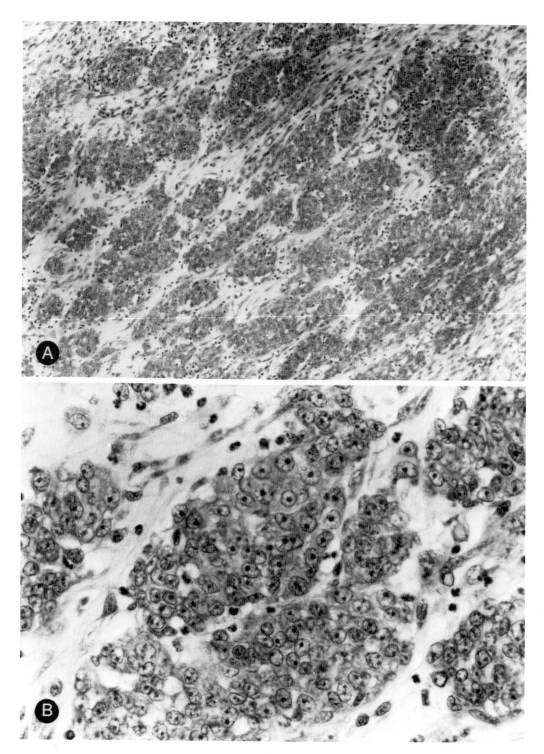

Figure 6.12.   Malignant Melanoma, Case 6.1. *A,* the neoplasm is composed of lobules and clumps of closely apposed tumor cells separated by a cellular fibrous stroma. *B,* at higher magnification, the cells have large vesicular nuclei and one, or a few, prominent nucleoli. Occasional neutrophils are present in the stroma.

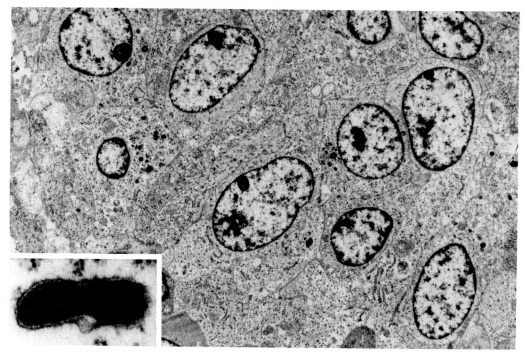

Figure 6.13.   Malignant Melanoma, Case 6.1. Neoplastic cells are closely apposed and form interwoven cytoplasmic processes. The cytoplasm contains a variety of organelles including electron-dense structures, which, at high magnification, can be seen to have features consistent with premelanosomes *(inset)*. (Micrograph courtesy of Dr. R. M. Minor and Louise Barr.)

that suggested by the histologic features and observed clinical behavior.

Malignant neoplasms often contain many cells in mitosis, and the mitotic figures may be abnormal (Fig. 6.11). Also, malignant neoplasms may be highly cellular. This is an important feature in classifying mesenchymal neoplasms in which the high cellular density may partly reflect the failure of the neoplastic cells to differentiate and produce extracelluar matrix.

The cytologic features of anaplasia can be recognized not only in histologic preparations, but also in touch preparations from tumor masses, smears of effusions, or aspirates from neoplasms (Fig. 6.14). This technique sometimes can provide a rapid diagnosis and assure prompt treatment.

Functional Differentiation

Well-differentiated neoplasms may retain the functional characteristics of the parent tissue. Logically enough, functional capacity is retained best in highly differentiated, benign neoplasms. Thus glandular adenomas may secrete mucus, and endocrine adenomas may secrete hormones. Malignant neoplasms may retain some functional capacity, and 'in some cases these functions may be very deleterious to the host, as discussed below. Functional activity is, in fact, the basis on which the origin of many neoplasms may be recognized. For instance, melanomas produce melanin, osteosarcomas produce osteoid, and adenocarcinomas of the thyroid gland produce colloid.

The Stroma of Neoplasms

The stroma (the supporting connective tissue) of neoplasms is important to the

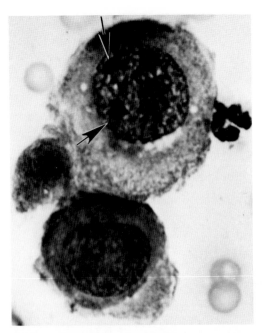

Figure 6.14. Cytology of Malignant Neoplasms. In this imprint from a malignant squamous cell carcinoma from the skin of a dog, the neoplastic cells are large, hyperchromatic, and have nuclei that contain prominent nucleoli *(arrows).*

survival of tumor cells, as it carries their blood supply. Benign tumors usually are well vascularized. Some malignant neoplasms, however, are poorly vascularized and, as a result, may contain areas of necrosis due to ischemia (Fig. 6.15).

Epithelial neoplasms usually have a connective tissue stroma of variable density. It is non-neoplastic but grows with and supports the neoplastic cells. Some carcinomas induce relatively abundant stromal proliferation, such neoplasms often being referred to as **scirrhous carcinomas.** This stromal induction appears to be a property of the neoplastic cells and is characteristic of certain neoplasms, such as carcinomas of the stomach or intestine. The presence of abundant stroma makes neoplasms firm to palpation.

Growth of Neoplasms

In general, benign tumors grow slowly, and malignant tumors grow rapidly. At first glance it would seem logical that the growth rate of neoplasms is exponential and a function of the length of the mitotic cycle. This is not generally true. The actual growth rate of a neoplasm, like that of a normal tissue, is determined by the length of the mitotic cycle, the growth fraction (or proportion of cells in mitosis), and the rate of loss of cells from the neoplasm.

The concept that neoplastic cells divide at a more rapid rate than normal tissue is, generally speaking, not true. In fact, the length of the mitotic cycle in some normal tissues, such as jejunal epithelial cells, is shorter than that of the fastest-growing neoplasms. Frequently the cell cycle time for neoplastic cells is longer than that of the normal germinal cells from which they are derived. Human bone marrow precursor cells, for instance, have a cell cycle time of about 18 h, while the neoplastic cells of acute myeloblastic leukemia have a cell cycle of about 80 h. In the case of chronic myelogenous leukemia, the cell cycle time has been measured at about 120 h. The length of the mitotic cycle, then, is relatively unimportant in determining the rate of growth of neoplasms. Of more importance is the growth fraction, which can vary widely. The factors determining the proportion of cells in mitosis are not well defined, but the most important may be the degree of differentiation of the neoplasm. In many cells, full differentiation precludes further mitotic division. Therefore, well-differentiated neoplasms contain a high proportion of cells unable to divide and so grow slowly. Conversely, poorly differentiated neoplasms often contain a high proportion of cells in the growth fraction and usually grow rapidly. The immune response, which will be discussed in more detail later in this chapter, apparently also can influence the number of cells in the growth fraction. At least, in some experimental systems, interference with the immune response allows an increased number of undifferentiated neoplastic cells

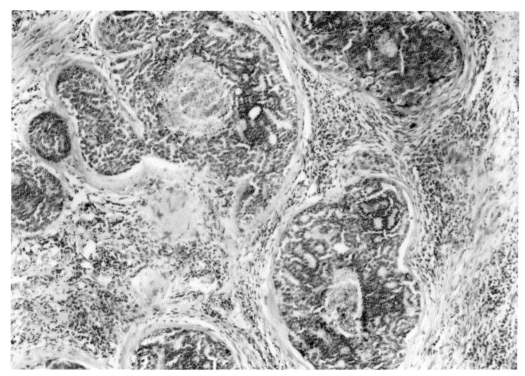

Figure 6.15.   Necrosis in a Malignant Neoplasm. In this carcinoma from the mammary gland of a dog central areas of necrosis are present in the larger lobules of neoplastic tissue.

to become mitotically active. Even the growth fraction, however, is not the only important factor in determining the rate of growth of neoplasms. The mitotic index, or proportion of cells in mitosis at any one time, is also an undependable measure of growth rate. Mitoses may take two or three times as long in some neoplasms as in normal tissues, producing a high mitotic index without a commensurate increase in cell growth rate.

The extent to which cells are lost from neoplasms, by necrosis or exfoliation, is the most important factor determining their overall rate of growth. In neoplasms the rate of cell loss by necrosis may be very high, approaching 100% of those produced in some cases. Although this may seem unlikely at first glance, it can be put in perspective by comparison with tissues that are normally continually replaced, where the rate of cell loss *is* 100% of those produced. Any rate of loss below 100% therefore represents actual growth.

Necrosis of tumor cells may be due to differentiation and cell aging, chromosomal and biochemical abnormalities, ischemia, inadequate nutrition, or immunologic attack. Ischemia is one of the most important causes of tumor cell necrosis. Cells further than about 100–150 μm from a small blood vessel will undergo necrosis. In addition, although the cell cycle length is not influenced by relative ischemia, the proportion of cells in the growth fraction is. Neoplastic tissue near a zone of ischemia therefore will have fewer cells in mitosis than that in a well-oxygenated area. Tumors have a variety of patterns of vascularization, including peripheral with penetrating vessels, peripheral without penetrating vessels, and central. The peripheral patterns tend to produce areas of central necrosis in growing tumors, whereas the central pattern is more often associated with single-cell necrosis throughout the tissue. One other factor that may influence rate of tumor growth is its location. It has been shown in mice, for example, that subcutaneous tumors in anterior locations grow more rapidly than those in posterior sites. These differences are thought to be mediated through differences in vascular supply.

Spread of Tumors—Invasion and Metastasis

Benign tumors are generally noninvasive (Fig. 6.10). They are localized, clearly demarcated from the surrounding tissue, and are often, but not invariably, separated from it by a **capsule** or rim of connective tissue. The latter may be derived from compressed, preexisting stroma or may be part of the stroma of the neoplasm. Benign neoplasms usually grow by expansion.

Malignant neoplasms, in contrast, usually exhibit local **invasiveness** or **infiltration.** In other words, they extend into and may cause considerable destruction of surrounding tissue (Fig. 6.16). Some malignant neoplasms may be encapsulated, but there is usually microscopically evident invasion of the capsular stroma. Some types of neoplasms are known to be characteristically **locally invasive** yet do not usually spread far from their original site. Examples are neurofibromas and hemangiopericytomas of the skin of the dog. Clinical knowledge of this property prompts the surgeon to attempt wide excision to avoid leaving foci of neoplastic cells in the tissue. However, such tumors are difficult to remove completely and tend to recur locally, thus necessitating a cautious prognosis.

Malignant neoplasms also have the potential to **metastasize,** or spread to distant sites not directly contiguous with the primary mass. Neoplasms that metastasize are unequivocally malignant, this process being the most dangerous property of malignant neoplasms. Metastasis may occur by several mechanisms. Invasion and transportation *via* **lymphatics** is one major mechanism by which neoplastic cells spread (Fig. 6.17 and Fig. 6.19*A*), and the site of metastasis tends to be influenced by the lymphatic drainage of the primary lesion. For example, adenocarcinomas of the mammary gland tend to spread to superficial inguinal and mammary lymph nodes, and malignant neoplasms of the mouth tend to spread to the submandibular and cervical lymph nodes. Further dissemination can occur along the secondary pathways of lymphatic drainage. Metastasis *via* **blood vessels** is equally important and perhaps even more serious, as the draining lymph node that might at least provide some barrier to widespread dissemination is not available. Vascular invasion, a prelude to hematogenous spread, occurs most commonly *via* veins, venules, and capillaries, as the thick walls of arteries are more resistant to penetration. The pattern of spread again reflects, at least to some extent, the distribution of the affected vessels. Thus, intestinal tumors may gain access to the portal circulation and spread to the liver. Many blood-borne tumor emboli metastasize to the lung because it is the first major capillary bed that they encounter (Fig. 6.18). For this reason radiographic examination of the lung often is carried out when metastasis is suspected, as it might be, for example, in the case of an osteosarcoma of the long bones. The histopathologic detection of vascular and lymphatic invasion (shown in Fig. 6.19) is therefore of great prognostic significance. Vascular invasion is definitive evidence of malignancy but, although it suggests a strong potential for metastasis, it does not confirm that metastasis has occurred or even that it will occur. For example, in some neoplasms, such as canine seminoma, vascular emboli often can be detected if a careful search is made but, despite this, these neoplasms rarely establish metastatic growths in distant sites.

Neoplasms also may metastasize by exfoliation and implantation. This occurs

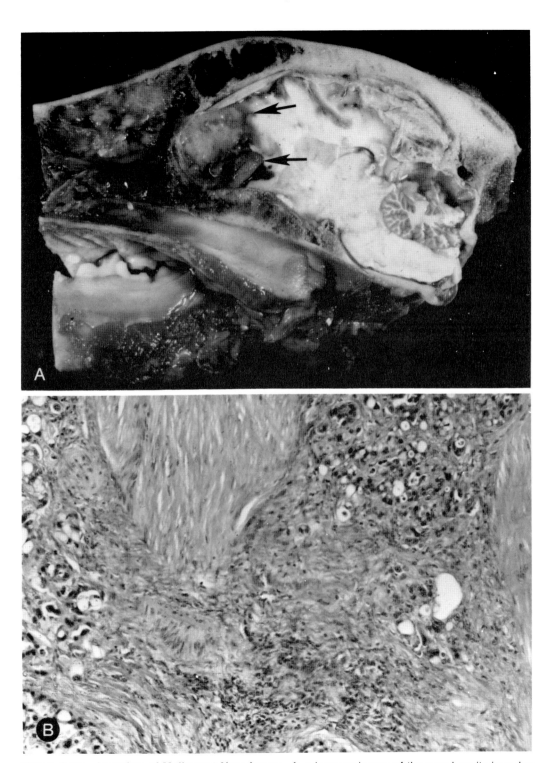

Figure 6.16. Invasion of Malignant Neoplasms. *A,* adenocarcinoma of the nasal cavity in a dog. Note that the neoplasm has invaded through the cribriform plate into the parenchyma of the brain *(arrows). B,* transitional cell carcinoma of the bladder in a dog. Groups of neoplastic cells have invaded the muscular wall of the bladder. The primary mass is at the *left.*

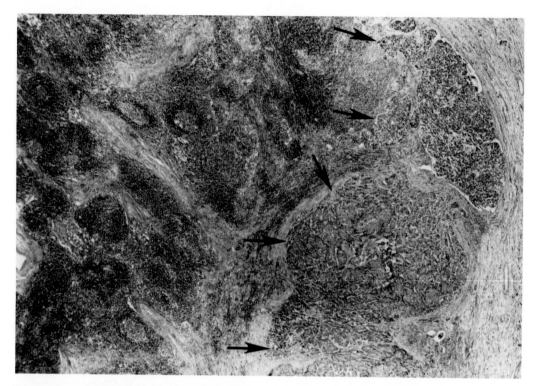

Figure 6.17. Metastasis to a Lymph Node. Neoplastic tissue with the characteristics of a carcinoma is growing in the subcapsular sinus and adjacent cortical tissue of the lymph node *(arrows)*. The primary neoplasm was a carcinoma of the mammary gland.

when neoplastic cells, usually from a carcinoma, gain access to a serosal surface and desquamate. These cells may spread throughout the body cavity, implant, and proliferate. This process commonly is encountered in cases of gastric or intestinal carcinoma (Fig. 6.20) and in canine ovarian adenocarcinomas. Direct transplantation of neoplastic cells *via* surgical instruments, gloved hands, or hypodermic needles may lead to the establishment of metastasis. For example, the use of a scalpel to first excise a tumor, then to perform a biopsy of a lymph node could lead to the growth of neoplastic tissue in the second surgical site.

Metastasis is a complex biological process that is clearly very important to understand, and it has formed the basis of intensive research. The factors that influence metastasis and the survival of tumor emboli will be discussed in more detail later in this chapter.

The criteria for malignancy discussed in this section are of obvious prognostic significance, and attempts have been made to quantitate them in order to more precisely define the prognosis. **Grading** of neoplasms represents an attempt to *quantitate* characteristics such as anaplasia and mitotic activity which form the basis of our subjective evaluation of malignancy. **Staging** of neoplasms attempts to classify them according to their progression, taking into account the size of the primary lesion, the presence of lymph node involvement, and distant metastasis. In man a number of such systems have been developed and are widely used for prognostic purposes. In animals, however, fewer such attempts have been made. One major reason for this is the difficulty of

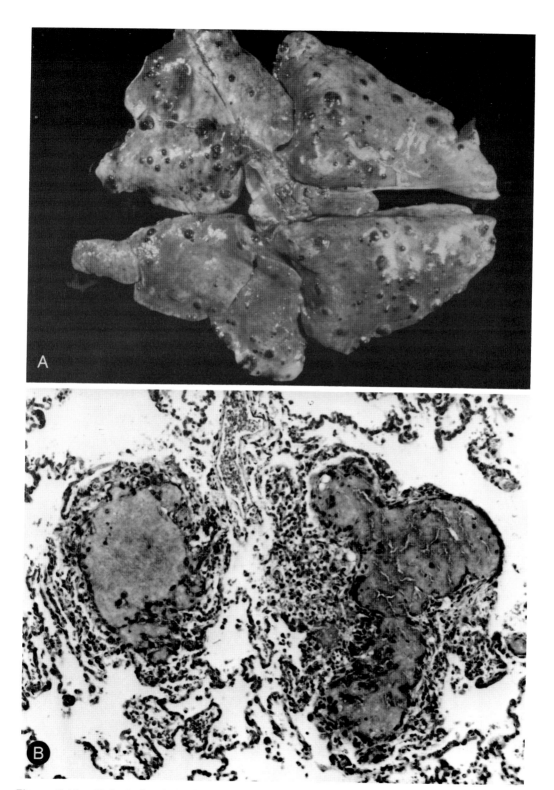

Figure 6.18. Metastasis. *A,* in this lung of a dog there are multiple, variably sized nodules of metastatic neoplastic tissue. In the fresh tissue these were dark red. *B,* histologically the neoplastic tissue formed spaces filled with blood, a feature characteristic of hemangiosarcoma.

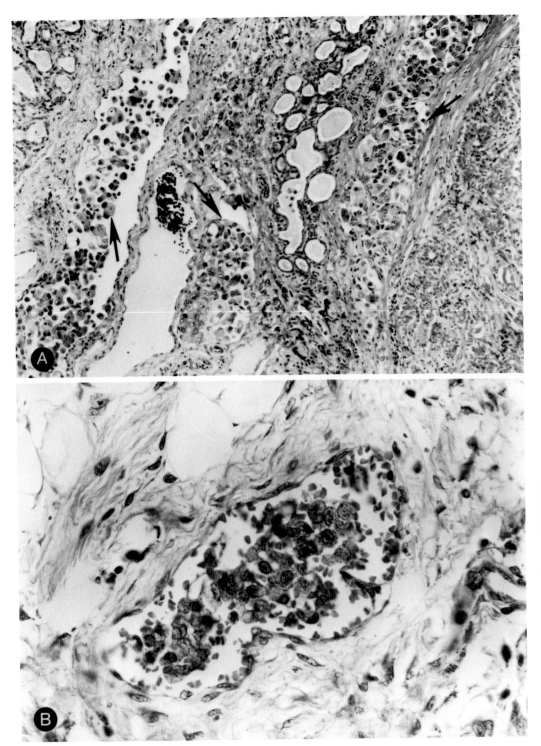

Figure 6.19.   Vascular Invasion by Neoplasms. *A,* many embolic cells from an adenocarcinoma of the mammary gland are present in lymphatic vessels *(arrows)*. Part of the primary neoplasm is visible on the *right. B,* embolic cells from a carcinoma of the esophagus are present in a venule. Erythrocytes are also in the lumen of the vessel.

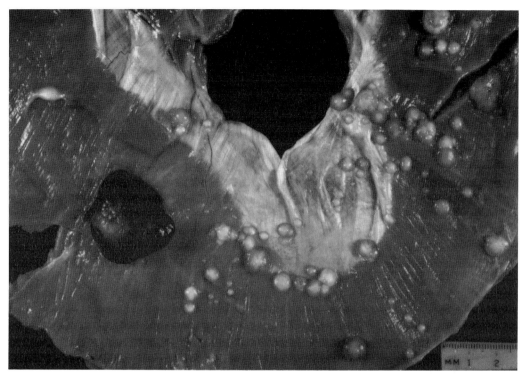

Figure 6.20.   Implantation. Neoplastic cells from a gastric carcinoma in a dog have implanted and are growing on the diaphragm. One mass is hemorrhagic.

obtaining good follow-up information on animal patients. Such systems are only useful if their ability to correlate morphologic characteristics with clinical behavior is established for each type of neoplasm in each animal species. However, grading and staging systems have been proposed for canine lymphomas and mast cell tumors. In the case of mast cell tumors, for example, clear differences in survival have been shown between low-grade and high-grade tumors.

PATHOGENESIS OF NEOPLASIA

In this section current knowledge of the mechanisms that underlie the development and subsequent behavior of neoplastic cells is discussed. The student probably will feel some frustration in reading this material because of a certain lack of dogma, which simply reflects the changing nature of our understanding of pathogenetic mechanisms in neoplasia. In view of this, it would be unrealistic to attempt to synthesize a single viewpoint that could, in only too few years, be proven wrong. Indeed, since the first edition of this book, major advances have been made in our understanding of the biology of neoplasia, in particular with regard to its genetic basis. Therefore, we will continue to outline the major theories that presently form the basis of our understanding of the biology of neoplasia.

Neoplasia is a disease that affects most, if not all, vertebrate species. With some exceptions, it tends to be a disease associated with aging. It is presumably partly for this reason that neoplasia is seen more frequently in dogs and cats than other domestic animals, dogs and cats being allowed to live out their natural lifespan, that is, to age. It is generally considered that aging *per se* is not a direct factor in the induction of tumors, but presumably allows increased opportunity to develop neoplasia, including cumulative exposure to environmental carcinogens. Furthermore, the development of neoplastic disease is a very prolonged process, often requiring half the normal lifetime of the animal (*see* below). This alone would bias the occurrence of neoplasia to older animals. However, there is some evidence that there is an increase in susceptibility to carcinogens in older animals. The basis for this phenomenon is at present unknown.

Control of Cell Growth

Given that neoplasms represent uncontrolled growth of certain cells, it clearly is important to attempt to understand those mechanisms that normally control growth. Study of these mechanisms usually is carried out using cell cultures. When normal cells are grown *in vitro* they spread out to form a single sheet, or monolayer, of cells. Growth ceases when the cells reach a certain density, and the cells remain quiescent but healthy. This process is known as cell **density-dependent inhibition,** or **contact inhibition,** of growth. In contrast, malignant cells grow in a haphazard way, pile up into multiple layers, and are much less responsive to cell density-dependent mechanisms of growth control. These cells tend to grow until they exhaust the medium of nutrients. These characteristics may be induced in cultures of normal cells by treatment with carcinogens, a process known as neoplastic **transformation.**

Growth Factors

It is now known that the most important signals regulating cell growth come from outside the cell, in the form of **growth factors (GFs).** These substances are defined as polypeptides that stimulate cell proliferation *via* interaction with specific receptors on the cell surface. A number of such GFs have been identified. They are hormone-like but act in a local, rather than an endocrine, manner. GFs are present in many kinds of tissues, both adult and embryonic, and in cultured cells. Receptors for GFs are also widespread. Most cells bear receptors for more than one GF, and multiple GFs are required for maximal stimulation of proliferation in most cell types. Different GFs act at different stages of the cell cycle. There is some specificity of action of GFs, some stimulating relatively specific cell populations, others affecting a wide variety of cells. Many of the differences in growth behavior of cultured neoplastic cells mentioned above can now be accounted for by reduced requirement for specific growth factors. This could be accounted for by autonomous synthesis of GFs (so-called autocrine stimulation), the expression of an abnormal receptor, or the activation of post-receptor pathways. The biological importance of GFs is further underscored by the fact that some **oncogenes** (discussed below) encode GFs, their receptors, or proteins involved in transduction of their signal. Table 6.3 summarizes some of the known important GFs discussed below.

EPIDERMAL GROWTH FACTOR (EGF). EGF is a small polypeptide first isolated from male mouse submaxillary gland, but which is expressed in a variety of tissues. It is mitogenic for a variety of cultured epithelial and mesenchymal cells. In some systems it acts synergistically with platelet-derived growth factor and/or insulin. EGF is also capable of inducing features of differentiation in some cells and *in vivo*. The receptor for EGF is expressed on a wide variety of cells. It is a transmembrane protein with an extracellular domain that serves to bind the GF, a transmembrane domain, and an intracellular domain that acts as a tyrosine protein kinase. As described below, the v-*erb*B oncogene encodes a homologue of the EGF receptor in which the extracellular GF binding domain has been lost. It is

Table 6.3
Cellular Growth Factors

GF[a]	Size	Major Source	Target
EGF	6 kDa	Submaxillary gland, Brunner's glands, parietal cells (?)	Many epithelial and mesenchymal cells
TGFα	5.6 kDa	Placenta, embryo, transformed cells	Same as EGF
TGFβ	25 kDa	Platelets, kidney, placenta, cultured cells	Fibroblasts, keratinocytes, mammary epithelium, carcinoma and melanoma cell lines
PDGF	32 kDa	Platelets, endothelial cells, placenta	Mesenchymal cells, smooth muscle cells, placental trophoblasts
IGF-1	7 kDa	Adult liver, smooth muscle	Epithelial and mesenchymal cells
IGF-2	7 kDa	Fetal liver, placenta	Epithelial and mesenchymal cells
IL-2	15 kDa	T helper cells	Cytotoxic T cells
FGFs	16 kDa	Brain, pituitary, macrophages, tumors	Endothelium and fibroblasts
β-NGF	26 kDa	Submaxillary gland	Sympathetic and sensory neurons
CSF-1	70 kDa	Mouse L cells	Macrophage progenitors
CSF-2	15–28 kDa	Endotoxin-treated lung, placenta	Macrophage and granulocyte progenitors
Multi-CSF (IL-3)	28 kDa	T cells	T cells, macrophage progenitors, granulocytes, eosinophils, mast cells
TNF	17 kDa (Monomer)	Activated macrophages	Fibroblasts

[a] The abbreviations used for the names of growth factors are explained in the text.

believed that this results in constitutive activation of the receptor, stimulating cellular proliferation.

TRANSFORMING GROWTH FACTOR TYPE α (TGFα). TGFα is also a small polypeptide which shows considerable sequence homology to EGF. It is expressed in placenta and embryonic tissues, and in a variety of transformed cells. However, it has not been found in non-neoplastic adult tissues and presumably it represents the embryonic form of EGF. It binds to the EGF receptor and therefore has effects essentially identical to EGF.

TRANSFORMING GROWTH FACTOR TYPE β (TGFβ). Despite the similarities in name, TGFβ is quite distinct from TGFα.

It is expressed in a wide variety of cell types. Depending on target cell type, TGFβ can either stimulate or inhibit cell proliferation. Some of its actions are probably mediated by induction of other growth factors, such as PDGF. The receptor for TGFβ is distinct and is expressed in essentially all cells.

PLATELET-DERIVED GROWTH FACTOR (PDGF). PDGF is a potent mitogen originally purified from platelets, but also expressed in endothelial cells and newborn rat aortic smooth muscle cells. Most neoplastic mesenchymal cells are thought to produce PDGF or a similar molecule. PDGF is a major mitogen in serum. It is a dimer of about 32 kDa. The B chain of

PDGF is encoded by the c-*sis* protooncogene. Receptors for PDGF are found on a wide variety of mesenchymal cells, and it is mitogenic for fibroblasts, endothelial and other cells. Receptors are also found on placental trophoblastic cells. The receptor is a protein tyrosine kinase, which is autophosphorylated by binding of the GF.

INSULIN-LIKE GROWTH FACTORS (IGF-1 AND IGF-2). These GFs are known also as somatomedin C and somatomedin A respectively. IGF-1 is produced in response to circulating growth hormone, is one of the major GFs in plasma and serum, and is mitogenic for a wide variety of cultured cell types. It has been suggested that IGF-2 is an embryonic counterpart of IGF-1, although each appears to have its own receptor. The receptor for IGF-1 is related to the insulin receptor and has protein tyrosine kinase activity. The tyrosine kinase domain shows sequence homology with the tyrosine kinases encoded by the *src* and *ros* oncogenes.

INTERLEUKIN 2 (IL-2). Originally called T cell growth factor, IL-2 is induced in T helper cells by antigen (or the lectin Con A) and acts on cytotoxic T cells. The expression of receptors for IL-2 in the latter is also induced by interaction with antigen (or lectin).

FIBROBLAST GROWTH FACTORS (FGFs). Two types of FGF, acidic and basic, have been described. They were originally extracted from brain tissue. The FGFs have also been referred to as endothelial growth factor, chondrosarcoma growth factor, and heparin-binding growth factors. Basic FGF now has been extracted from a wide variety of tissues, including vascular endothelium. Acidic FGF has been found only in brain, retina, bone matrix, and osteosarcoma. There is evidence that FGFs are stored in components of the extracellular matrix. Both interact with the same receptor. The FGFs are mitogenic for fibroblasts and endothelial cells. Basic FGF is a potent angiogenic factor *in vivo* and

appears to be identical to tumor angiogenesis factor (*see* below).

NERVE GROWTH FACTORS. NGF has been known for some time as a factor important in the maintenance and differentiation of sympathetic and sensory neurons. Receptors for NGF are found on these cells, as well as normal and neoplastic chromaffin cells. Generally, NGF inhibits proliferation and induces differentiation.

COLONY STIMULATING FACTORS (CSF-1, CSF-2, MULTI-CSF). These GFs regulate the growth and differentiation of hematopoietic precursor cells. CSF-1 is interesting in that it appears that the product of the c-*fms* protooncogene is its receptor, again a tyrosine kinase. The v-*fms* oncogene may encode an abnormal receptor. Furthermore, human patients with chromosomal deletions affecting the c-*fms* gene are predisposed to the development of myeloid leukemia or polycythemia vera.

TUMOR NECROSIS FACTOR (TNFα, CACHECTIN). TNFα is a polypeptide characteristically produced by activated macrophages, originally described for its ability to induce necrosis in certain types of tumors. It is closely related to lymphotoxin, sometimes called TNFβ. More recently it has been recognized that TNFα is a cytokine with a variety of activities. These include inhibition of lipoprotein lipase (cachectin activity), activation of neutrophils, and stimulation of fibroblast growth. Receptors for TNFα are found on a variety of cells.

Overview of GF Mechanisms in the Regulation of Cell Growth

Growth factors are the major external signals responsible for the regulation of growth in mammalian cells. Most stimulate cell growth, but a few, such as TGF-β, can inhibit it. GFs bind to receptors on the cell surface, and through transmembrane proteins, serve to transmit information *via* a complex, interactive network of intracellular signaling pathways

(Fig. 6.21). Components of this network include enzymes, in particular protein kinases, and second messengers. The latter include cyclic nucleotides, such as cAMP, phosphorylated proteins, diacylglycerol, inositol trisphosphate (IP$_3$), calcium ions, and hydrogen ions. Some of these signal transduction pathways are obviously important in activating genes encoding proteins important for entry into the mitotic cycle. They include the products of some oncogenes, such as c-*myc*, c-*fos,* and c-*myb*. However, many of these intracellular signals are shared and subserve a variety of cell functions. They are discussed in Chapter 4 in the context of activation of inflammatory cells. It is not surprising, therefore, that in neoplastic cells, where some of these signaling mechanisms are inherently altered, there

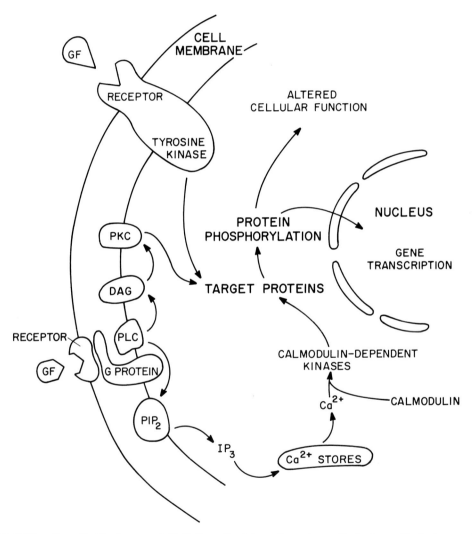

Figure 6.21.   Growth Factors and Cell Growth. Interaction of growth factors with their receptors can modulate a variety of cellular functions, included gene transcription. These activities are modulated through tyrosine-specific kinases forming part of the receptor complex, protein kinase C, or calcium-activated protein kinases. Abnormal expression of any of these signals can alter cellular proliferation. Many oncogene products are analogues of components of this system. The abbreviations used are GF, growth factor; PKC, protein kinase C; DAG, diacylglycerol; PLC, phospholipase C; PIP$_2$, phosphoinositol bisphosphate; IP$_3$, inositol trisphosphate.

are a wide variety of functional distur-bances. The important events in control-ling cell growth appear to occur prior to the onset of the S phase of the mitotic cycle, that is, during G_0 and G_1.

Both **autocrine** and **paracrine** mech-anisms have been proposed to account for the growth advantage of neoplastic cells. In the former it is proposed that neoplas-tic cells are stimulated by GFs that they themselves produce. It has been possible to show in one instance that cells of an osteosarcoma line produced both PDGF and its receptor. Antibody to PDGF in-hibited growth of these cells. Similarly, the gibbon ape leukemia cell line MLA-144 both produces and responds to IL-2. Antibody to IL-2 strongly inhibits the growth of these cells. However, it is not always possible to demonstrate similar mechanisms in other neoplasms.

Paracrine mechanisms, in which GFs produced by one cell type stimulate an-other, have also been proposed. For ex-ample, the production of GFs by neoplas-tic cells probably stimulates the proliferation of stroma, including its vas-cular elements. Angiogenesis, a neces-sary event in the growth of the neoplasm as a whole, has clearly been shown to depend on the production of growth fac-tors, including FGF, by neoplastic cells (*see* below). It also is quite likely that GFs produced by neoplastic cells are involved in the abundant stromal response seen in some carcinomas. Moreover, the stroma itself could serve as a source of GFs for tumor cells. One could even imagine a situation where the neoplastic and stromal cells support one another. Although not all of these interactions are proven, there is no doubt that GFs are important in the regulation of cell growth, and their links to oncogenes leave little doubt that they are important in the pathogenesis of neo-plasia.

Other Growth Control Mechanisms

In tissues that are continually renewed, substances called **chalones** apparently play an important role in the control of growth. Chalones are substances pro-duced by a subset of maturing cells which control the growth of the germinal cells of the same population. They have been best studied in the epidermis. In the skin, two chalones have been identified; G_1 chalone inhibits the transition from the G_1 to the S phase of the mitotic cycle, while G_2 chalone inhibits the transition from G_2 to the M phase. G_1 chalone is a glycopeptide that appears to be produced by the maturing keratinizing epidermal cells and acts on basal cells already com-mitted to differentiation (Fig. 6.22). G_2 chalone appears to be produced by a sub-set of differentiating basal cells before they lose the capacity to divide, and it acts on early noncommitted basal cells. These chalones are tissue, but not species, specific.

Although tumor-producing substances cause a loss of responsiveness to G_1 chal-one, this also occurs in nonspecific forms of hyperplasia, and no definite role of chalones in neoplasia has been proven. Nonresponsiveness to G_1 chalone is also a characteristic of fetal or neonatal cells. Nonresponsiveness may therefore reflect failure of differentiation, which would be expected to occur in neoplastic tissue.

Role of Intracellular Messengers

Growth factors and other signals acting at the cell surface must influence cell activity through intermediate molecules. Among these are the cyclic nucleotides, cyclic adenosine 3',5'-monophosphate (cAMP) and cyclic guanosine 3'5',-mono-phosphate (cGMP), calcium, inositol phos-phates, and intracellular proteins in-duced by the cell surface signal. There is a variety of evidence that cAMP can in-fluence cell growth. For example, there are measurable changes in levels of cAMP throughout the cell cycle, and for some cell types increased intracellular levels of cAMP stimulate cell growth. However, the growth of other cell types in culture is inhibited by cAMP. Furthermore,

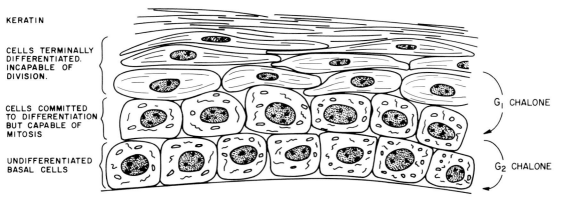

Figure 6.22.   Action of Chalones in the Epidermis. G_1 *chalone* is produced by differentiated cells that are no longer capable of division, and it acts on basal cells committed to differentiation but still capable of division. G_2 *chalone* is produced by the latter population and acts on basal cells not committed to differentiation.

mutations in cAMP-dependent protein kinases, through which the actions of cAMP are mediated, do not interfere with cell growth. It seems likely, therefore, that the effects of cAMP on cell growth are nonspecific. Similarly, binding of GFs is known to activate other second messenger systems, such as inositol trisphosphate (IP_3) and diacylglycerol, allow the influx of Ca^{2+} ions, and activate protein kinase C, but there is little evidence of specific defects in these systems in neoplasia. More interestingly, it is known that the expression of certain oncogene products is induced by the binding of growth factors to their receptors (*see* section on oncogenes). For example, the product of the *ras* oncogene may be an intermediate in transducing the growth factor signal, and the *myc* gene product is a nuclear-associated protein that may be involved in regulation of cell proliferation. The very fact that these proteins are the products of oncogenes suggests that they are important in control of cell growth, and that, when abnormal, they can lead to transformation.

Finally, contact inhibition of growth does seem to be important, at least under culture conditions. As cultures become confluent, cells cease growing and become quiescent. It is known that such cells have

a higher requirement for GFs than those growing at low density. This is not associated with any consistent change in the density of receptors for GFs, both increases and decreases having been reported in different cell types. The effect apparently depends on contact between cell membranes. In particular, the addition of membrane fractions to cells growing at low density can mimic the effect of contact inhibition of growth. Thus, it would appear that interaction of receptors on the surface of cells can function to oppose the effect of mitogens. Presumably, these effects are mediated by some intracellular mechanism, but the details remain to be elucidated.

Properties of Neoplastic Cells

Neoplastic cells, particularly those of malignant neoplasms, differ in many ways from normal cells. Some of these differences already have been discussed as they can be appreciated in the clinical situation. In addition, such cells may show loss of density-dependent control of growth and contact inhibition of movement *in vitro*, changes in biochemistry, antigenicity, karyotype, and cell surface characteristics. It should be kept in mind that many of these changes probably represent epiphenomena, or "noise," resulting from the fundamental changes underlying neoplastic transformation, but not causing it. This problem has made the analysis of the molecular basis of transformation extremely difficult.

Changes in the cell membrane in transformed cells have been studied extensively in an attempt to shed some light on the nature of the basic defect in cellular control which underlies neoplasia. A number of biochemical changes on the surface of transformed cells have been described. Among the most prominent is the consistent loss of a protein once referred to as LETS protein (large external transformation-sensitive), now called **fibronectin,** from transformed cells. In addition other proteins and polypeptides may be lost from, or reduced on, the cell surface. The mechanism of loss of these molecules is unknown but probably includes failure of synthesis or shedding from the cell surface.

Other proteins, usually glycoproteins, may be increased in amount or appear *de novo* in transformed cells. This is important, as some of these presumably include new antigens that appear on the surface of some transformed cells. Variable changes in sialic acid content, glycosylation of surface glycoproteins, and length of glycosyl chains on cell membrane gangliosides also may occur.

Many of these changes also occur in normal cells during mitosis. However, in transformed cells at rest there is no switch to the normal pattern. Therefore, there appears to be a loss of ability to carry out cell density–dependent modulation of the cell membrane in transformed cells.

Cell surface enzyme activities also may be altered in transformed cells. In particular there is usually an increase in activity of proteases and glycosidases. These may be of some pathogenetic importance, as treatment of normal cells with proteases induces in them many of the characteristics of transformed cells. Also, some of the altered growth properties of transformed cells *in vitro* and some of their altered surface characteristics can be modified by protease inhibitors.

Changes in the cell surface also may result in increased **agglutinability** of transformed cells by plant agglutinins. This apparently is due to the synthesis or unmasking of receptors for these substances. There is a strong correlation between the degree of agglutinability and transformation of the cells.

Thus a variety of cell membrane changes that appear to be related to mechanisms of control of growth occur in neoplastic and transformed cells. The various surface changes described in transformed cells may lead to failure to establish functional contact between cells which, through transmembrane cytoskeletal linkages, normally results in modulation of DNA synthesis and cell movement. The exact mechanism or mechanisms involved, however, remain to be fully elucidated.

Other biochemical changes, such as the absence of normal enzymes or the presence of abnormal ones, can occur in neoplastic cells. Although these are generally nonspecific, they tend to be more severe in anaplastic, malignant neoplasms than in benign tumors. Very anaplastic cells tend to revert to glycolytic energy metabolism even in the presence of oxygen. This is a general property of rapidly dividing cells.

The cells of many neoplasms, especially in man where they have been studied in detail, have **abnormal karyotypes.** These may involve alterations in chromosome number or morphology. Karyotypic abnormalities vary from tumor to tumor and tend to be more severe and more variable in anaplastic, malignant tumors. In a number of cases, however, karyotypic abnormalities are quite constant and are thought to be causally related to those particular neoplasms. In dogs, the transmissible venereal tumor (TVT) is consistently found to have an abnormal karyotype, the number of chromosomes, usually 59, differing from that of normal dog cells which have 78. Some variation in the karyotype of these tumor cells does occur, however. The relationship of specific chromosomal defects to the development of neoplasia is discussed in more detail later.

The Etiology of Neoplasia

In the great majority of cases of naturally occurring neoplasia, the specific cause of a particular tumor is unknown. However, for some, and in the case of experimentally induced neoplasms, predisposing or direct causes have been identified. Certainly, many agents have now been identified which can cause cancer. Substances which cause neoplasia are referred to as **carcinogens.** More specifically, a carcinogen may be defined as any substance or agent that produces, in exposed individuals, an incidence of neoplasia greater than that observed in those who are unexposed (controls). Known carcinogens fall into three categories, namely chemicals, physical agents, and viruses.

A wide variety of **chemicals** has been shown to be carcinogenic. Some of these act locally at the site of application, and some act remotely. A bewildering variety of chemical carcinogens is known, including polycyclic hydrocarbons, azo dyes, aromatic amines, and nitrosamines. Some of these are synthetic experimental compounds, but many occur in the environment, either naturally or as pollutants. One important group of naturally occurring chemical carcinogens is the aflatoxins. These substances, among which aflatoxin B_1 is the most important, are produced by a species of fungus, *Aspergillus flavus*. Aflatoxins are hepatotoxic and can produce hepatic neoplasms in birds, fish, primates, and rodents.

Many chemical carcinogens are, in truth, **procarcinogens** and must undergo cellular metabolism to produce **proximate** or **ultimate carcinogens.** For example, both polycyclic hydrocarbons and aflatoxins are metabolized to epoxides, which are the true carcinogens. This phenomenon explains, in many cases, the species or organ specificity of certain carcinogens. Species specificity depends on the metabolic capability of the cells of particular species, while organ specificity depends on the site of metabolism. The liver, therefore, is a frequent target organ of carcinogens, consistent with its role in metabolizing toxins. As well, the urinary bladder is often affected by carcinogens whose metabolites are excreted through the urinary tract. Some chemicals are **complete carcinogens,** that is, they can cause the development of neoplasms after a single dose. Others require interaction with other compounds, either **cocarcinogens** or **promotors** (*see* below). Some complete carcinogens, administered in low doses, can also require interaction with other compounds.

Simple **inorganic salts** can act as carcinogens. For example, in man, salts of nickel and beryllium are known to have carcinogenic potential. Proven cases with similar etiology are rare in animals, but there is some evidence that similar mechanisms may be involved in some cases of osteosarcoma. In dogs in which metal fixation devices having multiple parts have been implanted for long periods, an unexpectedly high number of osteosarcomas occurs. Moreover, these are usually in the midshaft region of the bone rather than at the usual predilection sites for this neoplasm. It is thought that electrolytic activity set up by slight differences in the composition of the components leads to relatively high local concentrations of metal ions, which in turn act as a carcinogen.

Hormones are known to be involved in the etiology of a number of tumors in domestic animals, rodents, and man. In many cases these arise in the target tissue of the hormone, as a consequence of continual hormonal stimulation. For example, if ovarian tissue is implanted into the spleen of previously ovariectomized experimental animals, the implanted ovary will eventually become neoplastic. In this experimental situation continued stimulation of the ovary occurs due to the destruction, in the liver, of the estrogens it secretes, with consequent loss of feedback on the pituitary gland. Apparently, continual stimulation of the ovary by gonadotrophins can cause neoplasia. In dogs it is known that long-term stimulation of the mammary gland by progesterone may result in the occurrence of mammary tumors. Other neoplasms in the dog also are known to be hormone dependent, and knowledge of this may be important to the clinician. For example, multiple adenomas of the circumanal glands occur frequently in old, male dogs. These neoplasms are influenced by testosterone, and castration of the affected animal will greatly reduce the incidence of recurrence.

The **physical state** of a carcinogen can be important. This is best illustrated by certain plastic films which, when implanted into the tissues, produce sarcomas. When these same plastics are implanted as a powder or a perforated film, they are not carcinogenic. Therefore, the physical state rather than the chemical nature of the material seems to be important in this case.

Exposure to **radiation** is one of the best-known causes of neoplasia and has received considerable publicity in recent years. Ultraviolet radiation, x-rays, and radiation from radioactive material all can cause neoplasms. In animals, the most striking example is the occurrence of squamous cell carcinomas resulting from excessive exposure to ultraviolet (UV) light. White cats living in hot, sunny climates commonly develop tumors on the ears or nose. Hereford cattle, which commonly have unpigmented eyelids, often develop ocular squamous cell carcinoma due to UV irradiation. Other forms of radiation are known to have caused neo-

plasms in man, and can induce neoplasms in experimental animals. Radiation also can cause transformation of cells *in vitro*.

Viruses, without doubt, can cause neoplasms, and the field of viral oncogenesis is one of the most exciting areas of research into the etiopathogenesis of neoplasia today. It is, in fact, from the study of viral oncogenesis that much of our current knowledge about oncogenes has arisen. Viral oncogenesis is discussed fully later in this chapter.

Mechanisms of Carcinogenesis

It should be stated from the outset that there is no generally accepted, unified concept of the biologic mechanisms that underlie the development of neoplastic disease. In this section some of the theories of carcinogenesis and the evidence supporting them will be discussed. Most models are based on studies of chemical carcinogenesis, but viral oncogenesis also will be considered, and an attempt will be made to relate these theories to naturally occurring neoplastic disease.

Whatever the fundamental cellular changes underlying carcinogenesis are, certain observations can be made about the process. It is, at least in the case of chemical carcinogenesis, a dose-dependent and cumulative process. Therefore, the quantity of chemical which will cause neoplasia may be administered singly or as multiple, sequential doses. This implies that progressive changes occur in the target cells during exposure to the substance. Whatever these changes are, they are retained in affected cells after cessation of treatment and may be expressed many cell generations later as neoplasia. It has been shown in several experimental systems that the changes brought about in cells exposed to a dose of a chemical carcinogen which is insufficient to produce tumors are retained. Therefore, the exposed individuals retain a higher than normal risk of developing neoplasia if again exposed to the same substance. This is of obvious importance to individuals who have been repeatedly exposed to a carcinogen.

Cellular proliferation enhances the process of carcinogenesis and probably is necessary for carcinogenesis. This may well reflect a necessity for changes to progress or become fixed in the altered cells. It is known that cells that are transformed either *in vivo* or *in vitro* must evolve in some way before they can express themselves as neoplasms. For example, if cells are transformed *in vitro* and immediately implanted in an experimental animal they usually are not tumorigenic. However, if they are transformed and allowed to proliferate *in vitro* before implantation, they do produce tumors. There is also evidence that some carcinogens interact preferentially with DNA in proliferating cells and at certain stages of the cell cycle.

Carcinogenesis is a chronic process, requiring long periods of time, sometimes amounting to more than half the lifespan of the animal. It is now generally believed that, in most cases, carcinogenesis involves changes in a small number of cells, occurring in many steps. The process is progressive, each step increasing the probability of the emergence of a malignant neoplasm. The appearance of recognizable neoplastic cells therefore occurs as a late event. Much of the evidence for this concept has come from the detailed study of chemical carcinogenesis in the skin, the liver, and other tissues. In these models it has been possible to dissect some of the steps involved.

Initiation and Promotion

Some of the first evidence that more than one process, or step, is involved in carcinogenesis was provided by experiments carried out years ago which led to the concept of two-stage induction of neoplasia. More recently this concept has been extended to include progressive changes that occur in transformed foci and in established neoplasms. In the original ex-

periments it was found that a single application of a carcinogen, such as benzopyrene, could sensitize skin without actually producing tumors. When a second agent, such as croton oil, was applied repeatedly to the same area, tumors appeared. These processes were called **initiation** and **promotion,** the first agent being the **initiator** and the second, the **promoter.** Initiation and promotion have been shown to occur in a number of organs *in vivo,* notably the skin, the liver, the colon, and the urinary bladder, as well as having been demonstrated *in vitro.* These processes are summarized in Figure 6.23.

Initiation involves a change in a target tissue, caused by a carcinogen, such that the altered cells can be induced (by a promotor) to develop focal proliferations, which in turn can act as sites for the further development of malignancy. Initiation is a rapidly occurring, heritable, essentially irreversible change that produces no permanent morphological changes or autonomous growth in the tissue. It is induced by a single exposure to the initiator. Although it is generally regarded as irreversible, there is some evidence that tumor yield may decrease after long periods indicating slow reversibility. Initiation therefore resembles direct carcinogenesis in that it apparently induces a change in the treated cells which is passed on from generation to generation. Initiation itself is believed to involve at least two steps. The first is the induction of a molecular lesion (or lesions) in rare target cells. The second is the fixing of such lesions by a round of cell proliferation. In models of carcinogenesis in the liver, for example, it is possible to show that the molecular lesion relevant to initiation has a relatively short lifespan, unless cell proliferation occurs. Thus, to induce initiation in the liver, the administration of the initiator must be accompanied or shortly followed by something that causes cell proliferation.

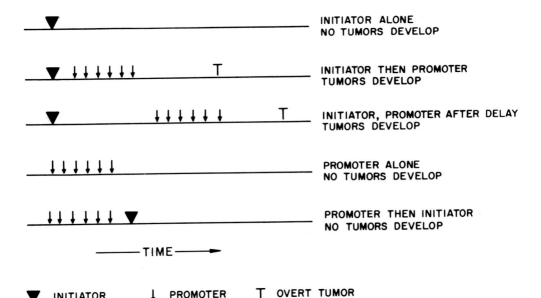

▼ INITIATOR   ↓ PROMOTER   T OVERT TUMOR

Figure 6.23 Actions of Initiators and Promoters. Production of tumors requires an initiator followed by a promoter. Initiator alone, promoter alone, or initiator preceded by promoter fail to produce tumors. There may be a considerable delay between applying initiator and promoter, and there is a delay, or latent period, between treatment and tumor development. (Adapted from H. C. Pitot: *Fundamentals of Oncology,* ed. 3, Marcel Dekker, New York, 1986.)

The nature of the molecular lesion responsible for initiation is unknown. Most initiators, like carcinogens in general, bind to DNA, RNA, and proteins, and it is generally held that DNA is a major molecular target in initiation. The stable nature of initiation, together with the requirement for a round of cell proliferation to "fix" the change, suggests that mutation-like alterations in DNA may be important. On the other hand, there are a number of known carcinogens that do not seem to interact chemically with DNA. Whether these compounds can induce more subtle genetic changes is yet to be established. The general question of the genetic basis of neoplasia is discussed later in this chapter.

Promotion is the process by which an initiated tissue is induced to develop focal proliferative lesions, some of which may later be the site of further changes leading to the development of full-fledged malignant neoplasms. After initiation, no proliferative lesions are present. Under the influence of the promotor, such lesions (in the skin, papillomas, in the liver, hepatocellular nodules) appear. These lesions result from the expansion by growth of cells phenotypically altered by initiation, and their constituent cells can be shown to have increased mitotic activity. At least in the liver, these proliferative lesions have been shown to be clonal in origin, that is, each nodule is derived from a single initiated cell. Promotors may therefore be regarded as providing a selection pressure allowing the emergence of clones of initiated cells.

In both the skin and liver models, many of these focal proliferative lesions undergo remodeling by differentiation and come to resemble the surrounding normal tissue. A small percentage of the nodules or papillomas, however, persist. Their constituent cells continue to proliferate, and they are believed to be the site in which further progressive changes occur during the development of true neoplasms.

Unlike initiation, promotion appears to

be a prolonged process which requires continual or repeated applications of the promoter over a certain period of time to produce tumors in the initiated tissues. After their application, there is a minimal latent period before tumors appear which is independent of the dose of promoter used. Because interruption of treatment with a promotor can result in the failure of development of tumors, promotion is sometimes said to be reversible. While this is true, it is also apparent that, at some point, the process of promotion is complete and the development of tumors, after the latent period, is irrevocable. Different promoters, with comparable effects in terms of inflammatory or hyperplastic responses, can produce different tumor yields. Promotion is, therefore, a complex phenomenon, and its mechanisms may vary with different promoters. It should be distinguished from **cocarcinogenesis,** that is, a simple additive effect with the initiator. Some substances that do act as cocarcinogens are not promoters, and some weak promoters are in fact anticarcinogenic when applied together with the initiator.

Again, the molecular basis of promotion is uncertain but several observed effects of promoters may be important. Promotors exhibit a wide variety of effects on normal tissues. They can cause inflammation, they induce hyperplasia, and they alter patterns of differentiation, as well as inducing a variety of biochemical changes. At least in the skin model, it is now known that promotion can also be separated into stages, a specific early stage and a later, less specific stage. These are referred to as **stage 1** and **stage 2 promotion** respectively. Stage 1 promotion is characterized by certain phorbol esters, the active ingredients of croton oil, the promotor used in the first initiation and promotion experiments. The development of tumors in initiated skin requires only a single exposure to stage 1 promotor, but prolonged or multiple exposures to a stage

2 promotor. Stage 1 promotion is thought to involve a rapidly induced change in cell differentiation with the acquisition of altered proliferative capacity. Stage 2 promotion involves the selective proliferation of these altered cells, and seems to be a result of the hyperplasia induced by stage 2 promotors.

Stage 1 promotors, such as the phorbol ester 12-O-tetradecanoylphorbol-13-acetate (TPA), interact with high-affinity receptors on the cell membrane. The specific binding site is a protein kinase, **protein kinase C.** In the presence of calcium ions and phospholipid, TPA activates this enzyme, resulting in the phosphorylation of serine and threonine residues in certain cellular proteins, including growth factor receptors. These protein phosphorylation reactions are crucial in both the regulation of cellular responses to hormones and growth factors, and in the regulation of many other cell functions including gene expression, that of certain oncogenes such as *myc* and *fos* included. The parallels between the actions of stage 1 promotors and the responses to growth factors should be apparent from our previous discussion of the latter. It is not yet known whether analogous stage 1 and stage 2 promotion can be demonstrated in tissues other than the skin.

Progression of Neoplasia and Tumor Latency

From our discussion of initiation and promotion it is evident that a number of sequential events are necessary for the development of preneoplastic proliferative lesions. Furthermore, these clones, although homogeneous at first, generally become progressively more heterogeneous with respect to a variety of phenotypic features, including proliferative capacity. As already discussed, these lesions eventually develop into malignant neoplasms. This evolution, which has been termed **tumor progression,** continues throughout the natural history of the neoplasm and may result in increasing malignancy. In other words, progression consists of a series of discrete changes in a population of cells, initiation being the first. Subsequent changes take place in the population of cells altered during the early events of tumor initiation. Evidence for this concept comes from observed changes in the nature of some neoplasms with time. Relatively benign tumors may gradually show more and more anaplasia and become more malignant in behavior. Other features change progressively as well. For instance, the karyotype of neoplastic cells may become increasingly abnormal with time. It is still debated whether all malignant neoplasms evolve through a transient, benign, focal proliferative lesion, as described in these experimental systems, or whether some malignant neoplasms arise *de novo.* Certainly some malignant neoplasms seem to arise in dysplastic lesions, and rare examples seem to arise without apparent preneoplastic changes. In the latter, however, it is difficult to rule out unobserved changes. In the case of preneoplastic dysplastic lesions, the differences may be more apparent than real, since dysplasia involves cellular proliferation and, presumably, alterations in differentiation.

Included within the concept of tumor progression is **tumor cell latency.** Latent tumor cells are those that have undergone some inherent change that makes them neoplastic, but which, at least for a while, fail to express this potential. Initiated cells, for instance, could be regarded as latent tumor cells which, under appropriate circumstances (*e.g.,* contact with promoter in the initiation-promotion model), progress to form overt neoplasms. Latency also has been documented in other experimental tumor systems, in particular the murine mammary tumor model. In this system carcinogens such as oncogenic viruses, chemical carcinogens, or

hormonal influences initially induce multiple hyperplastic nodules that fail to grow beyond a few millimeters in diameter. It has been shown that this failure to grow is due to control exerted by normal epithelial cells in nearby mammary ducts. The hyperplastic nodules are capable of more extensive growth when removed from this influence and therefore represent latent tumors. Autonomously growing neoplasms apparently arise as a result of subsequent changes, or progression, which occur in some of these cells. In the murine mammary tumor system these occur as multiple, morphologically distinct variants. The fact that such distinct lesions develop suggests that a variety of changes occur in a number of cells, each one different from the next. However, only those cells with changes enabling them to escape from growth controls are able to proliferate. Each of these then gives rise to a clone of heritably stable subtypes. Most such changes appear to be random and independent of selection pressures. There is evidence however that, at least in some cases, heritable changes in the neoplastic cell population can be induced by changes in the local environment.

The basis of progression, like that of carcinogenesis itself and initiation and promotion, is at present unknown. Arguments can be advanced to support multiple mutations (multiple "hits") or epigenetic phenomena (*i.e.,* abnormalities of regulation and differentiation) as the explanation for these changes.

Latent, or **dormant,** tumor cells are well known in clinical medicine. It sometimes happens, years after the surgical excision of a primary neoplasm, that tumors recur at the original site, or that metastases appear, presumably derived from cells "left behind" at the time of surgery. The emergence of these tumors usually is explained as being due to some poorly understood local environmental changes that allow them to grow. An equally viable explanation is that random changes equivalent to tumor progression have occurred in the dormant cells allowing them to escape the constraints to which they had been subjected for so many years.

Changes can also occur which result in reduced tumorigenicity in initiated cell populations. It has been mentioned that hyperplastic nodules induced in the liver by carcinogens can regress by differentiation to morphologically normal cells. Similarly, dysplastic lesions induced in tracheal mucosa by carcinogens can regress to a morphologically normal state. What is not known at present is whether these regressed lesions retain an increased susceptibility to neoplasia. Certainly, in the experimental tracheal mucosal model, regression of the dysplastic lesions is not accompanied by a reduced risk of neoplasia, but it is not clear whether this retained susceptibility resides in the cells derived from the original dysplastic lesions or in other altered cells.

Genetic Aspects of Neoplasia

In the recent past there has been considerable controversy about the genetic basis of carcinogenesis and neoplastic transformation. On the one hand is the argument that neoplastic transformation is due to **somatic mutation,** that is, a genetic change in cells of the body other than germ cells. Such mutations would be expected to be heritable in the sense that they would be passed on at mitosis to daughter cells. The counterargument is that neoplasia is caused by **epigenetic events,** those that involve changes in gene regulation and expression without actual damage or changes in the genes themselves. Over the last few years it has become clear that there is compelling evidence for a genetic basis to neoplasia.

Indeed, there is no doubt that damage to the host genome and mutations in certain genes can underlie neoplastic transformation, but mutational and epigenetic factors are not mutually exclusive, and both types of change can contribute to the development of a neoplasm. All in all, it is certain that genetic events play a consistent and important role. In the discussion that follows we will freely utilize evidence gained from human neoplasia, believing that human models of animal disease are as valid as the reverse.

There is a large body of indirect evidence supporting somatic mutation as the cause of neoplastic transformation. First, neoplasia obviously involves a heritable change in the affected cells. One neoplastic cell gives rise to others that continue to express the abnormalities characteristic of neoplasia. Heritable changes in cells usually are thought of as being genetic in nature. Furthermore, most carcinogens are mutagens. As already alluded to, most chemical carcinogens or their metabolites react with DNA. Most of them can, in suitable test systems, be shown to be mutagenic. Radiation also is known to be mutagenic. UV irradiation, for example, is known to cause DNA damage, including the formation of pyramidine dimers. Normally cells try to repair damage to DNA (*see* Chapter 7) but some of the mechanisms are error prone, and altered sequences may become incorporated permanently. There is evidence, in mammalian cells, that such errors may be significant in carcinogenesis. For example, if these error-prone mechanisms of repair are inhibited, the toxicity of mutagens is increased. However, the carcinogenicity of skin irradiation is *reduced* by the same treatment. In this situation, it seems that no repair is better than incorrect repair.

Individuals with mutations resulting in defective repair of DNA are prone to neoplastic disease. The most instructive of these diseases is **xeroderma pigmentosum** of man. This syndrome is known to be due to a specific defect in the ability of patients to repair damage to DNA induced by UV irradiation. Affected individuals can repair other types of damage to DNA, such as that caused by x-irradiation, indicating an exquisite level of specificity in these repair mechanisms. Patients with xeroderma pigmentosum have a very high incidence of skin neoplasms associated with exposure to sunlight. They occur at an early age, and the relative frequency of the various types of neoplasms parallels that of normal people who spend a lot of time in the sun. The absolute frequency is, however, about 10,000 times that of normal individuals. This suggests strongly that faulty repair of DNA can result in neoplasia. Additional evidence for the mutational basis of neoplasia is provided by the high frequency of cancer in humans with other hereditary chromosomal fragility syndromes. Some of these are associated with DNA repair deficiencies. Furthermore, there is now overwhelming evidence that chromosomal abnormalities are consistently found in neoplastic cells. The evidence that these are involved in the development of neoplasia are discussed below.

In addition to the syndromes referred to above, there are several well-known instances of hereditary neoplasia or hereditary predisposition to neoplasia. These include retinoblastoma, Wilms' tumor and others in man, and a hereditary form of renal carcinoma in rats. In the case of hereditary **retinoblastoma,** it has quite clearly been shown that individuals at risk are heterozygous (*i.e.,* carriers) for deletions or some other defect in a particular segment of chromosome 13. All cells of their body therefore carry one such defective chromosome. It has also been shown that tumors in most of these individuals are homozygous or hemizygous for the defective chromosome, the normal one having been lost or replaced by duplication of the defective one. Thus it seems that a particular gene and its product have been lost from these cells. The role that such a gene might play in the development of neoplasia is discussed further below. This disease not only contributes to the evidence for a mutational basis of

neoplasia, it provides a compelling example of the "multiple hit" phenomenon, whereby it is believed that more than one genetic event is required to induce a neoplasm. Here the first event is a germline mutation; the second event is a somatic mutation, often brought about by chromosomal rearrangement.

The fact that most neoplasms are clonal in origin (*see* below) is also consistent with a mutational basis for neoplasia. One could ask why more varied manifestations of somatic mutation do not become apparent. For the results of a mutation to be evident, however, a clone of recognizable size must develop, and only those events that confer a proliferative advantage, that is, cause a tumor, would become manifest.

The final, and perhaps most interesting, piece of evidence in this argument, is the fact that specific genes that can contribute to the development of neoplasia have now been identified. These are referred to as **oncogenes** and are discussed more fully below.

We have already pointed out that the development of most neoplasms is a prolonged process involving many steps during the evolution of a malignant neoplasm. Most investigators would argue that this implies multiple genetic changes. Epidemiological evidence has suggested that at least two genetic changes, and sometimes as many as six, may be required for the full development of the neoplasm. This has been referred to as the **"multiple hit"** phenomenon. We have already mentioned one well-known example, and further evidence will be presented below.

For completeness we should admit that there are also arguments against mutation as the basis of carcinogenesis. The alternative view is that neoplasia represents a defect in the epigenetic mechanisms involved in cellular differentiation and function. The evidence for this is drawn from several sources. For example, it may be argued that the characteristics of normal tissues are heritable, in the sense that liver cells produce liver cells, and that normal tissue cells can mimic many of the behavioral characteristics of neoplastic cells. For instance trophoblastic cells are invasive, and endometrial cells may implant in abnormal sites. Furthermore, there is evidence that the loss of control of growth and differentiation, which is characteristic of neoplasia, may, in some circumstances, be reversible. There are documented cases of neoplasms undergoing terminal differentiation with the loss of further capacity to grow. The most striking evidence comes from studies that have been carried out on teratocarcinomas of mice. These malignant neoplasms are believed to arise from primitive stem cells and show multiple pathways of differentiation. If teratocarcinoma cells are implanted into developing blastulae from normal mice, the baby mice that result are mosaics composed of cells from the blastula and cells from the implanted neoplastic cells. These mice do not develop teratocarcinomas. It therefore appears that the neoplastic cells can be induced to undergo normal differentiation if subjected to the appropriate environment. In this particular case epigenetic control mechanisms may underlie neoplastic transformation.

In summary, there are compelling arguments for the role of somatic mutation and genetic abnormalities in the etiology of neoplasia. The most impressive arguments against mutation depend on the fact that the neoplastic phenotype can sometimes be reversed. However, it is becoming apparent that the normal control of cellular growth and differentiation is extremely complex, involving many interactive processes, some of which counter others. Evidence is accumulating that the products of different genes can augment or counteract those of others, so that the final phenotype depends on the relative contributions of each. Evidence has even emerged of cancer-causing genes (oncogenes) and cancer-suppressing genes (so-called antioncogenes). These are discussed more fully below.

Tests for Carcinogenicity

Because of the potential hazards of any new chemical, including drugs and many other compounds used in modern society, methods are required to test for carcinogenicity. Some of the testing is done in animals, but this is obviously time-consuming, expensive, and controversial because it raises humane issues. The idea that most carcinogens are also mutagens has led to alternative methods of testing *in vitro* such as the **Ames test.** This test uses specific mutant strains of *Salmonella typhimurium* bacteria which are incubated with the test chemical. Liver microsomes are included to allow metabolic activation of the substance, and mutagenicity is measured by quantitating the number of bacterial revertants. The validity of this test depends on the assumption that a chemical proven mutagenic in a bacterial system will be carcinogenic in animals. Using this system, it already has been shown that many known carcinogens are mutagenic. However, the validity of the test is not yet generally accepted, and exceptions to the proposal that carcinogens are mutagens do occur, as discussed below. Tests similar to the Ames test using animal cells instead of bacteria have also been utilized to detect mutagenicity.

Chromosomal Abnormalities and Neoplasia

The fact that cancer cells have karyotypic abnormalities has been known for many years. However, it was generally believed that many of these changes represented secondary events occurring during the progression of the neoplasm. An exception to this belief was the so-called **Philadelphia chromosome** (Ph[1]), a cytogenetic marker for chronic myelogenous leukemia in humans. This marker chromosome is the result of a translocation between chromosomes 9 and 22. It is present in most patients with the disease, and has been observed in normal individuals who later developed the disease. It was therefore thought to play some causative role in this neoplasm.

With the advent of high-resolution cytogenetic banding techniques our view of the significance of chromosomal abnormalities in neoplasia has changed. It has now been recognized that nonrandom chromosomal abnormalities are a consistent feature of many neoplasms. Over 90% of human malignancies have clonal cytogenetic alterations. In many cases the abnormalities are specific and characteristic for a particular type of neoplasm. Although we will not discuss every example, a few of them have been particularly instructive in understanding genetic events that may underlie the development of neoplasia.

Study of chromosomal abnormalities in certain human lymphomas and leukemias has been particularly enlightening. One of the most instructive has been Burkitt's lymphoma, an aggressive B cell neoplasm usually affecting children. It is endemic in Africa, where it is associated with infection with Epstein-Barr virus (EBV), and occurs sporadically in other parts of the world without association with the virus. All cases of Burkitt's lymphoma have translocations between chromosome 8 and either chromosome 14, 22, or 2. Each of the latter three chromosomes carries a locus for parts of the immunoglobulin molecule. The breakpoint on chromosome 8 is close to the cellular oncogene c-*myc*, and the final result is that c-*myc* becomes juxtaposed to one of the immunoglobulin loci, and the oncogene comes under the influence of tissue-specific genetic enhancers at these sites. The net result of these translocations is believed to be that the transcription of the c-*myc* oncogene is deregulated, contributing to the neoplastic phenotype. (We will discuss the *myc* oncogene more fully later in this chapter.) Further weight is added to the significance of these findings by the fact that analogous translocations, involving immunoglobulin loci and *myc*, are associated with plasmacytomas in the mouse and the rat, and that translocations whose breakpoints interrupt the T cell receptor are involved in T cell neoplasms in man. Molecular analysis of chromosomal breakpoints in other lymphoid neoplasms has now been used to identify and clone putative new oncogenes.

In the case of chronic myelogenous leukemia (CML) and the Philadelphia chromosome, another known oncogene, c-*abl*, is transposed from chromosome 9 to chromosome 22, near a particular locus called *bcr*. The molecular mechanisms involved in this case are a little different from those of Burkitt's lymphoma and *myc*. In CML the juxtaposition of *abl* and *bcr* results in the transcription of a hybrid mRNA that codes for a fusion protein containing parts of each parent protein. This protein has protein kinase activity and functions at a high level of activity.

Chromosomal abnormalities tend to become progressively more extensive as tumors progress, contributing additional changes in the genetic makeup of the neoplastic cell population, part of the multiple hit hypothesis that we have already mentioned. The changes may include addition of chromosomes or their loss. Addition may cause increased expression of important genes, while chromosome loss could lead to the loss of important genes similar to that which occurs in retinoblastoma. As tumors progress, particular parts of the genome may become amplified and are seen as abnormal banding regions, so-called **double minutes,** or **homogeneous staining regions,** on cytogenetic examination. In some cases these amplified regions have been shown to involve oncogenes, leading to increased gene expression. This is thought to contribute to progressive increase in malignancy.

Unfortunately, specific chromosomal defects have not been studied in detail in most naturally occurring neoplasms of animals. In dogs, consistent chromosomal abnormalities occur in the **transmissible venereal tumor (TVT),** where tumor cells have an abnormal number of chromosomes, usually 59, rather than the normal 78. Nevertheless, the well-understood examples from human neoplasms discussed above document the significance of chromosomal abnormalities in the pathogenesis of neoplasia, and provide compelling evidence for the role of specific "cancer genes," the oncogenes.

Oncogenes and Cancer Suppressor Genes

The explosion in understanding of the genetic basis of neoplasia is due to dramatic advances that have been made in recent years in the identification and characterization of specific genes thought to be important in control of growth and differentiation and in the generation of the neoplastic phenotype. These genes are the **oncogenes.** The first indications of the existence of such genes came from the study of oncogenic retroviruses (discussed in more detail elsewhere in this chapter). Typical retroviruses contain three genes: *gag,* coding for capsid proteins, *pol,* coding for reverse transcriptase, and *env,* coding for envelope proteins. Viruses containing these genes are competent to replicate and include some slowly transforming retroviruses, such as murine leukemia virus (MuLV), avian leukosis virus, and feline leukemia virus (FeLV). These are infectious viruses capable of producing lymphomas or leukemias in their host. Characteristically, they require a long incubation period in which to produce neoplastic disease. In contrast, the acutely transforming retroviruses are capable of

inducing tumors very rapidly. They do not occur widely as infectious viruses, but are typically isolated from tumors. The archetype of this group is **Rous sarcoma virus,** originally isolated from a sarcoma in a chicken. In addition to the three genes already described, this virus was found to contain another gene, dubbed *src.* This gene is necessary and sufficient for cellular transformation. It is one of about 20 **viral oncogenes** (v-*onc*) known to be associated with acutely transforming retroviruses. Other such viruses are replication defective in that parts of the usual genome are deleted and replaced by the v-*onc.* They are therefore only able to replicate if cells are co-infected with a competent "helper" virus, which supplies the missing functions.

Knowledge of the viral oncogenes led to the discovery that tissue cells of normal animals contain homologous genomic sequences that have come to be known as **cellular oncogenes** (c-*onc*), or **protooncogenes.** These are highly conserved, ubiquitous genes, found in organisms widely separated on the evolutionary scale. It is now believed that the viral oncogenes arose by incorporation of host genomic sequences into the viral genome.

About 40 oncogenes are now known. Not all of these are associated with viral homologues. Alternative approaches, such as cloning chromosomal breakpoints and DNA transfection assays have identified these additional oncogenes. Table 6.4 summarizes some of the best characterized oncogenes.

What, then, is the normal function of these genes and how are they involved in the development of neoplasia? The term "oncogene" is really, in the light of current understanding, a misnomer. Obviously, these genes are not present to cause cancer. Rather, it is generally believed that oncogenes, or actually their products, play an important role in the regulation of cell growth and differentia-

Table 6.4
Some Oncogenes and Their Gene Products

Oncogene	Retrovirus	Tumor Type	Gene Product[a]	Cellular Location
src	Rous sarcoma	Fibrosarcoma	TK	Plasma membrane
yes	Avian sarcoma	Sarcoma	TK	Plasma membrane
ros	Avian sarcoma	Sarcoma	TK; GF receptor?	Plasma membrane
abl	Abelson murine leukemia	Leukemia	TK	Plasma membrane
mos	Moloney murine sarcoma	Sarcoma	S/TK	Cytoplasm
raf	Murine sarcoma	Sarcoma	S/TK	Cytoplasm
fgr	Feline sarcoma	Fibrosarcoma	TK	?
fes	Feline sarcoma	Fibrosarcoma	TK	Plasma membrane
kit	Feline sarcoma	Fibrosarcoma	TK; GF receptor?	
fms	Feline sarcoma	Fibrosarcoma	TK; CSF-1 receptor	Plasma membrane
erb-B	Avian erythroblastosis	Erythroleukemia Carcinomas (man)	TK; EGF receptor	
neu	—	Breast carcinoma	TK; GF receptor?	Plasma membrane
sis	Simian sarcoma	Sarcoma	PDGF-like	Secreted
H-ras	Harvey murine sarcoma	Many tumors (man)	G protein-like	Plasma membrane
K-ras	Kirsten murine sarcoma	Many (man)	G protein-like	Plasma membrane
N-ras	—	Many (man)	G protein-like	Plasma membrane
myc	Avian myelocytomatosis	Murine myeloma; Burkitt's lymphoma	DNA binding; Gene regulation?	Nucleus
L-myc	—	Human small cell lung carcinoma	As for myc	Nucleus
N-myc	—	Human neuroblastoma	As for myc	Nucleus
myb	Avian myeloblastosis	Leukemia	?	Nucleus
fos	Murine osteosarcoma	Sarcoma, osteosarcoma	?	Nucleus
ski	Avian carcinoma	Carcinoma	?	Nucleus

[a]The abbreviations used are: TK, Tyrosine-specific protein kinase; S/TK, Serine/threonine-specific protein kinase; GF, growth factor; CSF-1, colony stimulating factor 1; EGF, epidermal growth factor; PDGF, platelet-derived growth factor.

tion, and important information is beginning to emerge concerning their functions. These functions can be grouped loosely into those associated with the cell nucleus and those associated with the cytoplasm or cell membrane (*see* Table 6.4).

Oncogenes whose protein products are located in the nucleus are thought to be involved in regulation of transcription and gene expression. These include the *myc* family (c-*myc,* N-*myc,* and L-*myc*), c-*myb,* c-*fos,* and a cellular protein called p53. The exact role of their protein products is not known. It is interesting to note, however, that *myc* and *myb* share sequence homology with the E1a transforming gene of adenovirus. The latter is known to code for a nuclear protein that binds to regulatory regions in DNA to increase the transcription of a number of cellular genes. This, together with the known ability of the *myc* and *myb* proteins to bind to DNA, suggests that their protein products may play a similar role. The products of *myc* and *fos* are associated in the nucleus with small nuclear ribonucleoproteins that are involved in post-transcriptional splicing of RNA. These genes may therefore also play a role in regulating these events. Both *myc* and *fos* are expressed during the transition of cells from the G_0 to the G_1 phase of the cell cycle. Although the exact mechanisms are still not clear, all of this evidence suggests that these genes are involved in the regulation of expression of other genes important in mitotically active cells.

The picture is a little clearer concerning the probable functions of oncogenes whose protein products are expressed in the cytoplasm or at the cell membrane. Most of these code for proteins with protein kinase activity, phosphorylating their targets on either tyrosine or threonine/serine residues. As discussed in Chapters 4 and 5, and in this chapter in relationship to growth factors, such protein phosphorylation is known to be important in regulation of a wide variety of cellular functions. This group of oncogenes can be grouped in the *src* gene family, all showing some homology with the tyrosine kinase domain of *src*. Some of these oncogenes code for receptors for growth factors. For example, *erb*-B encodes the EGF receptor and *fms* encodes the CSF-1 receptor. The sequence of others, such as *kit, neu* and *ros* suggests that they encode similar membrane-spanning receptors. Each of these also demonstrates protein kinase activity in its cytoplasmic domain. The *sis* oncogene falls into a special class. Its normal gene product is PDGF which, as we have already mentioned, is a potent mitogen.

The *ras* family of oncogenes also forms a special group. It includes three genes, H-*ras* (related to the Harvey murine sarcoma virus), K-*ras* (related to the Kirsten murine sarcoma virus), and N-*ras* (a cellular oncogene discovered in neuroblastoma cells). These genes are very closely related and, again, are highly conserved, being found in yeast, for example. The proteins encoded by the *ras* genes are closely related to the G proteins. These are GTP-binding proteins located in the plasma membrane which have intrinsic GTPase activity. They are known to be important in the transduction of signals from certain receptors to cytoplasmic second messengers (*see* also Chapter 4).

Thus an intriguing thread begins to emerge with respect to the oncogenes that have been implicated in the pathogenesis of neoplastic transformation. One of these genes encodes a growth factor, several encode known or putative receptors for growth factors, some encode G proteins involved in transduction of surface signals to the interior of the cell, and others are involved in regulation of gene expression in the nucleus. They form an interactive network of regulatory mechanisms involved in controlling many aspects of cellular function, only part of which is control of growth and differentiation. If these genes, or their products, function abnormally in neoplastic cells, it is not surprising that the latter show a bewildering variety of phenotypic changes, even without the alterations of other genes that also presumably contribute. What then is the evidence that these genes do contribute to the development of neoplastic disease?

There is a massive literature pertaining to the role of oncogenes in the causation of cancer and it would be superfluous to review it in detail here. Discussion of a few well-studied oncogenes will illustrate why there is strong reason to believe that they can indeed act as cancer-causing genes. A primary piece of evidence, of course, comes from the fact that acutely transforming viruses such as Rous sarcoma virus are capable of transforming cells *in vitro* and of causing tumors *in vivo*. Fibroblasts transformed by RSV, for example, are tumorigenic when inoculated into chickens. The specific role of the v-*src* gene in this case is documented by the fact that mutations, such as deletions, within the gene result in loss of transforming capability. Furthermore, cloned v-*src* DNA has been shown to be capable of transforming cells into which it is introduced by transfection. The very rapid development of tumors which characterizes the acutely transforming viruses, however, is in marked contrast to the slow and progressive development of most naturally occurring neoplasms. Despite this there are several lines of evidence that oncogenes play a role in natural tumorigenesis.

Transfection assays, in which DNA from tumor cell lines or tumor tissue is introduced into rodent cells, have shown that about 15–20% of human tumors contain "activated" oncogenes, capable of transforming the recipient cells. The great majority of these have turned out to be members of the *ras* family.

In many cases it has been shown that oncogenes such as *myc* are expressed at high levels in certain neoplasms. We have already discussed one example where translocation of the *myc* gene to immunoglobulin loci is associated with the development of lymphoid neoplasms. Two points related to this phenomenon argue for a causative role of the oncogene in the development of the neoplasm; these are the consistency of the relationship between the deregulation of *myc* transcription resulting from juxtaposition to the immunoglobulin enhancers, and the development of neoplasms in the particular cell types in which the immunoglobulin enhancers would be expected to be active. The *myc* gene is expressed at high levels in several other kinds of tumors. This is true in small cell lung carcinoma of man, for example. It is interesting that this amplification of expression, which may be 20 to 80 times normal, is usually associated with the more highly malignant forms of the tumor. It should also be pointed out that amplification is often a late event in the progression of the tumor, so other factors must be involved in its development.

In many other cases mutations in the oncogene seem to be important in endowing transforming capacity. One of the best examples is provided by the *ras* oncogene family. The *ras* genes most commonly acquire their transforming capabilities by point mutations involving particular amino acids. As already mentioned, the *ras* protein product shares sequence homology with G proteins, and shares their ability to bind and hydrolyze GTP. Normal G proteins are activated by GTP binding and inactivated by its hydrolysis to GDP. The mutations that activate *ras* oncogenes block or greatly reduce the ability to hydrolyze GTP. In this way the transducing functions of the *ras* G protein are continually active, leading to activation of cellular functions that apparently affect the growth and differentiation of the cell. Further support for the role of activated *ras* genes in tumor development comes from studies of carcinogen-induced neoplasms in animals. In a high percentage of these, including mammary tumors, skin carcinomas, thymomas, and kidney tumors, one of the *ras* family of genes has been found to be activated. Furthermore, specific mutations in the gene have been found. Activated *ras* genes have also been found in early papillomas resulting from typical initiation/promotion protocols. This suggests that activation of *ras* contributes to the initiation of the tumor.

Other examples of activation of an oncogene by structural abnormalities is provided by the *abl* and the viral *erb*-B genes. As explained previously, the transposition between chromosomes 9 and 22, which is common in chronic myelogenous leukemia in man, results in a hybrid gene that produces a fusion protein. The *abl* gene product is a tyrosine kinase, whose activity is greatly enhanced in the fusion protein. Again, a structural abnormality in the gene product drives an important cell regulatory mechanism at abnormally high levels. The v-*erb*-B gene encodes a truncated form of the receptor for epidermal growth factor lacking its extracellular domain. In this case, it is thought that the tyrosine kinase activity of the cytoplasmic domain is constitutively activated.

It is generally accepted that, with the exception of the acutely transforming retroviral oncogenes, activation of a single oncogene is insufficient for complete tumorigenesis. Several pieces of evidence support this view. For example, mutated *ras* oncogenes transform rodent fibroblastic cell lines, but not rat embryonic fibroblasts established in primary culture. To explain this it is argued that the cell lines have already undergone some genetic changes accounting for their immortality. Activation of the *ras* gene is apparently sufficient for initiation of tumor development, but not for complete carcinogenesis. Similarly, activation of the *myc* gene alone does not seem to be sufficient for tumorigenesis. For instance, in transgenic mice carrying an activated *myc* gene driven by an immunoglobulin enhancer, the gene is expressed constitutively in the target lymphoid tissue. However, the neoplasms that develop are clonal, suggesting that additional events are required for complete transformation. Similar results have been obtained with *myc* genes constitutively expressed in mammary tissue. It has been proposed that cooperation between nuclear and cytoplasmic oncogenes is particularly important, the former contributing immortalization of the cells, the latter changes in growth control, reflected *in vitro* by properties such as anchorage-independent growth. In agreement with this concept, transformation of primary rat fibroblasts can be achieved by co-transfection with *ras* and a nuclear oncogene such as one of the *myc* genes. As well, several human tumors have been found to contain two activated oncogenes, one from each of these groups.

Some recent elegant experiments in a reconstituted organ system have clarified the cooperative role of *ras* and *myc* in tumorigenesis. When progenitor cells were infected with a retrovirus containing only the *ras* oncogene, the resultant tissue was either normal, or if sufficient numbers of cells were infected, it showed dysplastic changes. On the other hand infection with a virus carrying only *myc* produced hyperplastic changes. Neither oncogene alone produced any tumors. In contrast, infection with a virus carrying both *ras* and *myc* resulted in the development of malignant tumors. Most of the tumors were clonal, suggesting that even in this situation further genetic changes had contributed to the development of malignancy. Nevertheless, these studies confirm the potential for oncogenes, particularly multiple oncogenes acting in concert, to induce neoplastic disease.

The Role of Suppressor Genes

The oncogenes that we have just discussed are often referred to as dominant genes, or dominantly acting genes, because they encode a protein that, *when present,* has a positive action in the induction of cancer. In other words, their gene products promote abnormal cell proliferation or differentiation. There is strong evidence that these are not the only genes involved and that there are genes whose gene product, *when absent,* contributes to the development of neoplasia. Again, several lines of evidence support this view.

Early evidence for cancer-suppressor genes came from work in which transformed, tumorigenic cells were fused with normal cells. When this is done the hybrid cells that result often lose their tumorigenicity. Furthermore, some of these, if maintained in culture, can regain tumorigenicity, and it has been found that this phenomenon is associated with the loss of particular chromosomes derived from the normal parent cell, implying that suppression is the property of particular genes. Somatic cell hybridization can also suppress the tumorigenicity induced by oncogenic viruses and oncogenes. Tumorigenicity of cells transfected with a *ras* oncogene could be suppressed by fusion with normal cells, despite the continued elevated expression of the gene's protein product.

The most direct and compelling evidence for tumor-suppressor genes comes from the study of inherited cancers associated with chromosomal deletions. The best-characterized example is hereditary retinoblastoma in man. Individuals at risk for this tumor are heterozygous for a defect at a particular locus on chromosome 13. In some cases this is due to a deletion. Such individuals therefore carry the defect in all of their somatic cells. They are at high risk for development of retinoblastoma. Analysis of the karyotype of the tumor cells has shown homozygosity of the defect on chromosome 13. This results from either recombinational events leading to loss of the normal chromosome 13 or replacement of the normal by duplication of the defective chromosome. In these patients, therefore, the first genetic event is the inheritance of a mutation at a particular locus (termed the *Rb* locus) through the germ cells. The second event is loss of the normal chromosome in one or a few cells so that they become homozygous for the defective gene. This phenomenon strongly suggests that the product of the *Rb* gene is somehow important in suppressing neoplastic development. Again, the *Rb* gene presumably is not present just to prevent cancer. Undoubtedly it too plays some important regulatory role, perhaps in down-regulating other genes. The *Rb* gene has recently been cloned and its product shown to be expressed in essentially all tissue cells but its function is not yet fully understood. In the light of this widespread expression, it is interesting to note that carriers of retinoblastoma are also at high risk for the development of osteosarcoma. In this case too, the tumors are homozygous for the *Rb* locus. Observations very similar to those for retinoblastoma have been made

in Wilm's tumor and certain other tumors in man, suggesting that there may be a diverse group of so-called cancer-suppressor genes.

Other evidence for suppressor function includes the ability to induce terminal differentiation in some tumor cells by chemical or other signals. This includes cells carrying highly activated oncogenes, such as the myelomonocytic cell line, HL60. In this line granulocytic differentiation can be induced by retinoic acid, and is accompanied by down-regulation of *myc*. In the case of several oncogenes, linked regulatory sequences have been found which control the expression of the gene. It is apparent that the expression of the cellular oncogenes, like other genes, is under strict control. Finally, it is known that the growth of transformed cells, including cells transformed by *ras* or *myc*, can be suppressed by surrounding normal cells. This property appears to be mediated by small molecules that can diffuse through gap junctions, but the mechanisms are otherwise poorly understood.

To recapitulate, there is now overwhelming evidence that genetic mechanisms, including somatic mutation and chromosomal rearrangements, play an important basic role in the genesis of neoplastic disease. In many cases, these mechanisms involve the activation or mutation of oncogenes, which promote the development of neoplasia. Evidence is emerging, however, that another group of genes, whose products suppress the development of cancer, are also important. Since only about 20% of human tumors have been shown to contain activated oncogenes, it is possible that these so-called cancer-suppressor genes play a role at least equal in importance to that of oncogenes. This field is likely to continue to evolve rapidly.

Viral Oncogenesis

Both DNA and RNA viruses can cause neoplasia. As shown in Table 6.5, onco-

Table 6.5
Viruses Causing Neoplasia

Virus	Species	Neoplasm
DNA viruses		
Adenovirus		
Various strains	Hamster	Experimental tumors
Herpesvirus		
Marek's disease virus	Chicken	Lymphosarcoma (Marek's disease)
Rabbit Herpesvirus	Rabbit	Lymphosarcoma
Guinea pig Herpesvirus	Guinea Pig	Lymphosarcoma
Herpesvirus saimiri and	Nonhuman primates,	Lymphosarcoma
Herpesvirus ateles	abnormal hosts	
Epstein-Barr virus	Man	Burkitt's lymphoma (suspected)
		Nasopharyngeal carcinoma (suspected)
Lucké virus	Frog	Renal adenocarcinoma
Papovavirus		
Simian virus 40 (SV40)	Hamster	Experimental sarcoma
Polyomavirus	Mouse	Multiple experimental tumors
Papillomavirus	Dog, cow, man, rabbit	Papilloma
Poxvirus		
Yaba virus	Rhesus monkey	Histiocytoma
Shope fibroma virus	Rabbit	Fibroma (myxomatosis)
RNA viruses		
Retroviruses	Chicken	Lymphosarcoma, sarcoma
	Cat	Lymphosarcoma, leukemias, fibrosarcoma
	Mouse	Lymphosarcoma, leukemias, mammary tumors, sarcomas
	Gibbon ape	Lymphosarcoma
	Reptiles	Sarcomas
	Cow	Lymphosarcoma
	Man	T cell neoplasms

genic DNA viruses include adenoviruses, herpesviruses, papovaviruses, and poxviruses. Adenoviruses do not cause neoplasms in their natural hosts, but some are able to do so in experimental animals, in particular neonatal hamsters. Papovaviruses include the papilloma viruses which cause benign papillomas in dogs, cattle, man, and probably the horse, and which have been implicated in certain malignant neoplasms of man. Poxviruses cause the Shope fibroma of rabbits, and Yaba virus (also a poxvirus) causes histiocytomas in Rhesus monkeys. Herpes-

viruses are probably the most important oncogenic DNA viruses. They are known to cause renal adenocarcinomas in frogs (Lucké virus) and malignant lymphoid neoplasms in rabbits, guinea pigs, nonhuman primates, and chickens. In the latter species, the resultant neoplastic disease is called Marek's disease. One of the most extensively studied of the neoplasms caused by DNA viruses, it is discussed specifically later in this chapter to illustrate aspects of the pathogenesis of naturally occurring neoplastic disease caused by a virus. Herpesviruses have also been implicated in at least three forms of neoplasia in man (Table 6.5), but as yet their role is not fully proven.

All oncogenic RNA viruses belong to the **retrovirus** groups, so named because they possess an enzyme called **reverse transcriptase** or, more correctly, RNA-dependent DNA polymerase. This enzyme is capable of forming DNA using an RNA template, a feat that mammalian cells cannot normally accomplish. The retroviruses fall into two major groups, **endogenous,** those integrated into the host genome and transmitted vertically in a Mendelian fashion, and **exogenous,** those transmitted horizontally between host animals as true infectious agents. All of the retroviruses important in naturally occurring neoplastic disease belong to the latter group. It is important to realize that, although all oncogenic RNA viruses are retroviruses, not all retroviruses are oncogenic. Some, for instance, cause pneumonia, encephalitis, and other diseases in sheep and goats. Even most of those that can cause naturally occurring neoplasms do so in only a small percentage of infected hosts, and can also cause other diseases. Retroviruses cause lymphomas and sarcomas in a number of species including chickens, mice, and cats, lymphomas in cattle and Gibbon apes, and mammary carcinomas in mice. The viruses can be classified according to their ultrastructure into types A, B, or C. Type B retroviruses cause mammary carcinomas in mice, and type C viruses cause the other forms of neoplasia mentioned above. In cats, retroviruses cause lymphoma and, less often, myeloid neoplasia. They are implicated also in other diseases including thymic atrophy, enteric disease, immunosuppression, anemia, and abortion. The causative virus is called feline leukemia virus (FeLV). Besides the murine oncogenic retroviruses, FeLV is one of the most studied of the group. It too will be discussed in more detail later in this chapter.

Mechanisms of Viral Oncogenesis

DNA VIRUSES. In the case of potentially oncogenic DNA viruses, one of two consequences may follow infection. First, the infection may be **productive.** In other words, the cells produce infectious virus and are lysed as a result. Alternatively, the cells may be transformed, in which case the infection is nonproductive, and the cells are not killed. Such transformation does not require complete infectious virus; it can be produced by viral DNA or by portions of it. Therefore, transformation by DNA viruses appears to result from the introduction of specific gene sequences or gene products. Considerable advances have been made in understanding the nature and mechanism of action of these products.

Like the oncogenic retroviruses, oncogenic DNA viruses have been shown to contain oncogenes, that is, genes that can be responsible for neoplastic transformation of infected cells. In contrast to the former, however, the oncogenes of DNA tumor viruses are not closely related to cellular oncogenes, although their gene products may interact. Oncogenic gene products associated with some of the DNA tumor viruses are summarized in Table 6.6.

In the case of oncogenic adenoviruses, neoplastic transformation appears to involve the cooperation of two viral genes, E1A and E1B. Each of these encodes two proteins. The role of each of these domains in neoplastic transformation is not completely clear. However, E1A appears to confer on the cell the property of indefinite growth. Either of the two protein products can do this, but both are required for actual neoplastic transformation. E1A can regulate the transcription of viral, and probably cellular, genes. The E1B gene products alone do not appear to be able to alter cellular phenotype, although both proteins apparently contribute to the development of tumors. The

Table 6.6
Oncogenic Gene Products of DNA Viruses[a]

Virus	Gene Product	Proposed Function	Location
Adenovirus	E1A (26 kDa)	Transcriptional regulation (?)	Nucleus; cytoplasm
	E1A (36 kDa)	Transcriptional regulation	Nucleus; cytoplasm
	E1B (21 kDa)	?	Nuclear membrane
	E1B (55 kDa)	Binds cellular p53 protein, mRNA transport	Nucleus
Polyoma	Large T antigen	DNA synthesis, regulation of transcription	Nucleus
	Middle T antigen	Binds and enhances $pp60^{c-src}$	Plasma membrane
	Small T antigen	?	
SV-40	Large T antigen	DNA synthesis, regulation of transcription, binds p53 protein	Nucleus, plasma membrane
	Small T antigen	?	Cytoplasm
Poxviruses	Vaccinia growth factor	—	Binds to EGF receptor

[a] The abbreviations used are: $pp60^{c-src}$, protein product of the cellular *src* oncogene; EGF, epidermal growth factor.

larger of the two E1B proteins appears to be involved in the transport of mRNA from the nucleus to the cytoplasm.

Most information on papovaviruses has been obtained from the SV40 and polyoma viruses. Polyoma virus contains genes that code for three proteins referred to as **large, middle, and small T antigens.** The large T antigen confers on cells the properties of indefinite growth and a reduced requirement for growth factors. Middle T antigen contributes to other features of the transformed phenotype. SV40 encodes a large and a small T antigen, the former combining the actions of polyoma large and middle T antigens. These gene products may exert their effects through interaction with cellular genes or oncogenes. Polyoma middle T antigen becomes associated with the c-*src* protein product on the inner aspect of the plasma membrane, greatly enhancing its tyrosine kinase activity. SV40 large T antigen interacts with a cellular regulatory protein known as p53, itself a putative oncogene. Interestingly, the large adenovirus E1B protein also interacts with this

protein. The role of the small T antigens is unclear.

The oncogenic gene products of other DNA viruses are much less clearly understood. One other interesting example of interaction of a gene product of a DNA virus and a cellular oncogene is provided by the pox viruses. Some of these contain a gene coding for a growth factor related to EGF, and their ability to produce tumors is thought to be related to binding of this protein to the EGF receptor.

RETROVIRUSES. Through the agency of the enzyme reverse transcriptase, the retroviruses synthesize a DNA copy of their RNA genome. This DNA intermediate becomes incorporated into the genome of the host, where it is known as a provirus. Replication-competent retroviruses contain three genes, *gag*, which codes for the precursor protein of the four virion core proteins, *pol*, coding for the reverse transcriptase, and *env*, coding for the virion envelope glycoproteins. It is relevant to our later discussion to point out that the viral genome also contains regulatory sequences which, in the DNA provirus, are called **long terminal repeats or LTRs,** one being positioned at each end of the viral genome. The LTR contains the viral promotor and enhancing elements, and, as is discussed later, may be important for the abnormal expression of cellular oncogenes in transformed cells.

Two groups of oncogenic retroviruses exist, the acutely transforming retroviruses and those that may cause cancer after a long incubation period. The acutely transforming viruses are typically isolated from tumor tissue, but such isolates are relatively rare compared to the so-called chronic retroviruses. These viruses carry oncogenes that, when introduced into the infected cell, account for their ability to rapidly induce tumors. As we have mentioned before, the viral oncogenes (v-*oncs*) are derived from cellular genes (c-*oncs* or protoonocogenes) that have been transduced by the virus. Usually the proteins encoded by the v-*oncs* are abnormal, being fused to fragments of normal viral proteins or otherwise mutated. In most cases (Rous sarcoma virus being the exception) the acutely transforming retroviruses are replication defective due to loss of part of the normal viral genome during the transduction process. With the exception of Rous sarcoma virus, therefore, they require co-infection with a helper virus for productive infection to occur. The role of oncogenes in the induction of neoplasia has already been discussed and we will not repeat that discussion here.

From the point of view of naturally occurring neoplastic disease, the second group of oncogenic retroviruses, the chronically transforming viruses, are perhaps most important. This group includes feline leukemia virus (FeLV), bovine leukemia virus (BLV), avian leukosis virus (AVL), gibbon ape leukemia virus (GaLV), and murine leukemia viruses (MuLV). These viruses are infectious agents transmitted horizontally from animal to animal. They can cause lymphomas and leukemias in infected animals, but are also associated with a wide spectrum of other disease syndromes. The group also includes two viruses now known to cause certain kinds of T cell lymphomas in man, the human T cell lymphotropic viruses (HTLV I and HTLV II).

The chronically transforming retroviruses do not contain oncogenes, and mechanisms of neoplastic transformation different from those of the "acute" viruses must be involved. Several mechanisms have been proposed, one of the most important being the insertion of the virus close to cellular oncogenes, resulting in their alteration or activation. The provirus of retroviruses can be integrated into multiple sites in the host genome, and the insertion process is believed to be essentially random. However, if tumors caused by these viruses are examined, they are found to be clonal, with the virus integrated into the same site in each cell. This implies that each tumor is derived from a single cell, presumably one in which the provirus, by chance, inserted into a site critical to transformation. This site often appears to be related to a cellular oncogene. For example, in B cell lymphomas caused by AVL, the provirus has been found to be inserted near the c-*myc* gene, and in erythroblastomas caused by the same virus, the integration site is near the c-*erb* gene. Frequently the provirus present in these tumors is defective and may consist of little more than the viral LTR. It is thought that the regulatory sequences contained in the LTR are able to enhance the transcription of the nearby cellular oncogene. Insertion of a retroviral provirus could also disrupt a cellular gene, resulting in an abnormal gene product or abnormal regulation. However, these mechanisms have been less well documented.

Two of the viruses in this group, BLV and HTLV, which are distantly related and which share some biological characteristics, appear to transform cells by yet another mechanism. As in the case of other chronically transforming retroviruses, the individual tumors caused by BLV and HTLV are clonal, each cell having the same integration site. What is unique is that the insertion site differs in tumors from different patients. This suggests that for these two viruses the site of integration is not critical for the development of tumors and need not be close to a cellular oncogene. It appears that HTLV and BLV are able to influence host cell gene expression by **transacting** mechanisms (*i.e.,* mechanisms acting at a distance). A unique region *(X)* in the HTLV genome contains a gene now known as *tat*. In the virus the protein product of this gene appears to interact with sequences in the LTR to help regulate virus production. However, in the infected host T cell the *tat* gene product appears to influence host gene regulation and induces both the expression of IL-2 (interleukin 2) receptors and the production of IL-2. In this way the cells are induced to proliferate through an autocrine mechanism. Later, once the neoplasm is fully developed, the cells become independent of the need for IL-2 and cease to make it. This suggests that, consistent with the general scheme that we have described for tumor progression, further genetic alterations occur in the course of development of T cell neoplasms caused by HTLV.

Examples of Virus-Induced Neoplasms in Animals

In order to put some of the discussion of viral oncogenesis into the perspective of naturally occurring disease, three examples will be discussed. These are Marek's disease of chickens, caused by a DNA virus, feline leukemia, caused by a conventional chronically transforming retrovirus, and bovine leukemia, caused by a virus resembling HTLV.

MAREK'S DISEASE. This disease is a form of lymphoma, which occurs in chickens, caused by a *Herpesvirus* (Marek's disease virus, MDV). Its characteristic lesions include enlargement of peripheral nerves, and lymphoid tumors of T cell origin occurring in a variety of tissues (Fig. 6.24). Enlargement of nerves is due to neoplastic infiltration accompanied by demyelination, proliferation of Schwann cells, and a variable inflammatory infiltrate. Early in the course of infection, MDV causes degeneration of lymphoid tissue in the bursa of Fabricius, the thymus, and the spleen, and of the epithelium of the feather follicles. The degenerative lesions in the feather follicle epithelium are accompanied by the formation of intranuclear and intracytoplasmic inclusion bodies.

Chickens developing Marek's disease become infected at an early age. Infection is fully productive only in the epithelium of feather follicles, and virus is shed in dander, which serves as the source of infectious virus for susceptible chickens. In lymphoid cells, infection is essentially nonproductive, although limited production of viral DNA and antigens sometimes occurs. This nonproductive infection is accompanied by transformation. Tumor cells contain multiple copies of MDV DNA, the number varying between different chickens. The cellular location of viral DNA is not yet firmly established, although there is some evidence that viral DNA can be integrated into the host genome. Infection with MDV gives rise to a number of viral or virus-coded antigens in infected cells. One antigen, **Marek's associated tumor-specific antigen** (MATSA) was thought to be a virus-specific membrane antigen that could be used as a marker for neoplastic transformation in Marek's disease. However, recent data suggest that MATSA is expressed on non-neoplastic, activated T cells and that it is not specific for Marek's disease.

Resistance to Marek's disease is influenced by host genetic factors, and high-susceptibility and low-susceptibility strains of chickens have been developed. Resistance is not against initial infection

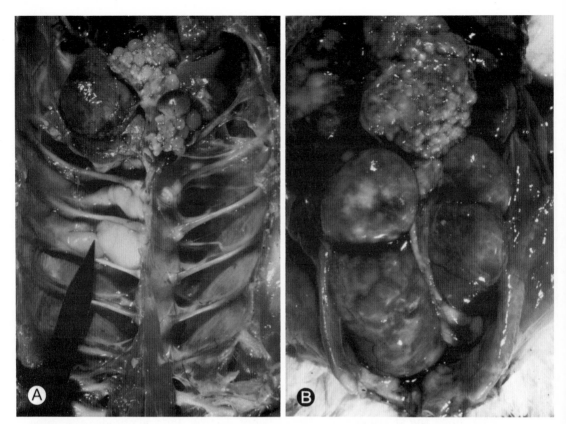

Figure 6.24 *A* and *B*.   Lesions of Marek's Disease. *A,* in this chicken, nerves infiltrated by neoplastic lymphocytes are enlarged *(pointer).* These intercostal lesions are very suggestive of Marek's disease. *B,* both the kidney and the ovary in this bird are enlarged due to infiltration by neoplastic lymphocytes. (Courtesy of Department of Avian and Aquatic Animal Medicine, Cornell University.)

but against later amplification of infection and tumor development. As thymectomy, but not bursectomy, reduces resistance, it seems to depend on intact T cell function, but not on antibody. However, antibody does develop to MDV antigens including, in some cases, MATSA. There is also some evidence that antibody may provide partial protection. For example, in chicks with maternal antibody the disease has a prolonged incubation period and the extent of lesions may be reduced.

Chickens may acquire active immunity to Marek's disease, and this disease provides one of the few instances, so far, in which vaccination against a neoplastic disease has been possible. Vaccination may

be carried out either with an attenuated or nonpathogenic MDV or with *Herpesvirus* of turkeys (HVT). HVT cross-reacts with MDV, but it is nonpathogenic for the chicken and may therefore be used as a vaccine. Vaccinated chickens remain susceptible to infection, although viremia and shedding of the virus from the feather follicles is reduced. Once again, immunity against development of tumors is involved. Vaccination appears to prevent the proliferation of transformed cells as well as reducing the extent of virus replication. The mechanisms involved in this antitumor immunity are not clear, but appear to be cell mediated. Cytotoxic T cells directed against both MATSA- and

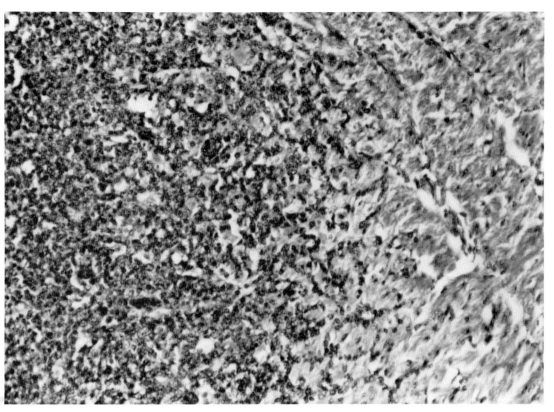

Figure 6.24 C.   Lesions of Marek's Disease. In this case, pleomorphic neoplastic lymphocytes infiltrate the myocardium.

MDV-specific antigens are present in vaccinated chickens. The success of vaccination against Marek's disease is probably due to a combination of antiviral and antitumor immunity, involving several mechanisms.

Mechanisms by which MDV causes neoplasia are poorly understood. Although viral DNA exists in multiple copies in host cells and possibly is integrated into the host genome, no definitive oncogenes have been identified.

To recapitulate, Marek's disease illustrates several important features of neoplasia induced by DNA viruses. Transformed cells do not produce virus, but viral DNA is present in multiple copies in the cells, perhaps in an integrated form. Natural susceptibility is under genetic influence. Transformed cells contain viral and membrane-associated antigens, and immunity can be induced against the development of tumors. What makes Marek's disease unique is the fact that it is the first neoplastic disease to be successfully controlled by vaccination.

FELINE LYMPHOSARCOMA. Feline leukemia virus (FeLV), as indicated earlier in this chapter, can cause a variety of diseases in cats, the one of interest to this discussion being lymphosarcoma (lymphoma). FeLV is one of the best studied of the oncogenic retroviruses. Its existence was first suggested by epidemiologic studies of clusters of feline lymphosarcoma, and its recognition was seminal to the realization that infectious viruses could cause naturally occurring cancers.

Infection by FeLV is common in random, outbred, cat populations, particularly where groups of cats live in close association. The virus is excreted in saliva and is spread primarily by horizontal transmission. Infection is usually followed by a mild, transient illness a few weeks after exposure. The majority of infected cats develop an immune response to the gp70 and p15E envelope proteins, clear the virus, and become immune. Those that do not become persistently infected, some developing lymphosarcoma months to years later, others dying of other FeLV related diseases. The lesions in feline lymphosarcoma consist of solid lymphoid tumors in a variety of organs (Fig. 6.25), or, less commonly, leukemia may occur. Neoplasms derived from T lymphocytes are most common, although B cell tumors also occur. FeLV can also induce myeloid and erythroid leukemias. Tumors may be either virus positive or virus negative. In other words, transformed cells may, or may not, replicate virus. Lymphosarcoma may also occur in cats in which FeLV cannot be detected, although these animals often have a history of exposure to the virus, and their tumor cells bear the tumor-specific antigen FOCMA (*see* below). This suggests that FeLV also plays an etiologic role in such "FeLV-negative" lymphosarcomas.

FeLV-transformed cells contain a number of virus-specific antigens. These include type-specific viral envelope antigens, group-specific internal virion antigens, and the virus-specified **feline oncornavirus cell membrane antigen, or FOCMA.** (Oncornavirus is an older name for oncogenic RNA viruses.) FOCMA, as its name implies, is expressed on the surface membrane of transformed cells but not on normal lymphocytes, even those infected with FeLV. It is therefore a tumor-specific antigen. The exact nature of FOCMA is unclear. It is not part of the virion, but it shows some relationship to the gp70 envelope protein of a particular group of FeLV, FeLV group C. Antibody may develop to viral envelope

antigens, to FOCMA, and to other viral antigens. Antibody to the envelope proteins, gp70 and p15E, is virus neutralizing and will protect against infection. Antibody to FOCMA does not protect against infection but, if present in significant titers, protects against the development of lymphosarcoma in infected cats, and against sarcomas induced by feline sarcoma viruses (*see* below). Thus, cats in a natural population exposed to FeLV may fail to become infected and therefore not develop immunity; may become infected, develop antiviral immunity and clear the virus; may fail to develop immunity to the virus but develop anti-FOCMA antibodies that protect against the development of tumors; or may fail to develop either form of immunity and develop lymphosarcoma or other form of FeLV-related disease. Chronically infected carrier animals also occur. The response of animals to infection depends, in part, on the dose of virus and age at exposure. Young kittens often do not mount an adequate immune response and thus acquire active infection, which may lead to the development of neoplasia.

The mechanism of transformation by FeLV has not been fully elucidated. Presumably, mechanisms related to viral integration, similar to those of other chronically transforming retroviruses, are involved. There is evidence of activation of c-*myc* in some feline lymphosarcomas.

FeLV also appears to be uniquely able to transduce cellular oncogenes to produce acutely transforming retroviruses, the **feline sarcoma viruses (FeSV).** Amongst the isolates of FeSV so far obtained from naturally occurring feline fibrosarcomas, seven different oncogenes, namely *fes, fms, sis, abl, fgr, K-ras,* and *kit,* have been shown to have been transduced. These FeSVs are associated with FeLV helper viruses. In each case so far examined, the gene product is a fusion of the product of the viral *gag* gene and the cellular oncogene. FeSV-induced fibrosar-

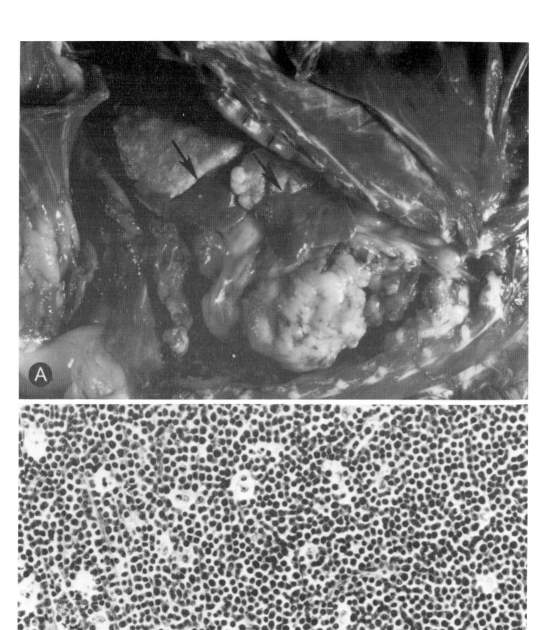

Figure 6.25   Lesions of Feline Lymphosarcoma. *A,* thymic lymphosarcoma in a cat. A large mass of neoplastic tissue displaces the lungs dorsally. The lungs are partially atelectatic *(arrows).* This is one of the more common lesions of feline lymphosarcoma. *B,* The mass consists of a sheet of relatively uniform neoplastic lymphocytes. The cells in the clear spaces are macrophages that have phagocytosed necrotic neoplastic cells.

comas do not occur in clusters, are apparently not transmitted horizontally, and presumably arise *de novo* in FeLV-infected cats.

Feline lymphosarcoma or leukemia therefore also demonstrates several biologic characteristics of virus-induced neoplasia, some of which it shares with Marek's disease. The disease is horizontally transmitted, infection may be productive of virus or not, and it is associated with specific viral and cell membrane antigens. The association of productive infection with cell transformation is characteristic of oncogenic retroviruses and contrasts with oncogenic DNA viruses. FeLV infection is also of interest because antibody against a tumor-specific antigen, FOCMA, can protect against the development of neoplastic disease. Tumor immunology will be discussed at some length later in this chapter, but the ability of an effective immune response to FOCMA to protect against neoplastic disease is one of the best-documented examples of effective tumor immunity.

BOVINE LEUKEMIA. Enzootic bovine leukemia has been recognized as a probable infectious neoplastic disease for many years. Its occurrence had been linked to the introduction of an animal from a herd containing affected animals to a naive herd, and it could be experimentally transmitted. The cause of the disease was revealed to be a retrovirus, bovine leukemia virus (BLV), when virus particles were recognized in cultures of lymphocytes from animals with persistent lymphocytosis, a second syndrome associated with the neoplastic disease. As already mentioned, BLV is now known to be closely related to the HTLV family of retroviruses.

BLV is an exogenous retrovirus that induces B cell leukemia or lymphosarcoma, as well as a non-neoplastic disease referred to as **persistent lymphocytosis.** Infection is thought to involve biting insects as vectors and can be iatrogenic, through the use of common hypodermic needles. BLV produces persistent infections, and infected animals develop a strong immune response to viral antigens. Development of neoplastic disease is a rare event in infected animals. Sheep can be infected experimentally and are very sensitive to the development of tumors, also usually of the B cell type. Goats can also be infected but are resistant to tumor development.

As discussed earlier, there are striking similarities between tumors induced by BLV and those induced by HTLV. Bovine tumors from a single animal have a clonal integration site, but this site varies from animal to animal. Tumor cells contain one to four integrated copies of the provirus, but they express no viral RNA or proteins. BLV contains a unique gene region, *px*, corresponding to the X region of HTLV. The product of this region is also thought to be transacting, and to be required at least for the initiation of transformation. As cultured transformed B cells do not express any part of the BLV genome, it appears that the product of the *px* region is not required for maintenance of the transformed phenotype. This is very reminiscent of the findings for HTLV and human T cell neoplasms, and again suggests that further genetic changes are required for development of the fully transformed cell.

Bovine leukemia and BLV therefore further illustrate the parallels that exist between neoplastic (and other) diseases in man and other animals. There is little reason to doubt that the study of such animal models is valuable to an understanding of mechanisms involved in human disease and, conversely, that many principles established for human disease can be applied to those of animals.

The Clonal Nature of Neoplasms

If carcinogenesis is the result of rare somatic mutations, and in particular if multiple "hits" are necessary, only rarely should an initially normal target cell acquire the changes that result in a neoplasm. Further, it would be expected that every cell in a tumor would be derived from that single altered cell. The tumor cells should, in other words, form a **clone,** or be **monoclonal.** Whether or not this is actually the case can be investigated by examining certain cell markers.

Such investigations indicate that the great majority of naturally occurring tumors, at least in man where they have been adequately studied, are monoclonal. For example, both in man and in dogs multiple myelomas, neoplasms of plasma cell origin, secrete a single class of immunoglobulin. This would not be expected if the tumors were derived from multiple plasma cells. Likewise the neoplastic cells in Waldenström's macroglobulinemia secrete only IgM and bear IgM on their surface.

A second useful marker system results from the process of **X-inactivation mosaicism.** In each somatic cell, during the early growth of the female embryo, one X chromosome of each pair is randomly inactivated. Some enzymes that occur in two forms (*i.e.,* isoenzymes) are coded for by genes carried on the X chromosome. If an individual is heterozygous for such an enzyme, then the form carried by any particular cell will be either one or the other, depending on which X chromosome is inactivated, but not both. In man, one such enzyme is glucose-6-phosphate dehydrogenase (G6PD). The two forms may be designated $G6PD^a$ and $G6PD^b$. In a particular cell, if the X chromosome carrying the gene for $G6PD^a$ is inactivated, the cell will contain $G6PD^b$, and *vice versa*. Because X chromosome inactivation is random, tissues, being made up of many cells, contain both enzyme forms, although each cell contains only one. If a neoplasm arises in a heterozygous individual from a single altered cell, then the neoplastic tissue should contain only one isoenzyme (Fig. 6.26). Using this system

in man, a number of types of tumors have been examined and, in almost all cases, tumors have proven to be monoclonal at the time of study. In the case of multiple tumors, such as multiple leiomyomas of the uterus, any one tumor has a single enzyme type, although different tumors in the same organ may have different isoenzymes. Similar studies, using chimeric animals produced in the laboratory, have yielded similar findings.

These results imply that most tumors are derived from a single altered cell. This is compatible with the "multiple hit" theory of carcinogenesis. It also argues against the idea, suggested in the past, that normal cells may be recruited into neoplasms.

Occasional neoplasms are found in man which contain cells of both enzyme types. In particular, the hereditary tumors neurofibroma and trichoepithelioma are usually of mixed enzyme pattern. This suggests that, in these cases, tumors are derived from a number of altered cells. This finding could be explained by arguing that the genetic defect carried by all of the patient's cells would make it more likely that several cells in a given area could undergo additional events leading to polyclonal neoplasms. Similarly, it has been shown in mice, using the marker enzyme phosphoglycerate kinase, that tumors induced by the carcinogen 3-methylcholanthrene are polyclonal. This effect is dose related, very low doses of carcinogen tending to produce monoclonal tumors. Therefore, it seems likely that the production of polyclonal tumors by high doses of chemical carcinogen are due to the initiation of many cells, making progression to multiple neoplasms relatively likely. The possibility that tumors arise as polyclonal populations with subsequent elimination of all but the most aggressive clones must be considered. However, there is little or no evidence for this.

Other information also can be obtained from this system. For example, in chronic

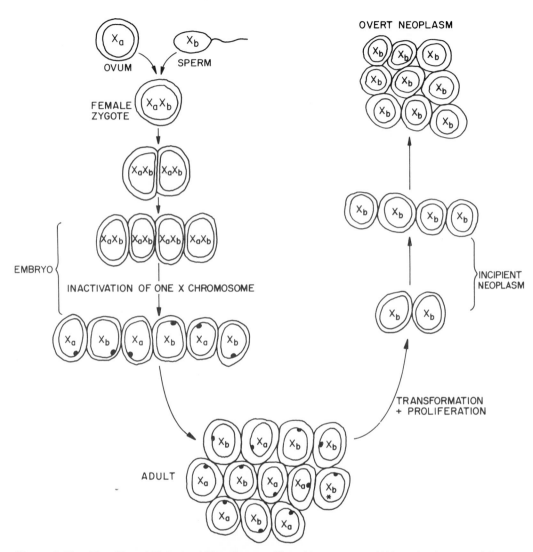

Figure 6.26.   The Clonal Nature of Neoplasms. The phenomenon of X-inactivation mosaicism can be used to test the hypothesis that neoplasms are clonal, or derived from a single transformed cell. During the early development of the female embryo, one X chromosome is inactivated. This is a random process and, if the individual is heterozygous for an isoenzyme (indicated here as $_a$ and $_b$) coded for by genes on the X chromosome, each cell in the adult will carry one or the other enzyme form. If only one cell, indicated by *asterisk* (*), undergoes neoplastic transformation, all of the cells in the resultant tumor will bear the same isoenzyme. This is usually the case, and most tumors are believed to be monoclonal in origin.

myelogenous leukemia of man, all red blood cells, as well as the neoplastic white blood cells, are of one isoenzyme type. This implies that the alteration leading to the neoplastic disease occurs in a primitive stem cell. Dysplastic lesions, and carcinoma *"in situ"* also appear to be monoclonal by this criterion. The latter finding makes the possibility of clonal elimination an unlikely explanation of monoclonality of tumors.

Vascularization of Neoplasms

Neoplastic cells, like all other cells, need a supply of nutrients and oxygen and a way to rid themselves of waste products in order to survive. Diffusion of oxygen and other substances can occur over a range of only about 150 μm, so cells need to be within this distance of capillary vessels. Tumors therefore must become vascularized in order to grow to a significant size. It has been known for many years that proliferation of blood vessels occurs in tissues adjacent to tumors, and that capillaries from those tissues penetrate and vascularize the neoplasm. It is only in recent years, however, that this process, known as **tumor angiogenesis,** has been recognized as a specific biological phenomenon.

Several lines of evidence support the contention that lack of vascularization limits the growth of neoplasms. For instance, when fragments of tumors are transplanted to avascular sites such as the anterior chamber of the eye, they do not grow beyond about 2 mm in diameter. At this stage, cells near the surface still proliferate, but the mass does not enlarge because of cell death in the center of the mass. Moreover, if neoplastic tissue is transplanted to the cornea it grows as a thin plate between the layers of corneal stroma until it nears the vascular bed at the limbus. At that stage, when neoplastic cells are within about 2 mm of the vascular supply, small vessels begin to grow into the cornea toward the mass, which they eventually reach and penetrate. Following vascularization, the rate of growth of the mass increases dramatically.

A number of steps are involved in the vascularization of tissue *in vivo*. New capillaries are formed by sprouting, mainly from venules. The basement membrane of the venule is locally degraded, probably due to secretion of collagenase and plasminogen activator by endothelial cells. Endothelial cells migrate toward the angiogenic stimulus, in this case a developing tumor, align to form sprouts, then develop lumina. Continued growth of the budding capillaries is accompanied by mitosis of cells near the leading edge of the sprout. The formation of anastomotic capillary loops is followed by the establishment of blood flow. It seems likely that signals are required to initiate these events in both physiological and pathological situations. This realization has led to the search for signals that might be involved in angiogenesis, including tumor angiogenesis.

It is now known that the vascularization of tumors is stimulated by diffusible substances secreted by neoplastic cells or other cells associated with the neoplasm, in particular, macrophages. A number of such substances have been demonstrated in tumor extracts, including one initially called **tumor angiogenesis factor (TAF).** It is now recognized that several well-characterized endothelial growth factors, which may be produced by neoplastic or normal cells, are involved in angiogenesis. Other mediators, less well characterized, probably also exist.

Amongst the most important of these substances is the family of **heparin-binding growth factors.** These have been referred to by a variety of names, but they correspond to the fibroblast growth factors, basic FGF and acidic FGF. These GFs, which have been discussed earlier in this chapter, are potent mitogens for endothelial cells and are angiogenic *in vivo*. Another potent angiogenic factor that has been isolated from tumor cells is **angiogenin,** a 14.4 kDa polypeptide that has been shown to be a ribonuclease. It is not known whether this activity is related to its angiogenic properties. It is not a mitogen for endothelial cells, suggesting that it acts through an intermediate mechanism, perhaps by causing release of other angiogenic factors from tissue cells such as macrophages. The transforming growth factors, **TGF-α** and **TGF-β,** also are angiogenic *in vivo*. TGF-α is an endothelial cell mitogen, but TGF-β inhibits proliferation of endothelial cells in culture. It too may act by stimulating macrophages to release mitogens. Macrophages have been demonstrated to secrete factors stimulating angiogenesis, including **tumor necrosis factor (TNF-αs).**

Based on these concepts, tumors can be considered to grow in two phases (Fig. 6.27). Avascular growth precedes tumor vascularization and during this phase a tumor can reach only 1–2 mm in diameter before it becomes dormant in terms of total tumor growth. This might provide one explanation for the clinical observation of dormancy, in which metastatic lesions develop many years after the removal of the primary mass. Carcinoma *in situ* also might be regarded as an example of growth in the avascular phase. It has been suggested that such lesions are limited in size until the basement membrane is breached and the neoplasm is vascularized. Whether the basement membrane is breached by tumor cells or by proliferating vessels is not yet established. Preneoplastic lesions have also been shown to have increased angiogenic capabilities.

In the vascular phase of growth, tumor cells initially grow exponentially. The growth of large tumors is, however, limited by necrosis as we have already discussed. It is often said that rapidly growing malignant neoplasms "outgrow their blood supply," but more plausible explanations are provided by the observations that the surface area of the vascular network relative to tumor mass decreases as

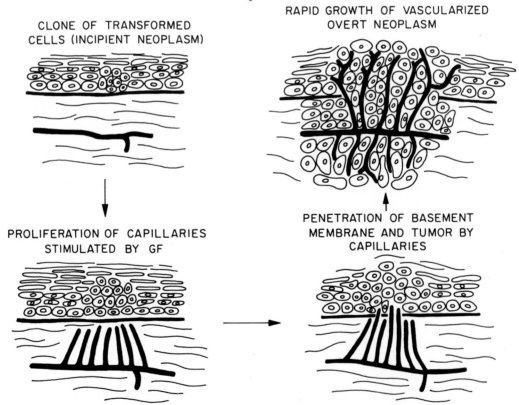

Figure 6.27. Effect of Angiogenesis on Tumor Growth. Prior to vascularization, the incipient tumor is limited in its ability to grow. Neoplastic cells produce endothelial growth factors, such as FGF, which stimulate the growth of blood vessels toward the tumor. Once the tumor is vascularized the neoplastic cells are able to proliferate to produce an overt tumor. The abbreviations used are: GF, growth factor; FGF, fibroblast growth factor.

the tumor grows, and that tumors develop high interstitial fluid pressure, which compresses capillaries within the mass. Necrosis is probably largely due to ischemia resulting from these phenomena.

Tumor angiogenesis also can be inhibited, one source of an inhibitor being cartilage. Normal hyaline cartilage is of course devoid of a blood supply in the adult animal. Furthermore, it is well known to resist invasion by neoplasms. For example, osteosarcomas rarely invade across joint spaces (Fig. 6.28), apparently due to resistance to invasion by the articular cartilage. Experimentally it has been shown that fragments of viable cartilage can inhibit the vascularization of transplanted tumors, for example, in the cornea. If the cartilage is first boiled this inhibition does not occur, suggesting that viable cartilage secretes some inhibitory substance. The nature of this substance is as yet unclear, although it has been reported to have protease-inhibiting properties. The significance of possibly being able to inhibit vascularization of tumors is obvious. Without vascularization the growth of neoplasms, in particular metastases, would be limited, and much of their clinical significance might be avoided. It is of some interest, therefore, that heparin or certain fragments of heparin, when administered with cortisone or some of its metabolites lacking glucocorticoid or mineralocorticoid activity, also inhibits angiogenesis. This combination of drugs has been shown to cause regression of tumors in experimental animals, and even to eradicate them completely in some cases. Thus, interference with

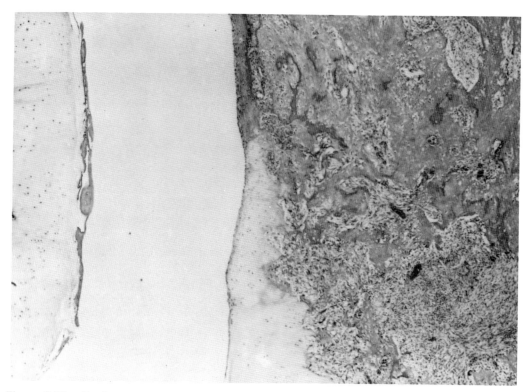

Figure 6.28.   Resistance of Articular Cartilage to Neoplastic Invasion. The osteosarcoma at the *right* of the micrograph has compressed but not invaded the articular cartilage, and the joint space in this cat is not involved. This is the usual finding in osteosarcomas and presumably reflects the general resistance of cartilage to neoplastic invasion.

tumor angiogenesis may prove to be a promising therapeutic approach.

MECHANISMS OF INVASION AND METASTASIS

The spread of neoplastic cells from a primary tumor by tissue invasion and metastasis is the most serious and life-threatening characteristic of malignant cells. It is important, therefore, to explore and understand the mechanisms by which cancer cells are able to invade and metastasize. In recent years some light has begun to be shed on these processes.

Tumor Heterogeneity

An important characteristic of neoplasms is that the cells making up the tumor are not identical. It is now well recognized that these cells vary considerably in a wide variety of characteristics including morphology, biochemical properties, cell surface antigens and receptors, growth rate, susceptibility to therapeutic interventions, and susceptibility to immune attack. Such morphologic variability is easily appreciated during histopathologic examination, when it is termed **pleomorphism** and forms one of the criteria for malignancy. This variation between cells making up a single neoplastic mass has been dubbed **tumor heterogeneity,** and it extends to the ability of tumor cell populations to invade and metastasize. We will have more to say about this when we discuss mechanisms of metastasis, but for now we will consider ways in which such heterogeneity arises.

It may be confusing to try to reconcile the fact that the majority of tumors arise from single altered cells with the fact that all tumors contain a heterogeneous cell population. Perhaps the best way to rationalize this is to consider that the whole organism arises from a single cell and is a clone, yet is made up of cells with markedly different characteristics. This analogy can be taken further because the properties that characterize tumor cell

heterogeneity are heritable in the sense that they are passed on as cells divide. Differences between tumor cells in a single neoplasm, therefore, arise during the evolution of the tumor, that is, during tumor progression.

As we have already discussed, tumor progression is generally considered to be the result of accruement of genetic alterations, and neoplastic cell populations are regarded as being genetically unstable. However, variants can arise very rapidly in tumors, and epigenetic mechanisms, rather than true mutations, have also been proposed to account for this. In particular, attention has been drawn to the role of methylation of DNA, a known mechanism of inactivation of gene expression which is heritable from cell to cell. Conversely, demethylation can reactivate genes. It has been proposed that progressive hypomethylation of DNA in tumors results in altered gene expression. On the other hand neoplastic cell populations are generally recognized as having high mutation rates. Since many genes can contribute to the characteristics that we are discussing, accumulated mutations in a number of genes could occur quite quickly. We do not wish to reopen the argument of mutation *versus* epigenetic change. Suffice it to conclude that both mechanisms most likely contribute to the generation of tumor cell heterogeneity.

A fascinating aspect of tumor heterogeneity concerns the interaction of subclonal cell populations within a neoplasm to stabilize the population as a whole. When clones have been isolated from heterogeneous tumor cell populations they have been found to be highly unstable. Passage either *in vivo* or *in vitro* generates variant cell populations much more quickly than such variants emerge in polyclonal, or heterogeneous, populations. When several clones are cultured together, however, the phenotype of the constituent cells is stabilized. This indicates that interactions between the tumor cells in polyclonal tumors is important in establishing an equilibrium in which the generation of new variants is limited. The mechanisms underlying these interactions are unknown, but they have some important implications. As mentioned later, individual metastases are believed to arise from single cells that become established at a site distant from the primary tumor, that is, they are clones. Although they are initially homogeneous, cellular heterogeneity quickly arises. It appears that the same phenomena occur *in vivo,* driving the emergence of new variants. Another implication is that the reduction of tumor cell burdens by therapeutic means presumably reduces tumor cell heterogeneity again driving the generation of new variants. Some of these may acquire increased resistance to the treatment, a possibility which forms part of the rationalization for the use of multiple drugs in the treatment of cancer.

Tumor Cell Invasion

Tissue invasion is important as a mechanism of local spread of neoplastic tissue and as a mechanism of local tissue destruction. It is also a prerequisite for metastasis, being necessary for neoplastic cells to gain access to, and to leave, the vasculature. In general, poorly differentiated neoplasms demonstrate more aggressive invasiveness than those that are well differentiated. Three basic mechanisms, **mechanical pressure, tumor cell motility,** and **enzymatic destruction of local tissue barriers,** have been proposed to account for the ability of malignant cells to invade normal tissues. It is possible that all three contribute.

It has been proposed that mechanical pressure resulting from rapid growth results in neoplastic cells being forced into the surrounding tissues. This is certainly an oversimplification because, although they are exceptions to the usual, some neoplasms which grow rapidly are noninvasive and some which are highly invasive grow slowly. It is possible also to inhibit tumor cell proliferation without preventing invasion. Furthermore, such a mechanism does not account for the fact that individual or small groups of neoplastic cells are commonly observed in the stroma removed from the main mass.

In studying malignant neoplasms histologically, one often observes cords of neoplastic cells apparently insinuating themselves between surrounding tissue elements, or individual tumor cells in the surrounding tissue completely detached from the main mass. Such appearances suggest that the neoplastic cells can actively migrate through the tissue. In fact, tumor cells have been directly observed, under experimental conditions, to migrate through tissues. This includes vessel walls, either between endothelial cells or through gaps created by endothelial cell necrosis. Ultrastructurally, invading neoplastic cells are seen to possess long, thin processes squeezing between tissue structures. Thus, it seems reasonable to assume that active migration by tumor cells is an important part of invasion. Unfortunately, there is conflicting evidence regarding the role of active cell motility in neoplastic invasion. Detailed studies of particular neoplastic cell lines show poor correlation between invasiveness and motility *in vitro,* and treatment with inhibitors of cell motility, such as cytochalasin B, apparently does not reduce tissue invasion or the rate of metastasis. We will proceed on the assumption, however, that neoplastic cells can be translocated from the primary mass into the surrounding tissue. Part of this process seems to involve detachment of tumor cells from the main mass, a phenomenon that can be observed consistently in malignant neoplasms. The mechanisms of cell detachment have not been well characterized, but the process seems to occur most readily in poorly differentiated tumor cells. It may involve changes in intercellular junctions, such as desmosomes, or in **cell adhesion molecules (CAMs)** expressed on the cell surface. The latter are exemplified by neural cell adhesion molecule (N-CAM) and liver cell adhesion molecule (L-CAM). The latter is found on a variety of epithelial cells. CAMs are now recognized to play an important role in intercellular recognition, inductive events during development, and maintenance of adult tissues. They are tempting targets, therefore, for speculation concerning some of the altered behavior of neoplastic cells. Few data exist on changes in CAMs on transformed cells. However, in certain cells transformed by the Rous sarcoma virus there is a dramatic reduction in the expression of N-CAM with a concomitant reduction in cellular adhesiveness. These cells also displays increased motility, but whether the two events are related is unclear. This seems not to be a generalized phenomenon either, as a different, chemically transformed cell line does not show any reduction in the expression of N-CAM.

There are considerably more data to support the role of various enzymes in the localized destruction of tissue surrounding a neoplasm. The main barrier that invading tumor cells must overcome is the **extracellular matrix.** This consists of a network of collagen and elastic fibers embedded in a gel containing proteoglycans, glycosaminoglycans, and various proteins. The invasiveness of some neoplastic cells has been correlated with their production of enzymes capable of destroying components of the matrix. The enzymes generally implicated in this process are proteinases (endopeptidases), hydrolyzing proteins in the matrix, and glycosidases, hydrolyzing carbohydrate components.

Collagen is the most abundant protein in the intracellular matrix. Because of this, particular attention has been paid to the role of collagenases in tumor invasion. These enzymes are capable of cleaving the triple helix of collagen at specific sites. A number of neoplastic and normal cells have been shown to secrete collagenases, and the production of collagenases has been positively correlated with tumor invasiveness. Despite this, there is some doubt about their role in the degradation of collagen *in situ.* In the extracellular matrix most of the collagen is assembled into fibers that are extremely resistant to the action of collagenases. It is more likely that collagen could be degraded by other proteolytic enzymes, including trypsin, plasmin, cathepsins, and elastase, which attack the non–triple helical region of collagen. This attack destabilizes the collagen fiber, making it susceptible to further degradation. Again, there is evidence that some tumor cells can secrete enzymes of this type, and that inhibitors of proteinases can reduce invasiveness.

Basement membranes present a special barrier against tumor invasion. They are thin, sheet-like structures that support certain tissue types, in particular epithelium, and separate them from connective tissues. Basement membranes are composed of type IV collagen associated with heparan sulfate proteoglycans, and specialized proteins including laminin. Although not strictly germane to the discussion of tissue destruction by invading tumor cells, it is worth mentioning that laminin is a molecule involved in cellular substrate recognition processes. It can induce changes in cell attachment, growth, migration, and morphology. Certain cells, including some neoplastic cells, bear specific receptors for laminin and interaction of tumor cells with laminin appears to play a role in metastasis. This is discussed below. Some neoplastic cells produce a specific collagenase capable of cleaving type IV collagen, that is, a type IV collagenase. Collagens of the basement membrane are also particularly prone to degradation by the proteinases that we have already discussed.

Another enzyme system worthy of specific mention is **plasminogen activator (PA)**. There is evidence that urokinase-PA (uPA) is involved in matrix degradation in the tumor invasion zone. u-PA converts plasminogen to plasmin, an enzyme with broad proteolytic activity and capable of activating latent collagenase. In at least one experimental system it has been shown that inhibition of u-PA by specific antibodies reduced metastasis, presumably by interfering with invasion by neoplastic cells.

Tumor cells themselves are not the only source of enzymes capable of degrading the intercellular matrix. Interactions of tumor cells with non-neoplastic host cells, in particular fibroblasts, has been shown to induce increased production of enzymes by the latter. Continuous interaction between the cells is required for this effect to be sustained. Endothelial cells probably also play a similar role. The ability of growing capillaries to invade an avascular tissue, such as the cornea, is well known, and vascularization of a growing tumor may promote local tissue destruction and invasion.

The action of these enzymes results in a drastically altered extracellular environment. Destruction of collagen fibers is thought to produce a marked expansion and hydration of the ground substance of the matrix, promoting invasion by neoplastic cells. Some of the cleavage products are also thought to have significant biological actions, including chemotactic and growth-promoting effects. For example, growth stimulatory activity has been associated with heparan sulfate fragments. Although not yet documented, this may be due to release of FGF. Substances other than enzymes also could promote invasiveness. Prostaglandins, for instance, are thought to be secreted by some neoplasms and to play a role in promoting lysis and consequently invasion of bone.

The destruction of intercellular matrix and growth of the tumor, in particular in the case of carcinomas, is accompanied by the deposition of new, abnormal connective tissue rich in glycosaminoglycans. This connective tissue and its matrix is thought to promote migration of tumor cells. Furthermore, compartmentalization of glycosaminoglycans in different concentrations is thought to lead to fluid streaming, which might also promote cellular translocation.

Interaction of certain tissues with the tumor also is important in limiting invasive behavior. This is particularly apparent in the case of hyaline cartilage and may be due to mechanical barriers provided by the tissue or to specific mechanisms such as inhibition of angiogenesis. Inflammation in tumors may either increase or reduce their ability to invade, depending on the balance between destruction of surrounding tissue and destruction of tumor cells.

Metastasis

Metastasis, the ultimate hallmark of malignancy, constitutes the greatest threat to the life of a patient suffering from neoplastic disease. It is therefore very important to understand why it occurs and what influences it. Here we will attempt to summarize current knowledge of the biologic mechanisms that influence the metastatic process.

The Metastatic Process

It is now clear that metastasis is an extremely complex, but inefficient, process. Even in a tumor capable of metastasis, only a fraction of a percent of neoplastic cells released into the circulation survive to form new growths. However, tumors are capable of shedding literally millions of neoplastic cells into the circulation each day, so that if even a tiny fraction survive, many metastases can be formed. To produce metastases, tumor cells must successfully accomplish a number of steps. They must detach from the primary mass, invade local tissue, penetrate blood vessels or lymphatics, and release emboli. The embolic tumor cells must survive in the circulation, be arrested in small vascular channels in distant sites, again penetrate the vessel wall and invade locally, proliferate, and become vascularized (Fig. 6.29). Metastasis is therefore a step-wise process. Because only those cells able to accomplish *all* of these feats can produce metastasis, it is also generally considered to be a selective process.

Vascular Invasion

We have already discussed in some detail the mechanisms that are thought to be involved in invasion of local tissue. Here we will simply reinforce some concepts that are particularly related to ways in which tumor cells penetrate vessels to gain access to the circulation.

A distinction is often made between the lymphatic and the hematogenous routes of metastatic dissemination. This concept is convenient for the purposes of discussion, but the final consequences are similar. Although tumor cells initially may enter either lymphatics or blood vessels, they readily exchange between the two systems. Lymph, of course, eventually drains into the vena cava, and venolymphatic anastomoses have been demonstrated in other tissues. Cells have been shown to pass from lymphatics to blood vessels and the reverse, sometimes migrating through tissue spaces to do so.

Despite these caveats, the early pattern of metastasis can be influenced by the route of dissemination. Neoplastic cells entering the lymphatic system tend to be carried to the regional lymph node. It is a common belief that, once there, tumor emboli will be filtered out. Although this can occur, the lymph node can be bypassed, either by cells moving through the lymph node to the efferent lymphatics or by passing through anastomosing vessels in the perinodal tissue. When embolic neoplastic cells do reach the draining lymph node they enter the subcapsular sinus where they may be arrested and grow (Fig. 6.30). As the metastatic lesion develops, cells grow into the cortical sinuses and medullary sinuses and eventually destroy and replace the normal nodal tissue. Well before the latter occurs, however, neoplastic cells are present in the efferent lymphatics, and these may establish metastatic lesions in more distant lymph nodes or in other organs.

The importance of the regional lymph node as a barrier to the dissemination of neoplastic cells is of more than academic interest because of clinical disagreement as to whether apparently normal lymph nodes should be removed during surgical treatment of neoplasms. Proponents argue that they should be removed and examined for the presence of micrometastases. Antagonists argue that they should be left to act as a filter. Current evidence indicates that the role of the lymph node as a filter in neoplasia is variable and at best it may serve only to delay dissemination of the neoplasm.

The lymph node draining a neoplasm may undergo hyperplasia of both T lymphocytic and B lymphocytic components, suggesting a possible immune response to the neoplasm. Experimental studies, however, fail to demonstrate a specific role for the regional lymph node compared to other lymphoid tissues. For example, in dogs with naturally occurring tumors, no difference in cytotoxicity to tumor cells could be demonstrated between lymphocytes from the regional lymph node, distant lymph nodes, and circulating lymphocytes. In addition, removal of the regional lymph nodes has not affected the rate of metastasis of neoplasms in other experimental studies. The subject of tumor immunology, including the role of immunologic events in limiting metastasis, will be discussed later in this chapter.

Metastasis *via* the hematogenous route occurs when competent neoplastic cells invade blood vessels or gain access to the

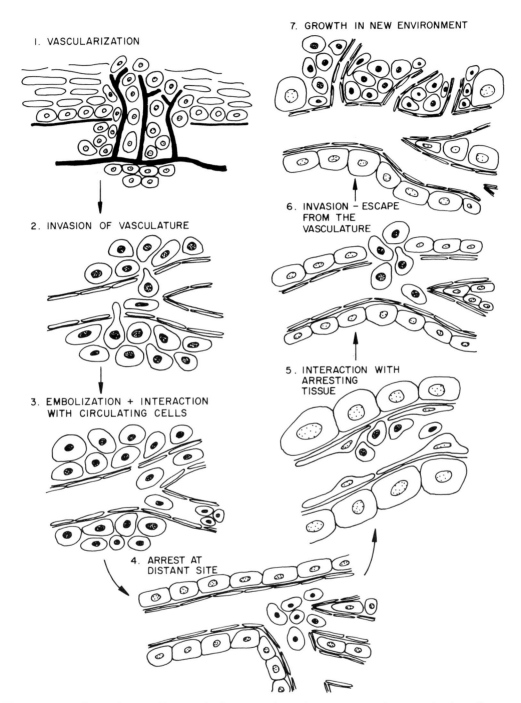

Figure 6.29.   Steps in the Metastatic Process. In order to metastasize, neoplastic cells must accomplish several processes. These are summarized graphically in this figure.

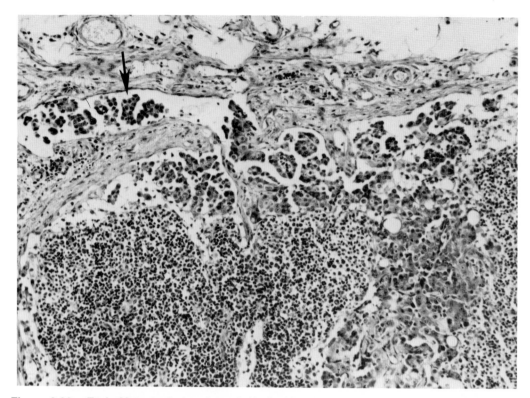

Figure 6.30. Early Metastasis to a Lymph Node. Neoplastic cells from a carcinoma are present in an afferent lymphatic *(arrow)* and in the subcapsular sinus. Proliferating cells have invaded the cortical tissue.

blood stream *via* the lymph. Direct penetration of blood vessels usually involves the capillaries and venules (as well as lymphatics, of course). Invasion of arterial vessels to gain access to the circulation is quite rare. However tumor cells gain access, when dissemination occurs *via* the hematogenous route metastatic lesions can occur in a variety of organs. Factors affecting patterns of metastatic spread are discussed below.

One of the first steps in the metastatic process, then, is the release of cells from the primary mass to form emboli (Fig. 6.31). The properties that enable tumor cells to do this are incompletely understood, but observations have been made which throw some light on this process. First, it seems clear that vascularization of the tumor is a prerequisite for tumor cell embolism. In experimental studies,

tumor emboli are never detected in the effluent blood before proliferating vessels penetrate the mass. Furthermore, lesions diagnosed as carcinoma *in situ* very rarely if ever metastasize before vascularization occurs. The penetration of vessels by neoplastic cells is probably influenced by factors similar to those involved in local invasion. The basement membrane of endothelial cells presents a particular barrier to the entry of neoplastic cells to the vasculature. As already mentioned, some tumor cells produce specific collagenases capable of attacking type IV collagen. It is worthy of note that several neoplastic cell lines show a positive correlation between this ability and the capacity to metastasize. Blood turbulence and manipulation of the tumor mass are known to increase the number of cells released into the circulation. This obser-

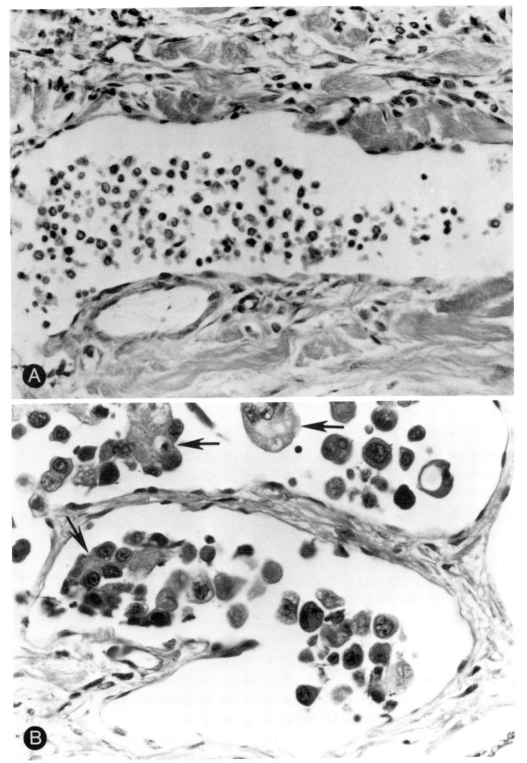

Figure 6.31.   Interaction of Embolic Tumor Cells. *A,* these embolic cells from a canine mast cell tumor are individualized and, therefore, may be less likely to be arrested. *B,* Some of these embolic cells from a canine mammary carcinoma are present as single cells, but many have formed multicellular clumps *(arrows).* The clumped cells are more likely to be arrested in a distant capillary bed.

vation has obvious potential clinical significance. It should be added however, that such manipulation has never been proven to result in increased numbers of metastases.

Dissemination of Embolic Tumor Cells

Embolism of tumor cells is probably a continuous process, and large tumors can release enormous numbers of neoplastic cells into the circulation. Quite obviously, not all of these cells result in metastatic neoplasms, and other factors must affect the success of the metastatic process. The great majority of cells released from the primary tumor die, many of them in the circulation. Factors involved in killing embolic tumor cells include mechanical shear forces, oxygen toxicity (mediated by reactive oxygen species), attack by host immune cells, and an unfavorable nutritional environment, including a lack of growth factors, which might be present in the environment of the primary tumor but not in the bloodstream. From this and discussions below, it is quite clear that the presence of tumor emboli in the circulation does not necessarily mean that metastatic lesions will develop. In fact, in man, careful comparisons of patients with otherwise comparable tumors show no difference in prognosis between those observed to have vascular invasion and those who do not. The presence of emboli is, however, definitive evidence of malignancy and hence affects the prognosis adversely.

Arrest of Embolic Tumor Cells

Most of the tumor cells that do survive the journey through the vasculature are arrested in the first capillary bed they encounter. Commonly this is in the lungs, but for intestinal neoplasms, for example, the usual primary site of arrest is the liver. The arrest of tumor emboli is partly dependent on their size, and aggregates of cells (such as shown in Fig. 6.31*B*)

survive longer at the site of arrest and are more likely to result in metastases than single cells. Neoplastic cells can be released in groups, or single cells may form aggregates in the circulation as the result of adhesive interactions amongst themselves or by interaction with platelets, lymphocytes, monocytes, or fibrin. Despite these interactions, experimental studies have demonstrated that most metastases are clonal in origin, that is, originate from single arrested embolic cells.

Endothelial damage may favor metastasis by providing a site at which platelets, fibrin and tumor cells can interact. Experimental studies have shown that depletion of platelets can reduce the incidence of metastasis, and inhibition of fibrin formation or stimulation of fibrinolysis have similar effects. Platelet aggregation by tumor cells may also result in secretion of important mediators. These include potential adhesion factors such as fibronectin, vasoactive substances that may enhance entrapment of embolic cells, and growth factors, in particular PDGF.

The fate of circulating cells has been studied by injecting labeled tumor cells into experimental animals, usually by the intravenous route. As observed in clinical cases, most of these cells are arrested in the first capillary bed they encounter, typically in the lung. Depending on the nature of the cells, including their deformability, some of them fail to be arrested and continue to circulate. The majority of the cells that are arrested quickly die. There also is evidence that some of the arrested cells are later released and recirculate. Pulmonary metastases develop from the relatively few cells that arrest and *remain* in the lung. Of those that escape arrest and those that recirculate, some may be arrested in other tissues, a proportion of which may develop into metastases at those sites. Some of the arrested cells apparently can remain dormant, although still viable. The main evidence for this is that patients may develop metastatic disease years after the removal of a primary tumor, but the phenomenon has been reproduced experimentally albeit on a shorter time scale. Dormancy can result from failure of arrested cells to become vascularized, lack of appropriate growth factors, or immunologic restraint. We have already discussed the possible role of tumor progression in altering the constituent cells so that these constraints would be overcome, releasing them from dormancy.

There is abundant evidence that the arrest and retention of embolic neoplastic cells in distant capillary vessels is not a chance event. Rather, it frequently involves specific interactions between the surface of the tumor cell and endothelial cells or the underlying basement membrane. Because these interactions can influence the site of arrest and metastatic growth, they are discussed separately.

Organ Preference of Metastasis

It is obvious from the study of clinical material that certain types of neoplasms show a characteristic distribution of metastatic lesions. In other words, they show organ preference. Recognition of this type of behavior is of obvious importance in evaluation of a patient with neoplastic disease. For example, osteosarcomas in the dog metastasize frequently and, when they do, they do so most commonly to the lung. Therefore, follow-up evaluation of a canine patient with an osteosarcoma should always include assessment of the possible existence of pulmonary metastases. Similarly, some lymphosarcomas in cats preferentially involve the thymus, some the intestine, and some the cortex of the kidney. In the cow, lymphosarcoma commonly involves the wall of the abomasum, the uterus, and/or the right atrium of the heart.

Two explanations, not mutually exclusive, have been proposed to account for patterns of metastatic spread. Distribution of metastases may be explained by **hemodynamic and anatomic factors** that determine the route of dissemination of neoplastic cells. According to this theory, embolic tumor cells are distributed according to patterns of lymphatic or venous drainage. In most cases this is a satisfactory explanation. It is consistent with the fact that the lung, the first organ encountered by most circulating neoplastic cells, or the regional lymph nodes are often the first sites of metastatic involvement. In many cases, however, patterns of metastasis cannot be explained in this way. The so-called **"seed and soil" theory,** proposed by Paget in 1889, suggests that peculiar properties of the embolic neoplastic cells (the "seed") and their preferred tissue (the "soil") determine preferred patterns of metastasis. There is now abundant experimental evidence to support Paget's view, even though the latter is a century old. Direct evidence is provided by observations of metastasis to ectopic tissue. For example, if neoplastic cells known to preferentially metastasize to the lung are injected into an animal bearing lung tissue implanted subcutaneously, they will colonize the ectopic tissue as well as the lung. They will not colonize similarly implanted kidney.

Cellular adhesion events are now recognized as important in the pathogenesis of metastasis. In the current context, interactions between circulating neoplastic cells and endothelial cells, basement membrane, and parenchymal cells in the arresting tissue are of interest. There is clear experimental evidence correlating adhesion between tumor cells and endothelial cells with capacity and site preference of metastasis. Highly metastatic cell lines have been shown to adhere avidly to microvascular endothelium, while low metastatic lines do not. Furthermore, B16 melanoma cells selected for high lung-colonizing capability (*see* below) adhere preferentially to lung microsvascular endothelium, while brain-colonizing variants prefer brain microvascular endothelium. Similar results have been obtained with a number of other tumor cell systems.

The surface components of endothelial cells responsible for these interactions have not been definitively identified, but several glycoproteins may be involved. Differences in adhesion may be associated with differences in the amounts of some of these components displayed on different endothelial cells. This situation is reminiscent of lymphocyte homing mechanisms in which glycoproteins (so-called **vascular addressins**) displayed on endothelial cells also have been identified. On tumor cells, lectins and glycoproteins have been implicated, but not fully characterized. In summary, it can be said that no single membrane component is responsible for adhesion between tumor cells and microvascular endothelium, but such interactions certainly do occur.

Neoplastic cells can also bind to the basement membrane underlying endothelial cells. Such interaction can occur when endothelial cells are injured or when they retract after interaction with tumor cells. Several components of the basement membrane, including fibronectin, laminin, proteoglycans, and type IV collagen may be involved. Antibodies to laminin-binding cell surface moieties or peptide fragments of laminin, for example, can interfere with the binding of certain neoplastic cells to basement membrane and can reduce metastatic capability. We should stress, also, that laminin is certainly not the only important recognition molecule in the basement membrane.

Recently, some fascinating findings have come to light linking specific interactions between tumor cells and endothelial cells to components of the extracellular matrix. When endothelial cells from bovine aorta are grown on extracellular matrix from particular organs, such as the lung or liver, they adopt characteristics that allow them to interact specifically with selectively metastasizing tumor cell lines.

For example, tumor cells that metastasize to the lung adhere preferentially to aortic endothelial cells grown on lung matrix. Similarly, tumor cells preferring the liver, adhere to endothelium grown on liver matrix. Nonmetastasizing tumor cells show no such preference. These findings indicate that the expression of components which are recognized by metastatic neoplastic cells on the surface of endothelial cells is modulated by extracellular matrix components. Finally, interactions between neoplastic cells and parenchymal cells are also probably important in determining metastatic preference, but fewer data are available and they will not be discussed further here.

Heterogeneity, Metastasis, and Cellular Interactions

In recent years a number of remarkable experiments have been carried out which examine the effect of phenotypic heterogeneity on the metastatic capabilities of neoplastic cells. They are worth considering in some detail as they have contributed significantly to our understanding of the properties that influence the behavior of malignant cells.

The hypothesis on which these experiments were based was that primary tumors, being heterogeneous, would contain some cells capable of metastasis and some not. If this is the case, it should be possible to select a line of cells more highly metastatic than those of the primary tumor. To test this, the B16 melanoma, which originally arose in a strain of syngeneic mice, was used. When unselected tumor cells were injected into mice, some of the cells produced metastatic lesions in the lung. Cells were harvested from pulmonary lesions, passaged *in vitro*, then again injected into mice. In this way cells that metastasized to the lung were repeatedly selected (Fig. 6.32). The cells resulting from ten such passages were dubbed B16 F10 cells, and the unselected cells were called B16 F1. These two populations were then compared, and B16 F10 cells had a much greater capacity to metastasize than B16 F1 cells. Furthermore, the B16 F10 cell line metastasized exclusively to the lung, in contrast to B16 F1 cells, which form metastases in several organs. Following similar procedures, another B16 melanoma line was developed which metastasized preferentially to the rhinal fissure of the brain. These experiments suggest that the primary tumor contained cells that had an enhanced ability to metastasize and that the selection procedure enriched them. Other interpretations are possible, however. In particular it could be argued that the cells that arrest in the lung or brain might adapt to growth in those tissues, thus producing a population better able to survive at those sites. This possibility was ruled out by serially transplanting cells directly to the brain. When cells were directly passaged in this way, rather than passaging metastases, no selection occurred. That cells with special capabilities for metastasis preexist in the primary tumor was confirmed by producing clones from single, unselected cells. When cloned cell suspensions were injected into recipient mice, a wide variation in the number of metastases resulted, some lungs having only a few and some having hundreds (Fig. 6.33). In contrast, cells from the original tumor not subjected to cloning produced a relatively constant number of pulmonary metastases.

These experiments have been repeated with other tumor cells. They provide compelling evidence that, within a primary neoplasm, component cells differ in their capacity to metastasize and to colonize particular tissues. The question can be asked: what are the differences between neoplastic cells which determine their ability to do this? A number of factors probably contribute. Highly metastatic, selected cell lines have been shown to be more invasive in the subcutaneous tissue, to form clumps more readily, and to be

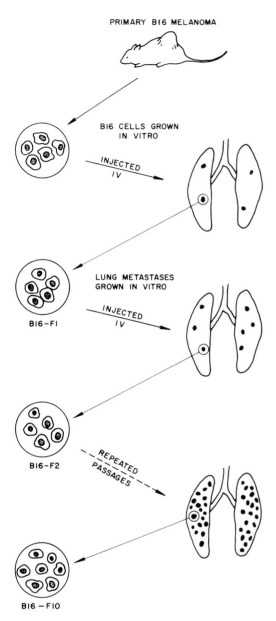

Figure 6.32. Selection of Highly Metastatic Neoplastic Cells. Cells from a primary tumor, in this case a B16 melanoma, are grown *in vitro,* then injected intravenously. Cells harvested from pulmonary metastases are again cultured and called B16 F1 cells. After the 10th such passage, the cultured cells are called B16 F10 cells. The latter metastasize much more readily than do B16 F1 cells, and they metastasize preferentially to the lung. (Adapted from G. L. Nicolson: Cancer metastasis. *Scientific American* 240:66–76, 1979.)

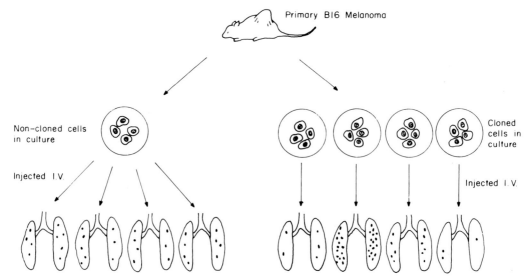

Figure 6.33. Cloning of Neoplastic Cells. If cells from a primary B16 melanoma are injected intravenously, they produce a relatively uniform number of pulmonary metastases in different mice. If clones are produced from single neoplastic cells, they will produce widely divergent numbers of pulmonary metastases. This is evidence that, within the original tumor cell population, cells exist which have a variable ability to metastasize. (Adapted from G. L. Nicolson: Cancer metastasis. *Scientific American* 240:66–76, 1979.)

more easily entrapped in the lung. They also are better able to adhere to cell culture monolayers, whether of the same or different cell type. More importantly, B16 F10 cells, which metastasize preferentially to the lung, adhere rapidly and strongly to lung cells, but less readily to cells of other tissues. In contrast B16 F1 cells are less adherent and nonselective. In addition, highly metastatic cell lines of several types, when compared to the corresponding low metastatic lines, adhere much more avidly to pulmonary endothelial basement membrane. As already discussed, they also adhere to the appropriate microvascular endothelial cells. Highly metastatic B16 cell lines also produce relatively high levels of type IV collagenase, suggesting an enhanced ability to lyse subendothelial basement membranes.

There is also evidence that these properties are associated with differences in the surfaces of the neoplastic cells. Highly metastatic B16 F10 cells shed vesicles that can be fused with the plasma membranes of B16 F1 cells. When this is done, an enhanced capacity to metastasize to the lung is conferred on the B16 F1 cells. Other properties of selected cells, such as resistance to cytotoxic lymphocytes, also can be transferred. Because the transferred vesicles persist in the recipient cells for only 18–24 hours, it appears that the properties transferred from F10 to F1 cells are important early in the metastatic process, probably in arrest or early invasion. Presumably then, some of the surface components discussed earlier in this chapter are important in determining their ability to metastasize. Despite all of these advances, no general property has been found that explains the metastatic ability of all malignant cells. In fact, given the wide variation in metastatic ability and the complexity of interactions between the host and neoplastic cells, it is unlikely that any single property will explain the ability of some cells or, conversely, the inability of others to metastasize. Undoubtedly though, our increasing knowledge of the biology of malignant cells eventually will lead to more effective control of the disease.

EFFECT OF THE TUMOR ON THE HOST

Obviously malignant neoplasms, because of their invasive nature and ability to metastasize, will cause more harm to the host than benign tumors. Even benign tumors, though, can have devastating effects. Any space-occupying lesion can lead to dysfunction of an organ. For example, a mass compressing the common bile duct can cause obstruction to bile flow, icterus, and eventually extensive liver damage. Tumors in the brain, even when histologically benign, cause local destruction of the parenchyma and can produce severe clinical illness and eventually death. Another example occurs in horses in which benign, pedunculated lipomas can become twisted around a segment of intestine producing intestinal obstruction or infarction and death of the animal. Malignant neoplasms can cause similar problems. For example ad-

enocarcinomas of the intestine often cause obstruction, particularly when associated with abundant sclerosis. Malignant neoplasms also have the ability to invade and destroy adjacent tissue, which is obviously detrimental to the host (Fig. 6.16).

Paraneoplastic Syndromes

Apart from their ability to injure host tissues directly, as just described, many neoplasms can cause illness by indirect mechanisms. The resultant diseases are known as paraneoplastic syndromes. In some of these (examples of which are included in Table 6.7) the underlying mechanisms are well understood. In others they are unknown. Benign tumors, being well differentiated, can retain functions characteristic of normal cells and excessive secretion of their products can cause clinical disease. This occurs most commonly in animals with tumors of endocrine origin. A well-known example is provided by tumors of the β-cells of the pancreatic islets, which occur relatively commonly in dogs. These tumors, when functional, secrete insulin and cause severe hypoglycemia, which results in syncope and sei-

Table 6.7
Some Paraneoplastic Syndromes

Tumor Type	Clinical Syndrome	Mechanism
B cell neoplasia	Hyperviscosity	Macroglobulinemia
	Coagulopathy	Paraproteinemia
Multiple myeloma	Nephrotoxicity	Bence Jones proteinuria
Lymphosarcoma	Hypercalcemia	Osteoclast activating factors
Carcinoma of glands of anal sac (dog)	Hypercalcemia	Unknown secreted product
Sertoli cell tumor	Feminization	Secretion of estrogens
Pulmonary neoplasms	Hypertrophic pulmonary osteoarthropathy	Unknown
Mast cell tumor	Coagulopathy, duodenal ulcers	Secretion of heparin and/or histamine
Pancreatic β-cell tumor	Hypoglycemia	Insulin secretion
Pancreatic islet cell tumor	Zollinger-Ellison syndrome	Gastrin secretion
Pituitary tumor	Cushing's disease	ACTH secretion
Adrenal tumor	Cushing's syndrome	Cortisol secretion

zure-like activity. Other neoplasms of endocrine origin also can secrete hormones. For example, functional tumors of the adrenal cortex or of the adenohypophysis can cause hyperadrenocorticism, and tumors of the α-cells in the pancreatic islets can secrete gastrin. Malignant neoplasms also can retain secretory functions and carcinomas of the β-cells of the pancreas can metastasize, yet still secrete insulin. In fact, monitoring of blood glucose levels is a useful way to detect metastasis after surgical removal of such neoplasms.

Sometimes neoplasms secrete hormones or hormone-like substances not usually associated with the cell of origin. A good example of this phenomenon is provided by **hypercalcemia of malignancy.** This syndrome has been associated with a number of neoplasms in man and animals, including lymphosarcoma, squamous carcinoma of the lung (in man), and carcinoma of the mammary gland. Hypercalcemia also has been reported in dogs as a frequent complication of carcinomas of the apocrine glands of the anal sacs. Although specific mechanisms have not been elucidated for this particular neoplasm, hypercalcemia of malignancy probably can result from the secretion of one of a number of substances. In the case of lymphoma and myeloma, osteoclast-activating factors have been implicated. This probably represents a group of cytokines, which may include lymphotoxin, colony stimulating factors, and interferons.

In other tumors, such as pulmonary carcinomas and canine carcinoma of the apocrine glands of the anal sac, substances that act at a distance appear to be produced. For a long time it was suspected that some of these tumors secreted ectopic parathyroid hormone (PTH). Recently, however, PTH-like peptides and their genes have been identified in certain human tumors causing hypercalcemia. These peptides share sequence homology with PTH at their amino-terminal

ends, compete with PTH for its receptors, and are inhibited by inhibitors of PTH. Like PTH they activate adenyl cyclase in bone cells and can cause resorption of bone in culture systems. They are therefore thought to play an important role in mediating hypercalcemia of malignancy. The PTH-like peptides resemble a factor normally produced by keratinocytes. This suggests that they are not "aberrant hormones," as was once thought, but normal cellular products that have unforeseen actions when secreted, perhaps in quantity, by neoplastic cells. Other substances, amongst them TGF-α, are also thought to play a role in hypercalcemia of malignancy. It is possible that different mediators participate in different kinds of tumors, or even that more than one mediator is involved in individual cases.

Other distant effects of neoplasms are less easy to rationalize. For example **hypertrophic osteoarthropathy** (pulmonary hypertrophic osteoarthropathy) can occur in dogs with neoplasms in the lung or bladder. In this syndrome the presence of the mass somehow causes the proliferation of osseous tissue in the bones of the distal limbs. The mechanisms involved are unknown but removal of the mass can result in the resolution of the osseous lesions. The syndrome also may be associated with non-neoplastic intrathoracic lesions, suggesting that the lesions are not the result of a specific function of the neoplastic cells. A variety of other relatively specific syndromes occurs, but they will not be explored in detail here.

Cancer Cachexia

Very often the most important indirect result of malignant neoplastic disease is cachexia. Affected animals are often anorexic, have generalized wasting, and are weak. Inadequate food intake probably contributes to this process in many cases, but it is certainly not the sole explanation, as many animals with neoplastic disease eat normally yet lose body condition. It also has been postulated that tumor tissue competes with the host for nutrients. Although this may again contribute, it is difficult to explain cachexia associated with relatively small tumors on this basis.

There is adequate evidence of profound changes in **energy metabolism** in animals with neoplasia. In general, neoplastic disease results in increased energy spending. Carbohydrate metabolism is altered, sometimes associated with changes in insulin sensitivity or secretion, as is lipid and protein metabolism. In addition there are alterations in the activity of many enzymes in animals with neoplasms, some being elevated and some decreased.

Many of the metabolic derangements associated with tumor cachexia have been attributed to **tumor necrosis factor (TNFα)**, also known as **cachectin.** This cytokine is produced by activated macrophages in a variety of chronic diseases, including neoplasia. Cachectin (as we will call it in this context) is capable of eliciting a variety of responses in the host. It has been implicated as a central mediator of wasting in chronic disease states. When administered to animals it induces a cachectic state, and it is capable of suppressing the expression of a number of important metabolic enzymes. For example, it drastically reduces lipoprotein lipase activity in adipocytes, as well as other enzymes contributing to lipogenesis. Beyond these effects, TNF/cachectin also appears to be responsible for many of the changes in endotoxic shock.

NEOPLASIA AND IMMUNITY

Observations made in naturally occurring cases of neoplasia sometimes suggest that the host can react against the presence of tumor cells. For example canine mammary tumors, seminomas, some mast cell tumors and, in particular, cutaneous histiocytomas often contain infiltrating lymphocytes (Fig. 6.34). In the case of canine mammary tumors, perivascular lymphocytic infiltrates have been associated with an improved prognosis and, in the case of canine cutaneous histiocytomas, the infiltrates have been associated with regression of the tumors. Other neoplasms, such as the canine transmissible venereal tumor (TVT), regress with some regularity, suggesting that the host can in some way defend itself against the neoplastic growth. The field of tumor immunology is, however, replete with contradictory results and controversy.

Tumor Antigens

There is no doubt that many tumors bear new antigens not found on normal host cells. These antigens are most common in experimentally induced tumors, and spontaneous neoplasms are less frequently antigenic. The antigens borne on the surface of the neoplastic cells are known by a variety of names, including **tumor-specific antigens** (TSA), **tumor-specific transplantation antigens** (TSTA), or **tumor-associated transplantation antigens** (TATA). Transplantation antigens are detected by the elicitation of an immune response to transplanted tumor cells in syngeneic normal animals. Thus, their detection depends on effective immunogenicity. This distinction is important, as not all antigens expressed on tumor cells are effectively immunogenic. Some antigens, therefore, would not be able to induce immune-mediated destruction of tumor cells. Nor are all antigens expressed on tumor cells strictly abnormal. For instance, many tumors in a number of animal species bear embryonic antigens. These are substances found normally on the surface of embryonic cells but not on normal adult cells. They do not usually function as transplantation antigens.

Neoplasms induced by oncogenic viruses bear antigens that are consistent and specific for the particular causative virus. These tumor-specific cell surface

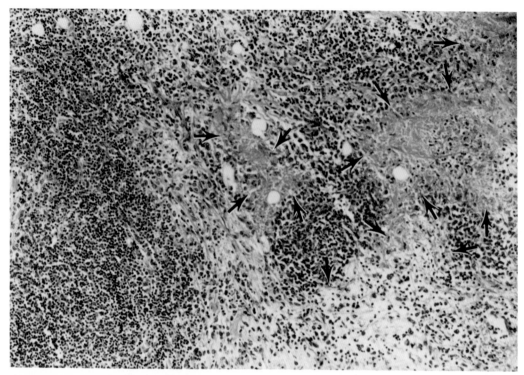

Figure 6.34.   Lymphocytic Infiltrate in a Canine Cutaneous Histocytoma. This tumor is infiltrated by large numbers of small, densely stained lymphocytes. Associated with the infiltrate are areas of tumor necrosis (delineated by *arrows*).

antigens are not part of the virion, although infected cells may, of course, contain antigenic viral material. The antigens are a consequence of cell transformation rather than infection and may represent the product of transformation-specific genes. One of the better known specific, virus-induced cell surface antigens is FOCMA (feline oncornavirus cell membrane antigen), which is found on neoplastic lymphocytes in feline lymphosarcoma (*see* the earlier discussion of FeLV) and on cells transformed by feline sarcoma virus (FeSV).

In contrast, neoplasms induced by chemical carcinogens bear antigens that are unique to each individual tumor. Different tumors induced by the same chemical bear different antigens, even when several tumors occur on the same animal. There is, apparently, almost unlimited diversity in the antigens that may be

expressed, and they vary widely in immunogenicity.

The first requirement for an immune-mediated attack on neoplastic cells, namely antigenicity, or more importantly, immunogenicity, is therefore often satisfied. Nevertheless, many of us and many of our animals will develop neoplastic disease. Clearly, immunologic rejection of neoplasms does not always occur. What must now be considered is the evidence that it can occur at all, and if it can, what allows some neoplasms to escape destruction.

The Concept of Immunologic Surveillance

Some years ago it was postulated that the immune system played an important role in preventing neoplastic disease. It was proposed that neoplasms arose frequently in all individuals and that the immune system of normal animals recognized the abnormal cells and destroyed them early in their development. Thus, clinically apparent neoplasms were thought to be due to a failure in the host's immune defenses. This theory, called **immunosurveillance,** was prompted partly by the fact that the only known function of T lymphocytes, at that time, was the rejection of foreign, grafted cells. The concept was inherently attractive and provided a believable explanation for the role of T cells.

Today it is known that T lymphocytes have a variety of functions, including defense against viruses and other intracellular parasites. The concept of immunologic surveillance, at least in its original form, is currently much less attractive, and a large body of evidence argues against it. Most of this evidence derives from the study of immunodeficient animals and people. If neoplasms do arise commonly and are usually rejected, immunoincompetence should consistently be associated with an increased incidence of neoplasia. The evidence is that this is not so. Nude mice, which lack a thymus and so have no T cells, do not develop unusual numbers of tumors. They are, however, as susceptible as normal mice to chemical carcinogenesis and, as would be expected, are more susceptible to virus-induced tumors. Similarly, mice whose immune function is experimentally suppressed or immunodeficient people develop no more tumors than usual. As a caveat, it must be added that in all immunoincompetent animals, including people, there is an increase in the incidence of neoplasms of lymphoid origin. This, however, is thought to be due to abnormal regulation of lymphoid precursor cells, which results from the immunosuppressed state, rather than failure of a surveillance mechanism. Immunosuppressed people also have a somewhat increased incidence of tumors of the lip, skin, and cervix. All of these are suspected of being of viral origin, which

might explain their increased occurrence in these individuals.

There is other evidence against a role for immunosurveillance. Immunologically privileged sites, such as the cheek pouch of the hamster, are not subject to an unusual number of neoplasms and, contrary to what would be expected, there is no increase in polyclonal neoplasms in immunosuppressed people.

All of these findings suggest that the concept of immunologic surveillance, as originally stated, is probably incorrect. The modern concept is that tumors arise very rarely and cellular immunity has not evolved specifically to combat them. Yet the rejection of the original hypothesis should not be taken as proof that the immune system plays no role in combating neoplasia. For instance, nude mice do possess other potent effector mechanisms that could destroy neoplastic cells. These include natural killer (NK) cells and macrophages. If neoplastic transformation occurs only rarely, there may not be a dramatic increase in the incidence of neoplasia in immunosuppressed individuals. It is well documented that, at least in some circumstances, neoplasms can elicit an immune response. Our task therefore is to understand why this response is not always effective and to learn to manipulate it.

Evidence for Immunity Against Tumors

There is evidence in a number of experimental systems that the immune response can influence the fate of a neoplasm. These experiments usually are carried out in syngeneic strains of animals, so as not to confuse responses to histocompatibility antigens with those to tumor antigens.

In the case of tumors induced by oncogenic viruses, there is clear evidence that the immune response can prevent the development of neoplasms. For example, polyoma virus, when injected into neonatal mice that are immunologically immature or into immunosuppressed mice, causes the development of a variety of neoplasms. These neoplasms, when transplanted to normal, immunocompetent syngeneic hosts, will survive and grow (Fig. 6.35). When the virus is injected into normal adult mice, it does not induce tumors. However, when polyoma virus–induced tumors are transplanted to syngeneic adult mice previously injected with the virus, the tumors fail to survive and grow. Similar results can be obtained using other viruses such as adenovirus or SV40 virus. As previously discussed, each of these viruses evokes antigens on the surface of transformed cells which are peculiar to the particular virus. Apparently, an immune response against these can prevent the development of neoplasms. In the polyoma virus system, it appears that infection of the immunocompetent adult mouse does induce surface antigens in some transformed cells that are recognized and destroyed. The resultant immunity prevents the subsequent establishment of transplanted tumors. This clearly demonstrates that effective antitumor immunity is possible, but it raises the question of why an effective response does not occur to the tumor transplanted to the previously unexposed host.

Effective immunity against naturally occurring virus-induced tumors is also well recognized, one of the better understood examples being feline lymphosarcoma. Like other virus-induced neoplasms, these tumors bear surface antigens, in this case FOCMA, against which an effective immune response can be mounted. In the cat, virus-neutralizing antibodies can protect against FeLV infection, and antibodies against FOCMA, although they do not prevent infection, do protect against the development of tumors.

The situation in the case of chemically induced tumors is, of course, more complex, because each tumor bears its own unique antigens. Immune-mediated rejection of such tumors can, however, be dem-

onstrated under appropriate experimental conditions. If, for instance, a tumor is induced in a mouse using a chemical carcinogen such as 3-methylcholanthrene, it can be transplanted to syngeneic animals where it will survive and grow. If the growing tumor is resected, the "cured" mouse that results is then resistant to further transplantation of neoplastic cells. This too indicates that immune rejection of tumor cells is possible, but, again, the primary tumor and the tumor transplanted to the nonimmunized host are not rejected. The reasons for failure of rejection of primary tumors are at present unknown, but some possibilities are discussed below. Furthermore, the whole question of tumor immunity is additionally complicated by the fact that, in many systems, tumors are unaffected by the immune response. In some systems, in fact, tumor growth can be stimulated by an immune response. Many questions remain to be answered before we can understand and exploit the nature and effects of immunity to tumors. Nevertheless it is worthwhile examining some of the effector mechanisms that are thought to be involved in tumor immunity and the ways in which the transformed cells may escape them.

Effector Mechanisms in Tumor Immunity

Potentially, tumor cells may be lysed or prevented from growing in a number of ways. Generally, it is difficult to examine these mechanisms directly *in vivo* and much of the available data has been obtained from *in vitro* assays, often correlated with *in vivo* behavior.

Cellular Cytotoxicity

This immune reaction, mediated by cytotoxic T lymphocytes, is thought to be one of the most important means by which the immune response can eliminate tumor cells. Sensitized T cells recognize antigens on the transformed cells and in-

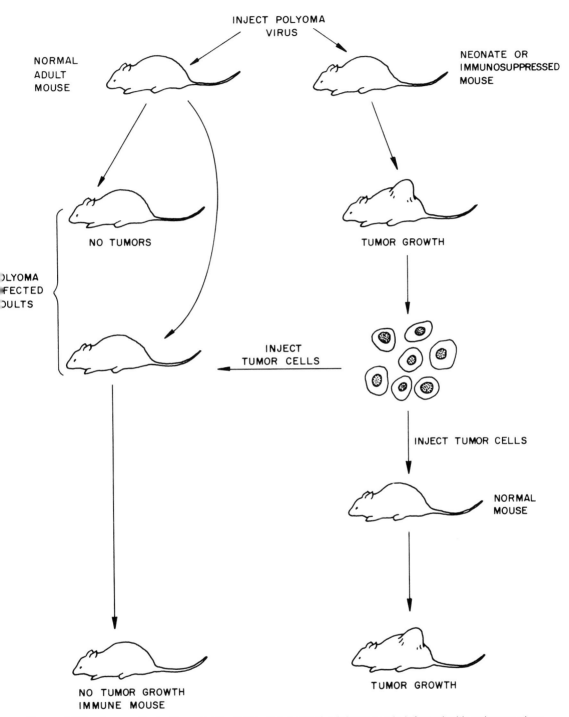

Figure 6.35. Immunity to Neoplastic Cells. If a normal adult mouse is infected with polyoma virus it does not develop tumors. If neonates or otherwise immunoincompetent mice are infected, they do develop tumors. The neoplastic cells may then be transferred to normal adult syngeneic mice, where they will grow and produce tumors. If cells are transferred to mice previously infected with polyoma virus, no tumors develop. These mice are immune to the development of the neoplasm. (Adapted from L. J. Olds: Cancer Immunology. *Scientific American 236*:62–79, 1977.)

teract directly with them to induce "leakiness" in the cell membrane and eventually lysis (*see* Chapter 5 for a discussion of this process). This mechanism may be involved in canine-transmissible venereal tumor (TVT), as peripheral blood lymphocytes (PBL) from dogs in which the neoplasm has regressed are cytotoxic for tumor cells *in vitro*. In contrast PBL from dogs with progressive tumors are not. Similar evidence has been obtained in other systems. For example, the role of cytotoxic T cells has been studied in progressing and regressing UV-induced sarcomas. Regressor tumors contained three times the number of T cells compared to progressor tumors, while the numbers of other potential effector cells were comparable. T cells from the regressor tumors showed antigen-specific cytotoxicity against tumor cells *in vitro,* while those from the progressor tumors did not. These data support a role for cytotoxic T cells in immune reactions against neoplasms. Unfortunately, similar studies in other tumor systems often produce conflicting results, indicating that the outcome depends on a number of events that are not always predictable.

Antibody

The role of antibody in tumor immunology is somewhat controversial. Certainly cytolysis by antibody and complement has been shown to occur in some systems. Activation of complement is *via* the classic pathway, the alternate pathway apparently being ineffective. This mechanism therefore requires that immunoglobulins bind to the surface of tumor cells in order to activate complement, following which the cell membrane is rendered "leaky," leading to lysis. Antibody also may play a role in tumor cell lysis by participating in **antibody-dependent cellular cytotoxicity (ADCC).** This mechanism has not been shown to occur *in vivo* but certainly is demonstrable *in*

vitro. The reaction is mediated by so-called **killer cells,** or K cells, lymphocytes that lack both T cell and B cell markers. K cells recognize the Fc portion of antibody molecules bound to the surface of target cells, which they lyse after direct contact is made.

Besides the potential for antibodies generated by the host against specific tumor antigens, there is also evidence that normal individuals carry natural antibodies. These may react with embryonic antigens or with cross-reactive antigens associated with infectious agents. In mice the antigens are often those of endogenous viruses. The potential of these antibodies to lyse tumor cells has been examined *in vitro,* where it has been found that several kinds of neoplastic cells could be lysed in the presence of complement. There is evidence that macrophage-dependent rejection of small tumor inocula may depend on natural antibodies. Immune reactions against tumors not dependent on specific cytotoxic T cells probably represent a mixture of mechanisms including natural antibodies, nonspecifically activated macrophages, and NK cells, depending on the type of tumor and the capacities of the host.

Natural Killer Cells

There is also evidence that certain tumor cells may be lysed by a form of natural immunity mediated by natural killer cells (NK cells). NK cells are a subset of lymphocytes, distinct from T cells and B cells. They fall within the group of lymphoid cells known as **large granular lymphocytes.** Cytotoxicity mediated by NK cells also requires contact with the target cell. Tumor cells apparently are distinguished from normal cells by nonimmunologic mechanisms. NK cell activity is enhanced by exposure to tumor cells, viruses, and certain adjuvants and chemicals. This phenomenon is not immunologically specific, however, and is thought to be mediated by interferons and interleukin 2 (IL-2). Experimental evidence for a role for NK cells in the control of tumor growth and metastasis *in vivo* has been obtained using strains of mice deficient in NK activity. In these animals, injection of tumor cells selected *in vitro* for enhanced susceptibility to NK-mediated lysis led to increased growth rate, shorter induction times, and increased metastatic capability of the resultant neoplasms compared to those in control mice. Conversely, induction of NK cell activity reduced the rate of growth and metastatic capability of tumors. Additional evidence is provided by the fact that tumors rarely metastasize in nude mice, which have high NK activity. Finally, adoptive transfer of NK cells to irradiated mice has been shown to increase the resistance of the recipients to NK-susceptible tumors. Most studies of the role of NK cells suggest that they are effective against small tumor loads, but that they have little effect on established tumors. They may therefore play a significant role in surveillance against incipient tumors and in removing circulating tumor cells.

Macrophages

Macrophages often form a major cellular component in neoplasms undergoing rejection, and they may be important effector cells in tumor immunity. Macrophages incubated with T lymphocytes sensitized to tumor cells become specifically cytotoxic for those cells. This activation of macrophages is mediated by a lymphokine known as **specific macrophage arming factor (SMAF)**. The cytotoxic action of armed macrophages depends on direct contact with the target cells. Ability of activated macrophages to kill tumor cells *in vitro* has been correlated with reduced tumor growth *in vivo*. Additionally, when specifically armed macrophages are transferred to experimental animals they are capable of preventing the growth of tumor cells injected intravenously or intraperitoneally. Macrophages also may be toxic to tumor cells to which antibody is bound.

Macrophages may be nonspecifically activated by a variety of substances such as endotoxin, aggregated IgG, and peptidoglycans from mycobacteria. Tumor cells may be lysed by such activated macrophages and are much more susceptible than normal cells. The mechanism by which such activated macrophages recognize tumor cells is not known, but apparently it is not dependent on immunologically specific mechanisms or the presence of strong neoantigens. Presumably they are able to recognize some alterations on the surface of the neoplastic cells.

Tumor Immunity and Metastasis

A number of observations suggest that immune mechanisms may be involved in reducing or delaying metastatic spread of tumors, despite the fact that the primary neoplasm is not controlled. It has been known for many years that, in an animal with a progressively growing primary tumor, the growth of small implants of the same mass could be suppressed. This is reminiscent of a clinical observation wherein incipient metastases can "take off" after removal of a primary tumor, apparently having been kept in check until that time. Nonspecifically activated macrophages are thought to be involved in this phenomenon. Circulating neoplastic cells are also thought to be vulnerable to destruction by immune effector mechanisms. There is a strong inverse correlation between levels of NK cells and the ability of tumors to metastasize in experimental animals. Enhanced resistance to metastasis has also been accomplished by transfer of NK cells.

Possible Escape Mechanisms

Given that a variety of mechanisms can mediate rejection of transformed cells, why do they fail to do so in naturally occurring neoplasms? A number of reasons, outlined below, have been proposed.

Modulation of cell surface antigens occurs in some tumor cells exposed to high-titer antibody. Those antigens that undergo such modulation are known to be relatively mobile in the cell membrane, leading to redistribution and in some cases to shedding. Under such circumstances specific effector mechanisms cannot be activated. Antigenic modulation is apparently a specific response, because transplantation of modulated tumor cells to seronegative syngeneic hosts leads to the reappearance of the antigens.

The rapid turnover and shedding of antigen may result in the presence of circulating antigen or immune complexes that may act as blocking factors and interfere with immune effector mechanisms. Antibody molecules themselves can act as blocking factors. In the case of canine transmissible venereal tumor, for instance, serum from dogs in which the tumor has regressed can inhibit the growth of tumor cells *in vitro*. Sera from dogs with progressive tumors can block this activity. In other words, sera of dogs with progressive tumors contain blocking activity. In this particular example, both tumor inhibitory and blocking activity are in the IgG fraction, and no immune complexes are apparently involved. More to the point, the importance of the interplay of these phenomena is illustrated by the strong correlation between the relative reactivities of inhibitory and blocking activity, and the clinical course of the neoplasm. In this particular neoplasm, therefore, both cytotoxic T cells and antibody may be important as effector mechanisms, and antibody may act as a blocking factor.

It also has been proposed that tumor cells may produce substances that are toxic to effector cells, suppress the function of effector cells, or destroy antibody. For example, some tumor cells can suppress the activity of macrophages. This activity appears to be mediated by a low molecular weight substance that can inhibit mononuclear cell chemotaxis *in vivo* and *in vitro* and which can, when administered to experimental animals, enhance the growth of transplanted tumors.

Another possible mechanism of escape is the emergence of cells resistant to immunologic attack. Tumor heterogeneity would suggest that such cells exist in any malignant neoplasm. It is possible, using selection procedures similar to those described earlier in this chapter, to select cells that are less susceptible to immune-mediated lysis. Conceivably then, an immune-mediated attack on a tumor could destroy susceptible cells, while allowing the emergence of a population resistant to the process.

The possibility of immunosuppression contributing to the *progression* of a neoplasm cannot be dismissed despite the evidence, cited earlier, that immunosuppression does not appear to lead to a dramatic increase in the incidence of nonlymphoid neoplasms. Many cancer patients (in humans and experimental animals, where it has been studied) are in fact immunosuppressed. It is probable, however, that in many cases this results from, rather than predisposes to, the tumor. Many carcinogens, such as irradiation, oncogenic viruses, and some chemicals are, however, immunosuppressive, and it is still possible that this contributes to the establishment of tumors.

It has been suggested that very small tumor cell loads could escape detection by the immune system, and that by the time the tumor cell load reaches the threshold required for an immune response the neoplasm is too well established to be rejected. Of course, in the case of naturally occurring tumors the initial tumor load is by definition small. This phenomenon has been referred to as "sneaking through." Recent evidence suggests that it is real, but that it is not a passive event in which transformed cells are just not noticed. It appears that it is due instead to the early generation of specific suppressor cells. This has been well documented in skin tumors induced by UV light and will be discussed below.

Finally, it has recently been shown that the ability to mount an immune attack on circulating tumor cells can be influenced by the nature of the antigens of the major histocompatibility complex (MHC) displayed on the cancer cell. The class 1 MHC genes are involved in the process of MHC restriction, regulating the ability of T cells to recognize antigens on cells. In mice, there are two class 1 MHC genes, called H-2K and H-2D. In comparing a highly metastatic carcinoma clone to a low metastatic clone, it was found that the highly metastatic clone displayed a high density of H-2D and little H-2K, while the reverse was true for the low metastatic clone. This was found to correspond to immunogenicity; the highly metastatic clone generated a poor cytotoxic response, while the low metastatic clone generated a strong response. A series of gene transfer experiments have shown that the ratio of H-2K to H-2D determines the vigor of the immune response to the tumor cells and, correspondingly, the degree of metastasis. Expression of high levels of H-2D with low levels of H-2K apparently suppresses the immune response. Similarly, the loss of the appropriate MHC class 1 antigens has also been shown to result in reduced immunogenicity and enhanced tumorigenicity.

Enhancement of Tumor Growth by Suppressor Cells

Recent studies have suggested a possibly important role for tumor-specific suppressor cells in inhibiting the immune-mediated attack on tumor cells and thus in enhancing tumor growth. For example, if cells are taken from a tumor growing in one mouse and transplanted to a syngeneic mouse previously immunized with tumor cells, they will fail to grow, due to immune-mediated rejection. If, however, the transplanted cells are given together with spleen cells from the tumor-bearing donor mouse, they will not be rejected but will survive and grow. Furthermore, if tumor-bearing mice are given antithymocyte antiserum there is a marked enhancement of tumor regression. These phenomena have been shown to be due to a population of suppressor T cells that are immunologically specific for antigens borne on the tumor cells. They apparently suppress the usual host effector mechanisms and allow enhanced growth of tumor cells.

Suppressor cells also may play a role in carcinogenesis. Evidence for this comes from studies of squamous cell carcinomas induced in mice by UV irradiation. These tumors are highly antigenic, and if transplanted to normal syngeneic mice they will be rejected. If, however, the recipient mouse is first subjected to a subcarcinogenic dose of UV light, a population of suppressor cells is induced which enhances the growth of the transplanted neoplasm. There is also evidence that suppressor cells may be produced as a response to very small doses of tumor cells. This observation, which can be regarded as a form of tolerance, may explain the "sneak through" phenomenon described earlier. In other words, the initially small number of tumor cells in a naturally occurring tumor could induce an effective suppressor cell population before any cytotoxic effector mechanisms were stimulated.

There is evidence from studies in man that suppressor cells may play an important role in influencing the outcome of naturally occurring neoplastic disease. It has been shown that patients with osteosarcoma may have circulating cells that are cytotoxic to tumor cells when tested *in vitro*. In some patients these cytotoxic cells can only be demonstrated when a suppressor cell population is first removed. The suppressor cells can inhibit the cytotoxicity reaction if returned to the incubation medium. The possible clinical importance of such observations is illustrated by one study in which all of a group of four patients with osteosarcoma who had significant suppressor cell function of this type had pulmonary metastases. Only one of a group of six patients who did not have demonstrable suppressor cell activity had pulmonary metastases.

Finally, it should be added that suppressor activity also resides in cells other than T lymphocytes, including macrophages and possibly B cells. Suppressor activity also may be nonspecific in nature and could account for the immunosuppression found in tumor-bearing patients and experimental animals.

An influence of suppressor cells on metastatic capacity also has been shown in the UV light–induced squamous cell carcinoma system already alluded to. Some tumors induced by this treatment produce a higher rate of metastasis when transferred to mice treated with subcarcinogenic doses of UV irradiation than in control mice. This enhanced capacity for metastasis is immunologically specific and can be transferred using lymphocytes, presumably suppressor cells, from UV-irradiated animals.

NEOPLASIA IN PERSPECTIVE

In this chapter we have explored the nature and pathogenesis of neoplastic disease in some detail. The reader may have reached this point wondering what all this has to do with real life and the practice of clinical medicine. In order to answer that question we will consider a clinical case which illustrates that the principles we have discussed *are* real and *do* have relevance to our understanding of neoplastic disease as we see it in our patients.

Case 6.2: Paraneoplastic Syndrome

Brandy, an 11-year-old, female Golden Retriever dog was presented with a history of depression, poor appetite, and obvious weight loss of about 1 week duration. Previous medical history was unremarkable. On questioning, the owner reported that the dog had recently had polydipsia (increased thirst) and polyuria (increased volume of urine). On physical examination the animal was lethargic and moderately weak, most noticeably in the rear limbs. A firm, nonpainful mass about 3 cm in diameter was palpated in the perineum adjacent to the rectum. A complete blood count (CBC) and blood chemistry panel was ordered. The CBC was unremarkable, but the chemistry panel showed mild elevations of serum enzymes (alanine amino transferase, aspartate aminotransferase, and alkaline phosphatase) suggestive of liver damage. The serum calcium was elevated to 14.4 mg/dl (normal = 9.8-12.0 mg/dl). Abdominal radiographs suggested enlargement of the liver, but abdominal detail was poor due to ascites. The mass was resected surgically and noted at that time to be very vascular, firm, tan in color, and locally invasive. It extended along the wall of the rectum but was not closely adherent to it. The mass was fixed in neutral buffered formalin and submitted for histopathologic evaluation. Two days after surgery, a second chemistry panel showed that the serum calcium had dropped to 10.3 mg/dl.

Histologically the mass was made up of cuboidal or polyhedral cells that were fairly regular in size (Fig. 6.36). They had uniform, round-to-oval nuclei and lightly stained, basophilic cytoplasm that was sometimes vacuolated. The cells were arranged into irregular-sized lobules, which were separated by coarse, densely collagenous connective tissue septae. Some areas had occasional acinar structures. Their lumens often contained eosinophilic secretory product *(arrow)*. Occasional small invasive foci of neoplastic cells were present in the capsule, and occasional emboli of neoplastic cells were found in lymphatics. Based on these characteristics, a diagnosis of adenocarcinoma of the apocrine glands of the anal sac was made. The pathologist commented that this type of tumor was usually highly malignant and that metastasis to the internal iliac lymph nodes was common. Close clinical surveillance was therefore advised.

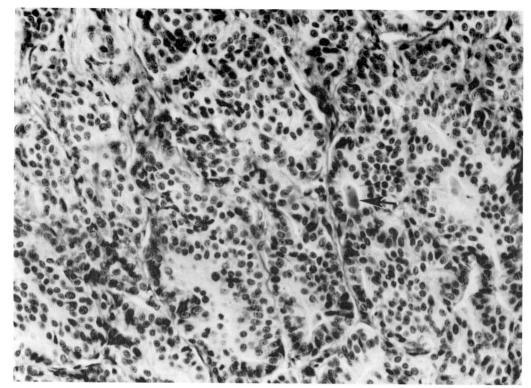

Figure 6.36.   Adenocarcinoma of the Apocrine Glands of the Anal Sac, Case 6.2. Neoplastic cells form solid lobules separated by collagenous stroma. Occasionally the cells form acini containing eosinophilic secretory product *(arrow)*.

Two months after initial presentation, the dog was again examined because of recurrence of clinical signs. No mass could be palpated in the perineum but the serum calcium was 16.2 mg/dl. Radiographs showed a number of dense masses in the lungs. Because of the poor prognosis the owners decided on euthanasia. At postmortem examination a large, irregular, firm mass was found in the caudal abdominal cavity. The internal iliac lymph nodes were greatly enlarged and firm. Variably sized metastatic lesions were also found in the lungs and in the liver. Histologically, all of these closely resembled the original biopsy.

Comments on Case 6.2.

This case documents the importance of several of the biologic phenomena discussed in this chapter. This neoplasm was diagnosed as an adenocarcinoma because it showed evidence of differentiation into acini

and because of definitive evidence of malignancy, in the form of tissue and vascular invasion. The lobular arrangement with coarse fibrous septae and occasional acini is highly characteristic of tumors derived from the apocrine glands of the anal sacs. The pathologist was therefore confident in making this specific diagnosis. Also, these tumors behave in a very consistent way. Almost all cases metastasize to the internal inguinal lymph nodes early in the course of the disease, and less commonly to other organs. This could be dependably predicted in this case and was confirmed at necropsy. Based on their knowledge of this neoplasm, the clinician and the pathologist had to offer a poor prognosis in this case.

This case is also a good example of a paraneoplastic syndrome. Hypercalcemia is a frequent complication of this neoplasm and is thought to be associated with the secretion of some biologically active substance. The fact that resection of the primary mass was followed by normalization of the serum calcium levels supports this. At present the nature of the substance is unknown. As in this case, the monitoring of serum calcium can be used as an indicator of recurrence or metastasis of the neoplasm when it is biologically active. This is true not only of neoplasms producing hypercalcemia but also of all those secreting some measurable biologically active compound.

Lastly, adenocarcinoma of the apocrine glands of the anal sac illustrates the likelihood of certain syndromes or lesions occurring in specific patient populations. This neoplasm occurs most commonly in old female dogs. Therefore, when such a dog presents with signs of weakness, depression, polydypsia, and polyuria, this condition should be suspected. Of course, there are other diseases that can produce such signs, but it is in this way that lists of differential diagnoses are constructed. In this case, serum chemistry revealed hypercalcemia, and physical examination revealed a perineal mass. With all this information the informed clinician can make a presumptive diagnosis of adenocarcinoma of the apocrine glands of the anal sac with a high degree of confidence. Our efforts to understand the basic biologic phenomena that accompany neoplastic disease, or other diseases for that matter, are not simply a matter of academic curiosity. They will, in the long run, provide the tools by which we can provide better patient care.

Reference Material

Becker, F.F.: Recent concepts of initiation and promotion in carcinogenesis. *Am. J. Pathol. 105*:3–9, 1981.

Bishop, J.M.: Viral oncogenes. *Cell 42*:23–38, 1985.

Cockerell, G.L., and Slauson, D.O.: Patterns of lymphoid infiltrate in the canine cutaneous histiocytoma. *J. Comp. Pathol. 89*:192–203, 1979.

Croce, C.M.: Chromosome translocations and human cancer. *Cancer Res. 46*:6019–6023, 1986.

Essex, M., McLane, M.F., Kanki, P., Allan, J., Kitchen, L., and Lee, T.H.: Retroviruses associated with leukemia and ablative syndromes in animals and in human beings. *Cancer Res. 45*:4534–4538, 1985.

Farber, E.: The multistep nature of cancer development. *Cancer Res. 44*:4217–4223, 1984.

Farber, E., and Sarma, D.S.R.: Hepatocarcinogenesis: a dynamic cellular perspective. *Lab. Invest. 56*:4–22, 1987.

Feldman, M., and Eisenbach, L.: What makes a tumor cell metastatic?. *Sci. Am. 259*:60–87, 1988.

Fidler, I.J.: Macrophages and metastasis—a biological approach to cancer therapy: Presidential address. *Cancer Res. 45*:4714–4726, 1985.

Folkman, J.: Tumor angiogenesis. *Adv. Cancer Res. 43*:175–203, 1985.

Folkman, J.: How is blood vessel growth regulated in normal and neoplastic tissue? G.H.A. Clowes memorial award lecture. *Cancer Res. 46*:467–473, 1986.

Folkman, J., and Klagsbrun, M.: Angiogenic factors. *Science 235*:442–447, 1987.

Goustin, A.S., Leof, E.B., Shipley, G.D., and Moses, H.L.: Growth factors and cancer. *Cancer Res. 46*:1015–1029, 1986.

Hanna, N.: Natural killer cell-mediated inhibition of tumor metastasis in vivo. *Surv. Synth. Pathol. Res. 2*:68–81, 1983.

Hansen, M.F., and Cavenee, W.K.: Genetics of cancer predisposition. *Cancer Res. 47*:5518–5527, 1987.

Hardy, W.D.: Feline retroviruses. In *Advances in Viral Oncology, Vol. 5. Viruses as the Causative Agents of Naturally Occurring Tumors*, edited by G. Klein. Raven Press, New York, 1985.

Hennings, H., and Yuspa, S.H.: Two-stage tumor promotion in mouse skin: An alternative interpretation. *JNCI 74*:735–740, 1985.

Heppner, G.H.: Tumor heterogeneity. *Cancer Res. 44*:2259–2265, 1984.

Herberman, R.B.: Natural killer cells and tumor immunity: 1985. In *The Year in Immunology, Vol. 2*, edited by J.M. Cruse and Lewis R.E., Jr. S. Karger, Basel, 1986.

Herrlich, P., and Ponta, H.: 'Nuclear' oncogenes convert extracellular stimuli into changes in the genetic program. *TIG 5*:112–115, 1989.

Hicks, R.M.: Pathological and biochemical aspects of tumor promotion. *Carcinogenesis 4*:1209–1214, 1983.

Hunter, T.: The proteins of oncogenes. *Sci. Am. 251*:70–78, 1984.

Klein, G.: The approaching era of the tumor suppressor genes. *Science 238*:1539–1545, 1987.

Klein, G., and Klein, E.: Evolution of tumours and the impact of molecular oncology. *Nature 315*:190–195, 1985.

Levine, A.J.: Oncogenes of DNA tumor viruses. *Cancer Res. 48*:493–495, 1988.

Liotta, L.A.: Tumor invasion and metastasis: Role of the basement membrane. *Am. J. Pathol. 117*:339–348, 1984.

Liotta, L.A.: Tumor invasion and metastasis—role of the extracellular matrix: Rhoads memorial award lecture. *Cancer Res. 46*:1–7, 1986.

Lugo, M., and de Klein, A.: Metaplasia. An overview. *Arch. Pathol. Lab. Med. 108*:185–189, 1984.

Marshall, C.J.: Oncogenes. *J. Cell Sci. Suppl. 4*:417–430, 1986.

Marx, J.L.: How cancer cells spread in the body. *Science* 244:147–148, 1989.

Meuten, D.J., Capen, C.C., Kociba, G.J., and Cooper, B.J.: Hypercalcemia of malignancy. Hypercalcemia associated with an adenocarcinoma of the apocrine glands of the anal sac. *Am. J. Pathol.* 108:366–370, 1982.

Moore, M.: Natural immunity to tumors. Theoretical predictions and biological observations. *Br. J. Cancer* 52:147–151, 1985.

Mundy, G.R.: Hypercalcemia of malignancy revisited. *J. Clin. Invest.* 82:1–6, 1988.

Mundy, G.R., Ibbotson, K. J., and D'Souza, S. M.: Tumor products and the hypercalcemia of malignancy. *J. Clin. Invest.* 76:391–394, 1985.

Nelson, D.S., and Nelson, M.: Evasion of host defences by tumours. *Immunol. Cell Biol.* 65:287–304, 1987.

Nicolson, G.L.: Cell surface molecules and tumor metastasis. Regulation of metastatic phenotypic diversity. *Exp. Cell Res.* 150:3–22, 1984.

Nicolson, G.L.: Organ specificity of tumor metastasis: role of preferential adhesion, invasion and growth of malignant cells at specific secondary sites. *Cancer Metastasis Rev.* 7:143–188, 1988.

Nusse, R.: The activation of cellular oncogenes by retroviral insertion. *Trends Genet.* 2:244–247, 1986.

Pauli, B.U., and Knudson, W.: Tumor invasion: A consequence of destructive and compositional matrix alterations. *Hum. Pathol.* 19:628–639, 1988.

Pauli, B.U., and Lee, C.-L.: Organ preference of metastasis. The role of organ-specifically modulated endothelial cells. *Lab. Invest.* 58:379–387, 1988.

Pitot, H.C.: *Fundamentals of Oncology*, ed. 3. Marcel Dekker, Inc., New York, 1986.

Poste, G., and Greig, R.: The experimental and clinical implications of cellular heterogeneity in malignant tumors. *J. Cancer Res. Clin. Oncol.* 106:159–170, 1983.

Powell, P.C.: Marek's disease virus in the chicken. In *Advances in Viral Oncology, Vol. 5. Viruses as the Causative Agents of Naturally Occurring Tumors*, edited by G. Klein. Raven Press, New York, 1985.

Prehn, R.T.: Tumor-specific antigens as altered growth factor receptors. *Cancer Res.* 49:2823–2826, 1989.

Ritz, J.: The role of natural killer cells in immune surveillance. *N. Engl. J. Med.* 320:1748–1749, 1989.

Rozengurt, E.: Signal transduction pathways in mitogenesis. *Br. Med. Bull.* 45:515–528, 1989.

Sager, R.: Genetic suppression of tumor formation: a new frontier in cancer research. *Cancer Res.* 46:1573–1580, 1986.

Sanchez, J., Baker, V., and Miller, D.M.: Basic mechanisms of metastasis. *Am. J. Med. Sci.* 292:376–385, 1986.

Santos, E., and Nebreda, A.R.: Structural and functional properties of *ras* proteins. *FASEB J.* 3:2151–2163, 1989.

Schat, K.A.: Marek's disease: a model for protection against herpesvirus-induced tumours. *Cancer Surv.* 6:1–38, 1987.

Schirrmacher, V.: Cancer metastasis: Experimental approaches, theoretical concepts, and impacts for treatment strategies. *Adv. Cancer Res.* 43:1–73, 1985.

Seemayer, T.A., and Cavenee, W.K.: Molecular mechanisms of oncogenesis. *Lab. Invest.* 60:585–599, 1989.

Sibbitt, W.L., Jr.: Oncogenes, normal cell growth, and connective tissue disease. *Ann. Rev. Med.* 39:123–133, 1988.

Sporn, M.B., and Roberts, A.B.: Peptide growth factors and inflammation, tissue repair, and cancer. *J. Clin. Invest.* 78:329–332, 1986.

Straus, D.S.: Somatic mutation, cellular differentiation, and cancer causation, *JNCI* 67:233–241, 1981.

Tachibana, T., and Yoshida, K.: Role of the regional lymph node in cancer metastasis. *Cancer Metastasis Rev.* 5:55–66, 1986.

Temin, H.M.: Evolution of cancer genes as a mutation-driven process. *Cancer Res.* 48:1697–1701, 1988.

Terranova, V.P., Hujanen, E.S., and Martin, G.R.: Basement membrane and the invasive activity of metastatic tumor cells. *JNCI* 77:311–316, 1986.

Van den Hooff, A.: An essay on basement membranes and their involvement in cancer. *Perspect. Biol. Med.* 32:401–413, 1989.

Verma, R.S.: Oncogenetics. A new emerging field of cancer. *Mol. Gen. Genet.* 205:385–389, 1986.

Waterfield, M.D.: Altered growth regulation in cancer. *Br. Med. Bull.* 45:570–581, 1989.

Weinberg, R.A.: The action of oncogenes in the cytoplasm and nucleus. *Science* 230:770–776, 1985.

Weiss, L.: *Principles of Metastasis*, Academic Press, New York, 1985.

Wheelock, E.F., and Robinson, M.K.: Endogenous control of the neoplastic process. *Lab. Invest.* 48:120–139, 1983.

Willman, C.L., and Fenogliopreiser, C.M.: Oncogenes, suppressor genes, and carcinogenesis. *Hum. Pathol.* 18:895–902, 1987.

Woodruff, M.F.A.: Tumor clonality and its biological significance. *Adv. Cancer Res.* 50:197–229, 1988.

7

Nature and Causes of Disease:
Interactions of Host, Parasite, and Environment

Understanding Disease
  Concepts of Disease
  Infection and Disease
  Factors Affecting Susceptibility and Resistance
  Resistance to Entry of Organisms
  Inflammation and Immune Response
    Phagocytosis and Microbicide
    Escape Mechanisms Used by Microorganisms
    Intracellular Parasitism
    The Immune Response
      Modification of Parasitic Antigens
      Immunosuppression
      Other Methods of Avoiding the Immune Response
  Nutrition and Resistance to Infection
Genetic Aspects of Disease
    The Tools of Molecular Biology
    Inherited Diseases
    Genetic Influence on Susceptibility to Disease

    Damage to DNA and Its Repair
  Age of Host
  Immune Deficiency States
  Environmental Effects
Mechanisms of Damage to the Host
  Damage Due to the Parasite
    Direct Damage
    Exotoxins
    Endotoxins
      Endotoxin and the Complement System
      Endotoxin and Arachidonic Acid Metabolism
      Endotoxin and the Clotting System
      Endotoxin and Neutrophils
      Endotoxin and Macrophages
      Endotoxin and the Endothelium
  Damage Due to the Host Response
    Inflammation and the Immune Response
    Fever and Other Systemic Reactions
Spread of Infection and Tissue Tropism
Persistence of Infection
Reference Material

UNDERSTANDING DISEASE

Concepts of Disease

What causes disease? The answer to this question has always been complicated, and it seems that the more we learn about disease, the more complicated it becomes. The infectious diseases form a good example. It was not so long ago that infectious diseases were regarded in a rather simplistic way: if a certain organism was present, then the patient had the disease that it was known to cause. For instance, if you were infected with *Bacillus anthracis*, then, by definition, you had anthrax. **Koch's postulates** grew from such a simple concept. They stated that, in order to be recognized as the cause of a disease, an organism should be consistently isolated from affected patients and should, when injected into unaffected animals, reproduce the disease. These principles grew from observations made on highly virulent organisms responsible for many of the major diseases that plagued man and animals in the past. Koch's postulates are still valid, but today many of the diseases for which the "one organism, one disease" paradigm held have been controlled. They have been replaced in order of importance by diseases for which Koch's postulates are not so easily satisfied.

In modern terms, it is important to recognize that the concept of **one cause** leading to **one disease** is almost always too simplistic. While it remains true that there would be no coccidiosis without coccidia and no mannosidosis without α-mannosidase deficiency, not all animals infected with coccidia or deficient in α-mannosidase develop the disease, or develop it at the same rate and severity. In contemporary terms, we tend to think of disease as **acquired** (such as coccidiosis) or **genetic** (such as mannosidosis), but it is equally clear that genetic factors can alter the outcome of acquired diseases and that, conversely, genetically determined diseases can be profoundly influenced by acquired factors. There are also a large number of diseases for which the **clinical** and **pathologic** manifestations are well established, but the various acquired or genetic factors responsible for the disease are poorly understood. Three of the major disease problems of modern man fit this category; cancer, degenerative arthritis, and arteriosclerosis.

Even for those diseases in which the etiology is fairly well established, it is increasingly clear that we must learn to think in terms of **multiple causation** of disease rather than a single cause. A good example might be an Arabian foal that died from the pulmonary complications of equine adenovirus infection and pneumocystosis. The virus, along with *Pneumocystis carinii,* are likely to be the etiologic agents responsible for the death of the foal, but the real story probably lies in the fact that the foal had genetically determined **combined immunodeficiency (CID).** This immunodeficiency in Arabian foals is inherited as an autosomal recessive trait and results in severe impairment of both cell-mediated and an-

tibody-mediated responses (*see also* Chapter 5). Since Arabian foals with normal immune function only rarely develop adenovirus infections and virtually never get pneumocystosis, it is fair to ask: what caused the disease? Was it the **acquired** infections themselves or the **genetic** predisposition to infection? Clearly, both were important factors in the death of the foal, which serves to underscore the importance of modern concepts of multiple causation.

The one constant thing about disease is its variability. The reasons for this become more clear when we recognize that there are an immense number of interdependent factors that influence the pathogenesis of a disease from inception to ultimate outcome. Some of these relate to the host and some to the various external causative factors such as bacteria and viruses. Many are also determined by alterations in the **environment** in which both the host and its parasites dwell. We are now forced to recognize that, although certain organisms can cause disease, they do not always do so. Conversely, not all hosts are equally susceptible to any one infectious agent. To make things even more confusing, diseases (or syndromes) that present with identical symptoms may be caused by different etiologies. Therefore, in order to understand the pathogenesis of diseases, it is essential to understand the way in which various host, parasite, and environmental factors interact to cause injury to the host. The collective effects of such injury are, after all, the basis for what we perceive as disease. In this chapter we will discuss some of the ways in which the host can influence its parasites as well as ways in which parasites influence the host. We will also consider the influence of factors external to both the host and its parasites.

We use the term **parasite** here in a generic sense; that is, any microorganism that lives in the host for at least part of its life cycle. It is important to remember that not all parasites cause disease. There are many parasites in the environment of the host, and all animals are colonized at an early age by a wide variety of microorganisms. Many of these establish an inoffensive relationship with the host and are referred to as **commensals.** They make up the normal flora of the skin, mucous membranes, and intestinal and respiratory tracts. In some cases the relationship may be mutually beneficial, one of the best examples of this being found in ruminants. The organisms in the forestomachs of these animals utilize nutrients ingested by the host and, in return, produce short-chain fatty acids and vitamins required by the host. Relationships that benefit both host and parasite are termed **symbiotic.**

Infection and Disease

What is **infection** or **parasitism?** They seem ubiquitous. Infectious **disease,** by contrast, is less common and only occurs when the activities of the organism, or of the host, or both, result in tissue damage. The mere presence of microorganisms does not imply the existence of disease. The organisms causing disease may be **exogenous,** not normally found in or on the host, or they may be **endogenous,** forming part of the animal's normal flora. Organisms vary in their ability to cause disease. Some, such as rabies virus, almost always cause severe illness. Others such as *Pneumocystis carinii* commonly parasitize animals but only occasionally cause disease, as in our example of the Arabian foal with CID. Organisms that usually are associated with disease are called **pathogens,** and, within a pathogenic species, different strains may vary in their ability to cause disease. Those that do so in a high proportion of infected hosts are referred to as **virulent** strains.

These various terms are useful in discussing infectious organisms and infectious disease, but they do have limita-

tions. No organism is known to cause disease in every infected animal, and, more importantly, there is no organism that never causes disease. The latter realization is becoming more and more important as clinicians manipulate their patients therapeutically and alter their ability to respond with normal defense reactions. Many organisms once considered harmless are now recognized to have pathogenic potential under the appropriate circumstances. Because infectious and parasitic diseases are still major causes of economic loss and fatality in domestic animals and man, it is of interest to review some of the ways in which parasitism results in disease.

FACTORS AFFECTING SUSCEPTIBILITY AND RESISTANCE

The production of infectious disease is a complex process involving a number of steps. The causative organisms must attach to the mucosa or skin, in many cases they must gain entrance to deeper tissues, and they must evade the defense mechanisms of the host, compete with other organisms, multiply, and produce tissue damage or malfunction. Parasites have evolved a variety of mechanisms to accomplish these goals, most of which are, after all, necessary for their survival. Host animals, on the other hand, have evolved defenses that may interfere with the parasite at a variety of levels. These defensive weapons provide resistance, either to infection or to disease.

Resistance to Entry of Organisms

The first line of defense against infectious disease is formed by the physical barriers that limit the access of organisms to the tissues. Organisms in the environment come into contact with the host through the skin and mucous membranes. The skin, of course, forms a relatively impermeable barrier to the entry of organisms. The superficial keratinized layer is relatively tough, and, although the skin is colonized by microorganisms, the turnover of the epithelium and the pH of the skin limit their numbers. In the stomach, the low pH of the gastric secretions is unfavorable for the survival of organisms. In the intestine, the presence of certain bacteria is essential for normal health. Abnormal accumulation is prevented by epithelial turnover (many of the bacteria adhere to epithelial cells), the protective barrier of mucus, and the continuous movement of the intestinal contents. In the urinary tract, the continuous flow of urine normally prevents access of bacteria to the kidneys, even when the urine in the bladder is contaminated.

In the respiratory tract a very elaborate physical mechanism has evolved for the clearance of inhaled particles, including microorganisms. In the bronchi and trachea, mucus secreted by globlet cells is continually moved toward the pharynx by the cilia of respiratory epithelial cells. Debris is therefore carried to the pharynx by this action, where it is swallowed. This mechanism very efficiently removes particles large enough to impact on the walls of the airways. Smaller particles such as bacteria (less than 2 μm) may reach the alveoli and escape mucociliary clearance by lodging in the lung at a level distal to the ciliated cells. Such small particles must be dealt with by other mechanisms, such as phagocytosis by alveolar macrophages. Once interiorized by phagocytosis, the particles are carried from the distal lung to this mucociliary escalator by the motile alveolar macrophages. It is known that various kinds of pulmonary injury which damage this mucociliary clearance mechanism or injure the alveolar macrophages have an adverse affect on lung clearance and defense mechanisms.

Parasitic organisms are able to overcome these physical host defenses in a variety of ways. Some overcome the barrier of the skin by utilizing insect vectors, so that, rather than having to make their own way, they are injected directly into the tissues. A number of important diseases are transmitted in this way. One of the most serious in man is malaria. The causative protozoal organisms, *Plasmodium* spp., are transmitted by the bite of certain mosquitoes. One approach to the control of malaria, therefore, has been to minimize the number of mosquitoes in the environment. Many other organisms are transmitted in this way. They include *Rickettsia* spp., spirochetes such as *Borrelia burgdorferi*, the cause of Lyme disease, trypanosomes, and many viruses. In many cases, the microorganism is obliged to spend part of its life-cycle in the vector, while in other cases the insect simply acts as a mechanical carrier.

Other microorganisms have evolved specific receptors for host cell membrane molecules, which allow them to adhere to host cells and avoid clearance mechanisms. Many viruses, for instance, specifically attach to cell membranes before entering the cell. This phenomenon not only explains the ability of these agents to overcome the host's barriers to infection but presumably explains their tissue tropism. A good contemporary example is the **acquired immunodeficiency syndrome (AIDS)** in man. Human AIDS is caused by a virus that specifically infects T helper cells and cells of the mononuclear phagocyte system (Langerhans cells of the skin and alveolar macrophages) carrying the CD4 cell surface receptor. It is the high affinity of the viral envelope glycoprotein gp120 for the CD4 molecule that enables the virus to bind to and enter the cells (*see also* Chapter 5).

Some bacteria also utilize specific receptors to attach to host cells. The importance of such mechanisms in disease production is well illustrated by many of the enteropathogenic strains of *Escherichia coli*. These bacteria cause disease by producing a toxin that acts locally on intestinal epithelial cells but, to produce disease, bacteria must accumulate in the intestine in large numbers. Some strains of *E. coli* can do this because they possess molecules that bind to receptors on host intestinal epithelial cells. These bacterial molecules are antigenic and are referred to as K antigens. In the pig, for instance, K88 antigens are important determinants of pathogenicity, while in the cow K99 antigens are important.

These antigens appear to be glycoproteins, and they form part of the fine filamentous structures, or pili, present on the surface of the organisms. The presence of these specific antigens are not the only determinant of bacterial adherence, however. In pigs, some strains of *E. coli* lacking K88 antigens are still able to adhere to and colonize the intestinal epithelium. This ability has been shown to depend on the presence of pili (not bearing K antigens), a capsule or, in some cases, both. The nature of the receptor on host cells to which bacterial adherence factors bind is still being defined. For instance, for some *E. coli* strains it appears to be a mannose-containing molecule, but in the case of some enteropathogenic porcine strains it is not.

Clearance mechanisms also may be interfered with by infectious organisms. Infection of the respiratory tract by certain viruses and *Mycoplasm* spp. can alter the function of ciliated cells, thus interfering with the mucociliary elevator. This is important in interfering not only with clearance of the primary infectious agent but also with that of other inhaled particles or microorganisms, especially bacteria, and it may result in secondary infections. This subject has been the object of extensive research using a variety of combinations of viruses and bacteria. Good examples are provided by Sendai virus infection in mice and parainfluenza 3 (PI-3) virus infection in cattle. The pulmonary inflammatory response elicited by many such respiratory tract agents can itself impair clearance mechanisms.

In mice it has been well documented that infection with Sendai virus (a parainfluenza virus) impairs clearance of bacteria from the lung. If mice are experimentally infected with both Sendai virus and potentially pathogenic bacteria, increased mortality occurs in those mice with the dual infection (Fig. 7.1). This

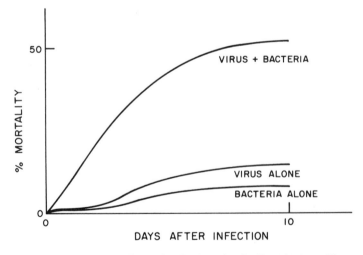

Figure 7.1. **Interaction of Viral and Bacterial Pathogens in Respiratory Disease.** The percentage mortality is much higher in animals infected with both pathogenic virus and pathogenic bacteria than in those infected with virus or bacteria alone. These experiments utilized combined infection in mice with parainfluenza virus and *Haemophilus influenzae*.

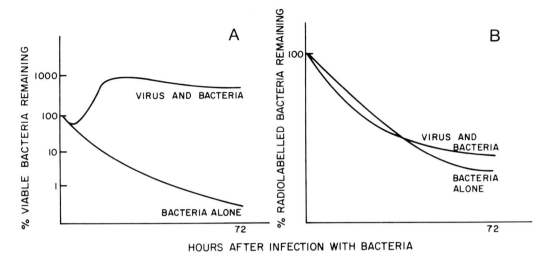

Figure 7.2.   Effect of Viral Infection on Clearance of Bacteria from the Lung. In dual infections with virus and bacteria, *A,* the population of bacteria in the lung progressively increases, rather than decreases as it does with infection by bacteria alone. *B,* When the bacteria used are radiolabeled, it can be shown that the introduced bacteria are removed from the lung as effectively in dual infections as in infections with bacteria alone. This type of data suggests that at least one effect of virus infections is to impair killing of bacteria by alveolar phagocytes.

has been shown to be associated with decreased clearance of viable bacteria from the lung. Two mechanisms could be involved, namely, impairment of mucociliary clearance mechanisms or, alternatively, impairment of phagocytic clearance from the deep lung by injury to the alveolar macrophages, causing diminished phagocytosis and killing. In this particular model system there is certainly a defect in phagocytosis and killing. If, for instance, mice are first infected with Sendai virus and then, about 6–7 days later, infected with pathogenic bacteria, the number of bacteria remaining in the lung exceeds that in mice infected with bacteria alone (Fig. 7.2A). In contrast, radiolabeled bacteria are cleared at similar rates in both groups (Fig. 7.2B). This suggests that it is not mucocilliary transport mechanisms that are disrupted but that phagocytosis and killing of the bacteria are impaired by the virus infection.

Other experiments have shown a reduced phagocytic capacity in virus-infected animals as well as an impairment

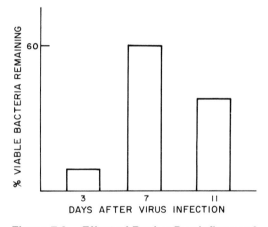

Figure 7.3.   Effect of Bovine Parainfluenza 3 Virus Infection on Bacteria. The time interval between viral injury and bacterial clearance is important. If *Pasteurella hemolytica* are administered 3, 7, or 11 days after virus infection, bacterial clearance is basically normal 3 days after virus infection but becomes severely impaired 7 days later, and the deficiency is still present 11 days after virus infection. (Adapted from the data of A. Lopez, R.G. Thomson, and M. Savan: The pulmonary clearance of *Pasteurella hemolytica* in calves infected with bovine parainfluenza-3 virus. *Can. J. Comp. Med.* 40:385–391, 1976).

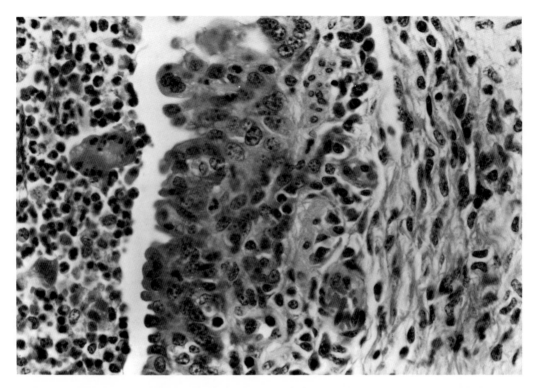

Figure 7.4. Morphologic Basis for Impaired Lung Clearance in Viral Infection. This lesion is from a case of bovine parainfluenza 3 virus infection. There is marked hyerplasia of bronchiolar epithelium. Note that the surface epithelium is immature and lacks cilia. Such a lesion would result in defective mucociliary clearance.

of killing of the bacteria that are phagocytosed. The latter defect apparently is due to impairment of fusion of phagocytic vacuoles with lysosomes. Similarly, PI-3 virus has been shown to impair the clearance of *Pasteurella haemolytica* from the lungs of calves (Fig. 7.3). This virus is known to infect alveolar macrophages and, as a consequence, to reduce their phagocytic capacity.

In most of these experiments, aerosols containing very small particles are utilized, and therefore most of the organisms are deposited in the deep lung where alveolar macrophages are most important for clearance. However, many viruses that infect the respiratory epithelium also are known to alter the function of the mucociliary apparatus. In PI-3 virus infections,

for instance, infected cells soon develop morphologic changes in the cilia and their basal bodies. Also, as a consequence of the hyperplasia of bronchiolar epithelium induced by this infection, immature cells line the bronchioles (Fig. 7.4). These cells lack the specialized functions of their mature counterparts, and this change is accompanied by changes in mucociliary clearance mechanisms.

Inflammation and Immune Response

The inflammatory and immune responses of the host are the most important of the host defense mechanisms (*see also* Chapters 4 and 5). The inflammatory response delivers phagocytes, serum products (including immunoglobulins and complement), cytotoxic cells, and degradative enzymes to the sites of infection. The nature of the host response varies and depends to some extent on the type of organism involved. Those that grow in an extracellular location tend to evoke a suppurative response. The inflammatory cells, chiefly neutrophils, are attracted by chemotactic factors produced either by the invading organisms or as a result of the complex mediator-generating pathways of the inflammatory response itself. At the site of infection these cells attempt to phagocytose and kill the organisms. Many phagocytes, especially neutrophils, may degranulate during the phagocytic process, releasing their enzymes into the tissues. Because this may result in local damage, the best outcome for the host is rapid killing of organisms with minimal tissue damage.

Organisms that have the ability to survive and grow inside host cells provide a special problem for the host in killing them. Such intracellular organisms are inaccessible to host effector cells, antibody, enzymes, and other host defense reactions. The inflammatory response in these cases tends to be chronic and granulomatous and is mediated in part through delayed-type hypersensitivity. Such lesion may persist for long periods of time, because the host cannot rid itself of the parasite. In such cases the likelihood of damage to the host is increased.

Phagocytosis and Microbicide

Part of the host response to infection is to mobilize phagocytes, chiefly neutrophils and macrophages, in an attempt to engulf and kill the invaders. In recent years the mechanisms by which phagocytes are able to actually kill microorganisms have been intensively studied. Emerging from this work is the realization that both **oxygen-dependent** and **oxygen-independent** mechanisms of bacterial killing are important, and that factors that adversely influence impor-

tant phagocyte biochemical activities, such as the **respiratory burst,** adversely affect host defense (*see* Chapter 4). The importance of oxidative mechanisms of bacterial killing is illustrated by **chronic granulomatous disease** of children. Patients with this disease lack the ability to generate a respiratory burst and therefore do not produce endogenous H_2O_2, superoxide anion, or the other bactericidal products we have discussed. They are very susceptible to infections, and their neutrophils cannot incorporate iodine into the bacterial cell wall. They are most susceptible to infections by catalase-positive organisms; catalase-negative organisms apparently produce enough H_2O_2 themselves to allow the system to function.

Nonoxidative bactericidal systems also are involved. Phagocytosed bacteria are exposed to a low pH in the phagolysosome, conditions that do not favor their growth. **Lysozyme** is also present in phagocytes. It acts on peptidoglycans in bacterial cell walls. With the exception of a few Gram-positive bacteria, however, it requires the cooperation of other effectors, such as antibody and complement, to unmask its substrate. **Lactoferrin** is found in neutrophils and serves to deprive bacteria of iron. As a result it is bacteriostatic.

Macrophages, in contrast to neutrophils, are long-lived cells and are capable of a number of activities that may be utilized in defense of the host. They are, of course, important as phagocytes but differ somewhat from neutrophils in the way in which they kill microorganisms. They have a poorly developed myeloperoxidase system, and their lysosomal enzyme content differs slightly from that of neutrophils. Killing of ingested organisms in macrophages depends primarily on fusion of the phagocytic vacuole with lysosomes and exposure of organisms to the nonoxidative mechanisms that we already have discussed.

Escape Mechanisms Used by Microorganisms

Because phagocytosis is such an important first line of defense against invading organisms, it is of great significance that many organisms have evolved methods of counteracting it. The ability to avoid phagocytosis is an important determinant of virulence in a number of bacterial species. One mechanism involved in a number of bacterial infections is the ability of the organism to kill the phagocyte. Some strains of streptococci can produce substances called **streptolysins,** which cause the degranulation of lysosomes inside intact cells. This kills the phagocyte. *Listeria monocytogenes* and some staphylococci utilize similar mechanisms. In cattle, certain strains of *Pasteurella haemolytica* also apparently are toxic to alveolar macrophages and kill the phagocytes which ingest them. The importance of such phenomena can hardly be overemphasized. *P. haemolytica,* for example, is a major cause of pneumonia in cattle, and bovine pneumonia is one of the greatest causes of economic loss in the cattle industry today. *Corynebacterium ovis,* an important pathogen of sheep, possesses a toxic surface lipid that enables it too to destroy phagocytes.

A second mechanism which may be used to interfere with the function of phagocytes is inhibition of chemotactic migration. Streptolysins, besides their ability to kill phagocytes, can interfere with chemotaxis. Relatively low concentrations are required to do this, and the production of streptolysins obviously confers some advantage on the bacteria.

Probably the single most important mechanism in preventing phagocytosis, however, is inhibition of the actual engulfment process. Many bacteria and some yeasts are able to do this. The ability to resist phagocytosis is commonly related to the possession of a capsule, and encapsulated (or smooth) strains of certain bacteria are pathogenic, while unencapsulated (or rough) strains often are not. *Streptococcus equi, E. coli, Pasteurella multocida,* and the yeast *Cryptococcus neoformans* are examples of organisms in which capsules are considered to enhance pathogenicity. In some cases the thickness of the capsule correlates with the degree of virulence. Surface components other than capsules also can confer resistance to phagocytosis. For example, some strains of streptococci bear a surface protein called M protein, which also is able to confer resistance to phagocytosis.

The mechanisms by which capsules and other surface components confer resistance to phagocytosis are poorly understood. Phagocytes, particularly macrophages, are able to recognize abnormal cells, including organisms, without involving specific immunologic mechanisms. Presumably cell surface interactions are important in this process, and it is likely that capsules mask potential recognition sites on the organisms. In some cases it is thought that the strong negative surface change conferred by the capsule repels the negatively charged surface of the phagocyte. In the case of *C. neoformans,* however, where the presence of a polysaccharide capsule (Fig. 7.5) is strongly correlated with resistance to phagocytosis, the negative charge can be neutralized without enhancing phagocytosis. Even when a capsule is present, coating of the surface of organisms by antibody (opsonization) greatly enhances the ability of phagocytes to ingest them. This supports the concept that the efficacy of phagocytosis depends on the ability of the phagocytes to recognize the organism, whether it be *via* inherent surface components or *via* antibody that has combined with surface antigens.

Since the complement system is one of the most important means of host defense against infection, it should not be surprising that pathogens have developed a number of different strategies for its ev-

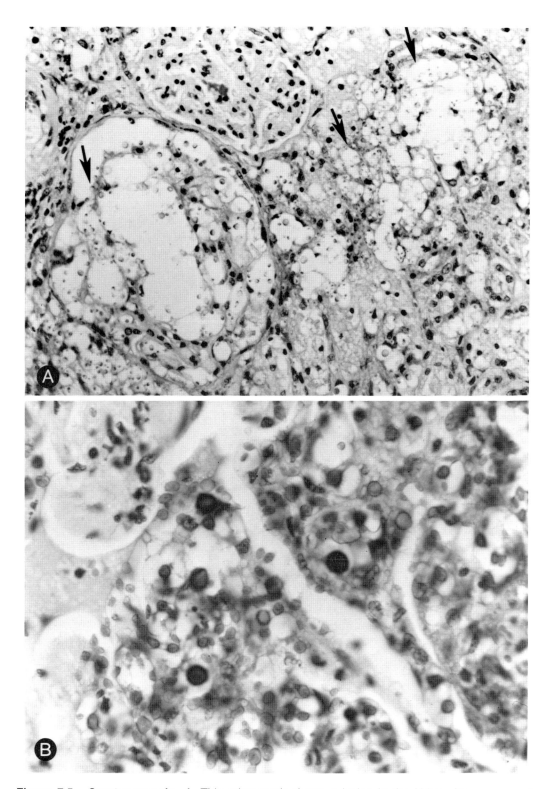

Figure 7.5. Cryptococcosis. *A,* This micrograph shows a lesion in the kidney from a case of disseminated cryptococcosis in a dog. Cystic spaces contain many organisms *(arrows),* but there is minimal inflammation. *B,* A mucicarmine stain for acid mucopolysaccharides clearly shows the dark capsule surrounding the organisms. This capsule is believed to confer resistance to phagocytosis.

asion. Evasion may occur on the surface of the organism itself because the complement cascade is not activated, because of complement inhibitors or inactivators released by the microorganisms, or because the **membrane attack complex (MAC)** either fails to form or does not lyse the organism. The binding of C1q may also actually facilitate entry into host cells of some organisms such as *Trypanosoma cruzi*, while certain of the membrane proteins of *Campylobacter fetus* interfere with the deposition of C3 on the bacterial surface. The high concentrations of ammonia produced by *Pseudomonas aeruginosa* may inactivate C3, and the same organism is known to produce elastase-like enzymes that can cleave a number of complement proteins. Lastly, certain microorganisms have developed sophisticated strategies for complement evasion based on such clever maneuvers as the generation of an inactivator of the C5a chemotaxin (group A streptococci), the proteolytic cleavage of bound C3 *(Leishmania donovani)*, or the formation of a non-lytic C5b-9 complex (certain strains of *Salmonella* spp. and *E. coli*). In this latter escape mechanism, long-chain surface endotoxin (LPS) molecules apparently impart a steric barrier prohibiting access of the C5b-9 MAC to the hydrophobic domains of the membrane. Studies of the means by which such microorganisms evade the complement system have been very instructive in improving our understanding of the complicated interface between the host and its parasites.

Intracellular Parasitism

Some organisms are able to enter cells and somehow survive and grow. Protozoa, such as *Toxoplasma gondii* and *Sarcocystis* spp., bacteria such as *Mycobacterium tuberculosis* and other mycobacteria (Fig. 7.6), rickettsiae, *Listeria monocytogenes* and *Brucella abortus*, fungi such as *Blastomyces dermatitidis* (Fig. 7.7), *Histoplasma capsulatum* and *C. neoformans*

(Fig. 7.5), and of course all viruses, can live inside host cells. Some of these organisms, including viruses and rickettsiae, have specific requirements for host cell products and therefore are **obligate** intracellular parasites. Others are **facultative** intracellular parasites and can live in the extracellular environment when necessary. Clearly, these organisms have evolved ways to avoid the ability of the host cell to kill them, and for many of them the macrophage provides a home rather than a site of destruction. Life in the intracellular environment does, of course, offer some advantages. The parasite is to some extent protected from the effector components of host defenses and is free of competition from other organisms. Its only problems are to compete with the host cell for essential nutrients and to avoid being killed by the cell itself.

The ways in which organisms avoid the attack mounted by the host cell are understood only incompletely, but a few mechanisms have been defined. Some strains of *M. tuberculosis*, for example, appear to be able to prevent fusion of the phagocytic vacuole, in which they entered the cell, with lysosomes. This is true only of intact, living organisms, as dead *M. tuberculosis* are phagocytosed and digested in the normal way. In mycobacteria, there is relatively good correlation between the ability to resist lysosomal fusion and virulence. *T. gondii* is also somehow able to prevent fusion with lysosomes. How these organisms accomplish this remarkable feat remains incompletely understood. In addition, this phenomenon is not the only way in which organisms can escape destruction. When mycobacteria are coated with antibody before phagocytosis occurs, fusion of lysosomes with the phagocytic vacuole does occur, but the bacteria still survive. In contrast, opsonization renders *T. gondii* susceptible to lysosomal fusion and kill-

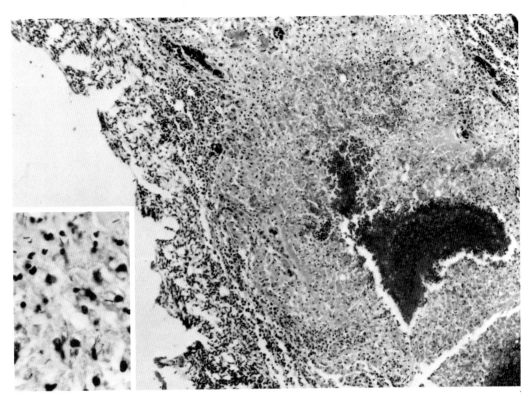

Figure 7.6.   Avian Tuberculosis. This micrograph shows a granuloma in the lung of a chicken with tuberculosis. A Ziehl-Neelsen stain for acid-fast bacteria clearly demonstrates the causative organisms in macrophages *(inset)*.

ing. Obviously, a number of different mechanisms of resistance must be involved.

Like *M. tuberculosis* that have been opsonized, *Mycobacterium avium* and *Mycobacterium lepraemurium* resist killing, despite the fact that fusion of the phagocytic vacuole with lysosomes does occur (even in the absence of antibody). The reason that these organisms can resist killing within the phagolysosome is poorly understood but probably it is related to the peculiar composition of their cell wall. Mycobacteria contain, in their walls, a high content of lipids, including true waxes. Certainly in the case of *B. abortus*, which also resists killing within the phagolysosome, there is evidence that a component of the cell wall is responsible. An additional mechanism that may be im-

portant in intracellular survival is escape from the phagolysosome. Rickettsiae, for instance, exist free in the cytoplasm of parasitized cells, but it is not clear whether this is due to escape from the phagocytic vacuole or from the phagolysosome, or to entry to the cell by some means other than phagocytosis.

The Immune Response

We do not intend in this discussion to fully reiterate the intricacies of the immune response (*see* Chapter 5). It is necessary, however, to consider its relevance to defense against parasitic disease and, as we have done for other defense mechanisms, to discuss the ways in which parasitic organisms avoid it.

The immune response is an extremely important defense mechanism against

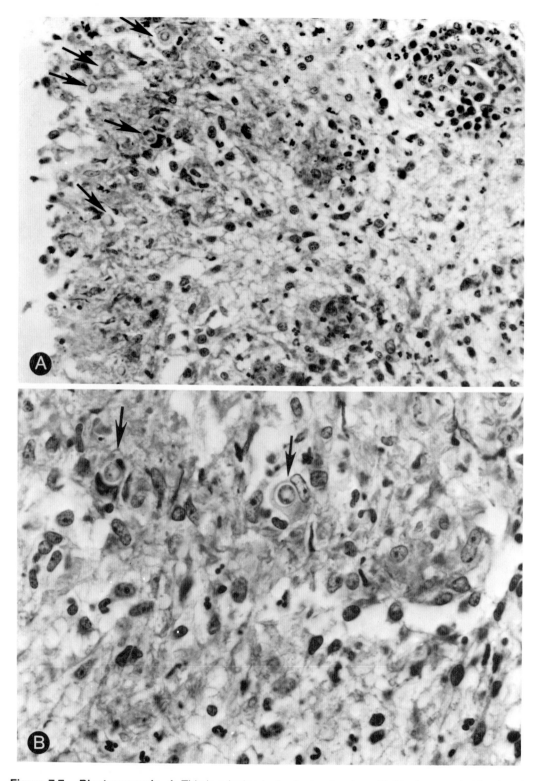

Figure 7.7.   Blastomycosis. *A,* This is a lesion in the brain of a dog with blastomycosis. The fourth ventricle is at *left.* There is necrosis of ependyma and of the parenchyma of the brain and infiltration by macrophages and neutrophils. Several organisms are present *(arrows). B, Blastomyces derma-titidis* organisms can be seen in macrophages *(arrows).*

parasitic disease, especially against infectious disease. Both humoral and cell-mediated responses play a role. Antibody can opsonize organisms, facilitating their phagocytosis as discussed above. It can inactivate toxins and surface receptors and can activate complement, resulting in lysis of target organisms or infected cells. The activation of complement also produces chemotactic substances that promote inflammation. Antibody is particularly important in protecting against extracellular organisms, but it also can limit infections by some intracellular organisms. For example, immunity to a number of viruses appears to be due to antibody, which probably inactivates circulating free virus and limits dissemination of infection.

Cell-mediated immunity (CMI) is mediated by T cells. It is a crucial mechanism for protection against intracellular parasites such as viruses, some bacteria, and fungi. Sensitized T cells can be directly cytotoxic to infected cells, or they can produce lymphokines that attract and activate other types of effector lymphocytes and macrophages. It should come as no surprise that many parasitic organisms have evolved ways to deal with the immune response. Although our knowledge of the methods they use is undoubtedly incomplete, a number of mechanisms that may be involved are known.

MODIFICATION OF PARASITIC ANTIGENS. In order to evoke an immune response, of course, parasitic organisms have to bear antigens to which the host can respond. The immunogenicity of organisms varies, and those that elicit a relatively weak response are at an advantage. It should be pointed out immediately that immunogenicity cannot be considered as simply a property of the organism. As discussed later in this chapter, genetic factors in the host can influence the immune response and the degree to which disease develops.

One way in which organisms might re-

duce their immunogenicity is by synthesizing antigens that imitate those of the host. This phenomenon, called **antigenic mimicry,** has been postulated to be an explanation for the observation that in certain parasitic infections, such as schistosomiasis, adult forms of the parasite persist in the host despite evoking an immune response. The immune response, in contrast, *is* effective against immature forms of the parasite (cercariae). True synthesis of host-like surface antigens by the parasite has, however, never been clearly established, and is now considered unlikely to occur even in schistosomiasis. A number of animal species can act as host for this parasite, and it is unlikely that it can mimic antigens of several different host species at will. A more likely explanation of its resistance to the immune response is that the adult parasites can adopt, or coat themselves, with host-derived material. This appears to be true at least for *Schistosoma mansoni*. If adult *S. mansoni* are grown in mice, then transferred to monkeys, they are killed as long as the recipient animals are immunized against mouse erythrocytes. They are not killed by nonimmunized animals. In this case, the parasites apparently mimic host tissues by adopting actual host components.

Another possible mechanism for avoiding the immune response of the host is the redistribution and possibly the shedding of surface antigens. This is similar to the phenomenon of **antigenic shedding,** which can occur in tumor cells (*see* Chapter 6). In this process surface antigens usually distributed diffusely on the parasitic cell surface become concentrated at one end, a process known as **capping.** Following this, the antigens may be shed. This mechanism has been demonstrated to occur *in vitro*, but its role *in vivo* is unclear.

Other organisms may *mask* their inherent antigens by producing a capsule. Some organisms, such as *S. equi*, have

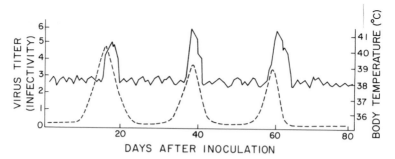

Figure 7.8.   Antigenic Variation in Equine Infectious Anemia (EIA) Virus. The clinical course of EIA is characterized by periodic exacerbations of anemia and fever *(solid line)* which are accompanied by surges of viremia *(dashed line).* Each increase in viremia is associated with the emergence of a new antigenic type of virus. (This is a hypothetical case adapted from the data of Y. Kono: Recurrences of equine infectious anemia; approaches to an understanding of the mechanisms. *Proceedings of the Third International Conference on Equine Infectious Diseases,* pp 175–186, 1972. Paris, 1973).

capsules composed predominantly of hyaluronic acid, which is nonantigenic. It is possible that this protects against an immune response to deeper antigens. In many cases, though, capsular components themselves are antigenic and may elicit an effective immune response.

One tactic that does seem to be of considerable importance, being utilized by a number of organisms, is **antigenic variation.** It has been documented in African trypanosomiasis, for instance, that there are fluctuations in the degree of parasitemia, which correspond to changes in the antigens carried by the parasite. Following each antigenic change in the organism, antibody specific for the new variant is generated by the host. The question then arises, is the appearance of new antigenic variants due to selection for small numbers of antigenic subtypes that already existed, or is the change induced by the presence of antibody against the parasite? The evidence is in favor of the latter. If immunosuppressed animals are infected with these trypanosomes, antigenic variation does not occur. Furthermore, if clones derived from a *single* parasite are used to infect host animals, antigenic variation still occurs. Therefore antigenic variation appears to occur as a consequence of an immune response and

to involve changes, presumably the synthesis of new antigens, in individual organisms. Currently it is thought that these parasites have genes coding for a finite number of surface antigens, which can be varied in a regular sequence as a result of exposure to the host immune response. Antibody probably has both an inductive role (bringing about the change), and a selective one (destroying organisms with "old" antigens against which antibody is directed). Antigenic variation also occurs in babesiosis in cattle and, at the other end of the biologic spectrum, in the virus diseases visna and equine infectious anemia (Fig. 7.8). The net result of antigenic variation is persistent infection. There are other diseases, such as Aleutian mink disease and African swine fever, in which persistent infection occurs despite the presence of large amounts of antibody. In such cases, although the antibody is directed against the virus, it is ineffective in ridding the host of infection. The mechanisms enabling the virus to persist in the face of specific antibody are essentially unknown.

IMMUNOSUPPRESSION. A number of infectious agents can impair the defense mechanisms of the host by causing immunosuppression (Table 7.1). This is usually a relatively nonspecific effect, and

Table 7.1
Examples of Immunosuppression Caused by Infection in Animals

Species	Agent	Effect
Canine	Distemper virus	Lympholytic infection; depletion of B and T cells from lymphoid tissues; thymic atrophy; reduced PHA[a] responsiveness
Canine	Parvovirus	Lympholytic infection; thymic atrophy; lymphopenia; functional deficiency unproven
Canine	*Demodex canis*	Serum factor suppressing PHA responsiveness of lymphocytes
Feline	Feline leukemia virus	Thymic atrophy; lymphoid depletion; depressed T cell function
Feline	Panleukopenia virus	Lympholytic infection; thymic atrophy, lymphoid depletion; suppressed T cell function in infected neonates
Bovine	Bovine virus diarrhea virus	B and T cell suppression
Equine	*Herpesvirus* type I	Lympholytic infection in neonates; thymic atrophy, lymphoid depletion

[a] The abbreviation used is: PHA, phytohemagglutinin.

the host becomes hyporesponsive to a variety of antigenic stimuli. Canine distemper virus (CDV) provides a good example. This virus infects and kills host lymphocytes, and infected animals have been shown to have depressed immune responses. Such immunosuppression may be important not only in reducing the efficacy of the host's defenses to the primary agent, in this case CDV, but to other agents as well. For instance, dual infections with CDV and *T. gondii* used to occur when distemper was more widespread. Presumably, this was because CDV-infected dogs were unable to mount an effective immune response to the second organism. More recently, dual infections with CDV and canine parvovirus (CPV) also have been seen. This also might be due to immunosuppression by the organisms involved. As CPV is also a lympholytic virus, even though no immunosuppressive effects have yet been properly documented, it is difficult to decide in this case which virus infection predisposes to the other.

As a final comment on this subject it should be pointed out that not only classical infectious agents cause immunosuppression. Dogs with generalized **demodicosis,** caused by the mite *Demodex canis,* have been shown to have a circulating serum factor that is able to suppress the responses of canine lymphocytes to phytohemagglutinin (PHA) *in vitro.* This effect does not occur in dogs with localized demodicosis, and it is possible that immunosuppression plays a role in the pathogenesis of the generalized form of the disease. This possibility remains to be proven.

OTHER METHODS OF AVOIDING THE IMMUNE RESPONSE. Some bacteria are capable of inactivating specific components of the immune response. Some produce proteases that are able to cleave antibody molecules. Their activity may be very specific. For example the human pathogens *Hemophilus influenzae* and *Streptococcus pneumoniae* produce enzymes that can cleave IgA_1, but not IgA_2, IgG, or IgM molecules. Staphylococcal protein A inhibits the function of antibody by competing for the Fc portion of the immunoglobulin molecule. Because the fixation of complement and phagocytosis of opsonized organisms each involves the recognition of the Fc fragment of bound antibody molecules, protein A interferes with both of these important defense mechanisms. Other bacteria, including some strains of *E. coli,* interfere with the effectiveness of complement fixation. This results from the presence of polysaccharide O antigens that project from the cell and cause complement activation to occur at a distance from the cell wall. Consequently, the bacterial cell is not lysed by the activated complement. We have already discussed some other means by which microorganisms escape the complement system.

Finally, some organisms, which are notably unusual in their properties, seem to completely avoid the host immune response. These are the agents that cause the so-called **neurodegenerative diseases** and **spongy encephalopathies;** scrapie of sheep, transmissible mink encephalopathy, and, in man, kuru and Creutzfeld-Jakob disease. In these diseases there is no apparent recognition of the agent by the host for reasons that remain, for the most part, unknown. The name **prion** has been given to these unusual agents, based on their alleged definition as small *proteinaceous infectious* particles that resist inactivation by procedures that modify nucleic acids. These prions are apparently not true viruses. It now seems likely that studies of prions will raise fundamental questions about how some infectious, environmental, and genetically programmed events may represent some form of conversion of normal, necessary proteins into lethal molecules. There is seemingly always something new under the microbiological sun.

Nutrition and Resistance to Infection

Severe malnutrition in the host, particularly undernutrition, interferes with the generation of antibody and the cellular immune response. Also, phagocytic function is depressed, and the integrity of physical barriers such as the skin and mucous membranes may be altered. These findings are not surprising and may predispose the malnourished animal to infectious disease. Less commonly considered, however, is the question of bacterial nutrition and the ability of the host to affect it. Bacteria, like their hosts, require certain essential nutrients. If the host could deprive the organism of some of these, it might provide a potentially important general means of defense against infection. That the host can, in fact, protect itself using such tactics is best illustrated by the requirement of bacteria for iron and the ability of the host to withhold this nutrient.

Iron is probably the single most important trace element required for bacterial growth. If it is lacking, bacteriostasis results, and suboptimal levels of iron interfere with the production of a number of bacterial products including toxins. Host animals, of course, also have a requirement for iron, and both animals and bacteria have evolved specific mechanisms for acquiring it. Bacteria produce iron-binding substances called **siderophores** that allow them to compete for the small amounts of free iron in the plasma and tissues. These products are synthesized and secreted, bind iron, and then are reabsorbed as iron chelates. Animals synthesize a number of iron-binding glycoproteins, the most important of which are **transferrin** and **lactoferrin.**

Host animals can limit the availability of iron to bacteria in a variety of ways. There is evidence that animals with infectious or inflammatory disease can selectively reduce intestinal iron absorption. Also, there is a redistribution of iron from plasma to storage pools. Plasma iron begins to fall early in the incubation period of infectious diseases and may become reduced by 50% or more. It returns to normal levels after recovery. Studies of the **anemia of inflammatory disease** in dogs have shown, for instance, that there is a modest anemia involving a reduction in hematocrit from about 50 to about 38, and a reduction in hemoglobin concentration from about 17 g/dl to about 12.5 g/dl. Associated with this, plasma iron may be reduced from about 113 μg/dl to about 62 μg/dl. Further study showed this to be due to increased storage of iron in a relatively less labile form, presumably in ferritin and hemosiderin. In other words, in inflammatory disease iron was sequestered in storage pools, and serum iron concentrations fell dramatically. This is a nonspecific effect that occurs in inflammatory disease of both noninfectious and infectious origin. It is tempting to speculate, however, that its purpose is to limit the availability of iron to bacteria that might infect the host.

In animals, iron-binding proteins are found not only in the plasma but also at sites prone to infection such as in milk, bronchial and intestinal secretions, and other body fluids. **Transferrin** is the major iron-binding protein in the plasma and **lactoferrin** is important in secretions, especially in milk. It also is released from the specific granules of neutrophils and thus may be secreted locally at sites of infection. Animals can modulate the synthesis of these compounds in response to infection. For instance, mice with experimental infections increase their rate of synthesis of transferrin, and infectious mastitis results in increased synthesis of lactoferrin in the bovine mammary gland. Within 90 h of the onset of experimental *E. coli* mastitis there is a 30-fold increase in the concentration of lactoferrin in the gland. Lactoferrin also is increased in the involuting gland.

Apparently the host also can interfere with the bacterial siderophore system. The synthesis of siderophores by bacteria is less efficient at high temperatures, such as are found in animals with fever, and antibody directed against bacteria also can reduce the synthesis of siderophores.

So, again, a contest has emerged between the host and its parasites, this time for iron. The host attempts to limit its availability, and the bacteria have developed methods to obtain it. It is generally accepted that the ability to produce adequate siderophores and the presence of iron-chelate binding sites, which may reside in the lipopolysaccharide component of the cell wall in some bacteria, are important determinants of bacterial virulence. There is experimental evidence that hyperferremia can enhance susceptibility to infection, and that hypoferremia can reduce it. This is a system, however, that is dangerous to manipulate. Because iron also is essential to the host, overzealous withdrawal of iron can adversely affect the susceptibility of the host to infection, presumably due to effects on other defense systems.

GENETIC ASPECTS OF DISEASE

It would be entirely inappropriate to leave our discussion of disease without saying something about the role of genetic factors in either producing disease directly, or in influencing its outcome. Truly dramatic advances have been made over the last few years in understanding genetic disorders and in applying molecular genetic techniques to understanding many other types of disease. These advances have been possible because of the development of new tools in molecular biology. There is a danger here of trying to write a text in molecular medical genetics rather than simply providing the perspective that we intend. This discussion will therefore be brief. We will discuss the nature of the new technology, then summarize in tabulated examples the types of genetically determined diseases that animals have. We will discuss some examples that demonstrate how genetic factors influence other types of disease, and end by briefly reviewing mechanisms of DNA repair and their potential role in mutagenesis.

The Tools of Molecular Biology

The advances that we have mentioned are commonly referred to as **recombinant DNA technology.** The major reason that these techniques are now possible is the availability of **restriction endonucleases.** These bacterial enzymes cleave DNA at specific nucleotide sequences, allowing it to be cut into relatively small fragments. It is now possible to identify, clone, and amplify genes directly from DNA or to produce clones from mRNA. The latter procedure exploits **reverse transcriptase** from retroviruses to make a DNA copy of the mRNA molecule. Because it is a complementary copy the product is referred to as cDNA. In either case the cloned molecules can be used as probes to look for the presence of a gene and its mRNA, and to assess their quantity. Furthermore, a variety of techniques allow the normalcy of the gene to be studied.

Yet another remarkable dividend has been the new-found ability to quickly determine the sequence of a protein. It is much easier to sequence DNA than to sequence protein. Frequently these days investigators who are interested in a particular polypeptide or protein will clone its gene, produce cDNAs, and sequence them. Because the genetic code is known, the sequence of the protein can very quickly be predicted. We have mentioned throughout this book many instances of knowledge that would not have been available without this technology. During our discussion of the genetic basis of neoplasia, we made passing reference to many such examples. The structure of the growth factors, for example, would be mostly unknown. The alterations in gene structure and the expression and amplification of oncogenes could not be measured. The nature of protein products encoded by the oncogenes would not be known.

These molecular techniques also pro-vide the ability to produce large quantities of purified protein products relatively easily and cheaply. The impact of this will be felt in all branches of the medical sciences. It is now possible, for example, to produce human insulin in bacteria. This will free patients from having to use insulin of porcine origin, avoiding the risks of adverse immunologic reactions. Similar benefits will come to veterinary medicine and agriculture. As an example, bovine growth hormone is already being produced in quantity, and is being tested for its capacity to improve production.

Another impact of molecular genetic technology has been the ability to search for the specific abnormal gene responsible for particular inherited diseases. Even when the gene product is unknown, specific defective genes can be tracked down. This approach has been dubbed **reverse genetics.** Briefly, to search for the gene causing a particular disease investigators generate DNA probes of known chromosomal location. Often the chromosomal location of a particular defect is known, and appropriate probes can be chosen. If not, random probes can be used, although the task becomes very much larger. What is done is to look for genetic linkage between the particular probe and the disease of interest. Without delving too deeply, the technique of **linkage analysis** depends on the occurrence of genetic recombination between loci on the same chromosome. The further apart two loci are, the more likely they are to recombine. During linkage analysis, if two loci (e.g., the disease locus and the probe in use) recombine less often than expected, they are said to be in **linkage disequilibrium.** When this occurs, it indicates that the probe is relatively close to the disease locus, and the hunt begins. Additional probes can be generated, and by "chromosomal walking" the gene can be found.

One of the most dramatic successes in "reverse genetics" has been the identification of the gene defect responsible for Duchenne muscular dystrophy, a devastating X-linked myopathy affecting young male children. We will briefly describe how this gene was located to demonstrate the extraordinary progress that can be made. The story also has a specific veterinary interest because it has been possible to demonstrate that certain myopathies of dogs are due to a defects in the same gene. Duchenne muscular dystrophy was known to frequently be associated with deletions of a particular part of the X chromosome. Investigators took advantage of this to identify a piece of DNA missing from one such patient. Briefly, normal DNA and patient DNA were mixed so that strands from each could bind to one another, then nonhybridized fragments were isolated as putative probes. It was soon shown that the probes recognized DNA missing from the patient. Linkage analysis showed that the probe was very close to the Duchenne locus. Then it was found that one of several probes generated could recognize mRNA present in normal muscle but not in dystrophic muscle. cDNA probes could then be made, the full length of the cDNA was sequenced, protein fragments were generated in bacterial hosts, and antibodies to **dystrophin** (as the newly recognized protein was called) were made. Dystrophin is now known to be a large protein with the characteristics of a cytoskeletal protein. It is located on the cytoplasmic face of the plasma membrane of the muscle cell, and its function is being actively investigated. Its sarcolemmal location is consistent with the findings of many pathologists who studied Duchenne muscular dystrophy, coming to the conclusion that some defect in the plasma membrane was responsible for the disease. Finally, using probes for the human gene and antibodies to its product, it has been possible to show that a myopathy of dogs, known as canine X-linked muscular dystrophy, is also due to absence of dystrophin. Advances in understanding of a human disease have thus helped to clarify a canine counterpart. Study of the disease in both species will be mutually beneficial.

Inherited Diseases

Hereditary disease are very commonly encountered in the practice of veterinary medicine, particularly in pet species such as the dog and the cat. One reason for this is the inbreeding that inevitably occurs in purebred animals. Because the gene pool is small, the chances of inadvertently breeding two animals carrying the same genetic defect are relatively high. Table 7.2 lists a small sample of known inherited disease in animals to illustrate their diversity.

Inherited diseases, of course, are due to mutations in particular genes and are passed on through the germ-line. A number of kinds of mutation can occur. These include point mutations, that is, a change in a single base, deletions or duplications of variably sized segments of the genome, gene rearrangements, or a variety of chromosomal abnormalities. Mutations can occur in the coding portions of the gene or in regulatory elements. The end result is the production of a defective protein or absence or reduction in the quantity of the protein product.

Many of the inherited diseases that we see are inherited as simple Mendelian traits. These include autosomal recessive (a very common mode of inheritance), autosomal dominant, or X-linked. They are usually the result of a mutation in a single gene, although syndromes occur where large deletions disrupt a number of adjacent genes. A clinician is often alerted to the possibility of an inherited disease by certain events. For example, inherited diseases occur most commonly in purebred strains. When a characteristic syndrome occurs in a number of animals of the same breed, an inherited problem might be suspected. Even more damning is the occurrence of more than one animal

Table 7.2
Some Genetic Diseases of Animals

Disease	Species	Inheritance[a]
Myasthenia	Dog	AR
Globoid cell leukodystrophy	Dog, mouse	AR
GM1 gangliosidosis	Cat, dog, cow	AR
GM2 gangliosidosis	Dog, cat, pig	AR
Mannosidosis	Cow	AR
Muscular dystrophy	Dog, mouse, cat	XR
Collie eye anomaly	Dog	AR
Progressive retinal atrophy	Dog	AR
Hepatic copper storage	Dog	AR
Chondrodysplasia of Malamutes	Dog	AR
Hip dysplasia	Dog	P
Patent ductus arteriosus	Dog	P
Subaortic stenosis	Dog	P
Persistent right aortic arch	Dog	P
Cyclic neutropenia	Dog	AR
Hemophilia A	Dog	XR
Hemophilia B	Dog	XR
Combined immunodeficiency	Horse	AR

[a]The abbreviations used are: AR, autosomal recessive; XR, X-linked recessive; P, Polygenic.

with the disease from the same litter, or from the same breeding, or from breedings of closely related animals. The nature of the disease can also be a clue to inheritance. For example, if a single case is shown by clinical or pathologic examination to be a **lysosomal storage disease,** it would be immediately suspected to be inherited. As a group, storage diseases are one of the most common of inherited diseases, and affected animals often present with neurologic signs. These occurrences, then, should raise a warning flag.

When a disease is inherited as a simple Mendelian trait, it is usually relatively easy to determine the mode of inheritance by pedigree analysis. Relatively large litter sizes in dogs and cats facilitate this. However, it must be borne in mind that the **penetrance** of a genetic disease may vary, so that not all animals with the defect are clinically apparent, and the **expressivity** of the disease may vary. A

further complicating factor is possible expression of signs in heterozygotes due to gene dosage effects. Finally, a number of diseases with a clear-cut genetic contribution are inherited as polygenic disorders. In other words, they are controlled by a number of genes acting in concert. Veterinarians are often consulted for advice on how to eliminate an inherited disease. This involves identifying the mode of inheritance, which may involve further test breedings for confirmation, testing of potential breeding animals as possible carriers, and identification of animals unlikely to be implicated as carriers, based on statistical methods. It is therefore essential to be aware of the pitfalls when attempting to set up eradication schemes. Identification of a biochemical defect often eliminates the need for these time-consuming and unpopular trials, as carriers can sometimes be identified by their intermediate expression of the gene product. Readers are referred to genetics texts for a fuller discussion of the various strategies that can be adopted.

Genetic Influence on Susceptibility to Disease

The outcome of interactions between the host and its parasites may be influenced dramatically by genetic factors in either party. In the case of microorganisms, genetic changes may greatly alter virulence. A good example is provided by encapsulated bacteria. We already have explained how the capsule of certain bacteria can enhance pathogenicity by enabling the organism to resist phagocytosis and, perhaps, by masking surface antigens. Genetic variants of such bacteria occur in which the capsule is lost, and this change usually is associated with loss of virulence. Genetic variation in viruses also may result in loss of virulence. This often occurs when viruses are passaged repeatedly in an abnormal environment, the process being known as **attenuation.** Attenuated strains of virus, usually produced by repeated passage in tissue culture, have been widely exploited as vaccines. Genetic changes in organisms also can enhance virulence. There is also some evidence, in the case of canine distemper virus for example, that attenuated virus strains can regain virulence when passaged through their normal host.

Bacteria can obtain new genetic information in two additional ways. Plasmids can transfer genetic information from one bacterial cell to another. The information sometimes codes for products such as toxins, which can be important determinants of pathogenicity. Later in this chapter we will discuss the importance of bacterial toxins in injuring the host. One important example is the production of enterotoxins by some strains of *E. coli*. The production of these toxins, which exert their effect on the intestine, is coded for by plasmids. In a similar vein, diphtheria toxin is produced only by strains of *Corynebacterium diphtheriae* that are infected with a bac-

terial virus, or bacteriophage. In this case, the information required for the production of the toxin is acquired by the bacterial cell when it is infected by the phage.

Genetic variation in organisms obviously can be very important. Microorganisms have an additional advantage since their short generation period gives them a capacity for rapid change not enjoyed by the host. Nevertheless, the genetic characteristics of the host are just as important. Genetic characteristics of the host presumably are involved in determining the susceptibility of species to particular infectious agents. Most microorganisms can infect only a limited range of host species. The reasons for this are not clear. We do not know why, for example, canine distemper virus can infect dogs and mink, but not cats, when feline panleukopenia virus infects cats and mink, but not dogs. Why, in contrast, can rabies virus infect all warm-blooded animals including birds? Even within species, there are often dramatic differences between strains or breeds in the way in which they respond to various parasites or organisms. Zebu cattle, for instance, are more resistant to ticks than European breeds. African swine fever virus causes devastating disease in domestic pigs but inapparent infection in the warthog.

Clearly, more than one mechanism is involved in these different processes. Species susceptibility to infection is poorly understood but presumably involves interactions between the surface of the organism and that of the host cells. Similar mechanisms probably underlie the tissue tropism shown by many infectious agents. Recent studies of interactions of viruses with their hosts has shown that surface changes in the virus induced by genetic manipulation can alter both host and tissue tropism.

Differences in susceptibility to disease in infected animals of different strains presumably is due to other mechanisms. Susceptibility to disease can be manipulated in the laboratory, and strains of mice can be selected which are resistant to specific diseases such as mouse pox, salmonellosis, or mouse hepatitis. Very often, of course, such variations are determined by alterations in immune responsiveness, which is, in turn, controlled by **immune response (Ir) genes.** A vigorous immune response usually correlates with protection from disease, but this is not always the case. The "usefulness" of the immune response depends on how effectively and how quickly it eliminates the agent, and how much tissue damage is incurred during the process. This can be exemplified by a couple of instances in which different strains of mice differ in their ability to respond to infectious agents.

Mouse pox virus, in the C57Bl mouse, induces a vigorous immune response that limits spread of the virus. As a result, lesions are minimized and the animal usually recovers. In contrast, other strains are, because of their genetic makeup, less able to mount an effective immune response. Virus is disseminated widely, and severe and usually fatal disease results. This is the way we expect things to work. A good immune response is protective, its absence is not. However, if mice of the same C57Bl strain are infected with lymphocytic choriomeningitis (LCM) virus, they develop only a very modest immune response, yet they do not develop severe lesions or disease. Other mouse strains *do* develop a strong immune response, but they also develop lesions and severe disease. In this case it is apparent that the immune-mediated attack on infected cells is associated with tissue damage and disease. The C57Bl mouse remains persistently infected but is not directly injured by the virus. Therefore, due to its genetic characteristics, this strain of mice is protected from one disease by being able to produce a vigorous immune response and from a second disease by not being able to respond. Such specificity of response and susceptibility demonstrates the ex-

quisite sensitivity of control of the host immune response to infectious organisms and other antigens.

Perhaps surprisingly, attempts to identify the mouse genes responsible for resistance to bacterial infection have produced results suggesting that a single gene is responsible. Furthermore, resistance is dominant. Similar results have been obtained with several different organisms. Interestingly enough, after our discussion of the role of genetically regulated immune responses, resistance to at least three organisms maps to the same region of chromosome 1 in the mouse. The evidence is that classical immune responses are not involved, but macrophages have been implicated in this genetically determined resistance. The results, at any rate, demonstrate that resistance and susceptibility to infectious agents are determined by a number of genetic influences.

Damage to DNA and Its Repair

It is beyond the scope of this discussion to consider in detail the biochemistry of DNA injury and repair. We will, however, briefly consider this subject with emphasis on the consequences of DNA injury. In part, this will complement our discussion of genetic aspects of carcinogenesis presented in Chapter 6.

DNA can be damaged in a variety of ways. These include damage to individual bases, strand breaks (single or double), altered base sequences, and cross-links between base pairs. The causes of such alterations are numerous and include radiation of various kinds and chemicals. In many cases the nature of the damage caused by a particular agent is unknown. In other cases it is understood in detail. For example, ultraviolet (UV) irradiation is known to cause the formation of pyrimidine dimers in the DNA molecule.

A number of mechanisms apparently are available to the cell for the repair of damaged DNA molecules. In some cases single-strand breaks may be repaired by the enzyme **polynucleotide ligase,** which simply rejoins the broken ends of the strand. **Excisional repair** (Fig. 2.33) is a more complex and important mechanism for repair of DNA, which involves several steps and the participation of a number of enzymes. It is used to repair DNA segments in which abnormal bases occur. It is likely that, despite the singular names used, the enzymes involved are part of complexes of cooperating enzymes and proteins that carry out the various steps. In the first step, an endonuclease causes a break in the DNA molecule adjacent to the defective base. An exonuclease then peels off, or excises, the segment in which the defect occurs, and DNA polymerase catalyzes the synthesis of a replacement strand using as a template the complementary bases on the opposite strand. The "patch" is then joined to the rest of the strand by a ligase. This method of repair is capable of repairing defects in bases such as the dimers formed by UV irradiation. It is relatively error free. However there is some evidence that, at least under some circumstances, it can exacerbate existing DNA damage. It apparently can generate double-strand breaks in DNA in which single-strand breaks already have been produced by some other agent. Double-strand breaks are considered to be more serious for the cell and more difficult to repair, since no intact complementary strand is available as a template.

Postreplication repair is a second method of restoration of the damaged DNA molecule. This type of repair process takes place during the replication of DNA. The mechanisms involved are not clearly understood, but it is considered to be more error prone than excisional repair. The repair of double-strand breaks is also probably error prone.

The importance of discussing DNA damage at all is that faulty repair *can* occur, and, when it does, it can result in **mutation.** When this occurs in a germ cell and is compatible with survival of the cell it leads to an **inherited mutation** that may be expressed as a defect in the progeny. In non-germ cells, faulty repair results in **somatic mutation.** A variety of phenotypic expressions may result from such mutations. When a structural gene is affected there may be enzyme defects and the synthesis of abnormal proteins. When regulatory genes are involved there may be changes in the rate or control of synthesis of gene products. Cells affected by somatic mutations may die or may remain viable.

Age of Host

Some diseases show a striking propensity to affect particular age groups. Canine *Herpesvirus* infection, for example, causes disease only in very young puppies, even though previously unexposed older dogs also are susceptible to infection. The reasons for this are poorly understood, although one possible explanation is that this virus prefers to grow at slightly lower temperatures than most. The relatively low body temperatures of young puppies, compared to that of adults, may enhance virus replication resulting in more extensive tissue damage. Another possible explanation might be that the immune response in such young animals is poorly developed.

In other cases, the reasons for age-related susceptibility are better defined. Transmissible gastroenteritis (TGE) virus causes disease only in very young piglets. This virus infects and damages epithelial cells on the intestinal villi. In very young pigs, the turnover of intestinal epithelial cells is rather slow compared to the adult, and the damaged cells cannot be quickly replaced. As a result villus atrophy occurs and severe diarrhea is the end result.

Young animals may also be more susceptible to infection due to relative immunologic immaturity or to lack of previous exposure to the agent. This becomes

Table 7.3
Examples of Immune Deficiency Diseases in Domestic Animals

Species	Disease	Nature of Defect
Equine	Combined immunodeficiency	Lack of functional T cells and B cells
Equine	Agammaglobulinemia	Lack of functional B cells
Equine	Selective IgM deficiency	Inability to synthesize or secrete IgM
Equine	Transient hypogammaglobulinemia	Delay in onset of antibody synthesis
Bovine	Lethal trait A-46	Defective T cell function; abnormal zinc metabolism
Bovine	Selective IgG_2 deficiency	Reduced IgG_2 synthesis
Canine	Cyclic neutropenia	Cyclic abnormalities of hematopoiesis
Canine	Granulocytopathy syndrome	Abnormal bacterial killing by neutrophils
Feline, bovine	Chédiak-Higashi syndrome	Abnormal granule containing cells; possible microtubular defect (by analogy to man)

particularly important in animals that fail to receive adequate maternally derived antibody.

Immune Deficiency States

A number of inherited immune deficiency states have been described in man, and there is growing evidence that a similar spectrum of such diseases is present in animals (Table 7.3, *see also* Chapter 5). Inherited defects in immunity in animals have been best characterized in the horse and the cow. Reports suggesting such disorders in sheep and dogs also have been published.

In the horse the best-characterized inherited immunodeficiency state is **combined immunodeficiency** (CID), a disease of the Arab breed. Lymphoid organs essentially lack lymphocytes (Fig. 7.9), and there is almost no circulating antibody. In other words, there is combined dysfunction of both T cell and B cell systems. Other immunodeficiency disorders in horses, probably inherited, include agammaglobulinemia, in which there is a lack of B cells and an inability to synthesize antibody, and selective IgM deficiency, in which the only abnormality is the absence of IgM.

In the cow an inherited defect has been described in which there is a loss of T cell function but normal B cell function. The disease also is associated with hyperkeratosis and can be corrected by treatment with zinc. It is inherited as an autosomal recessive trait and is postulated to involve an unusually high requirement for zinc, so that normal dietary levels are insufficient for normal T cell development. Another condition that is apparently inherited in cattle is selective deficiency of IgG_2.

All of these conditions are associated with some degree of increased susceptibility to infection. Foals with CID, for example, never live beyond a few months of age because of infectious diseases. Most commonly they succumb to pulmonary infections with equine adenovirus (Fig. 7.10), bacteria, or the protozoan organism *Pneumocystis carinii* (Fig. 7.11). The latter organism is ubiquitous and probably is present in the lungs of many animals. Normally it does not cause disease, but in the presence of immunodeficiency, whether primary or secondary, it can proliferate and cause pneumonia. In the other immunodeficiency states, infectious diseases are again the usual cause of death,

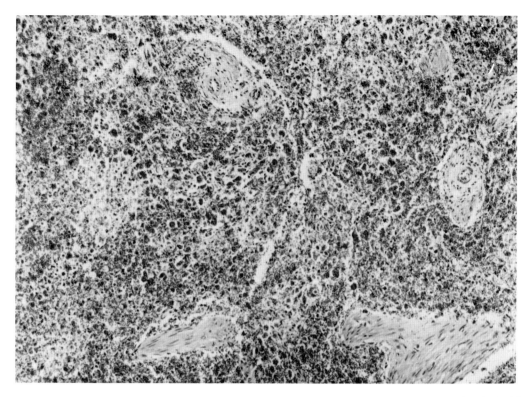

Figure 7.9.   Combined Immunodeficiency Disease (CID). In this spleen from an Arabian foal with CID there is no evidence of normal lymphoid follicle development (B cell areas), and the periarteriolar sheaths (T cell dependent regions) are sparsely cellular.

but affected animals tend to survive longer than is the case in CID.

Inherited immune deficiencies also occur in laboratory animals. The nude mouse, for instance, is congenitally athymic and lacks T cells, and a similar defect occurs in rats. These disorders, and those of man, will not be further discussed here.

The ability to mount an immune response is, of course, affected by many nongenetic influences. The most important of these is simple failure to obtain passive immunity *via* colostrum. Because most domestic animals obtain their maternally derived antibodies from this source, deprivation of colostrum will result in immunodeficiency, and the animals are at increased risk for infectious diseases. Other causes of immunosuppression are too nu-

merous to deal with here but include neoplasia, treatment with drugs (especially with the commonly used corticosteroids), and infections. In dogs, for instance, neoplasia, canine distemper, and generalized demodicosis all have been associated with immunosuppression. In cats, infection with feline leukemia virus (FeLV) is associated with immunosuppression, and this and other feline viruses are being intensely studied as models for human **AIDS (acquired immunodeficiency syndrome)** (*see also* Chapter 5).

Heritable defects in defense mechanisms other than classical immune responses also occur. In particular a number of defects in neutrophil function have been described. One of these, the **Chédiak-Higashi syndrome** in which abnormalities of lysosomes are prominent,

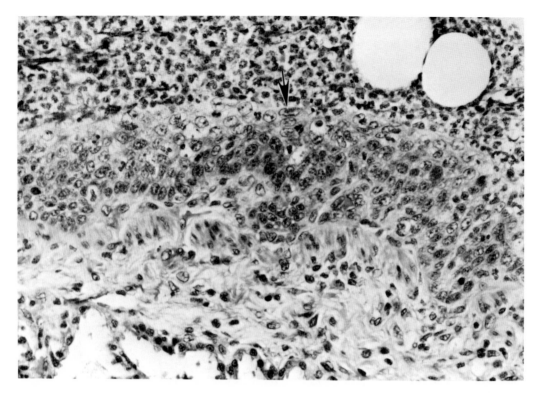

Figure 7.10.   Adenovirus Infection in Combined Immunodeficiency Disease (CID). This micrograph shows suppurative bronchiolitis and dramatic hyperplasia of the bronchiolar epithelium in a foal with CID. One epithelial cell contains a viral inclusion body *(arrow)*. The bronchiolar lumen is at the *top* and is filled with necrotic debris and inflammatory cells.

occurs in man, mice, cats, cattle, and mink. It is associated with giant granules in all granule-containing cells and, although they are able to phagocytose normally, neutrophils exhibit defects in chemotactic migration and in lysosomal degranulation. There is evidence to link these abnormalities to defects in microtubular function, which in turn may be due to dysregulation of the intracellular cyclic nucleotides cGMP and cAMP. Agents which elevate cGMP levels can correct the functional defects in this disease, and one of them, ascorbic acid (vitamin C), has been used successfully to treat human patients with Chédiak-Higashi syndrome. Hence, Chédiak-Higashi syndrome appears to involve a defect in control of the cytoskeleton. Whether this is due to abnormal cyclic nucleotide metabolism,

to defects at the cell surface, or to other abnormalities is as yet unknown. Chédiak-Higashi syndrome *does* show that information obtained in the laboratory by researchers interested in the biology of the disease can be applied in the field to help affected patients. This is no less true of diseases of animals than it is of man. In some species, including man and cattle, individuals with Chédiak-Higashi syndrome are abnormally susceptible to infections. In others, such as the cat, the disease does not predispose to infection, apparently reflecting differences in functional impairment of neutrophils.

In man there are a number of other neutrophil granulocytopathies. These include **chronic granulomatous disease,** in which there is a failure to generate a respiratory burst following phagocytosis.

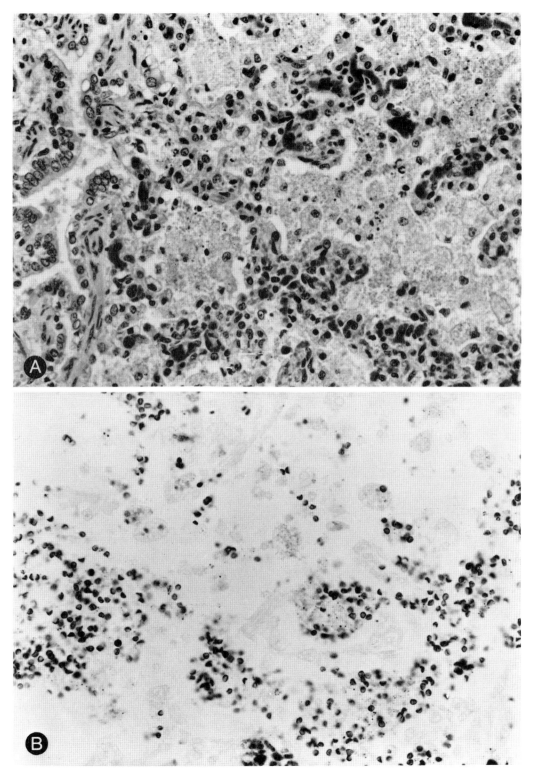

Figure 7.11. Pulmonary Pneumocytosis. *A,* In this lung there is a mild mononuclear cell infiltrate and the alveoli contain macrophages and exudate. This lesion is from an immunosuppressed horse. *B,* A silver stain reveals numerous *Pneumocystis carinii* organisms.

This in turn is associated with a failure to generate microbicidal oxidizing agents. Defects in the myeloperoxidase system and other enzymes, and lysosomal abnormalities also have been described. All of these result in abnormal susceptibility to infection. In dogs a disease called **canine granulocytopathy syndrome** has been described in which there is normal phagocytosis by neutrophils but defective intracellular killing of bacteria. The molecular basis of this disease is as yet undetermined, but it may be related to recently described deficiencies of the **leukocyte adhesion molecules (LeuCAMs)**. In **cyclic neutropenia** of collie dogs there is a periodic failure to produce neutrophils and other blood cells. In both of these canine diseases there is a greatly increased susceptibility to infections.

Environmental Effects

Although this discussion has concentrated on contributions of the parasite and the host in determining susceptibility to infection and disease, it would be incomplete without a brief discussion of the role of the environment. There are many environmental factors that can alter host resistance. Here only a few relatively important ones will be discussed.

Host defense mechanisms may be altered by environmental factors. Important in this respect are the alterations in the mucociliary elevator which can be brought about by excessively dry or cold air or, more importantly, by atmospheric pollutants. Ammonia, generated by bacterial breakdown of urea, can be an important pollutant in the environment of animals kept under intensive conditions. In pigs, ammonia contamination has been shown to impair bacterial clearance from the lungs, and in rats is has been shown to be an important predisposing agent to respiratory *Mycoplasma* infections. Similarly, a cold environment impairs pulmonary bacterial clearance in young pigs, and, presumably, a great variety of low-grade insults could predispose to pulmonary infection through similar mechanisms.

Changes of feed can be important in animal husbandry in increasing susceptibility of animals to infections. Ruminants, in particular, are very sensitive to such changes. As an example, changing a cow's diet to one rich in grain, especially crushed grain, can cause accumulation of lactic acid in the rumen. This local environmental change results in mucosal damage and secondary infections often caused by fungi (Fig. 7.12).

The nature of the microbial flora might itself be regarded as part of the environment of the host animal. The components of the microbial flora are in a finely balanced state that depends on the fact that various species of organisms can inhibit the growth of others. This occurs through nutrient competition and the production of antibiotic substances. Disturbances in the flora can lead to predominance of abnormal microbial species and to disease in the host. For example, antibiotic treatment, especially in ruminants, can kill off normal flora, allow the proliferation of resistant species, and may result in mycotic infections.

MECHANISMS OF DAMAGE TO THE HOST

As already stated in this chapter, disease only results when infection produces significant tissue damage or malfunction in the host. All of the defense mechanisms discussed above can be thought of as having evolved to protect the host from disease. This is, in fact, true from the point of view of the host *species,* but the *individual,* in combatting parasitism, may suffer a certain amount of damage. The significance of the damage, of course, depends on its extent and the site at which it occurs. Clearly, a lesion such as an abscess in the subcutis might be uncomfortable, but it can be resolved and does not impair the function of the host greatly.

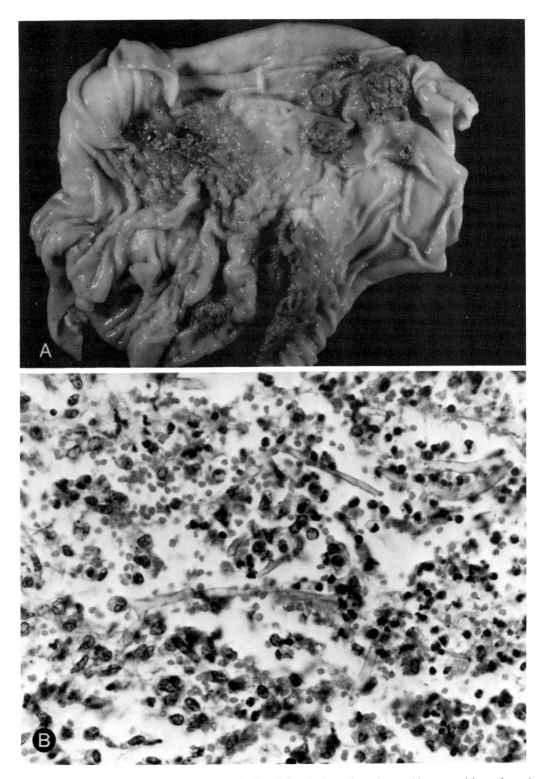

7.12. Mycotic Abomasitis. *A,* This cow had multifocal ulcerative abomasitis caused by a fungal infection associated with a sudden change of feed. *B,* Histologically, fungal hyphae can be seen associated with an inflammatory infiltrate and hemorrhage.

In contrast, an abscess in the brain probably would be fatal. Damage to the host can occur as a direct result of the activity of the parasite, or it may be a consequence of the attempt of the host to eliminate it.

Damage Due to the Parasite

Direct Damage

Some agents damage host cells directly. This is true of many viruses. After infecting the cell they shut down normal cellular metabolism and divert the activity of the cell to the production of virus. This results in alteration of membranes, dysfunction in homeostatic mechanisms, and eventually degeneration and cell death. There are many examples of virus-induced necrosis (Fig. 7.13). When viruses are grown *in vitro,* their cytotoxic effect often can be appreciated and is referred to as **cytopathic effect** (CPE).

In infected tissues, it can be difficult to separate the effect of the virus from that of the host's own attack on infected cells. For example, in some *Herpesvirus* infections, such as **Pachekos' disease,** which occurs in certain parrots, there are foci of cell necrosis with essentially no cellular inflammatory response. Presumably such lesions are due to direct effects of the virus. Poxvirus infections also are often characterized by cell degeneration and necrosis with little or no inflammatory response. In other virus infections, as in **infectious bovine rhinotracheitis,** also caused by a *Herpesvirus,* there is a marked inflammatory response. Presumably, in such cases, host cytotoxic effector mechanisms contribute to the destruction of tissue.

Exotoxins

In the case of other organisms, toxins often are postulated to be instrumental in damaging the host. Certainly many bacteria elaborate toxic substances, but only in a few cases can disease manifestations be attributed to one or a few tox-

ins. Bacterial toxins fall into two groups, exotoxins and endotoxins.

Exotoxins are specific secretory products of living bacteria and, unlike endotoxins, are not the product of bacterial autolysis. They are usually proteins, are produced by either Gram-positive or Gram-negative bacteria, and may act locally or systemically. Among the better known examples are the toxins produced by a number of clostridia.

Both *Clostridium tetani* and *Clostridium botulinum* produce potent neurotoxins, and **tetanus** and **botulism** are among the classic diseases in which clinical signs are attributable to the action of a single toxic bacterial product. Tetanus toxin is produced by organisms growing locally in the anaerobic environment that occurs in wounds. It acts both centrally and at the neuromuscular junction, but the spastic paralysis characteristic of tetanus is attributable to its ability to inhibit inhibitory interneurons in the central nervous system. *C. botulinum* produces a neurotoxin that is among the most potent toxins known. It is usually ingested with food in which the organism has been growing but, less commonly, the disease may result from contamination of wounds. The toxin acts solely at the neuromuscular junction and inhibits the release of acetylcholine from the nerve terminal. Botulism therefore is characterized by flaccid paralysis.

Other clostridia produce toxins that cause tissue damage. *Clostridium haemolyticum, Clostridium chauvoei,* and *Clostridium novyi* all produce toxins of this type. Some of them, at least, are phospholipases and presumably act by damaging cell membranes. The diseases they produce, such as **blackleg** in cattle, are characterized by massive tissue necrosis (Fig. 7.14). There is some advantage in this for the bacteria, as the necrotic tissue provides a suitable anaerobic environment in which the organisms can grow. Most of these clostridial diseases are produced by organisms that infect the

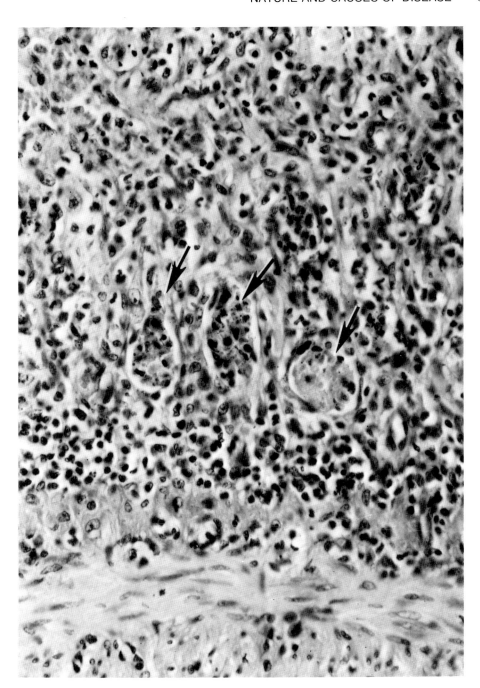

Figure 7.13.   Necrosis due to Viral Infection. This lesion is from a case of parvovirus infection in a dog. There is a loss of intestinal glands (crypts) and three remaining glands contain necrotic cellular debris *(arrows)*. The necrosis of epithelial cells is considered to be a direct effect of the virus.

tissues and act locally, but some, such as *Clostridium perfringens*, inhabit the intestinal tract where they produce toxins that are absorbed and act systemically.

Other bacteria, such as *Fusobacterium necrophorum* are also thought to produce necrosis due to toxins (Fig. 7.15).

Some bacteria that inhabit the intes-

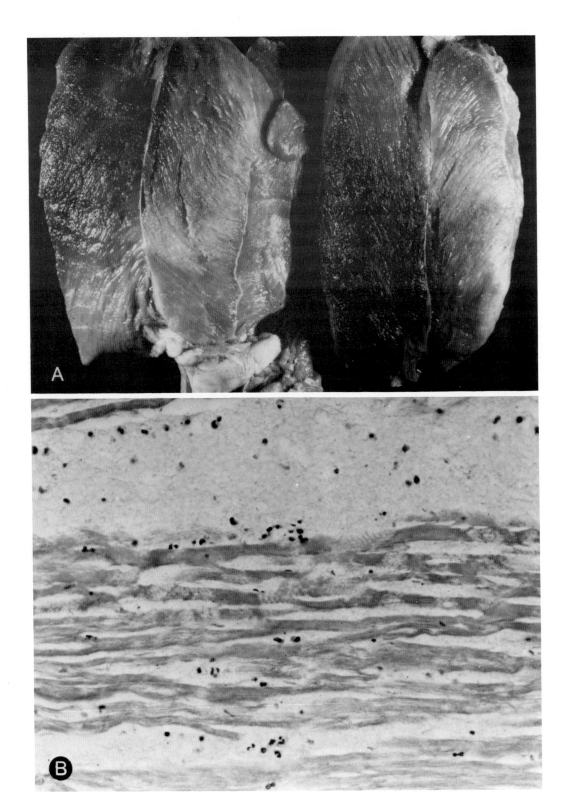

Figure 7.14. Necrosis due to Bacterial Toxins. These are lesions from a case of blackleg in a cow. *A,* The necrotic muscle tissue is dark and hemorrhagic. *B,* The muscle fibers are necrotic and separated from one another by protein-rich edema fluid. There is minimal inflammation.

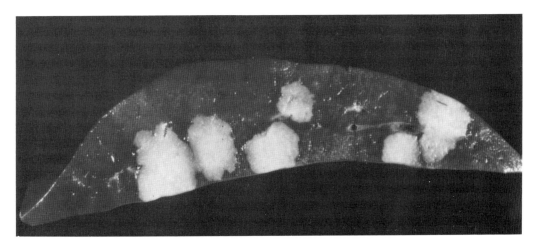

Figure 7.15. Necrosis due to Bacterial Infection. This photograph shows multifocal hepatic necrosis in a case of necrobacillosis in a cow. This lesion is thought to be due to toxins released by the causative organism, *Fusobacterium necrophorum.*

tine produce **enterotoxins** that act locally on the intestinal epithelium and cause diarrhea. The classic example is *Vibrio cholerae*, which causes the disease **cholera** in man. The organism produces **cholera toxin,** which seems to function by interference with GDP-GTP coupling *via* ADP-ribosylation of the α-subunit of one of the **G proteins** (G_s), thus providing rather steady activation of adenyl cyclase in intestinal epithelial cells, which in turn increases intracellular levels of cyclic AMP (cAMP). This results in a net secretion of water into the lumen of the small intestine rather than net absorption. The production of diarrhea depends on the accumulation of large numbers of organisms in the bowel lumen, and the massive secretion of water and electrolytes in the small intestine overwhelms the ability of the large intestine to absorb it. **Pertussis toxin** appears to function similarly (via ADP-ribosylation) but affects a different G protein (G_i). These toxins have been used extensively in studies of experimental cell biology since their influence on G proteins was discovered.

Some strains of *E. coli* produce enterotoxins that apparently act in a similar way and cause diarrhea in pigs, calves, and other species. Two toxins, one heat labile and one heat stable, have been identified. The labile toxin resembles cholera toxin. It is immunologically cross-reactive with cholera toxin, and it activates adenyl cyclase. It is, however, less potent. The actions of the stable toxin are less well understood. A number of other bacteria, including some strains of *Staphylococcus aureus* and *C. perfringens*, also produce enterotoxins, but their mechanisms of action are less well understood than those already discussed.

In summary, many bacteria specifically produce toxic substances that are apparently involved in the production of disease. Some, such as the examples discussed above, clearly are responsible for the major signs of the disease. In most cases, however, the production of bacterial disease is multifactorial, and the role of toxins is poorly elucidated. For example, *Pseudomonas aeruginosa* produces a number of substances that may be of pathogenetic significance. These include pigments, exotoxin A, phospholipase, proteolytic enzymes, so-called "slime," and endotoxin. The relative role of each of these products in causing disease is still unclear.

Endotoxins

Endotoxins basically are lipopolysaccharide complexes that form an intrinsic component of the cell wall of Gram-negative bacteria and can be released from both live and dead organisms. Isolated endotoxin consists of the lipopolysaccharide (LPS) together with variable amounts of protein and loosely bound lipids. LPS contains a lipid moiety, known as **lipid A,** tightly bound to the polysaccharide components. The latter consist of a core polysaccharide and the polysaccharide making up the O antigens that are specific for each species of bacteria. Lipid A is a unique molecule that is always very similar in structure (but not identical) regardless of the species of bacteria from which it is derived. Lipid A is considered to be responsible for many of the biologic effects exerted by endotoxin, although the other components also contribute.

When released into the circulation, endotoxins cause profound and adverse biologic effects involving many vital organ systems. Once in the bloodstream, peripheral blood leukocytes and the vascular endothelial cells are directly exposed to LPS.

The general effects of endotoxins are well known and include the induction of fever, shock-like reductions in systemic blood pressure, and changes in peripheral blood count and the blood coagulation system. It is also now readily apparent that endotoxins induce the production, synthesis, and/or secretion of a vareity of potent mediators and cytokines from other cell types. The diversity of the mediators that can be mobilized by endotoxin has made it difficult to define a unifying hypothesis for the mechanism(s) of action of endotoxin. It has also confounded attempts to provide specific therapy for endotoxin-related diseases.

Many interactions of endotoxin with host systems have been described (Table 7.4). These include effects on the complement system, coagulation systems, platelets,

Table 7.4
Summary of Effects of Endotoxin[a]

Tissue/System	Effect
Whole animal	Fever, leukopenia followed by leukocytosis, microvascular injury, disseminated coagulation
Complement	Classical/alternate pathway activation; anaphylatoxin generation; many secondary effects
Neutrophils	"Primes" PMN for various enhanced functions; prostaglandin/leukotriene production; oxyradical generation; secretion; aggregation; enhanced adhesion *via* Leu-CAMs
Clotting System	Intrinsic/extrinsic activation; enhance TF expression on cell surfaces; DIC
Platelets	Aggregation; sequestration; secretion
Macrophages	Activation; "primes" for enhanced function; secretion of cytokines (GM-CSF, IL-1, TNFα)
Endothelium	Direct damage (bovine); enhanced ELAM expression; mediator release

[a] Abbreviations used are: PMN, neutrophil; Leu-CAMs, leukocyte cell adhesion molecules; TF, tissue factor; DIC, disseminated intravascular coagulation; GM-CSF, colony stimulating factor; IL-1, interleukin-1; TNFα, tumor necrosis factor; ELAM, endothelial cell adhesion molecules.

neutrophils, monocytes and macrophages, and endothelial cells. How all of these fit into the total picture of the effect of endotoxins on the whole animal is as yet not fully elucidated. Some of the various effects of endotoxin on host systems are briefly discussed below.

ENDOTOXIN AND THE COMPLEMENT SYSTEM. One property of endotoxin which is probably of pathogenetic importance is its ability to activate complement. Endotoxin can activate both the classical and alternate complement pathways *in vitro*, and in each case activation may be independent of antibody. In addition, if antibody to endotoxin is present, complement may be activated in the usual way by the interaction of antigen with antibody. The usual mechanism of classical and alternate pathway complement activation by endotoxin appears to be different, however, as the classical pathway is activated by the lipid A region of the endotoxin molecule through direct binding and activation of complement component C1, while alternate pathway activation depends upon the polysaccharide portion of the endotoxin molecule. Complement activation, of course, leads to the generation of the potent anaphylatoxins C3a and C5a, but these and other complement-derived mediators have been difficult to implicate in clinical endotoxic shock because of the complexity of overlapping *in vivo* events. Some experiments, for example, have shown that depletion of complement reduces the effects of endotoxin on the host, while other studies have shown no effect. Variation in results from similar experiments on the actions of endotoxin is common and probably relates to the type of bacteria used as a source of toxin, the method of extraction, and other methodological differences. As a result, it is difficult to formulate unifying theories on the actions of endotoxins in the host.

ENDOTOXIN AND ARACHIDONIC ACID METABOLISM. Clinical studies have established that selective inhibitors of ar-

achidonic acid metabolism (nonsteroidal antiinflammatory drugs) or inhibitors of the products of arachidonic acid metabolism can have a beneficial influence on the pathophysiologic consequences of endotoxemia. More recent studies of both *in vivo* and *in vitro* situations have clearly established that endotoxins can elicit the production of both prostaglandins and leukotrienes. Macrophages and monocytes seem to be particulary sensitive targets for endotoxin-induced arachidonic acid metabolism, but neutrophils can respond similarly.

ENDOTOXIN AND THE CLOTTING SYSTEM. One of the key clinicopathologic features of Gram-negative sepsis with endotoxemia is the development of diffuse microvascular thrombosis. Some of this microvascular thrombosis is certainly related to the effects of endotoxin on endothelial cells, but endotoxin may also directly activate both the intrinsic and extrinsic coagulation pathways, and leads to enhanced expression of tissue thromboplastin (factor III, tissue factor) on the surfaces of monocytes and macrophages. As we may recall (*see also* Chapter 3), tissue factor serves as a form of binding site for factor VII, which becomes activated to cleave factors X and IX *via* the extrinsic coagulation cascade. Most investigators agree that the highly procoagulant tissue factor activity remains largely cell-associated with little released into the local microenvironment.

When two doses of endotoxin are administered to rabbits 24 h apart, bilateral renal cortical necrosis results. This is known as the **generalized Schwartzman reaction** and has been shown to be due to intravascular blood coagulation. Thrombi form in the renal glomerular capillaries and, in this model, result in cortical necrosis of the kidneys. The generalized Schwartzman reaction therefore is a consequence of **disseminated intravascular coagulation** (DIC), which is discussed later in this chapter.

Platelets also are affected dramatically by endotoxin. Administration of endotoxin to some animal species causes thrombocytopenia with aggregation and trapping of platelets in vascular spaces. It causes secretion of platelet-derived mediators, which may in turn contribute to changes in blood pressure and to vascular permeability changes. Complement appears to be important in platelet aggregation, and endotoxin has relatively little effect on platelets in species in which these cells have no immune adherence receptors. The action of endotoxin on platelets may, however, be important in DIC and endotoxin-induced tissue injury.

ENDOTOXIN AND NEUTROPHILS. It has been known for some time that either intravenous endotoxin administration or Gram-negative bacterial sepsis were likely to produce a precipitous neutropenia followed later by leukocytosis due to release of neutrophils from the bone marrow. This initial shift of neutrophils (PMN) from the circulating to the marginal pool is related to LPS-induced increased PMN adhesiveness to endothelium. LPS may interact with the PMN by simply binding to it, as a specific receptor for LPS on PMN has been difficult to identify. It has recently been suggested that LPS may interact with part of the same CR3 receptor that recognizes C3bi and Mo-1. LPS may also indirectly activate PMN by liberation of the potent anaphylatoxin and PMN agonist C5a *via* complement activation.

Multiple PMN functions are known to be altered upon LPS exposure including increased adhesiveness to endothelium, PMN-PMN aggregation, lysosomal granule release, and enhanced respiratory burst activity. LPS seems to act as a PMN primer for some of these functions; enhanced release of toxic oxygen metabolites such as superoxide anion (O_2^-) and hydrogen peroxide (H_2O_2) and increased release of PMN lysosomal contents occurs following low-dose priming of PMN with endotoxin. The release of such PMN constituents as toxic oxygen radicals and lysosomal granule contents by adherent neutrophils may be an important feature of the pathogenesis of microvascular injury in endotoxemia. To complicate the picture, however, we must point out that some studies suggest that animals depleted of neutrophils still react to endotoxin with the usual shock-like responses, so it may be that under certain conditions PMN are not essential to endotoxin-induced injury.

ENDOTOXIN AND MACROPHAGES. It has now been clearly established that monocytes and macrophages are very important in the pathogenesis of tissue injury produced by endotoxin. These cells are exquisitely sensitive to endotoxin and respond to it with changes in morphology, such as ruffling, increased phagocytic activity, and increased secretory activity. In short, endotoxin is capable of activating macrophages. Such activated cells secrete lysosomal enzymes such as collagenase, up-regulate expression of surface tissue factor for activation of the extrinsic coagulation pathway, and release potent cytokines like **colony stimulating factor (GM-CSF), tumor necrosis factor (TNFα),** and **interleukin-1 (IL-1).** GM-CSF is in turn capable of stimulating the proliferation of granulocytes and mononuclear phagocytes, and IL-1 and TNF_α have a plethora of biological effects (*see also* Chapters 4 and 5).

Endotoxin is one of the most potent known inducers of interleukin-1 (IL-1). Much of the released IL-1 is of mononuclear phagocyte origin, but other cell types may also contribute. The biological activities of IL-1 are as complex as is the activity of endotoxin, and include a variety of effects on diverse cell types (*see also* Chapters 4 and 5). Two classical IL-1 activities are the induction of fever (many of the activities of IL-1 were once attributed to a less well characterized "factor" known as **leukocyte endogenous**

pyrogen, now known to be IL-1) and the activation of lymphocytes. IL-1 also interacts with endothelial cells to enhance procoagulant (tissue factor) expression, enhances endothelial cell adhesiveness, and interfaces with the fibrinolytic system by inducing an inhibitor of tissue-type plasminogen activator (t-PA). Endotoxin-stimulated macrophages also produce **tumor necrosis factor (TNFα),** a potent mediator that has many related and overlapping biological functions with IL-1 (*see also* Chapters 4 and 5).

ENDOTOXIN AND THE ENDOTHE-LIUM. It is now well established that endothelial cell damage occurs *in vivo* in endotoxemia as evidenced by microvascular lesions as well as endothelial sloughing and the detection of endothelial cells in the circulation. The mechanisms of this injury, however, have been more difficult to define. Bovine endothelial cells seem to be particularly sensitive to endotoxin and can be directly injured by LPS *in vitro* in the absence of other factors. This may explain some of the sensitivity of cattle to diseases in which endotoxemia is involved. In most other species, however, endotoxin does not seem to play such a direct role, and several recent studies have implicated the neutrophil as a cellular intermediary. Under normal conditions, PMN marginated against the vascular endothelium or migrating through it toward tissue sites do not cause endothelial damage, but this picture may be quite different under the influence of endotoxin. In addition to causing enhanced adhesiveness of PMN to endothelium, endotoxin "primes" PMN for increased secretory and biochemical activity, possibly leading to endothelial cell damage *via* elaboration of toxic oxygen metabolites or lysosomal granule contents. Interestingly, direct contact and adhesion between the PMN and endothelium is apparently necessary for such injury to occur; when monoclonal antibodies

are utilized to block up-regulation of the leukocyte cell adhesion molecule (Leu-CAM) Mo1 on activated PMN, markedly reduced injury occurs *in vitro*.

Not only do the PMN become stickier, but the endothelium itself exhibits enhanced adhesiveness under the influence of endotoxin, due to increased expression of **endothelial cell adhesion molecules (ELAM).** In recent years, there has been a high level of interest in the role of the endothelial cell itself, apart from any other influences. One interesting observation is that the perfusion of one kidney by endotoxin, followed 24 h later by systemic administration, produces a Schwartzman reaction limited to one kidney. This suggests a role for local sensitization, which might be important in the pathogenesis of endothelial injury.

In conclusion, endotoxin produces a wide variety of effects on humoral and cellular mediation systems in the host. The contribution of each of these to the totality of effects of endotoxin in the intact animal is not entirely clear, but the remarkable sensitivity of monocytes and macrophages to endotoxin, and the diversity of biologic phenomena that they mediate, makes these cells likely to be among the most important targets for endotoxin *in vivo*. It is also important to recognize that endotoxins are certainly not the only determinant of pathogenicity in Gram-negative bacteria. Endotoxins may be present on bacteria that are not pathogenic, and, in some of known pathogenic bacteria, factors other than endotoxin are clearly involved. In the case of **typhoid fever** of man, for instance, endotoxins derived from the causative organism, *Salmonella typhi*, can produce signs similar to those seen in the naturally occurring disease. However, the induction of tolerance to the endotoxin does not provide protection against the disease when individuals actually are infected.

As a final word on toxins we should not

leave the impression that only bacteria produce toxins that damage the host. Certain ectoparasites, in particular some ticks, cause a toxicosis in their hosts. Some ixodid ticks such as *Dermacentor andersoni* in North America and *Ixodes holocyclus* in Australia produce a potent neurotoxin that is capable of paralyzing and killing the host. In the case of *I. holocyclus,* the toxin apparently acts at the neuromuscular junction and inhibits the release of neurotransmitter. It is interesting to speculate on the various ways by which such parasites have developed these sophisticated mechanisms of interaction with the host.

Damage Due to the Host Response

Inflammation and the Immune Response

The host response to parasitism is aimed basically at removing the invader from the host. Unfortunately the effector mechanisms employed to do this do not completely spare the host's own tissues, and damage may occur as a result of either local or systemic responses. Both the immune response and the inflammatory response can result in damage to the host. These mechanisms are discussed in detail in Chapters 4 and 5 and will be touched upon here only briefly in considering their contribution to the disease manifestations of parasitism.

Neutrophils, which abound in acute, suppurative, inflammatory reactions release a variety of substances, including enzymes, that can damage host tissues. The importance of this to the host clearly depends on both the site and the persistence of the inciting cause. Obviously an abscess in the brain is of far greater consequence to the host than the same lesion in the subcutis or even in the lung or liver. Chronic inflammatory lesions, especially granulomatous lesions such as those caused by mycobacteria or pathogenic fungi, also can injure the host by

acting as space-occupying lesions. Again, the significance of such a lesion varies with its site. Essentially all inflammatory lesions cause some damage, but the ideal outcome for the host is the rapid elimination of the inciting organism and minimal tissue damage. Fortunately for all of us this is usually the case.

Damage due to an immune response to a parasite usually is mediated by the final effector, the inflammatory response. This is not always a local event, and the various immunopathologic mechanisms by which the host can be damaged have been discussed in Chapter 5. Here it suffices to mention some examples that illustrate that the immune and inflammatory responses of the host may be responsible for the majority of the damage to the host. A good case in point is lymphocytic choriomeningitis (LCM) virus infection in mice. If mice are infected *in utero* or as neonates, before they are immunologically competent, a minimal immune response is mounted and infection persists. No significant damage to the host occurs. Similarly, in certain strains of mice that are genetically unable to mount a vigorous immune response to LCM virus, infection of adults does not produce significant disease. In contrast, mice able to mount a normal, vigorous, immune response develop inflammatory lesions and, as a result, severe disease. In this case, then, the virus itself is apparently relatively innocuous, and only the attempts of the host to get rid of it are responsible for tissue damage. Examples of naturally occurring diseases of domestic animals in which this is the case are less well defined, but they no doubt occur. **Aleutian mink disease** is one case in which essentially all of the lesions are immunologically mediated. Mink with this disease are persistently infected with the virus and develop high antibody titers. As a result, immune complexes are deposited in vessels and in glomeruli, resulting in vasculitis and glomerulonephritis. In the case of **feline infectious peritonitis,** recent evidence suggests that cats with the most vigorous immune response develop the most severe lesions, suggesting that in this disease too, it is the immune response and associated inflammatory lesions that mediate tissue damage (*see also* Chapter 5).

Fever and Other Systemic Reactions

One of the most characteristic systemic reactions associated with infectious diseases is **fever.** Fever is an alteration or adaptation of normal thermoregulation. It is therefore distinguished from hyperthermia, in which there is an uncontrolled elevation of body temperature. In fever, body temperature is still under control, but the so-called set point (or setting of the biological thermostat) is altered upwards. The control center for body temperature appears to be in the hypothalamus, where both cold-sensitive and heat-sensitive neurons reside. These neurons sense local temperature as well as integrating information from peripheral receptors. In mammals, when body temperature needs to be changed, heat is generated or lost as required by both physiologic and behavioral means. The former include shivering and vasoconstriction to elevate body temperature and sweating, panting, and vasodilation to lower it. Behavioral means essentially consist of seeking a warm or a cool environment. In poikilotherms, only behavioral means are used to regulate body temperature.

Fever is caused by a variety of stimuli known collectively as **exogenous pyrogens.** These include bacteria (both Gram-positive and Gram-negative), viruses, fungi, antigen-antibody interactions, some drugs, and, of course, endotoxin. However, all fevers, of any cause except direct brain damage, are now thought to be mediated primarily by a cytokine originally described as **leukocyte endogenous pyrogen,** now known to be **interleukin-**

1. Other cytokines and lymphokines also appear to contribute to the pathogenesis of fever including tumor necrosis factor (TNFα), γ-interferon (γ-IFN), and possibly lymphotoxin. Accordingly, even the rather recent consensus that fever might be largely due to a single endogenous pyrogen (IL-1) must now be modified, since no fewer than 3 cytokines (IL-1, TNFα, and γ-IFN) and possibly others (lymphotoxin) are apparently involved. It seems likely that even this current, more complicated view of the pathogenesis of fever will become even more elaborate.

The general characteristics of interleukin-1 (IL-1) have already been discussed (*see* Chapters 4 and 5). IL-1 is a multifunctional factor synthesized and released primarily by macrophages, but it can be produced by virtually all nucleated cells. Two distinct forms of IL-1 have been identified, IL-1$_\alpha$ and IL-1$_\beta$, which have similar if not identical functional activities and bind to the same receptor, but have somewhat distinct functional site sequences. IL-1 is thought to act on the thermoregulatory center in the hypothalamus to raise the "set-point" as previously described. A difficult concept to rationalize has been that there remains little solid evidence to document that IL-1 produced in peripheral tissues can penetrate the blood-brain barrier to enter the brain tissue itself. The most plausible explanation to date is that IL-1 exerts its major effects on the rich vascular network close to a cluster of neurons in the preoptic cranial hypothalamus. This site, known as the **organum vasculosum laminae terminalis (OVLT)** apparently manifests little if any of the typical characteristics of the blood-brain barrier. The best evidence for involvement of the OVLT is that its ablation prevents fever when IL-1 is injected systemically but has no effect on the fever induced by intracerebral injection of IL-1. This complicated story will no doubt be clarified in the future.

Of particular interest in this discussion

is the role of fever in the host. Fever occurs in all mammals, in birds, and, through behavioral adaptations, in poikilotherms such as lizards, snakes, and fish. In response to infection, for instance, a number of lizards and other poikilotherms have been shown to acquire a fever by seeking a warmer than usual environment. This suggests that fever has some beneficial effect, as such an adaptation would not be expected to be so well preserved during evolution if it did not. In mammals, it is difficult to study the role of fever in host defense, as any drugs or other means used to modify it might directly affect host defenses. On the other hand, fever can be prevented in poikilotherms simply by denying them access to a warmer environment. The use of this technique has shown that fever is probably beneficial. When lizards infected with *Aeromonas hydrophila* (a Gram-negative pathogenic bacterium) were held at two temperatures, 35°C and 42°C, those at the higher temperature generally survived whereas most of those at the lower temperature died. Furthermore, it has been shown that lizards with fever have a more efficient inflammatory response than those held at normal temperatures. Similarly, mammalian leukocytes exhibit maximum phagocytic activity at temperatures equivalent to moderate fevers. Another advantage of fever might involve the utilization of iron by bacteria. As discussed earlier, pathogenic bacteria ensure a supply of iron by synthesizing iron-binding siderophores. Bacteria can synthesize siderophores much less efficiently at relatively high temperatures, and fever may therefore interfere with bacterial growth by limiting the availability of iron. There is little direct evidence documenting a beneficial role for fever in mammals, but studies in rabbits correlating fever and survival have shown that modest fevers may be beneficial while high fevers apparently are not.

Cardiovascular changes resembling

Table 7.5
Underlying Disease Entities Often Associated with Disseminated Intravascular Coagulation (DIC)

Septicemia, endotoxemia
Malignant neoplasia, including leukemia
Obstetrical complications
Some forms of hepatic disease
Severe trauma/tissue injury, including burns
Intravascular immune reactions (anaphylaxis)
Systemic vascular disorders
Certain venoms and toxins

shock may complicate infectious disease. Most commonly this is seen with severe infections by Gram-negative bacteria and may, as suggested already, be due to the action of endotoxins.

Disseminated intravascular coagulation (DIC) is a potentially catastrophic systemic reaction in which there is generalized activation of the blood coagulation system. DIC has many possible causes including extensive tissue injury, neoplasia, systemic immunologic reactions (including anaphylaxis), and acute infections, especially those in which septicemia occurs (Table 7.5). In the latter case, coagulation is possibly activated by endotoxin or by widespread damage to the endothelium of vessels, and the implication that endotoxin is involved either by direct activation of the coagulation system or through microvascular damage has become axiomatic. Coagulation may be initiated by either the intrinsic or extrinsic pathways or, under some circumstances, by direct conversion of prothrombin to thrombin (*see also* Chapter 3). DIC may prove to be an important pathogenetic factor in many infectious diseases. For example, it recently has been suggested that DIC may be involved in the pathogenesis of **feline infectious peritonitis** and **infectious canine hepatitis,** a disease in which the causative virus can cause endothelial damage.

The immediate result of diffuse acti-

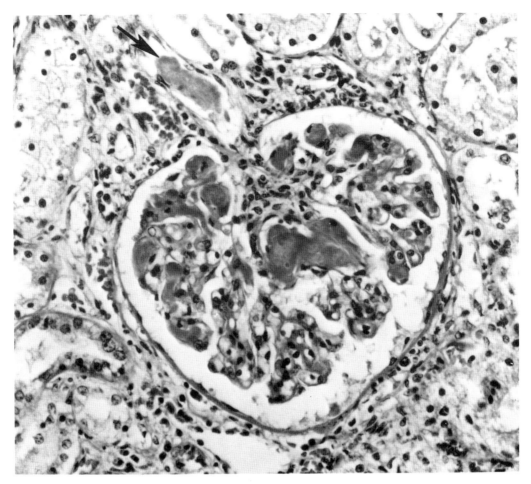

Figure 7.16. Disseminated Intravascular Coagulation. Several fibrin thrombi are present in the capillaries of this glomerulus. A thrombus also is present in the afferent arteriole *(arrow)*. Similar thrombi were present in many tissues from this dog.

vation of the blood coagulation system is the deposition of microthrombi in small vessels of many tissues, including the renal glomeruli (Fig. 7.16). Tissue ischemia and infarction can result. The thrombi are rapidly removed by the fibrinolytic system as a consequence of which breakdown products of fibrin and fibrinogen (**fibrin degradation products, FDPs**) can be detected in the circulation (*see also* Chapter 3). Such massive activation of the coagulation system results in the consumption of platelets and a number of coagulation factors, the end result of which

may be a defect in coagulation. Because this is due to the utilization of clotting factors to the extent that normal coagulation cannot occur, it is referred to as a **consumptive coagulopathy.** Some FDPs can further inhibit blood coagulation and exacerbate the tendency to bleed. Patients with DIC may therefore develop a **hemorrhagic diathesis** manifested by petechiae and ecchymoses in many tissues. Thus, regardless of its specific etiologic background, DIC develops through a sequence of events in which the seemingly paradoxical development of wide-

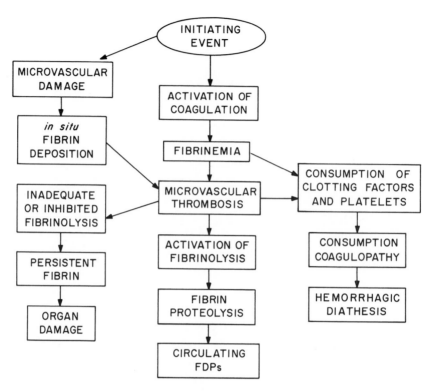

Figure 7.17.   Pathogenesis of Disseminated Intravascular Coagulation (DIC). The sequence of events in DIC includes initiation of coagulation followed by fibrin microthrombosis, consumptive coagulopathy, and eventual hemorrhagic diathesis. The tissue outcome can be influenced by how effectively the fibrinolytic system operates. (FDPs, fibrin degradation products)

spread microvascular thrombosis may lead to bleeding tendencies and the emergence of a hemorrhagic diathesis (Fig. 7.17).

SPREAD OF INFECTION AND TISSUE TROPISM

Simple, localized infections may be of little threat to the host but can become much more consequential when local extension or, more importantly, dissemination to other tissues occurs. Local extension of infection may follow the line of least resistance along tissue planes. It may be aided by tissue breakdown caused by proteolytic enzymes secreted by inflammatory cells and by tissue necrosis caused by the organisms themselves.

Organisms also may be disseminated to other tissues *via* the lymphatics and the blood. Organisms entering lymphatics may be removed by phagocytes in the regional lymph node, but this filtering capacity can be overwhelmed when the number of organisms is large, especially when the flow of lymph is rapid as may occur in an inflamed site.

Hematogenous dissemination is potentially the most rapid and effective way that organisms can spread to other organs. **Bacteremia** is quite a common event, but in most cases it is transient, organisms being removed by phagocytes in the liver and spleen. In some cases, however, organisms that lodge in the tissues survive and grow, producing secondary lesions (Fig. 7.18). Like neoplastic cells, organisms that spread in this way can show tissue tropism. For example, bacteremia commonly follows infection of young foals with *Actinobacillus equuli*, and secondary inflammatory lesions occur in other tissues. The kidneys and the lungs are the most common sites of such embolic lesions. In some cases organisms, in particular bacteria, may be carried in relatively large emboli that break off from primary inflammatory lesions. This is a particularly common consequence of bacterial endocarditis of the heart valves (Fig. 7.19). Such emboli lodge easily in secondary sites and establish additional lesions.

Viremia, the presence of virus in the blood, is a very important mechanism for dissemination of viruses from the primary site of infection to other tissues. Without viremia, many viral infections would be relatively innocuous. Virus may be carried free in the blood or may be associated with blood cells.

Many organisms, when they become disseminated, show a preference to infect certain tissues. In other words, they show tissue or organ tropism; parasites of many types demonstrate this phenomenon. The reasons for tissue tropism are often not understood, but in some cases explanations are known. One mechanism probably of general importance is that organisms may bear specific components that interact with receptors on target cells. This probably explains the tropism of some viruses for the respiratory tract and of others, such as rotaviruses, for the intestinal epithelium. Bacteria also may interact with tissues in their way, one of the best examples, already discussed in this chapter, being the interaction of certain strains of *E. coli* with the epithelial cells of the ileum.

In other cases, cells possess special

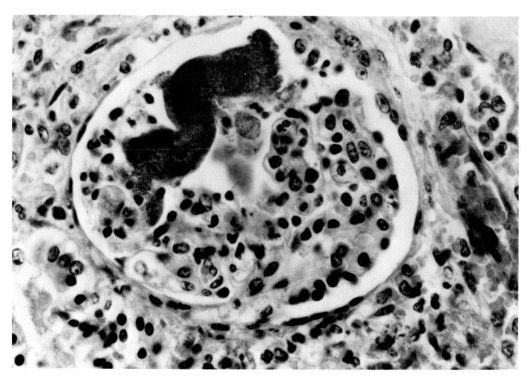

Figure 7.18. Bacterial Emboli. Embolic bacteria have lodged and proliferated in a glomerulus. Eventually these would cause an inflammatory response. This lesion is from a case of actinobacillosis in a foal.

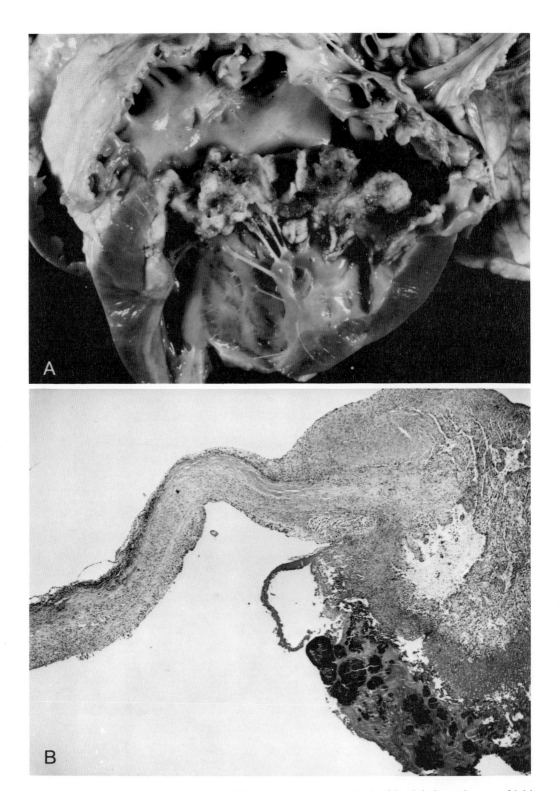

Figure 7.19. Valvular Endocarditis. *A,* The atrioventricular valve in this pig's heart bears a friable inflamed mass caused by bacterial infection. *B,* The histologic appearance of part of the mass is shown. The very dark material represents masses of bacteria embedded in necrotic inflammatory debris. Such masses often break off to form emboli that can establish infection at other sites.

properties that make them the specific target of infectious agents. For example, canine and feline (and other) parvoviruses require host cells in the S phase of mitosis in order to replicate. Thus tissues that contain many mitotically active cells, such as the intestinal glands (crypts), the lymphoid tissues, and bone marrow, are susceptible. In both panleukopenia of cats and canine parvovirus infection, therefore, there is often lymphopenia and neutropenia, and clinical disease is associated with enteric lesions that result from necrosis of crypt epithelium (Fig. 7.13). In other cases, the tissue involved contains unique nutrients required by the organisms. In ungulates, *Brucella abortus* shows a particular affinity for the placenta, fetal fluids, and chorionic tissue. In contrast, in other susceptible species, including man, it shows no particular tissue tropism. The tissue affinity of *B. abortus* is explained by the fact that the fetal fluids and placental tissues of susceptible ungulates contain significant amounts of **erythritol,** a nutrient for which the organism has a special requirement. In those animals in which *B. abortus* does not cause abortion, the placenta does not contain erythritol. Similarly, particular metabolic capabilities of the organism also may influence the site at which infections become established. *Corynebacterium renale* possesses the enzyme urease, which allows it to metabolize urea, giving this organism a special affinity for the urinary tract. This organism is a common cause of pyelonephritis in cattle. Evidence for the importance of this metabolic capability in the pathogenesis of the disease is the observation that mutants lacking urease still colonize the renal medulla but fail to flourish and therefore produce little damage.

Taking a broader view than tissue specificity, we might ask why organisms so often demonstrate strict host preferences. A few, such as rabies virus, are particularly nonselective, but most organisms have only one or a few host species in which they can establish infection. Generally speaking, the basis for this in particular cases is unknown but, again, the presence of cellular receptors for the organisms probably plays a part.

PERSISTENCE OF INFECTION

Many organisms are able to establish persistent infection. This may produce chronic disease, such as is seen in tuberculosis or Johne's disease, or intermittent disease, such as that seen in latent infections with some herpesviruses. Persistently infected animals often can act as sources of infection and thus be of considerable epidemiologic importance.

The mechanisms by which infections persist are in general poorly understood. Certainly the avoidance of the immune response, as already discussed, plays some role but it is equally certain that it is not the only factor involved. In both visna and equine infectious anemia, virus undergoes periodic antigenic changes that allow a burst of replication and infection of new cells, which probably is important in the progression of the disease. Infection persists, however, in the quiescent stages when circulating antibody is able to neutralize free virus. In the case of these retroviruses, integration of the viral genome into the DNA of the host is probably of great importance in maintaining infection. Herpesviruses frequently produce persistent, latent infections. Usually virus persists in neural ganglia, and those of us who suffer from common "cold sores" know that under certain circumstances, usually some form of stress, such infections can be activated. Lesions then appear in tissue innervated by infected neurons. A *Herpesvirus* of cattle, **infectious bovine rhinotracheitis virus,** can show similar behavior. The virus can cause lesions in the genitalia, which resolve but leave the animals with a latent infection. When stress is mimicked by treating such animals with corticosteroids, genital le-

sions reappear. In such *Herpesvirus* infections, free virus cannot be detected in
infected ganglia during the latent stages,
although viral DNA is present. It is likely
therefore that viral DNA is incorporated
into the cell in some way, although its
exact form is not yet known.

In this chapter we have discussed a
number of important ways in which the
host and its parasites, as well as their
common environment, may interact to
produce the disturbances of homeostasis
which we call disease. This knowledge
can be extremely useful in the study of
clinical medicine, and it serves as a basis
for understanding why animals respond
as they do to parasitic or infectious disease and why so many challenging variations in response exist.

Reference Material

Anderson, D.C., and Springer, T.A.: Leukocyte
adhesion deficiency: an inherited defect in the
Mac-1, LFA-1, and p150,95 glycoproteins. *Ann.
Rev. Med.* 38:175–194, 1987.

Arbuthnott, J.P.: Role of exotoxins in bacterial pathogenicity. *J. Appl. Bacteriol.* 44:329–345, 1978.

Babior, B.M.: Oxygen-dependent microbial killing
by phagocytes. *N. Engl. J. Med* 298:659–666, 1978.

Bachner, R.L.: Neutrophil dysfunction associated
with states of chronic and recurrent infection.
Pediat. Clin. N. Am. 27:377–401, 1980.

Barclay, R.: The role of iron in infection. *Med. Lab.
Sci.* 42:166–177, 1985.

Bernheim, H.A., Block, L.H., and Atkins, E.: Fever:
Pathogenesis, pathophysiology and purpose. *Ann.
Intern. Med.* 91:261–270, 1979.

Beutler, B., and Cerami, A.: Tumor necrosis, cachexia, shock, and inflammation: a common mediator. *Ann. Rev. Biochem.* 57:505–518, 1988.

Bloom, B.R.: Games parasites play: how parasites
evade immune surveillance. *Nature* 279:21–26,
1979.

Brubaker, R.R.: Mechanisms of bacterial virulence.
Ann. Rev. Microbiol. 39:21–50, 1985.

Bullen, J.J., Rogers, H.J., and Griffiths, E.: Role of
iron in bacterial infection. *Curr. Top. Immunol.*
80:1–35, 1978.

Cerami, A., and Beutler, B.: The role of cachectin/
TNF in endotoxin shock and cachexia. *Immunol.
Today* 9:28–31, 1988.

Cheevers, W.P., and McGuire, T.C.: Equine infectious anemia: Immunopathogenesis and persistence. *Rev. Infect. Dis.* 7:83–88, 1985.

Cooper, K.E.: The neurobiology of fever: Thoughts

on recent developments. *Ann. Rev. Neurobiol.*
10:297–324, 1987.

Cybulsky, M.I., Chan, M.K.W., and Movat, H.Z.:
Biology of Disease: Acute inflammation and microthrombosis induced by endotoxin, interleukin-
1, and tumor necrosis factor and their implication
in gram-negative infection. *Lab. Invest.* 58:365–
378, 1988.

Dinarello, C.A.: Induction of acute phase reactants
by interleukin-1. *Adv. Inflamm. Res.* 8:203–225,
1984.

Dinarello, C.A.: An update on human interleukin-
1: from molecular biology to clinical relevance. *J.
Clin. Immunol.* 5:287–296, 1985.

Dinarello, C.A., Cannon, J.G., and Wolff, S.M.: New
concepts on the pathogenesis of fever. *Rev. Infect.
Dis.* 10:168–189, 1988.

Donelson, J.E., and Turner, M.V.: How the trypan-
osome changes its coat. *Sci. Amer.* 252:44–51,
1985.

Elsbach, P., and Weiss, J.: Phagocytosis of bacteria
and phospholipid degradation. *Biochem. Biophys.
Acta* 947:29–52, 1988.

Evans, A.S.: Causation and disease: The Henle-
Koch postulates revisited. *Yale J. Biol. Med.*
49:175–195, 1976.

Fearson, D.T.: Cellular receptors for fragments of
the third component of complement. *Immunol.
Today* 5:105–112, 1984.

Finkelstein, R.A., Sciortino, C.V., and McIntosh,
M.A.: Role of iron in microbe-host interactions.
Rev. Infect. Dis. 5:S759–S777, 1983.

Forman, H.J., and Thomas, M.J.: Oxidant production and bactericidal activity of phagocytes. *Ann.
Rev. Physiol.* 48:669–680, 1986.

Gabay, J.E.: Microbicidal mechanisms of phagocytes. *Curr. Opinion Immunol.* 1:36–40, 1988.

Gallin, J.I., Goldstein, I.M., and Snyderman, R.:
*Inflammation: Basic Principles and Clinical Cor-
relates.* Raven Press, New York, 1988.

Giger, U., Boxer, L.A., Simpson, P.J., Lucchesi, B.R.,
and Todd, R.F. III.: Deficiency of leukocyte surface
glycoproteins Mo1, LFA-1, and Leu M5 in a dog
with recurrent infections: an animal model. *Blood,*
69:1622–1630, 1987.

Gordon, D.L., and Hostetter, M.K.: Complement and
host defence against microorganisms. *Pathology*
18:365–375, 1986.

Gordon, S.: Biology of the macrophage. *J. Cell Sci.*
4:267–286, 1986.

Gotschlich, E.C.: Thoughts on the evolution of strategies used by bacteria for evasion of host defenses.
Rev. Infect. Dis. 5:S778–S783, 1983.

Horwitz, M.A.: Phagocytosis of microorganisms. *Rev.
Infect. Dis.* 4:104–123, 1982.

Horwitz, M.A.: Intracellular parasitism. *Current
Opinion Immunol.* 1:41–46, 1988.

Horzinek, M.C.: Molecular pathogenesis of virus
infection. *Experentia* 43:1193–1196, 1987.

Hostetter, M.K., and Gordon, D.L.: Biochemistry of C3 and related thiolester proteins in infection and inflammation. *Rev. Infect. Dis. 9*:97–109, 1987.

Hurst, N.P.: Molecular basis of activation and regulation of the phagocyte respiratory burst. *Annals Rheum. Dis. 46*:265–272, 1987.

Joiner, K.A., Brown, E.J., and Frank, M.M.: Complement and bacteria: chemistry and biology in host defense. *Ann. Rev. Immunol. 2*:461–491, 1984.

Joiner, K.A.: Complement evasion by bacteria and parasites. *Ann. Rev. Microbiol., 42*:201–230, 1988.

Kampschmidt, R.F.: The numerous postulated biological manifestations of interleukin-1. *J. Leukocyte Biol. 36*:341–355, 1984.

Larrick, J.W., and Kunkel, S.L.: The role of tumor necrosis factor and interleukin-1 in the immunoinflammatory response. *Pharmaceut. Res. 5*:129–139, 1988.

Le, J., and Vilcek, J.: Tumor necrosis factor and interleukin 1: cytokines with multiple overlapping biological activities. *Lab. Invest. 56*:234–248, 1987.

Lehrer, R.I.: Neutrophils and host defense. *Ann. Int. Med. 109*:127–142, 1988.

Letendre, E.D.: Iron metabolism during infection and neoplasia. *Cancer Metas. Rev. 6*:41–53, 1987.

Levine, M.M.: *Escherichia coli* that cause disease: Enterotoxigenic, enteropathogenic, enteroinvasive, enterohemorrhagic, and enteroadherent. *J. Infect. Dis. 155*:377–389, 1987.

Linscott, W.D.: Biochemistry and biology of the complement system in domestic animals. *Progr. Vet. Microbiol. Immunol. 2*:54–77, 1986.

Mackowiak, P.A.: Microbial synergism in human infections. *N. Engl. J. Med. 298*:21–26, 1978.

Mathison, J.C., and Ulevitch, R.J.: Mediators involved in the expression of endotoxin activity. *Surv. Synth. Pathol. Res. 1*:34–48, 1983.

Mauel, J.: Effector and escape mechanisms in host-parasite relationships. *Progr. Allergy 31*:1–75, 1982.

Mauel, J.: Mechanisms of survival of protozoan parasites in mononuclear phagocytes. *Parasitol. 88*:579–592, 1984.

Mills, E.L.: Viral infections predisposing to bacterial infections. *Ann. Rev. Med. 35*:469–479, 1984.

Mims, C.A.: *The Pathogenesis of Infectious Disease*, ed. 2, Academic Press, London, 1982.

Mizok, B.: Septic shock: A metabolic perspective. *Arch. Int. Med. 144*:579–585, 1984.

Morrison, D.C., and Ryan, J.L.: Endotoxins and disease mechanisms. *Ann. Rev. Med. 38*:417–432, 1987.

Moulder, J.W.: Intracellular parasitism: life in an extreme environment. *J. Infect. Dis. 130*:300–306, 1974.

Movat, H.Z., Cybulsky, M.I., Colditz, I.G., Chan, M.K.W., and Dinarello, C.A.: Acute inflammation in gram-negative infection: endotoxin, interleu-kin 1, tumor necrosis factor, and neutrophils. *Fed. Proc. 46*:97–104, 1987.

Muller-Berghaus, G.: Pathophysiologic and biochemical events in disseminated intravascular coagulation: Dysregulation of procoagulant and anticoagulant pathways. *Semin. Thromb. Hemostas. 15*:58–87, 1989.

Murray, H.W.: Cellular resistance to protozoal infection. *Ann. Rev. Med. 37*:61–70, 1986.

Murray, H.W.: Interferon-gamma, the activated macrophage, and host defense against microbial challenge. *Annals Int. Med. 108*:595–608, 1988.

Murray, H.W.: Survival of intracellular pathogens within human mononuclear phagocytes. *Semin. Hematol. 25*:101–111, 1988.

Nathan, C.F.: Secretory products of macrophages. *J. Clin. Invest. 79*:319–326, 1987.

Oppenheim, J.J., and Jacobs, D.M. (eds): *Leukocytes and Host Defense*. Alan R. Liss, New York, 1986.

Ordnoff, P.E.: Genetic implications of pilation in *Escherichia coli:* implications for understanding microbe-host interactions at the molecular level. *Pathol. Immunopathol. Res. 6*:82–92, 1987.

Pestka, S., Langer, J.A., Zoon, K.C., and Samuel, C.E.: Interferons and their actions. *Ann. Rev. Biochem. 56*:727–778, 1987.

Petersen, P.: A perspective of infection and infectious disease. *Perspect. Biol. Med. 23*:255–272, 1980.

Peterson, P.K., and Quie, P.G.: Bacterial surface components and the pathogenesis of infectious disease. *Ann. Rev. Med. 32*:29–43, 1981.

Prusiner, S.B.: Prions and neurodegenerative diseases. *New Engl. J. Med. 317*:1571–1581, 1987.

Prusiner, S.B., Gabizon, R., and McKinley, M.P.: On the biology of prions. *Acta Neuropathol. 72*:299–314, 1987.

Rappolee, D.A., and Werb, Z.: Secretory products of phagocytes. *Current Opinion Immunol. 1*:47–55, 1988.

Reynolds, H.Y.: Lung inflammation: normal host defense or a complication of some diseases? *Ann. Rev. Med. 38*:295–323, 1987.

Roberts, R., and Gallin, J.I.: The phagocytic cell and its disorders. *Ann. Allergy 50*:330–343, 1983.

Rossi, F., Berton, G., Bellavite, P., and Della Bianca, V.: The inflammatory cells and their respiratory burst. *Adv. Inflamm. Res. 3*:329–340, 1982.

Rotrosen, D., and Gallin, J.I.: Disorders of phagocyte function. *Ann. Rev. Immunol 5*:127–150, 1987.

Skamene, E.: Genetic regulation of host resistance to bacterial infection. *Rev. Infect. Dis. 5*:823–832, 1983.

Slauson, D.O., Lay, J.C., Castleman, W.L., and Neilsen, N.R.: Acute inflammatory lung injury retards pulmonary particle clearance. *Inflammation 13*:185–199, 1989.

Smith, H.: The development of studies on the determinants of bacterial pathogenicity. *J. Comp. Pathol. 98*:253–273, 1988.

Sparling, P.F.: Bacterial virulence and pathogenesis: An overview. *Rev. Infect. Dis. 5*:S637–S646, 1983.

Spitznagel, J.K.: Microbial interactions with neutrophils. *J. Infect. Dis. 5*:S806–S822, 1983.

Templeton, J.W., Smith, R., III, and Adams, L.G.: Natural disease resistance in domestic animals. *J.A.V.M.A. 192*:1306–1315, 1988.

Van der Ploeg, L.H.T.: Control of variant surface antigen switching in trypanosomes. *Cell 51*:159–161, 1987.

Wannamaker, L.W.: Streptococcal toxins. *Rev. Infect. Dis. 5*:S723–S732, 1983.

Weinstein, L.: Gram-negative bacterial infections: A look at the past, a view of the present, and a glance at the future. *Rev. Infect. Dis. 7*:S538–S544, 1985.

Wilson, M.E.: Effects of bacterial endotoxins on neutrophil function. *Rev. Infect. Dis. 7*:404–422, 1985.

Woolcock, J.B.: *Bacterial Infection and Immunity in Domestic Animals.* Elsevier North-Holland, Amsterdam, 1979.

Wright, S.D., and Griffin, F.M., Jr.: Activation of phagocytic cells' C3 receptors for phagocytosis. *J. Leukocyte Biol. 38*:327–339, 1985.

Index

Page numbers in *italics* denote figures; those followed by "t" denote tables.

Absorption pressures
  edema and, 154
  Starling equilibrium and, 156
Acid-hematin, 81
Acquired immunodeficiency syndrome, 361
  animals models of, 362
  human, pathogenesis of, 361
  tropism for CD4 cells, 475
Actin
  chemotaxis and, 229
  in microfilaments, 31
  phagocytosis and, 232
Actin-binding proteins, 229
Activated partial thromboplastin time, 108
Acumentin, 229
Acute inflammation
  manifestations of, 190
  permeability changes and, 192
  vascular events in, 191
Acute phase reaction
  IL-1 and, 256
  proteins of, 256
ADCC *see* antibody-dependent cellular cytotoxicity
Adenocarcinoma
  definition of, 387
Adenoma
  definition of, 387
Adenylate cyclase
  cell activation and, 244
Adhesion molecules
  endothelial cells and, 218
  fibronectin and, 151
  leukocytes and, 217
  lymphocytes and, 304
AEF *see* Amyloid-enhancing factor
Afibrinogenemia
  congenital, platelet aggregation and, 127
Agammaglobulinemia, 360
Age
  and susceptibility to infection, 495
Agenesis
  definition of, 379
AIDS *see* acquired immunodeficiency syndrome
Albumin
  edema and, 157
Aleutian mink disease
  as immune-mediated disease, 510
Allergic contact dermatitis, 356
Alternate pathway
  complement activation and, 263, 264

components of, 268
  reaction sequence of, 269
Ammonia
  effect on respiratory clearance, 500
Amplification systems
  humoral, in inflammation, 260
Amputation neuroma, 278
Amyloid, 83
  degradation of, 86
  endocrine, 86
  formation of, 85
  molecular conformation of, 83
  staining of, 83
Amyloid P component, 86
Amyloid-enhancing factor, 86
Amyloidosis, 83
  familial, 86
  morphology of, *84*
  primary, 83
  secondary, 83
  ultrastructure of, 85
Anaphylactic trigger
  immune complex deposition and, *349*
Anaphylatoxins
  as chemical mediators, 249
  cellular range of, 250
  functions of, *250*
  inflammatory functions of, 270
  receptors for, 241
  vascular permeability and, 349
Anaphylaxis, 307
  bovine, 337
  type I hypersensitivity and, 332
Anaplasia
  in malignant neoplasms, 390
Anasarca, 162
Anemia of inflammatory disease, 489
Angioedema
  hereditary, 269
Angiogenesis
  growth of neoplasms and, 441
  inhibition of, 443
Angiogenin
  and vascularization of neoplasms, 441
Annulus
  of nuclear pore, 24
Anomalies
  developmental, 379
Anoxic cell injury
  free radicals and, 66

Anthracosis, 78
Anti-idiotypic antibodies, 363
Anti-receptor antibody diseases, 339, 341
Antibody
  isotypes of, 311
  opsonization and, 231
  role in immune response, 310
Antibody (B cell) deficiency diseases, 360
Antibody avidity
  immune complexes and, 343
Antibody excess
  immune complex formation and, 343
Antibody production
  assessment of, 369
Antibody-dependent cellular cytotoxicity, 311
  hypersensitivity and, 328
  lymphocyte cytolysis and, 323
  neoplasia and, 464
Antigen charge
  immune complexes and, 343
Antigen excess
  immune complex formation and, 343
Antigen presentation
  helper T cells and, 309
  immune induction and, *310*
Antigen presentation and recognition, 309
Antigen recognition
  by B cells, 309
  by cytotoxic T cells, 309
Antigen-antibody complexes
  pathogenetic potential, 342
Antigen-presenting cells, 309
  immune response and, 307
Antigen-specific T cell factor, 333
Antigenic mimicry
  in avoidance of immune response, 485
Antigenic shedding
  in avoidance of immune response, 485
Antigenic variation
  in avoidance of immune response, 486
  in equine infectious anemia, 486
Antigens
  in neoplasms, 459
  in virus-induced neoplasms, 459
Antihemophilic Factor
  intrinsic activation and, 110
  protein C and, 116
  Stuart-Prower Factor activation and, 112
Antithrombin III
  deficiency of, 116
  regulation of coagulation and, 115
Aplasia
  definition of, 379
Apoptosis, 316, 325
  and tissue atrophy, 37
  definition of, 49
  morphology of, *53*
Arachidonic acid
  biochemistry of, 251
  cyclooxygenase pathway, 252
  endotoxin and, 507
  lipoxygenase pathway, 252
  metabolism, *251*
  metabolites as mediators, 251
Arachidonic acid metabolism, 251
Arteriothromboses, 130
Arteritis
  thrombosis and, 120

Arthus reaction
  description of, 345
  mechanisms of, 345
  neutrophils and, 345
Ascorbate
  as cellular antioxidant, 66
Atherosclerosis
  cholesterol deposits in, 76
  morphology of, 77
Atopic dermatitis, 338
Atrophy
  cellular, *36*
  definition of, 35
  due to necrosis, *35*
  mechanisms of, 37
  of cells and tissues, 35
Autacoids, 251
Autoantibody
  definition of, 338
Autoantigens
  autoimmunity and, 363
  spectrum of, 366
Autocrine theory of transformation
  transforming growth factor and, 292
Autoimmune disease
  characteristics of, 363
  definition of, 359, 363
  examples of, *366*
  type II hypersensitivity and, 328
Autoimmune hemolytic anemia
  acquired, 339
  characteristics of, 341
Autoimmune reactions
  definition of, 338
Autoimmune skin disease
  Pemphigus (case report), 366
Autoimmune thrombocytopenia, 341
Autoimmunity
  definition of, 363
  induction mechanisms in, 364, *364*
  mechanisms of tissue injury in, 364
  physiological, 363
Autolysis
  definition of, 40
Autophagy
  definition of, 29, *29*
Avidin-biotin complex
  immunohistochemistry and, 371

B cell growth factors
  immune response and, *314*
B cells
  definition of, 306
B-cell growth factors, 314, 315
B16 melanoma
  in study of metastasis, 454
Bacteremia
  and spread of infection, 514
BALT *see* Bronchial-associated lymphoid tissue
Bacteria
  embolic, *515*
  interaction with viruses, *476, 477*
Band 3 antigen
  physiological autoimmunity and, 363
Basal lamina
  composition of, 151
Basement membrane
  and vascular invasion by neoplasms, 450

as barrier to tumor invasion, 446
  interaction with metastatic cells, 454
  wound repair and, 288
Basophils
  immune system and, 307
  inflammation and, 204
  morphology of, *207*
Benign neoplasms
  definition of, 386
Bile pigment, 80
Bilirubin
  as a tissue pigment, 80
Biopsy
  value of, 371
Blastomycosis, *484*
Blood coagulation
  clotting factors and, 105
  extrinsic activation and, 110
  intrinsic activation and, 108
  mechanisms of, 105
  mediator generation and, 258
  overview, *109*
  pathways, *110*
Blood flow
  characteristics of, 123
  importance in thrombosis, 124
  laminar, 123
Blood groups
  in animals, *340*
Blood stasis
  thrombosis and, 124
Blood turbulence
  thrombosis and, 124
Blood viscosity
  thrombosis and, 124
BLV *see* bovine leukemia virus
Botulism
  as toxic disease, 502
Bovine anaphylaxis, 337
Bovine leukemia, 438
Bovine leukemia virus
  carcinogenesis and, 438
  mechanism of transformation by, 432
  relationship to HTLV, 438
Bovine platelets
  open canalicular system and, 130
Bradykinin, 248
  generation of, 249
Bronchial-associated lymphoid tissue, 308
Bullous dermatoses, 341

C-kinin, 249
C-*onc see* cellular oncogenes, 423
C-reactive protein, 256
C1
  activation of, *265*
  trimolecular structure of, 265
C1 esterase inhibitor
  intrinsic pathway regulation and, 109
C1-inhibitor, 269
C1q
  structure of, 265
C1r, 265
C1s, 265
C2
  activation of, *266*
C3
  activation of, *266*

C3 convertase
  alternative pathway form, 269
  classical pathway form, 265
  complement activation and, 265
C3 receptors
  leukocytes and, 240
C3a, 249
  functions of, *250*
C3a receptors, 241
C3b
  immune adherence and, 265
  opsonization and, 231
C3bi
  ligand binding and, 217
C3e
  leukocyte immobilization and, 271
C4
  activation of, *266*
C4a 249
C5
  activation of, *267*
C5 convertase
  complement activation and, 267
C5a, 249
  functions of, *250*
C5a receptors, 241
C6
  blood coagulation and, 271
Cachectin
  as growth factor, 408
  in cancer cachexia, 459
  TNF and, 257
Cachexia
  in neoplasia, 458
Calcification
  dystrophic, 81
  metastatic, 82
  of tissues, 81
Calcium
  cell membrane damage and, 70
  divalent, as second messenger, 244, 245
  divalent, coagulation and, 110
  divalent, mast cell activation and, 333
  divalent, platelet activation and, 126
  divalent, Stuart-Prower Factor activation and, 111
  enzyme release and, 236
  in membrane damage and cell injury, overview, 71
  role in cell injury, 69, *72*
Calcium-calmodulin-dependent kinase, 242
Calcium paradox
  cell injury and, 70
Canalicular system
  open, of platelets, 129
Cancer, 377
  definition of, 385
Cancer suppressor genes, 427
Canine granulocytopathy syndrome, 500
  defective inflammation and, 172
Capsule
  bacterial, and avoidance of phagocytosis, 480
Carbon tetrachloride
  membrane damage and, 63
  metabolism of, and cell injury, 63
Carcinogen, 414
  definition of, 413
Carcinogenesis

Carcinogenesis—*continued*
  mechanisms of, 414
Carcinogenicity
  tests for, 421
Carcinogens
  chemical, 413
  metabolic activation of, 413
  physical state of, 414
Carcinoma
  definition of, 387
Carcinoma *in situ*
  dysplasia and, 384
  definition of, 389
Cardiac cirrhosis
  chronic hyperemia and, 96
Cardiac edema, 164
Cardiac failure
  edema and, 159
Cardiac thrombosis, 131
Cartilage
  as inhibitor of tumor angiogenesis, 443, *443*
Caseous necrosis
  definition of, 48
Catarrhal exudation, 187
Cathepsin G, 234
CD2 adhesion receptor
  lymphocyte binding and, 308
CD2 receptor
  lymphocytes and, 305
CD3 molecule complex, 304
Cell
  typical features of, *20*
Cell adhesion
  in metastasis, 453
Cell adhesion molecules
  leukocytes and, 217
  role in tumor cell detachment, 446
Cell biology
  pathology and, 16
Cell cycle, 378, *378*
Cell death
  definition of, 40
Cell injury, 39
  causes of, 54
  consequences of, 51
  definition of, 39
  hypoxia and, 54
  irreversible, 40
  mechanisms of, 53
  membrane damage and, 62
  morphology of, 40
  pathogenesis of, 53
  reversible, 40
  sequence of events in, 55, *57, 74*
  ultrastructure of, 43, *44*
Cell membranes
  movement of, 33
Cell proliferation
  wound repair and, 290
Cell swelling
  in cell injury, 40
  mechanisms of, in cell injury, 59
  morphology of, *41, 42*
Cell volume
  a regulation of, 59
Cellular adaptation, 19
  cell injury and, 34
Cellular atrophy, 35, *36*

Cellular oncogenes, 423
Cellular pathology, 19
Cellular regenerative capacity
  healing and, 275
Celsus, Cornelius, 168
Cerebrovascular accident
  stroke and, 101
Ceroid, 79
Chalones
  control of cell growth and, 410, *411*
Chédiak-Higashi syndrome, 360, 497
  microtubular function and, 32
  defective inflammation and, 172
Chemical mediators
  acute hyperemia and, 92
  definition of, 246
  hypersensitivity and, 326
  newly synthesized, 246
  preformed, 246
  vascular actions, *198*
Chemicals carcinogens, 413
Chemokinesis, 223
Chemotactic factors
  complement activation and, 250
  DTH and, 357
  list of, *224*
  lymphokines as, 254
Chemotaxis, 223
  actin and, 229
  actin-binding protein and, 229
  avoidance, by bacteria, 480
  biochemical basis of, 228
  cations and, 226
  cell deactivation and, 230
  complement activation and, 271
  cytoskeletal elements and, 228
  gradient orientation and, 228
  locomotor activity and, 228
  mechanisms of, 225, *227*
  mediators of, 223
  morphology of, 225
  myosin and, 229
  proteins important to, *228*
Chicken-fat clot, 132
Cholera toxin
  mechanism of action, 505
Cholesterol
  tissue accumulation of, 76
Christmas factor
  intrinsic activation and, 109
  Stuart-Power Factor activation and, 112
Chromatin
  staining of, 24
Chromosomal abnormalities
  in neoplasia, 421
  oncogene activation and, 422
Chronic granulomatous disease, 479, 498
  defective inflammatory defense and, 172
Chronic inflammation
  features of, 183
  macrophages and, 183
CID
  see combined immunodeficiency, 473
Classical pathway
  complement activation and, 263, 264
Clathrin
  coated pits, and, 31
Clearance

impaired, morphologic basis for, *478*
impairment by organisms, 476
Clinical immunology
definition of, 303
Clonality
of neoplasms, 438, *440*
Clostridia
production of toxins by, 502
Clotting factors
list of, *105*
Coagulation
activation processes and, 108
clinical evaluation of, 108
clotting factors and, 105
endotoxin and, 507
extrinsic pathway and, 108
intrinsic pathway and, 108
of blood, mechanisms of, 105
of blood, overview, 104, *109*
of blood, pathways, *110*
Coagulation factors
list of, *105*
Coagulation necrosis
definition of, 47
ischemic, thrombosis and, 145
Coated pits
receptor-mediated endocytosis and, 31
Cohnheim, Julius, 168
Collagen
platelet activation and, 127
extracellular matrix and, 150
structure of, 288
subendothelial types, 107
wound repair and, 286, 288
Collagenases
in tumor cell invasion, 446
wound repair and, 286
Colloidal-osmotic pressure
edema and, 157
of plasma, 157
Colony stimulating factors, 408
Combined immunodeficiency disease, 360
of Arabian horses, 360, 473, 496, *497, 498*
Commensal
definition of, 474
Complement
avoidance of, by organisms, 480
endotoxin and, 507
host defense and, 269
inflammation and, 269
Complement activation
alternate pathway, 263
biochemical pathways of, 265
central role of C3 in, 269
classical pathway, 263
general features of, 264
terminal sequence, *267*
Complement cytolysis
characteristics of, *319*
colloid-osmotic lysis and, 321
controls over membrane attack, 321
lipid-bilayer target of, 319
membrane attack complex, 319, *321*
one-hit kinetics of, 319, *319*
sequential events in, *322*
transmembrane channel formation, 319, *320*
Complement fixation
assays for, 370

Complement fragments
as inflammatory mediators, 249
Complement lysis
formation of membrane defects and, 268
mechanisms of, 267
Complement receptors
leukocytes and, 240
Complement system
components of, *264*
cytolytic attack mechanism of, 318
inflammation and, 263
inflammatory amplification and, 260
Complement-derived mediators
biological functions of, *270*
Complement-mediated cytotoxicity
hypersensitivity and, 328
Complement-mediated killing
mechanisms of, 318
Congenital lesions
causes of, 379
Congestion
definition of, 90
passive, 90
Congestive heart failure
hyperemia development and, 93
Connective tissue framework
importance in healing, 274
Connective tissue mast cells, 307
Connective tissue replacement
healing and, 273
healing by, 279
Consumptive coagulopathy
and DIC, 513
Contact activation
inflammation and, 261
regulation of, 109
Contact system
kinin generation and, 249
Coombs test
autoimmune hemolytic anemia and, 341
Copper
as a tissue pigment, 80
CR-1 receptors, 240
CR-2 receptors, 240
CR-3 receptors, 240
Cryptococcosis, *481*
CSF *see* Colony stimulating factor
Cutaneous basophil hypersensitivity, 206
Cyclic AMP
as second messenger, 244
Cyclic nucleotides
control of cell growth and, 410
Cyclooxygenase pathway
arachidonic acid metabolism and, 252
Cytocavitary network, 33
components of, *27*
Cytokeratins, 32
Cytokine
definition of, 252
Cytoplasmic organelles
structure and function of, 24
Cytoskeleton
in membrane movement, 33
role in chemotaxis, 228
role in phagocytosis, 232
structure and function of, 31
Cytosol
definition of, 24

Cytotoxic hypersensitivity
    ADCC and, 338
    characteristics of, 327
    complement mediated lysis and, 338
    features of, *329*
    hematologic disease and, *339*
    mechanisms of, 338
Cytotoxic T cells
    definition of, 306
    type I MHC antigens and, 306

Damage to host
    due to inflammation, 510
    mechanisms of, 500
Degeneration, cellular
    definition of, 40
Degranulation
    phagocytosis and, 231
Delayed-type hypersensitivity
    antigenic specificity of, 354
    cellular basis for, 352
    cellular infiltrates characteristic of, 355
    cellular transfer of, 354
    characteristics of, 328
    chemical mediators of, 356
    comparisons to cell-mediated immunity, 354
    effector T cells and, 356
    features of, *331*
    infectious agents and, *359*
    initiation of, 355
    lymphokines and, 356, 357
    mechanisms of, 352
    perspectives on, 358
    T-cell dependency of, 354
    T-cells and, 352
    typical causes of, *355*
    typical lesions of, 355
Dense granules
    of mitochondria, 26
Dermatitis
    atopic, 338
Desmin, 32
Diacylglycerol, 242
    as second messenger, 244
    mast cell activation and, 333
Diagnosis
    terminology and, 9
DIC *see* disseminated intravascular coagulation
Differentiation
    in benign and malignant neoplasms, 390
Diphtheritic exudation, 187
Disease
    causes of, 472
    concepts of, 472
    infection and, 474
Disseminated intravascular coagulation, 512, *513*
    causes of, *512*
    endothelial injury and, 120
    endotoxin and, 507
    pathogenesis of, *514*
DNA, repair of, 494
DNA viruses
    and carcinogenesis, 429
    mechanisms of carcinogenesis, 430
    oncogenes of, *431*
Dormancy
    of metastatic neoplasms, 453
    of neoplasms, 418

Dye exclusion tests
    for cell viability, 60
Dysplasia
    carcinoma in situ and, 384
    as preneoplastic lesion, 384
    definition of, 383
    epithelial, *385*
    pleomorphism in, 384
    reversibility of, 384
Dystrophic calcification, 81, *81*

E. coli
    enterotoxins of, 505
    mechanisms of adherence, 476
Ecchymotic hemorrhage
    morphology of, *99*
Edema, 149
    appearance of, 161
    cardiac failure and, 159
    clinical forms of, *164*
    clinical significance of, 163
    decreased colloidal osmotic pressure and, 157, *158*
    definition of, 89, 149
    dependent, 161
    description of, 149
    extracellular matrix and, 149
    gross appearance of, 162
    hydrostatic pressure and, 158
    hypoalbuminemia and, 157
    increased hydrostatic pressure and, *159*
    increased vascular permeability and, 160, *161*
    inflammatory, 160, *161*
    lymphatic blockade and, *160*
    lymphatic obstruction and, 160
    pathophysiology of, 156
    pitting, 161
    protein rich, 161
    pulmonary, *163*
EGF *see* epidermal growth factor, 406
Ehrlich, Paul, 169, 204
ELAM-1
    cell adhesion and, 218
Elastic fibers
    extracellular matrix and, 151
Elastin
    extracellular matrix and, 151
Electrocardiogram
    in myocardial ischemia, *61*
Electron microscopy
    in pathology, 7
ELISA *see* Enzyme-linked immunosorbant assay
Emboli
    definition of, 90
Embolism, 135
    definition of, 103, 135
    pulmonary, *133*
Embolus
    definition of, 103, 135
    generation of, 135
Endocarditis
    bacterial, 516f
Endocytosis
    definition of, 30
    receptor mediated, 31
Endogenous pyrogen
    IL-1 and, 256
Endoplasmic reticulum

in cell injury, 60
structure and function of, 26
ultrastructure, in cell injury, 44, *46*
Endothelial cells
adhesiveness and, 218, 509
contractility of, 221
endotoxin and, 509
inflammation and, 215
wound healing and, 289
Endothelial continuity
thrombosis and, 120
Endothelial Surface
clotting regulation and, 115
Endothelium
active metabolic functions and, 121
extracellular matrix and, in metastasis, 454
anticoagulant properties of, 121, *121*
endotoxin and, 509
leukocyte adhesion and, 218
morphology of, *194*
procoagulant properties of, 121, *121*
role in metastasis, 453
role in wound repair, 290
surface charge and thrombosis, 120
thrombosis and, 120
Endotoxin
arachidonic acid metabolism and, 507
clotting system and, 507
complement system and, 507
DIC and, 507
effects of, 506, *506*
endothelium and, 509
interleukin-1 and, 508
macrophages and, 508
neutrophils and, 508
Schwartzman reaction and, 507
nature of, 506
neutralization by complement, 271
TNF and, 257, 508
Enterotoxins
role in enteric disease, 505
Environment
influence on infectious disease, 500
Enzyme-linked immunosorbant assay, 370
Enzymes
in diagnosis of cell injury, 52, *54*
in tumor cell invasion, 446
Eosinophil chemotactic factor
mast cells and, 336
Eosinophils
as anti-parasitic cells, 204
characteristics of, *203*
description of, 201
functions of, 202
helminthotoxicity, *205*
hypersensitivity and, 307
immune system and, 307
morphology of, *203*
regulatory role of, 204
Epidermal growth factor, 406
wound repair and, 291
Epigenetic mechanisms
tumor heterogeneity and, 444
in carcinogenesis, 419, 420
Epistaxis, 98
Epithelioid cells
DTH reactions and, 356
granulomatous inflammation and, 188

ER, *see* endoplasmic reticulum
Erythroblastosis fetalis, 340
Escape mechanisms
in tumor immunology, 465
Esophageal varices
passive hyperemia and, 93
Esotropy
definition of, 33, *34*
Euchromatin
staining of, 24
Excisional repair of DNA, 495
Exogenous antigens
hypersensitivity and, 338
Exotoxins
role in injury to host, 502
Exotropy
definition of, 33, *34*
Extracellular matrix
as a barrier to neoplasms, 446
collagen and, 150
components of, 150
composition of, *150*
edema and, 149
elastic fibers in, 151
elastin in, 151
fibronectin and, 150, 151
glycosaminoglycans and, 150
proteoglycans and, 150
Extracellular matrix components
fibroblast elaboration and wound healing, 285
Extracellular matrix remodelling
wound repair and, 286
Extrinsic coagulation
activation speed and, 111
Extrinsic coagulation pathways
activation of, 110
initiation by tissue factor, 110
regulation of, 111
Exudate, 190
Exudates and transudates, *190*
Exudation
catarrhal, 187
diphtheritic, 187
fibrinonecrotic, 187
fibrinous, 185
inflammation and, 184
leukocytes and, 197
mucopurulent, 187
nonsuppurative, 188
serous, 186
suppurative, 185

F-actin, 229
Factor X
activation of, *111*
Fatty change
definition of, 42
in cell injury, 42, 72
morphology of, *43*, 73, *73*
Fcε receptors
aggregation, and mast cell activation, 333
FDPs *see* Fibrin degradation products
Feed
influence on infectious disease, 500
Feline immunodeficiency virus, 362
Feline infectious peritonitis
as immune-mediated disease, 511
Feline leukemia virus

Feline leukemia virus—*continued*
  carcinogenesis and, 435
  transduction of oncogenes by, 436
  disease spectrum of, 361
Feline lymphosarcoma, 435
  lesions of, *437*
Feline oncornavirus cell membrane antigen, 436
  tumor immunology and, 460, 462
Feline sarcoma viruses
  oncogenes and, 436
FeLV-FAIDS mutant
  immunosuppression and, 362
Fever
  mechanisms of, 511
  role in host, 512
FGF *see* Fibroblast growth factors, 408
Fibrin
  cross-linking and stabilization, 114
  formation of, *113*
  phases of formation in coagulation, 113
Fibrin degradation products
  clinical significance of, 142
  fibrinolysis and, 141
  in diagnosis of DIC, 513
  inflammation and, 259
Fibrin monomer, 114
  polymerization of in coagulation, 114
Fibrin polymers
  formation of in coagulation, 114
  soluble forms in coagulation, 114
Fibrin stabilizing Factor
  fibrin formation and, 114
  mechanisms of action, 114
Fibrinogen
  molecular structure, 113, *114*
  proteolysis of, 113
Fibrinoid, 76
Fibrinolysis, 140
  cleavage products of, 140
  clot resolution and, 135
  endothelium and, 122
  fibrin removal and, 137
  generation of FDPs and, *141*
  regulation of coagulation and, 115, 118
Fibrinonecrotic exudation, 187
Fibrinonecrotic tracheitis, *188*
Fibrinopeptides, 114
  inflammation and, 259
Fibrinous exudation, 185, *186*
Fibrinous pneumonia, *187*
Fibroblast growth factor, 408
  vascularization of neoplasms and, 441
  wound repair and, 292
Fibroblast interferon
  inflammation and, 255
Fibroblasts
  extracellular matrix elaboration and healing, 285
  functions in healing, 285
  inflammation and, 215
  role in wound repair and healing, 284
Fibronectin
  function of, 23
  in extracellular matrix, 150, 151
  neoplastic cells and, 412
  opsonization and, 231
  roles in wound healing, 288
  wound repair and, 286, *288*

Fibrous lamina
  of nucleus, 23
Filtration pressures
  edema and, 154
  Starling equilibrium and, 156
Flow cytometry
  analysis of equine neutrophils and, *374*
  principles of, 372, *373*
  usefulness as a tool, 371
Fluid mosaic model
  of plasma membrane, 22
Fluorescein-labeled antibodies
  diagnostic usefulness of, 371
Fluorescence microscopy
  in immunopathology, 7
fMLP
  chemotaxis and, 225
FOCMA
  see feline oncornavirus cell membrane antigen, 436
Free radicals
  cell injury and, 63
  cellular defenses against, 65
  cellular sources of, 63, *64*
  in anoxic cell injury, 66
Function activity
  in neoplasms, 397
Functional end arteris
  infarction and, 146

G-actin, 229
G-proteins
  cholera and pertussis toxins and, 505
  leukocyte activation and, 242
  mast cell activation and, 333
  transmembrane signaling and, 243
Galen, 168
GALT *see* Gut-associated lymphoid tissue
Gangrene
  definition of, 48
  dry, 48, *53*
  wet, 49
Gelsolin, 229
Gene amplification
  in neoplasia, 422
General pathology
  definition of, 4
Genetic factors
  influence on disease, 489
  neoplasia and, 419
GFAP *see* Glial fibrillary acidic protein
Giant cells
  DTH reactions and, 356
  granulomatous inflammation and, 188
Glanzmann's thrombasthenia
  hemostasis and, 107
Glial fibrillary acidic protein, 32
Glomerulonephritis
  immune-complex type, 342
  membranous, 344
  proliferative, 344
  type III hypersensitivity and, 328
Glucocorticoids
  mechanisms of action, 228
Glutathione
  as cellular antioxidant, 66
Glutathione peroxidase
  in cellular antioxidant reactions, 66

Glycocalyx, 23
  thrombosis and, 120
Glycogen
  depletion in cell injury, 62
Glycosaminoglycans, 152
  antithrombin III and, 115
  extracellular matrix and, 150
  link proteins and, 152
  wound repair and, 286
GM-CSF *see* Granulocyte-macrophage stimulating
    factor
Golgi apparatus
  structure and function of, 28
Grading
  of neoplasms, 402
Granulation tissue
  characteristics of, 279
  contractility of, 289
  differentiation from granulomatous
      inflammation, 279
  healing and, 279
  histologic appearance, *281*
  histologic zones in, 279, *280*
  major cell types in, 282
  morphology of, 279
Granulocyte-macrophage colony stimulating factor,
    316
Granulocytes
  types of, 197
Granuloma, 188
Granulomatous inflammation, *189*
  description of, 188
Growth
  contact inhibition of, 406
  control of, 406
  density-dependent inhibition of, 406
  factors affecting, 379
  of neoplasms, 398
  of tissues, 377
Growth factors
  growth of neoplasms and, 410
  importance in wound healing, 290
  in control of cell growth, 406, *407*, *409*
  vascularization of neoplasms and, 441
  wound repair and, 284
Gut-associated lymphoid system, 308

H_2O_2-myeloperoxidase-halide system
  bacterial killing and, 233, 479
  functions of, 234
Hageman Factor
  biochemical structure of, 108
  inflammatory activation of, 261
  intrinsic activation and, 108
  kinin generation and, 249
Hageman factor pathways, 260, *261*
  amplified inflammation and, *263*
Healing
  definition of, 293
  introduction to, 272
Healing and repair
  perspectives on, 294
  routes to normalcy in, *295*
Heart failure cells, 96
  morphology of, *95*
Helper T cells
  definition of, 305
Hemagglutination, 370

Hemarthrosis, 98
Hematogenous route of metastasis, 448
Hematoma
  definition of, 97
  morphology of, *98*
  organizing, 103
  subdural, 101
Hematopoiesis, 103
Hemolytic disease of the newborn, 340
Hemopericardium, 98
  morphology of, *102*
Hemoperitoneum, 98
Hemoptysis, 98
Hemorrhage
  by diapedesis, 97
  by rhexis, 97
  causes of, 100
  clinical significance of, 98, 101
  clotting deficiency and, 100
  definition of, 90, 97
  ecchymotic, 98
  ecchymotic, *99*
  gastric, *100*
  importance of amount, 98
  importance of location, 98, 101
  organization of, 103
  outcome and resolution, 101
  petechial, 98, *99*
  purpura, 100
  rate of accumulation, 98, 102
  reabsorption of blood, 103
  resolution of, 103
  trauma and, 100
Hemorrhagic diathesis
  and DIC, 513
Hemorrhagic Shock, 101
Hemosiderin, 79, 80
  at sites of hemorrhage, 103
  in macrophages in chronic hyperemia, 96
Hemostasis
  regulatory mechanisms in, 115
  thrombosis and, 104
Hemothorax, 98
Heparin
  inhibition of tumor angiogenesis and, 443
Hepatic cirrhosis
  passive hyperemia and, 93
Hereditary angioedema, 109
  complement system and, 269
Heterochromatin
  staining of, 24
Heterogeneity
  of neoplasms in metastasis, 454
Heterophagy
  definition of, 29, 30
Heymann nephritis, 347
High amplitude mitochondrial swelling, 56
High endothelial venules
  lymphocyte homing and, 210, 305, 308
High molecular weight kininogen
  intrinsic activation and, 108
  kinin generation and, 248
Histamine, 247
  mast cells and, 335
Histamine releasing factor, 333
Histiocytoma
  canine, immune reaction to, *460*
Histopathology

Histopathology—*continued*
  diagnostic usefulness in immunopathology, 370
HMW kininogen
  kinin generation and, 248
Homeostasis
  and cell injury, 35
Hormones
  in carcinogenesis, 413
Human T cell lymphotropic virus
  mechanism of transformation by, 432
Hyalin, 76
Hyaluronic acid
  wound repair and, 286
Hydrogen peroxide
  respiratory burst and, 233
Hydropericardium, 162
Hydrostatic pressure
  edema and, 158
Hydrothorax, 162
Hydroxyl radical
  bacterial killing and, 233
Hypercalcemia of malignancy, 458
Hyperemia
  active, definition of, 90
  acute, 91
  acute inflammation and, *193*
  acute local active, 91
  acute local active and inflammation, 191
  acute local passive, 92
  acute, morphology of, *92*
  appearance of, 95
  chronic, 91
  chronic generalized passive, 93
  chronic local passive, 93
  chronic passive and liver, 96
  chronic passive and lungs, 95
  chronic passive, of liver, *96, 97*
  chronic passive, of lung, *95*
  classification of, *91*
  congestive heart failure and, 93
  definition of, 90
  distribution of, 91
  duration of, 91
  generalized, 91
  generalized passive, routes to, *94*
  in acute inflammation, 92
  local, 91
  mechanisms of, 91
  physiological, 90
  venous obstruction and, 92, 93
Hyperplasia
  biliary, *382*
  bronchiolar, *382*
  definition of, 379
  endometrial, *381*
  nodular, 380
  pathologic, 380
  physiologic, 380
  reversibility of, 380
Hypersensitivity
  definition of, 303
  mechanisms of, 330
  types of, *326*
Hypersensitivity and immunity
  similarities and differences between, 303, 325
Hypersensitivity reactions
  classification of, *327*
Hypertrophy

definition of, 37
  of myocardium, 38
Hypoalbuminemia
  clinical background to, 157
  edema and, 157
Hypochlorite
  bacterial killing and, 234
Hypoplasia
  definition of, 379
  renal, *380*
Hypothyroidism
  atherosclerosis and, 76
Hypoxia
  cell injury and, 54, 55, *72*

IAPP *see* Islet amyloid polypeptide
ICAM-1
  cell adhesion and, 218
Idiopathic thrombocytopenic purpura, 341
IgA nephropathy, 348
IgE
  hypersensitivity and, 326
IGF, *see* Insulin-like growth factors
IL-1, 255
  DTH and, 358
  functional similarities to TNF, 257
Iliac thrombosis
  morphology of, *136*
Immediate-type hypersensitivity
  atopy and, 337
  bovine anaphylaxis and, 337
  cells involved in, 307
  characteristics of, 326
  features of, *327*
  IgE antibody response and, 333
  initiation of, 333
  lesions of, 337
  mechanisms of, 331
  milk allergy and, 337
Immune adherence
  C3b and, 265, 269
Immune complex deposition
  vascular permeability and, 348
Immune complex-mediated injury
  sequences in, *342*
Immune complexes
  circulating, 342
  deposition process for, 348
  formation and deposition, 342
  importance of antigen, 344
  in situ formation, 342
  intramembranous deposition of, 343
  pathogenicity of, 328
  persistent infectious antigens and, 344
  size and pathogenicity of, 343
  subendothelial deposition, 343
  subepithelial deposition, 343
Immune cytolysis
  similarities between complement and
    lymphocytes, 326
Immune deficiency, 496
  in animals, *496*
Immune interferon
  inflammation and, 255
Immune response
  avoidance by organisms, 485
  role in host defense, 478, 483
Immune system

cellular components of, 304
cellular components of, *305*
diseases of, 358
evaluation of, 368
Immune-complex disease
case report; glomerulonephritis, 351
characteristics of, 328
complement functions in, *350*
experimental basis of, 344
features of, *330*
importance of amount of antibody produced in, 347
major features of, *347*
mechanisms of, 341
mediation of lesions, 348
role of complement, 348
role of neutrophils, 350
tissue destruction in, 350
type III hypersensitivity and, 328
virally-induced, *345*
Immune-complex glomerulonephritis
histopathology of, *353*
immunofluorescence findings in, *353*
ultrastructural findings in, *354*
Immune-mediated tissue injury
characteristics of, 325
Immunity
definition of, 303
in neoplasia, 459
to neoplasms, evidence for, 461
Immunity and hypersensitivity
similarities and differences between, 303, 325
Immunobiology
definition of, 303
Immunochemistry
definition of, 303
Immunodeficiencies
acquired, virus infection and, 362
combined, 360
Immunodeficiency
and neoplasia, 461
Immunodeficiency diseases
acquired, 361
characteristics of, 359
definition of, 359
Immunodeficiency virus
feline, AIDS-like, 362
human (HIV), AIDS and, 361
Immunofluorescence
immunopathology and, 369
usefulness in diagnosis, 369
Immunogenetics
definition of, 303
Immunoglobulin classes
properties of, 311, *311*
Immunoglobulin deficiencies
selective, 360
Immunoglobulins
role in immune response, 310
Immunohematologic diseases, 339
examples of, *340*
Immunohematology
definition of, 303
Immunohistochemistry
diagnostic usefulness of, 371
in diagnosis of neoplasms, 390
principles in use, *372*
use in immunopathology, 346

Immunopathologic reactions
inflammatory basis of, 304
Immunopathology
definition of, 303
disciplinary scope of, 303
Immunoperoxidase techniques
immunopathology and, 370
Immunosuppression
by infectious agents, 486, *487*
Immunosurveillance
tumor immunology and, 460
Indirect immunofluorescence, 371
Infarct, *50*
definition of, 143
of spleen, *146*
Infarction, 143
cardiac, *149*
cardiovascular function and, 148
clinical significance of, 148
definition of, 54, 90
determinants of, 145
ischemic susceptibility of tissue and, 145
vascular anatomy and, 146
Infection
disease and, 474
persistence of, 517
spread of, 514
susceptibility and resistance to, 474
Inflammation
acute, *178*, 180
acute manifestations of, 190
as a surface phenomenon, 175
bovine pneumonia and, 176
cardinal signs of, 168
cellular and humoral participants in, *174*
cellular events of, 215
chemical mediators of, 246
chronic, 180
chronic, *182*
chronic, fibrosis and, 181
classical signs of, *169*
classification of, 178, *179*
definitions of, 169
degree of severity and, 179
distribution patterns of, 184
duration of, 180
exudate types and, 184
general features of, 170
generalities about, *170*
granulomatous, 188
hemodynamic changes and, 191
history of, 168, *168*
leukocytic events in, *216*
mechanisms of chronicity, 181
perspectives on, 271
role in host defense, 478
sequence of events in, *192*
subacute, 180, *181*
types of, 177
vascular events in, 191
vascular, thrombosis, 120
Inflammatory exudate
cell types in, 197
classification of, 184
Inflammatory lesions
distribution of, 184, *184*
Inflammatory lymphokines, 253
Inherited diseases

Inherited diseases—*continued*
  of animals, *492*
  study of, 491
Initiation
  in carcinogenesis, 415
  mechanisms of, 415
Initiation and Promotion, 415
Initiation and promotion, *416*
Innocent bystander lysis, 341
Inorganic salts
  as carcinogens, 413
Inositol trisphosphate, 242
  as second messenger, 244
  mast cell activation and, 333
Insulin-like growth Factors, 408
Integrins, 152
Interferon-α
  inflammation and, 255
Interferon-γ
  inflammation and, 255
Interferon-β
  inflammation and, 255
Interferons
  Interferon-γ, 315
  as inflammatory mediators, 255
  DTH and, 357
  effects on immune system, *316*
  immune system and, 315
  structure and function of, 255
  types of, 315
Interleukin-1
  biological activities of, 256, *256*
  characteristics of, 312
  endotoxin and, 508
  immune response and, 312, *313*
  inflammation and, 255
  macrophage secretion of, 307
  role in amyloidosis, 85
  role in fever, 511
Interleukin-2
  as growth factor, 408
  characteristics of, 312
  immune response and, 312
  role in transformation by HTLV, 433
Interleukin-3
  characteristics of, 313
  immune response and, 313
Interleukin-4
  characteristics of, 314
  immune system and, 314
Interleukin-5
  characteristics of, 315
  immune system and, 315
Interleukin-6
  characteristics of, 315
  immune system and, 315
Interleukins
  definition of, 255
  DTH and, 357
  immune response and, 312
Intermediate filaments
  cytoskeleton and, 32
  as markers in neoplasia, 32
Interstitial fluid pressure, 153
Interstitium
  components of, 149
  definition of, 149
  edema and, 149

Intracellular messengers
  control of cell growth and, 410
Intracellular organisms
  resistance to killing, 479
Intracellular parasitism
  mechanisms of, 482
Intradermal testing
  hypersensitivity and, 370
Intrinsic coagulation pathways
  activation of, 109
Intrinsic coagulation system
  activation of, 109
  initiation by Hageman Factor, 109
Invasion
  in neoplasia, 400, 445
  mechanisms of, 444
Ionic homeostasis
  in cell injury, 59
Iron
  infection and, 488
Irreversibility of cell injury
  determinants of, 68
Ischemia
  definition of, 54
Islet amyloid polypeptide, 86
Isoimmune reactions
  hematologic disease and, 340
Isotype switching, 311

K88 antigen
  role in bacterial adherence, 476
K99 antigen
  role in bacterial adherence, 476
Karyolysis
  definition of, 46
Karyorrhexis
  definition of, 46
Karyotype
  of neoplastic cells, 412
Killer (K) cells, 306
Killing
  avoidance of, by intracellular organisms, 482
Killing of organisms
  oxygen-dependent mechanisms, 479
  oxygen-independent mechanisms, 479
Kinins
  as mediators, 248
  functions of, 249
  inactivation of, 249
Koch, Robert, 169
Koch's postulates, 472
Kupffer cells, 306

Labile cells
  definition of, 275
  healing and, 275
Lactoferrin
  infectious disease and, 489
  in host defense, 479
Laminar blood flow
  disruption of and thrombosis, 124
Laminin
  metastasis and, 454
  basement membranes and, 288
  role in metastasis, 446
  wound repair and, 288
Langerhans cells, 306
Large granular lymphocytes, 306

Latency
  in neoplasia, 417
Lectins
  antigenic crosslinking and, 306
Lesion
  definition of, 8
Lesions
  causes and classes of, 13
  evolution of, 15
Leu M5, 217
Leu-CAMs, 217
Leukocyte activation
  mechanisms of, 239, *239*
Leukocyte adhesion molecules, 217
  deficiency of, 218
  in canine granulocytopathy syndrome, 500
Leukocyte emigration
  cell types and, 222
  description of, 219
  interendothelial route, *221*
Leukocyte endogenous mediator
  IL-1 and, 256
Leukocyte endogenous pyrogen
  role in fever, 511
Leukocyte immobilization factor
  C3e and, 271
Leukocyte inhibitory factor, 254
Leukocyte interferon
  inflammation and, 255
Leukocyte membrane activation, *226*
Leukocyte secretion
  frustrated phagocytosis, *238*
  regurgitation during feeding, *237*
Leukocytes
  accumulation of, 223
  adhesion and, 216
  adhesion molecules and, 217
  aggregation and, 216
  bacterial killing mechanisms, 233
  emigration of, 222
  inflammatory secretions and, 235
  kinetics of accumulation, *223*
  mechanisms of activation of, 239
  membrane activation, *226*
  secretion in inflammation, 237
  thrombosis and, 120
Leukokinins, 249
Leukotriene B4
  biochemistry of, 252
Leukotrienes
  generation of, 252
  inflammation and, 252
  mast cells and, 336
Lewis, Sir Thomas, 169
LFA-1, 217, 305
LFA-3, 308
Link proteins
  glycosaminoglycans and, 152
Linkage analysis
  in study of inherited disease, 490
Lipid
  intracellular accumulation of, 75
Lipid peroxidation
  and membrane injury, 63
  consequences of, 65
  definition of, 64
Lipid storage diseases, 76
Lipidoses

see lipid storage diseases, 76
Lipofuscin
  as tissue pigment, 78, *78*
  nature of, 28
Lipomodulin, 228
Liposomes, 319
Lipoxygenase pathway
  arachidonic acid metabolism and, 252
Liquefaction necrosis
  definition of, 47
Liver
  mechanisms of fatty change in, 74
  metabolism of lipid in, 75
Low amplitude mitochondrial swelling, 56
LTB 4
  as inflammatory mediator, 252
Lymph node permeability factor, 254
Lymphatic route of metastasis, 448
Lymphatic obstruction
  edema and, 160
Lymphatics
  edema and, 156
Lymphocyte blastogenesis assay, 370
Lymphocyte cytolysis
  cell types involved in, 322
  cytotoxic cell activation and, 323
  recognition of target cell and, 322
  release of cytotoxic activity and, 323
  sequential events in, 322
  target cell killing, *324*
Lymphocyte function tests, 370
Lymphocyte function-associated antigen, 305
Lymphocyte function-associated molecule 3
    (LFA-3), 308
Lymphocyte homing
  high endothelial binding factors and, 308
  high endothelial venules and, 211
  mechanisms of, 308
  receptors for, 308
Lymphocytes, 306
  B cells, 306
  cytotoxic T cells, 306
  description of, 210
  effector T cells, 356
  helper T cells, 305
  inflammation and, 210
  killer (K) cells, 306
  large granular, 306
  morphology of, *211*
  natural killer (NK) cells, 306
  null cells, 306
  suppressor T cells, 306
  T cells, 304
  types of in immunity, 304
Lymphoid system
  functional anatomy of, 308
Lymphokine
  definition of, 252
Lymphokines
  activities of, 253
  DTH reactions and, 355
  general features of, 252
  immune network and, 306
  immune response and, 311
  inflammation and, 252, 253
Lymphosarcoma
  feline, lesions of, 437
Lymphotoxins

Lymphotoxins—*continued*
  immune system and, 316
  TNF and, 316
Lysl-bradykinin, 248
Lysosomal enzymes
  as chemical mediators, 259
  leakage of, in cell injury, 61
  mechanisms of release, 236
  tissue injury and, 236
Lysosomal suicide, 236
  description of, 236
  mechanisms of, *236*
Lysosomes
  enzyme profile, *201*
  in cell injury, 44, 61
  lysosomal suicide, 236
  structure and function of, 28
Lysozyme, 234
  in host defense, 479

MAC *see* Membrane attack complex
Macrophage activation factor, 254
Macrophage chemotactic factor, 254
Macrophage procoagulant inducing factor, 357
Macrophage-derived growth factor
  wound repair and, 290
Macrophages
  description of, 207
  emigration through basement membrane, *220*
  endotoxin and, 508
  function in wound repair, 282
  functions of, 209
  immune response and, 306
  in granulation tissue, 282
  in tumor immunology, 465
  inflammatory functions and, 207
  morphology of, *208*
  procoagulant activity and, 140
  pulmonary intravascular, 209
MAF *see* Macrophage activation factor
Major histocompatibility complex
  tumor immunology and, 467
Malacia
  definition of, 46
Malformations, 379
Malignant neoplasms
  definition of, 386
Marek's associated tumor-specific antigen, 433
Marek's Disease, 433
  lesions of, *434*
Margination and pavementing
  of leukocytes, 216
Mast cells
  activation and mediator release, 333, 335
  activation of, *334*
  connective tissue type, 206, 307
  description of, 205
  functions in inflammation, 205
  immune system and, 307
  inflammation and, 204
  mediators of hypersensitivity and, *332*
  morphology of, *206*
  mucosal type, 206, 307
  stimulus-response coupling and, 333
Masugi nephritis, 347
MATSA *see* Marek's associated tumor-specific
    antigen
MCF *see* Macrophage chemotactic factor

Mediators
  newly synthesized, 335
  preformed, 335
Melanin
  as a tissue pigment, 79
Melanoma
  histopathology of, *396*
  ultrastructure of, *397*
Membrane attack complex
  complement lysis and, 267
  mechanisms of action, 267
  mechanisms of cell lysis and, 267
Membrane Damage
  cell injury and, 62
  cell injury and, *72*
  calcium and, in cell injury, 70
  causes of, 62
  consequences of, 67
  lipid peroxidation and, 65
  mechanisms of, 63
  morphology of, 67
Membrane lipid remodeling
  leukocyte activation and, 241
Metabolism
  in cancer cachexia, 459
Metaplasia
  definition of, 381
  osseous, of lung, *384*
  squamous, *383*
Metastasis, 447
  by implantation, *405*
  cell adhesion in, 453
  definition of, 400
  mechanisms of, 400, 444
  of neoplasms, 400
  organ preference of, 453
  patterns of, 453
  seed and soil theory of, 453
  steps in, 447, *449*
  to lymph node, *450*
  tumor immunology and, 465
  vascular invasion in, 448
Metastatic calcification, 82, *82*
Metastasis
  embolic tumor cells in, 450
Metchnikoff, Elie, 168, 260
Methionyl-lysl-bradykinin, 248
MHC antigens, class II
  lymphocyte activation and, 305
Microcirculatory bed
  schematic morphology of, *154*
Microfilaments
  cytoskeleton and, 31
  chemotaxis and, 228
  phagocytosis and, 232
Microtubule associated proteins
  cytoskeleton and, 32
Microtubules
  and cytoskeleton, 31
  chemotaxis and, 228
  phagocytosis and, 233
Microvascular physiology
  edema and, 153
MIF, *see* Migration inhibitory factor
Migration inhibitory factor, 253
  DTH and, 357
Milk allergy, 337
Mitochondria

high amplitude swelling of, *45, 56*
in cell injury, *58*
low amplitude swelling of, 56
structure and function of, 24
structure of, *25*
ultrastructure, in cell injury, 44, *45*
Mitochondrial-dense granules, 26
Mixed function oxidase enzymes
in cell injury, 63
Mixed lymphocyte reaction, 370
Mixed mammary tumor, *386*
Mixed neoplasm
definition of, 386
MLR *see* Mixed lymphocyte reaction
Mo1, 217
CR-3 receptor binding and, 240
Molecular biology
in study of disease, 490
Monoclonal antibodies
usefulness as a tool, 371
Monokine
definition of, 252
Monokines
immune response and, 311
Mononuclear phagocyte system
defects in, 360
immune response and, 306
MPIF *see* Macrophage procoagulant inducing
factor
Mucopurulent exudation, 187
Mucosal mast cells, 307
Mural thrombosis, 131
Muscular dystrophy
identification of gene defect, 491
Mutation
carcinogenesis and, 419
tumor heterogeneity and, 444
Myasthenia gravis, 341
Mycobacteria
avoidance of killing by, 483
Mycosis
due to feed change, *501*

Myelin figure
in necrosis, 47
Myelin figures
in cell injury, 44, 62
Myocardial infarction
morphology of, *149*
Myofibroblasts
wound contraction and, 289
Myosin
chemotaxis and, 229

N-formylated oligopeptides
chemotaxis and, 225
NADPH-oxidase
respiratory burst and, 233
Natural killer (NK) cells, 306
in neoplasia, 464
Necrosis
caseous, 48
classification of, 47
coagulation, 47
coagulation, *51, 52*
definition of, 40
due to bacterial infection, 505
due to bacterial toxins, *504*

due to viral infection, *503*
gangrenous, 48
gross appearance of, 46
gross appearance of, *50*
liquefaction, 47
morphology of, 45
morphology of, *48, 49*
vascular reaction to, 49
Neonatal isoerythrolysis, 340
Neoplasia, 377
chromosomal abnormalities in, 421
definition of, 384
effect on host, 457
etiology of, 413
genetic aspects of, 419
genetic predisposition to, 420
histogenesis and, 385
immunity in, 459
immunity in, mechanisms, 462
immunity, and antibody, 464
immunity, and escape mechanisms, 465
immunity, and MHC, 467
immunity and macrophages, 465
immunodeficiency and, 461
NK cells in, 464
nomenclature of, 385
pathogenesis of, 405
progression of, 417
suppressor cells in, 467
Neoplasms
behavior of, 386
benign, characteristics of, 389, *389, 392*, 393
benign, definition of, 386
benign, differentiation in, 390
classification of, 385, 386, 388
clonal nature of, 438
clonal nature of, *440*
cloning of, 456
dormancy of, 453
function in, 397
grading of, 402
growth of, 398
invasion by, 400, 445
invasion by, *401*
ischemic necrosis in, 399
ischemic necrosis in, *399*
malignant, characteristics of, 389, *389*, 394, 395
malignant, cytology of, 398
malignant, definition of, 386
malignant, differentiation in, 390
mechanisms of invasion and metastasis in, 444
metastasis by implantation, *405*
metastasis of, 400, *402, 403*
metastatic, selection of, *455*
mixed, definition of, 386
spread of, 400
staging of, 402
stroma of, 397
vascular invasion by, 404
vascularization of, 440
Neoplastic cells
dissemination of, 452
embolic, arrest of, 452
embolic, fate of, 452
embolism of, *451*
interaction of clones of, 444
properties of, 411
Neovascularization

Neovascularization—*continued*
  healing and, 277
Nephrotoxic nephritis, 347
Nerve growth factor, 408
Neurofilaments
  as intermediate filaments, 32
Neutrophils
  description of, 198
  endotoxin and, 508
  functions of, 200
  granule contents, 200
  granule contents, *200*
  important characteristics of, *200*
  in granulation tissue, 282
  inflammation and, 200
  injurious constituents of, 351
  morphology of, *199*
  role in immune-complex disease, 350
Newly synthesized mediators
  mast cells and, 335
NGF *see* Nerve growth factor
NK cells *see* Natural killer cells
NKCF *see* NK cytotoxic factor
NK cytotoxic factor, 316
Nonsuppurative exudation, 188
Normal cell
  structure and function of, 19
Nuclear envelope, 23
  nuclear pores of, 24
  structure of, *24*
Nucleoid
  of peroxisomes, 33
Nucleolus
  function of, 24
Nucleus
  in necrotic cells, 45
  structure of, 23
Null cells, 306
Nutmeg liver, 96
Nutrition
  resistance to infection and, 488
Nutritional edema, 164

Oncogenes
  activation by chromosomal abnormalities, 422
  gene products of, *424*
  function of, 424
  role in carcinogenesis, 423
Opsonins, 231
Opsonization
  phagocytosis and, 231
Organization
  healing processes and, 277
  of thrombi, 142
  of thrombus, *143*
Oxygen free radicals
  in cell injury, 64
Oxygen radicals
  bacterial killing and, 233
  tissue injury and, *351*
Oxygen-dependent bacterial killing, 233
Oxygen-independent bacterial killing, 233, 234

PAF *see* Platelet-activating factor
Paraneoplastic syndromes, 457, *457*
Parasitic edema, 164
Parathyroid hormone-like peptides
  in hypercalcemia of malignancy, 458

Parenchymal regeneration
  healing and, 273
Pasteur, Louis, 169
Pathogen
  definition of, 474
Pathogenesis
  definition of, 8
Pathology
  cell biology and, 16
  definition of, 2
  general, 4
  language of, 8
  specialties in, 3
  study of, 1, 10
  terminology of, 8
  tools of, 5
PDGF *see* Platelet-derived growth factor
Pemphigus
  histopathology, *367, 368*
  immunofluorescence findings, *369*
Perforins, 324
  lymphocyte cytolysis and, 324
Pericardial effusion
  edema and, 162
Perinuclear cisterna, 23
Permanent cells
  characteristics of, 277
  healing and, 275, 277
Peroxidase anti-peroxidase method, 371
Peroxisomes
  enzymes of, 33
  structure and function of, 33
Pertussis toxin
  mechanism of, 505
Petechial hemorrhage
  morphology of, *99*
Phagocytosis
  avoidance of, 480
  cytoskeleton and, 232
  definition of, 30
  degranulation and, 231
  description of, 230
  microbicidal mechanisms, 233
  morphology of, *231*
  role in host defense, 479
  sequential events in, *232*
Phagolysosome
  definition of, 260
  formation of, 231
Phagosome, 260
  definition of, 30
  formation of, 231
Philadelphia chromosome
  in chronic myelogenous leukemia, 421
Phlebitis
  thrombosis and, 120
Phlebothromboses, 130
Phosphoinositol
  metabolism of, 242
Phosphoinositol cycle, 243
Phosphoinositol turnover
  leukocyte activation and, 242
Phosphoinositols, 242
Phospholipase A2
  arachidonate metabolism and, 335
Phospholipase C, 242
  mast cell activation and, 333
Phosphoprotein phosphatases

dephosphorylation and, 245
Physiological autoimmunity, 363
Pigments
  in tissues, 76
Pinocytosis, 230
  definition of, 30
Planar lipid bilayers, 319
Plasma cells
  inflammation and, 210
  morphology of, *212*
Plasma membrane
  fluid mosaic model of, 22
  in cell injury, 58
  in cell interactions, 23
  proteins of, 22
  role in metastasis, 456
  structure and function of, 20
  structure of, *22*
  ultrastructure, in cell injury, 43
Plasma proteins
  edema and, 157
Plasma thromboplastin antecedent
  intrinsic activation and, 108
Plasmin, 137
  proteolysis and, 137
Plasminogen, 137
  activation of, 137
  incorporation into clots, 115
Plasminogen activator
  role in invasion and metastasis, 447
Plasminogen activators
  cellular and humoral sources of, *138*
  clot resolution and, 137
  extrinsic, 139
  Hageman Factor and, 138
  intrinsic, 138
  single chain urokinase-type, 139
  tissue type, 139
  urokinase-type, 139
  various types, 137
Platelet Factor 3, 129
Platelet Factor 4, 129
Platelet-activating factor
  effects on immune system, *318*
  functions of, 258
  general features of, 258
  immune system and, 317
  inflammation and, 258
  mast cells and, 336
Platelet-derived growth factor, 407
  wound healing and, 291
Platelets
  adhesion and aggregation, *128*
  adhesion to collagen, 127
  adhesion to substrates, 126
  aggregation and release reaction, *130*
  aggregation of, 126
  aggregation responses and, 127
  aggregation stimuli, 127
  alpha granules and, 129
  as inflammatory cells, 215
  as inflammatory cells, *215*
  blood coagulation and, 125
  endothelial surveillance and, 125
  fibrinogen receptor, 107
  GP IIb-IIIa complex, 107
  in hemostasis and thrombosis, *126*
  inflammation and, 212

mechanisms of adhesion, 126
  mediators and thrombosis, 120
  membrane glycoproteins, 107
  membrane phospholipids and aggregation, 129
  morphology of, *214*
  open canalicular system and, 129
  phases of aggregation, 127
  phospholipids and coagulation, 110, 112
  release reaction, 126
  release reaction and, *213*
  role in hemostasis and thrombosis, 126
  secretory components, *214*
  secretory responses in aggregation, 129
  thrombospondin and, 128
  von Willebrand factor receptors and, 121
Pleomorphism
  as expression of tumor heterogeneity, 444
  in dysplasia, 384
Pneumocystosis, *499*
Poly C9
  complement lysis and, 268
Polycythemia
  definition of, 90
Polyperforins, 324
  lymphocyte cytolysis and, 324
Polysomes
  definition of, 27
Postmortem autolysis
  definition of, 40
Postmortem thrombi, 132
Postreplication repair of DNA, 495
Preformed mediators
  mast cells and, 335
Prekallikrein
  inflammation and, 260
  intrinsic activation and, 108
Preneoplasia
  dysplasia and, 384
Primary lysosomes, 260
  definition of, 28
Proaccelerin
  intrinsic activation and, 110
  protein C and, 116
Proconvertin
  extrinsic coagulation and, 111
  Stuart-Prower Factor activation and, 111, 112
Profilin, 229
Prognosis
  definition of, 52
Progression
  in neoplasia, 417
  of neoplasms, and tumor heterogeneity, 444
Promotion
  in carcinogenesis, 415
  mechanisms of, 416
  stage 1 and stage 2, 417
Properdin
  alternate pathway and, 268
Properdin system
  components of, 268
  reaction sequence of, 269
Prostacyclin, 252
  anticoagulant functions of, 122
  cytokine induction of, 122
Prostaglandin endoperoxides, 252
Prostaglandins
  inflammation and, 252
  mast cells and, 336

Protein
    intracellular accumulation of, 76
Protein AA
    in amyloid, 83
Protein AL
    in amyloid, 83
Protein C
    tPA and, 117
    antihemophilic factor and, 116
    mechanisms of action, *117*
    proaccelerin and, 116
    regulation of coagulation and, 107, 115, 116
Protein kinase C
    leukocyte activation and, 242
    mast cell activation and, 335
Protein kinases
    phosphorylation and, 245
Protein S
    as cofactor for protein C, 117
Protein SAA
    in amyloidosis, 85
Protein-A method
    immunohistochemistry and, 371
Proteins
    of plasma membrane, 22
Proteoglycan
    structure of, 152
Proteoglycans
    extracellular matrix and, 150
    wound healing and, 287
Prothrombin
    conversion to thrombin, 112
    description of, 112
    vitamin-K dependency and, 112
Prothrombin time, 108
Protooncogenes, 423
Pseudoepitheliomatous hyperplasia
    healing and, 282
    morphology of, *283*
Pseudomelanosis, 79
Pulmonary embolism
    morphology of, *133*
Pulmonary thrombosis
    morphology of, *131*
Purpura
    idiopathic thrombocytopenic, 341
Pyknosis
    definition of, 46

Radial immunodiffusion, 369
Radiation
    cell injury and, 54
    as a carcinogen, 414
Radioimmunoassay
    immunoglobulin detection and, 369
Rb gene
    osteosarcoma and, 428
    retinoblastoma and, 428
Recanalization
    of thrombi, 142, *143*
Receptor-ligand binding
    cell activation and, 238, 245
Receptor-mediated endocytosis, 31
Receptors
    for entry of organisms, 475
    leukocyte activation and, 240
Recombinant DNA technology
    in study of disease, 490

Regeneration
    definition of, 293
    epithelial, *274*
    parenchymal, healing and, 273
    requirements of, 274
    requirements of, *274*
Renal edema, 164
Repair
    definition of, 293
    introduction to, 272
Reperfusion injury
    oxygen free radicals in, 66
RER, 27
    see rough endoplasmic reticulum, 26
Residual bodies
    definition of, 28
Residual bodies, *30*
Resistance
    to entry of organisms, 474
    to infection, factors affecting, 474
Respiratory burst
    features of, *233*
    phagocytosis and, 233
Restriction endonucleases
    in recombinant DNA technology, 490
Retinoblastoma
    cancer suppressor genes and, 428
    predisposition to neoplasia and, 420
Retroviruses
    acutely transforming, 432
    and carcinogenesis, 430
    chronically transforming, 432
    mechanisms of carcinogenesis, 431
Reverse genetics
    in study of inherited disease, 490
Reversibility of cell injury
    determinants of, 68
RGD sequences, 152
Rheumatoid arthritis
    autoimmunity and, 366
Ribosomes
    in RER, 27
    structure and function of, 27
RNA viruses
    carcinogenesis and, 430
Rough endoplasmic reticulum, 26
    synthesis of secretory proteins and, 27
Rous sarcoma virus, 423

S-protein, 321
SALT *see* Skin-associated lymphoid tissue
Sarcoma
    definition of, 387
Satellite cells
    muscle healing and, 278
Scarring
    healing and, 273
Schwartzman reaction
    endotoxin and, 507
Scu-PA, 139
Second messengers
    leukocyte activation and, 244
Secondary lysosomes
    definition of, 28
Seed and soil theory
    metastasis and, 453
Selenium
    in cellular antioxidant reactions, 66

Self tolerance
  autoimmunity and, 363
Self-antigens
  autoimmunity and, 363
Sequestered antigens
  autoimmunity and, 364
SER *see* smooth endoplasmic reticulum
Serology
  definition of, 303
Serotonin, 247
Serous exudation, 186
Serum protein electrophoresis
  immune evaluation and, 369
Serum sickness
  description of, 345
  glomerulonephritis in, 347
  pathogenesis of, 345
  sequential events in, *346*
Shock
  circulatory failure and, 102
  hemorrhagic, 101
  hypovolemic, 102
Signal transduction
  leukocyte activation and, *239*
Silicosis, 78
Single chain urokinase-type plasminogen
    activator, 139
Singlet oxygen
  bacterial killing and, 233
Skin reactive factor, 254
Skin testing
  DTH and, 370
Skin-associated lymphoid tissue, 308
Slow reacting substance of anaphylaxis, 252
  mast cells and, 336
Smooth endoplasmic reticulum, 26
  metabolism of toxins and, 63
  proliferation of, 38, *39*
  structure and function of, 28
Sodium pump
  in cell injury, 59
Somatic mutation
  carcinogenesis and, 419
Splenic infarct
  morphology of, *146*
Stable cells
  characteristics of, 276
  healing and, 275, 276
Staging
  of neoplasms, 402
Stains
  commonly used, 6
  in histopathology, 5
Starling equilibrium
  edema and, 154
  forces influencing, *155*
Stimulus-response coupling
  leukocyte activation and, 238
  leukocyte responses and, 235
  mast cell activation and, 333
  mechanisms of, *239*
Streptolysins
  in avoidance of phagocytosis, 480
Stress fibers
  cytoskeleton and, 31
Stroma
  of neoplasms, 397
Stuart-Prower Factor

activation of, 111, *111*
  cleavage of, 112
  coagulation and, 110
  extrinsic activation and, 112
  intrinsic activation and, 111
  linking intrinsic and extrinsic coagulation, 111
Suicide bag hypothesis
  cell injury and, 61
Superoxide anion
  respiratory burst and, 233
Suppressor cells
  tumor immunology and, 467
  effect on tumor growth, 467
Suppressor T cells
  definition of, 306
Suppurative exudation, 185
  morphology of, *185*
Susceptibility to infection
  factors affecting, 474
Susceptibility to disease
  genetic influence on, 493
Swelling
  cellular, 40
Symbiosis
  definition of, 474
Systemic lupus erythematosus
  autoimmunity and, 366
Systemic reactions
  effects of, 511

T cell deficiency diseases, 360
T cell receptor, 304
T cells
  characteristics of, 304
TCR2 molecule
  lymphocytes and, 304
T-dependent antigens, 306
T-independent antigens, 306
t-PA, 139
T3 molecule, 304
Tamponade
  cardiac, 101
Target cell killing
  immune system and, 318
Teratoma
  definition of, 386
Tetanus
  as toxic disease, 502
TGFα *see* Transforming growth factor type α, 407
TGFβ *see* Transforming growth factor type β, 407
Thixotropy
  edema and, 152
Thrombi
  fates after formation, 133
  morphogenesis of, 130
  morphology of, 131
  organization of, 142
  postmortem, 132
  recanalization of, 142
  resolution of, 142
Thrombin
  fibrinogen cleavage and, 114
  formation of, 112, *113*
  site of action, 112
Thrombocytopenic purpura
  idiopathic, 341
Thromboembolic colic
  morphology of, *147*

Thrombomodulin
    as endothelial thrombin receptor, 116
    thrombin and, 116
Thromboplastin
    coagulation and, 110
    extrinsic activation and, 110
    role as "tissue factor", 110
    structure of, 110
    Stuart-Prower Factor activation and, 111
Thrombosis
    arterial, 131
    blood composition and, 124
    cardiac, 131
    definition of, 90, 103
    general background to, 103
    hemodynamic mechanisms and, 122
    iliac, *136*
    mural, in heart, 131
    of cardiac valves, 131
    of vena cava, *136*
    organization of, *144*
    pathogenesis of, 118
    pulmonary, *131*
    recanalization of, *143*
    regulatory mechanisms in, *116*
    rheological factors and, *123*
    rheological mechanisms in, 122
    vascular injury and, 119
    vascular mechanisms in, 119
    venous, 132
Thrombospondin
    platelet aggregation and, 129
Thromboxanes
    coagulation and, 121
    inflammation and, 252
    prostacyclin and, 122
Thrombus
    definition of, 103
    degradation of, *145*
    fates of, *134*
    propagation of, *119*, 132, 134
Thymic permeability factor, 254
Tissue architecture
    importance in healing, 276
Tissue deposits, 75
Tissue edema, 149
Tissue factor
    thromboplastin and, 110
Tissue regeneration
    healing and, 273
Tissue-type plasminogen activator, 139
TNF *see* Tumor necrosis factor, 408
Tolerance
    autoimmunity and, 363
Trait A-46 of cattle
    immunodeficiency and, 360
Transferrin
    infectious disease and, 489
Transforming growth factor Type α, 407
Transforming growth factor Type β, 407
Transforming growth factors
    vascularization of neoplasms and, 441
    wound repair and, 292
Transfusion reactions, 339
Transmembrane signaling
    leukocyte activation and, 243
Transmembrane signalling
    mast cell activation and, *334*

Transmissible venereal tumour
    chromosomal abnormalities in, 423
    immunity to, 464
Transudate, 190
Traumatic neuroma, 278
Triple response of Lewis, 169
Tropism
    of infectious agents, 514
Tuberculosis
    avian, *483*
Tumor
    definition of, 385
Tumor angiogenesis, 441
    inhibition of, 443
Tumor angiogenesis factor, 441
Tumor Antigens, 459
Tumor heterogeneity, 444
    metastasis and, 454
Tumor immunity
    evidence for, 461
Tumor immunology, 459
    metastasis and, 465
    cellular cytotoxicity in, 462
    in virus-induced neoplasms, *463*
    mechanisms in, 462
    role of antibody in, 464
Tumor necrosis factor
    vascularization of neoplasms and, 442
    as growth factor, 408
    cachectin and, 257
    DTH and, 358
    effects on immune system, *317*
    endotoxin and, 257
    functional similarities to IL-1, 257
    general features of, 257
    immune system and, 315
    in cancer cachexia, 459
    lymphotoxin and, 254
    role in inflammation, 257
Tumor progression
    tumor heterogeneity and, 444
Turbulence
    thrombosis and, 123
TVT *see* transmissible venereal tumor
Type I collagen
    wound repair and, 288
Type III collagen
    wound repair and, 288
Type IV collagen
    basement membranes and, 288
    wound repair and, 288

u-PA, 139
Urokinase-type plasminogen activator, 139

V-onc *see* viral oncogenes, 423
Vane, John, 251
Vascular invasion
    in metastasis, 448
Vascular permeability
    acute inflammation and, 192
    edema and, 160
    histamine and, 194
    leukocyte dependent, 197
    leukocyte independent, 196
    mechanisms of, 196
    mediators of, *195*, *196*
    phases of, *195*

phases of in inflammation, 194
Vascularization
  growth of neoplasms and, 441, *442*
  of neoplasms, 440, 441
  role in metastasis, 450
  role in neoplastic invasion, 447
Vasculitis
  thrombosis and, 120
Vasoactive amines
  as mediators, 247
Vegetative valvular endocarditis
  thrombosis and, 131
Venous stasis
  thrombosis and, 123
Vimentin, 32
Viral oncogenes, 423
  mechanisms of, 430
Virchow, Rudolf, 118, 168
Virchow's Triad
  pathogenesis of thrombosis and, 118
  thrombosis and, *118*
Viremia
  spread of infection and, 515
Virulence
  definition of, 474
Virus neutralization
  complement and, 269
Viruses
  carcinogenesis and, 428, *429*
  as carcinogens, 414
  interaction with bacteria, *476, 477*
Vitamin E
  as cellular antioxidant, 66

Von Willebrand Disease, 107
Von Willebrand Factor
  collagen binding and, 107
  hemostasis and, 107
  platelet adhesion and, 127
  procoagulant functions and, 121

Water homeostasis
  in cell injury, 59
Weibel-Palade bodies
  von Willebrand factor and, 121
Wound contraction, 289
Wound healing
  features of, *287*
  general features of, 293
  role of macrophages in, 283

X-inactivation mosaicism
  tumor clonality and, 439
Xanthine oxidase
  role in anoxic cell injury, 66, *67*
Xeroderma pigmentosum
  predisposition to neoplasia and, 419

Zahn, lines of, 132
Zone of capillary proliferation
  granulation tissue and, 279
Zone of capillary sprouts and arches
  granulation tissue and, 280
Zone of mature connective tissue
  granulation tissue and, 279
Zone of necrotic debris
  granulation tissue and, 282